W9-BDB-099

The Medical Management of

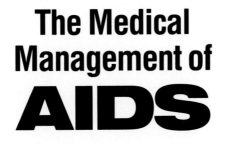

The Medical Management of

AIDS

THIRD EDITION

MERLE A. SANDE, M.D.

Professor and Vice-Chairman, Department of Medicine,
University of California, San Francisco;
Chief, Medical Service, San Francisco General Hospital
San Francisco, California

PAUL A. VOLBERDING, M.D.

Professor, Department of Medicine,
University of California, San Francisco;
Director, AIDS Program, San Francisco General Hospital
San Francisco, California

W.B. SAUNDERS COMPANY

Harcourt Brace Jovanovich, Inc.

Philadelphia / London / Toronto / Montreal / Sydney / Tokyo

W.B. SAUNDERS
Harcourt Brace Jovanovich, Inc.

The Curtis Center
Independence Square West
Philadelphia, Pennsylvania 19106

Library of Congress Cataloging-in-Publication Data

The Medical management of AIDS/[edited by] Merle A. Sande,
   Paul A. Volberding. — 3rd ed.
      p.   cm.
   Includes bibliographical references and index.
   ISBN 0-7216-6752-X
   1. AIDS (Diseases) — Treatment. I. Sande, Merle A.
II. Volberding, Paul.
   [DNLM: 1. Acquired Immunodeficiency Syndrome. WD 308 M489]
RC607.A26M43   1992
616.97'92 — dc20
DNLM/DLC   92-15451

THE MEDICAL MANAGEMENT OF AIDS   ISBN 0-7216-6752-X

Copyright © 1992, 1990, 1988 by W.B. Saunders Company

All rights reserved. No part of this publication may be reproduced or transmitted in any form or by any means, electronic or mechanical, including photocopy, recording, or any information storage and retrieval system, without permission in writing from the publisher.

Printed in Mexico

Last digit is the print number: 9   8   7   6   5   4   3   2   1

This book is dedicated to the many health care workers around the world who have provided unselfish and compassionate care for HIV-infected individuals and especially to those health care providers, including our own nurse Jane Doe, who have become infected while caring for AIDS patients. All of us owe these individuals a great debt for their true heroism in facing this epidemic.

CONTRIBUTORS

DONALD I. ABRAMS, MD
Associate Professor of Clinical Medicine, University of California, San Francisco;
Assistant Director, AIDS Activities Program, San Francisco General Hospital, San
Francisco, California
Dealing with Alternative Therapies for HIV; Hematologic Manifestations of HIV Infection

TIMOTHY G. BERGER, MD
Associate Professor of Clinical Medicine, University of California, San Francisco; Chief,
Dermatology Service, San Francisco General Hospital, San Francisco, California
Dermatologic Care in the AIDS Patient

GAIL BOLAN, MD
Assistant Professor of Clinical Medicine, University of California, San Francisco;
Director, STD Control Program, San Francisco Department of Public Health, San
Francisco, California
Management of Syphilis in HIV-Infected Persons

WILLIAM BUHLES, PhD
Department Head, Department of Immunology and Antiviral Therapy, Institute of Clinical
Medicine, Division of Syntex, Inc., Palo Alto, California
Management of Herpes Virus Infections (CMV, HSV, VZV)

JOHN P. CELLO, MD
Professor of Medicine and Surgery, University of California, San Francisco; Chief,
Gastroenterology Service, San Francisco General Hospital, San Francisco, California
Gastrointestinal Tract Manifestations of AIDS

RICHARD E. CHAISSON, MD
Assistant Professor of Medicine, Epidemiology, and International Health, Johns Hopkins
University; Director, AIDS Service, Johns Hopkins Hospital, Baltimore, Maryland
Bacterial Infections in HIV Disease

MICHAEL CLEMENT, MD
Assistant Professor of Clinical Medicine, University of California, San Francisco; Medical
Director, AIDS Clinic, San Francisco General Hospital, San Francisco, California
Natural History and Management of the Seropositive Patient

MOLLY COOKE, MD
Associate Professor of Clinical Medicine, Division of Internal Medicine, University of California, San Francisco; Attending Physician, AIDS Clinic, San Francisco General Hospital, San Francisco, California
Supporting Health Care Workers in Treatment of HIV-infected Patients

DAVID A. COOPER, BSc(Med), MD, FRACP, FRCPA, FACVen, FAFPHM
Associate Professor and Director, National Centre in HIV Epidemiology and Clinical Research, University of New South Wales; Director, HIV Medicine Unit, St. Vincent's Hospital, Sydney, Australia
Primary HIV Infection

BONNI BROWNLEE CROY, MPH
Crosby, Heafey, Roach, and May, San Francisco, Oakland, and Los Angeles, California
AIDS Litigation for the Primary Care Physician

JAMES W. DILLEY, MD
Associate Professor of Clinical Psychiatry and Project Director, AIDS Health Project, University of California, San Francisco; Senior Consulting Psychiatrist, AIDS Activities Program, San Francisco General Hospital, San Francisco, California
Management of Neuropsychiatric Disorders in HIV-Spectrum Patients

BASIL DONOVAN, MB, BS, FACVen, FAFPHM
Director, Sexual Health Clinic, Sydney Hospital, Sydney, Australia
Primary HIV Infection

W. LAWRENCE DREW, MD, PhD
Associate Professor, Laboratory Medicine and Medicine, University of California, San Francisco; Director, Clinical Microbiology and Infectious Disease, Mount Zion Medical Center of The University of California, San Francisco, San Francisco, California
Management of Herpes Virus Infections (CMV, HSV, VZV)

KIM S. ERLICH, MD
Assistant Professor of Clinical Medicine, University of California, San Francisco; Consultant in Infectious Diseases, Northern Peninsula Infectious Diseases, Daly City, California
Management of Herpes Virus Infections (CMV, HSV, VZV)

MARGARET A. FISCHL, MD
Professor of Medicine, University of Miami School of Medicine, Miami, Florida
Treatment of HIV Infection

JULIE LOUISE GERBERDING, MD, MPH
Assistant Professor of Medicine and Infectious Diseases, University of California, San Francisco; Director, HIV Prevention Services, San Francisco General Hospital, San Francisco, California
HIV Transmission to Providers and Their Patients

PHILIP C. GOODMAN, MD
Professor of Clinical Radiology, Duke University Medical Center, Durham, North Carolina
The Chest Film in AIDS

DEBORAH GREENSPAN, BDS, DSc, ScD(hc)
Clinical Professor of Oral Medicine, Department of Stomatology, School of Dentistry, University of California, San Francisco, San Francisco, California
Oral Complications of HIV Infection

JOHN S. GREENSPAN, BSC, BDS, PhD, FRCPath, ScD(hc)
Professor of Oral Biology and Oral Pathology and Chairman, Department of Stomatology, School of Dentistry; Professor of Pathology, School of Medicine, University of California, San Francisco, San Francisco, California
Oral Complications of HIV Infection

MOSES GROSSMAN, MD
Professor of Pediatrics Emeritus, University of California, San Francisco; Chief Pediatric Service, San Francisco General Hospital, San Francisco, California
Pediatric AIDS

JULIE HAMBLETON, MD
Fellow, Cancer Research Institute, University of California, San Francisco, San Francisco, California
Hematologic Manifestations of HIV Infection

HARRY HOLLANDER, MD
Associate Professor of Clinical Medicine, University of California, San Francisco; Attending Physician and Director, AIDS Clinic, H.C. Moffitt–J.M. Long Hospitals, San Francisco, California
Natural History and Management of the Seropositive Patient

PHILIP C. HOPEWELL, MD
Professor of Medicine, University of California, San Francisco; Chief, Chest Service, San Francisco General Hospital, San Francisco, California
Pneumocystis carinii *Pneumonia: Current Concepts*

ALLISON IMRIE, BSc
Senior Scientific Officer, Centre for Immunology, St. Vincent's Hospital, Sydney, Australia
Primary HIV Infection

DENNIS M. ISRAELSKI, MD
Assistant Clinical Professor, Stanford University School of Medicine, Stanford, California; Chief, Division of Infectious Diseases, San Mateo County General Hospital; Medical Director, San Mateo County AIDS Program, San Mateo, California
AIDS-associated Toxoplasmosis

MARK A. JACOBSON, MD
Assistant Professor of Medicine in Residence, University of California, San Francisco; Director of Clinical Research, AIDS Activities Program, San Francisco General Hospital, San Francisco, California
Mycobacterial Diseases: Tuberculosis and Disseminated Mycobacterium avium *Complex Infection*

HAROLD W. JAFFE, MD
Deputy Director for Science, Division of HIV/AIDS, Center for Infectious Diseases, Centers for Disease Control, Atlanta, Georgia
Acquisition and Transmission of HIV

LAWRENCE D. KAPLAN, MD
Assistant Professor of Clinical Medicine, University of California, San Francisco; AIDS Program, Oncology Division, San Francisco General Hospital, San Francisco, California
Malignancies Associated with AIDS

JOHN McDOUGALL KERN, JD
Crosby, Heafey, Roach, and May, San Francisco, Oakland, and Los Angeles, California
AIDS Litigation for the Primary Care Physician

BELLE L. LEE, PharmD
Assistant Professor of Medicine and Pharmacy, University of California, San Francisco; San Francisco General Hospital, San Francisco, California
Drug Interactions and Toxicities in Patients with AIDS

JAY A. LEVY, MD
Professor of Medicine and Research Associate, Cancer Research Institute, University of California, San Francisco, San Francisco, California
Viral and Immunologic Factors in HIV Infection

DONALD W. NORTHFELT, MD
Assistant Professor of Clinical Medicine and Cancer Research Institute, University of California, San Francisco; AIDS Activities Program, Oncology Division, San Francisco General Hospital, San Francisco, California
Malignancies Associated with AIDS

THOMAS R. O'BRIEN, MD, MPH
Medical Epidemiologist, Division of HIV/AIDS, Center for Infectious Diseases, Centers for Disease Control, Atlanta, Georgia
Acquisition and Transmission of HIV

RONALD PENNY, MD, DSc, FRACP, FRCPA
Professor of Clinical Immunology, University of New South Wales; Director, Centre for Immunology, St. Vincent's Hospital, Sydney, Australia
Primary HIV Infection

RICHARD W. PRICE, MD

Professor and Head, Department of Neurology, University of Minnesota School of Medicine, Minneapolis, Minnesota

Management of Neurologic Complications of HIV-1 Infection and AIDS

JACK S. REMINGTON, MD

Professor of Medicine, Stanford University School of Medicine; Professor of Medicine and Consultant in Infectious Diseases, Stanford University Medical Center, Stanford, California

AIDS-associated Toxoplasmosis

MICHAEL S. SAAG, MD

Assistant Professor of Medicine, The University of Alabama at Birmingham; Assistant Chief, Medical Service, Veterans Administration Medical Center, Birmingham, Alabama

AIDS Testing: Now and in the Future

SHARON SAFRIN, MD

Assistant Professor of Clinical Medicine, Epidemiology, and Biostatistics, University of California, San Francisco; Attending Physician, San Francisco General Hospital, San Francisco, California

Drug Interactions and Toxicities in Patients with AIDS

MERLE A. SANDE, MD

Professor and Vice-Chairman, Department of Medicine, University of California, San Francisco; Chief, Medical Service, San Francisco General Hospital, San Francisco, California

Cryptococcal Infection in AIDS

GEORGE A. SAROSI, MD

Professor of Clinical Medicine, University of Arizona College of Medicine; Chairman, Department of Medicine, Maricopa Medical Center, Phoenix, Arizona

Endemic Mycoses in HIV Infection

NATHAN SHAFFER, MD

Medical Epidemiologist, Pediatric and Family Studies Section, Epidemiology Branch, Division of HIV/AIDS, Center for Infectious Diseases, Centers for Disease Control, Atlanta, Georgia

Acquisition and Transmission of HIV

JOHN D. STANSELL, MD

Assistant Professor of Clinical Medicine, University of California, San Francisco; Director, Inpatient AIDS Service, San Francisco General Hospital, San Francisco, California

Cryptococcal Infection in AIDS

BRETT TINDALL, BAppSc, MSc
Senior Project Scientist, National Centre in HIV Epidemiology and Clinical Research,
University of New South Wales; Scientific Officer, Centre for Immunology, St. Vincent's
Hospital, Sydney, Australia
Primary HIV Infection

PAUL A. VOLBERDING, MD
Professor, Department of Medicine, University of California, San Francisco; Director,
AIDS Program, San Francisco General Hospital, San Francisco, California
Clinical Care of Patients with AIDS: Developing a System

JAMES R. WINKLER, DMD
Assistant Professor of Periodontology, Department of Stomatology, School of Dentistry,
University of California, San Francisco, San Francisco, California
Oral Complications of HIV Infection

CONSTANCE B. WOFSY, MD
Professor of Clinical Medicine, University of California, San Francisco; Co-Director,
AIDS Activities Program, and Assistant Chief, Infectious Diseases, San Francisco General
Hospital, San Francisco, California
Therapeutic Issues in Women with HIV Disease

JOHN M. WORLEY, DO
Chief Resident, Department of Neurology, University of Minnesota School of Medicine,
Minneapolis, Minnesota
Management of Neurologic Complications of HIV-1 Infection and AIDS

PREFACE

No disease in modern times has had quite the impact on the civilized world that the acquired immunodeficiency syndrome (AIDS) has. The disease has rapidly afflicted nearly a quarter of a million persons in the United States, and between 1 and 2 million more are believed to be infected with the causative agent, the human immunodeficiency virus (HIV). The scope of the epidemic is even more dramatic in equatorial Africa, where millions of people are already infected. The social and political instability engendered by the impact of tens of millions of HIV-related deaths can be expected to be enormous. Although the outlook in the near future for curative treatment or effective vaccine is still grim, some measure of success in responding to the epidemic has been achieved. The medical and scientific communities have effectively cooperated to quickly accumulate epidemiologic, clinical, and basic science knowledge about this pandemic. We have rapidly expanded our knowledge of retrovirology and have turned many of our most creative minds toward unraveling the biology of HIV. We have also developed highly efficient mechanisms for treating HIV-infected individuals.

Amid the social and political upheaval precipitated by the AIDS epidemic, a critical problem has silently but steadily emerged: Who is to provide care for the increasing numbers of afflicted individuals? There is a desperate need for physicians, nurses, and other health care workers to provide skilled care for these patients. Although few practitioners have denied their responsibility to provide care, there is a reluctance on the part of some to actively participate. In some the reluctance is undoubtedly due to fears of acquiring the infection through patient-care activities. This concern will likely be compounded if the Public Health Service is successful in restricting practice privileges of HIV-infected health care workers. This proposed policy recommendation is just the sort of disincentive to caring for AIDS patients that will further impede access of infected patients to care. For others, inadequate reimbursement schedules for HIV-related problems reduce the economic incentive to devote the time and resources required to treat HIV-infected patients. Perhaps most importantly, the relative newness of AIDS and the rapid evolution of knowledge about the complications of HIV infection have made it difficult for practitioners not directly involved in AIDS research or associated with large medical centers to keep abreast of new developments in the field. It is common for individual physicians, especially those who have limited opportunities for immediate consultation, to feel poorly equipped to handle AIDS patients.

For these reasons we believe that an important contribution to the medical literature can be made by continuing to publish an up-to-date text that addresses the clinical issues commonly encountered by practitioners who accept the challenges that AIDS provides. In our third edition we have again compiled contributions from many of the world's leading authorities on AIDS. The biology and epidemiology of HIV infection and approaches to reduce sexual and nosocomial transmission of the virus are reviewed. The initial diagnostic evaluation of HIV-infected patients is outlined, a new chapter describing the various tests available has been included, and a summary of the multidisciplinary approach to treating these patients within the community is provided. The chapter on antiretroviral chemotherapy has been expanded to include discussion of both the new drugs and combination chemotherapy. A new chapter on alternative therapies—drugs available through various "buyers' clubs" patronized by many HIV-infected patients—details these compounds, which have their own set of side effects and which sometimes confuse the therapy administered by the patient's physician. In this edition we have also addressed the controversies attendant on HIV testing and have discussed some of the legal ramifications that the physician must face when caring for this patient population.

The infectious complications of HIV infection, including diagnosis and treatment of *Pneumocystis carinii* pneumonia and other protozoal, mycobacterial, fungal, bacterial, and viral infections, have been reviewed from a clinical perspective, as have the AIDS-associated malignancies, including Kaposi's sarcoma and lymphomas. We have also included a review of the hematologic, endocrine, renal, and cardiac complications of AIDS. In each chapter, information is presented in a practical format that should allow the primary care physician dealing with the disease for the first time to attack the problem in a logical and up-to-date fashion. Chapters addressing the special problems faced by HIV-infected children and women and, for the first time, the psychological manifestations of HIV infection and management of them have also been included.

We hope that this text will again provide a useful update and review of contemporary clinical issues relevant to caring for individuals with HIV-related illnesses. We also hope that it will help alleviate some of the apprehensions elicited when patients with HIV infection and its myriad complications are encountered for the first time, so that patients can be approached with confidence and compassion.

We would like to thank The Burroughs Wellcome Company for again providing an educational grant that helped make this publication, and the associated conference, possible. Also, special thanks are extended to Jan Rogerson and her staff at the University of California, San Francisco (UCSF), Department of Medicine's medical service at San Francisco General Hospital and to Kathy Mello and her staff at the UCSF Department of Medicine's Office of Continuing Medical Education for their valued assistance and to our publisher, the W.B. Saunders Company, who with the third edition has again set a record in completing publication 6 months from the time the chapters were completed. This rapid turnaround has allowed us to provide the most up-to-date review possible of the clinical aspects of caring for patients with AIDS.

MERLE A. SANDE, M.D.

Department of Medicine, UCSF School of Medicine
Medical Service, San Francisco General Hospital

COLOR PLATES

COLOR PLATE IA. Maculopapular rash on trunk of an individual with acute HIV infection. (See page 69.)

COLOR PLATE IB. Hairy leukoplakia on tongue. (See page 167.)

COLOR PLATE IC. Giemsa stain of induced sputum demonstrating cysts and trophozoites of *Pneumocystis carinii*. There is no uptake of stain by cyst wall; therefore, walls appear as clear-to-white circles. Trophozoites appear as dark dots. ($\times 960$.) (See page 266.)

COLOR PLATE ID. Acid-fast stain of lymph node tissue demonstrating large numbers of red-staining *Mycobacterium avium-intracellulare*. (See page 290.)

COLOR PLATE IE. Severe edema complicating advanced lower extremity cutaneous Kaposi's sarcoma. (See page 401.)

COLOR PLATE IF. Cytomegalovirus-associated retinitis. Note characteristic hemorrhages and exudates. (See page 360.)

COLOR PLATE IG. Widespread cutaneous Kaposi's sarcoma in a Caucasian individual: typical violaceous appearance of skin lesions. (See page 401.)

COLOR PLATE IH. Typical appearance of early Kaposi's sarcoma involving the palate. (See page 401.)

PLATE I

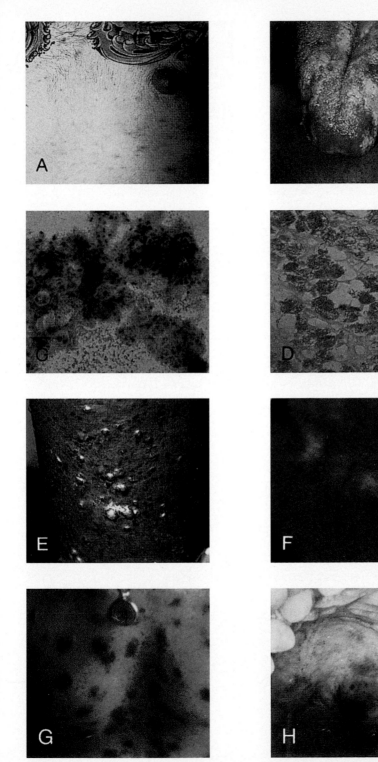

PLATE II

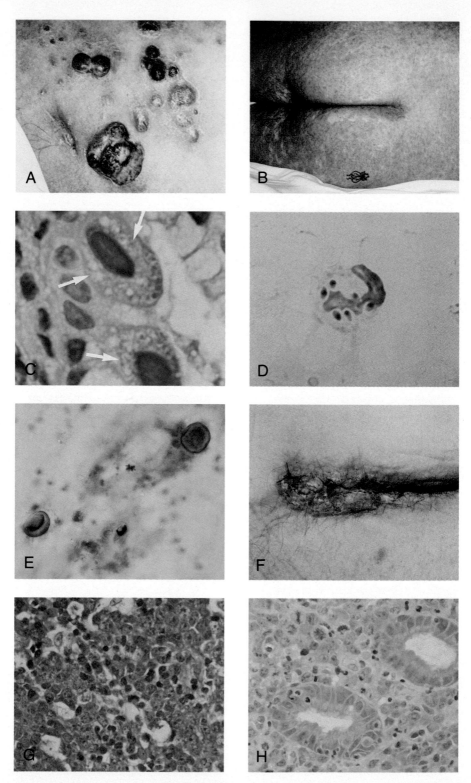

COLOR PLATE IIA.   Bacillary angiomatosis of the upper thigh in an AIDS patient who was seen initially 6 months earlier with subacute cellulitis. (See page 149.)

COLOR PLATE IIB.   Widespread maculopapular eruption typical of rashes seen with trimethoprim-sulfamethoxazole and other antibiotics. (See page 152.)

COLOR PLATE IIC.   Ampullary biopsy—AIDS papillary stenosis. Note large cells with intranuclear inclusions characteristic of cytomegalovirus *(arrows)*. (See page 186.)

COLOR PLATE IID.   Wright-Giemsa stain of circulating phagocyte with intracellular *Histoplasma capsulatum*. (See page 314.)

COLOR PLATE IIE.   Papanicolau stain of sputum demonstrating spherules (one intact, one partially collapsed) of *Coccidioides immitis*. (See page 317.)

COLOR PLATE IIF.   Atypical chronic HSV infection at the gluteal cleft in a patient with AIDS. Note the clinical resemblance to a pressure decubitus. (See page 371.)

COLOR PLATE IIG.   Small noncleaved-cell Burkitt's lymphoma involving lymph node. (Original magnification, × 100.) (See page 411.)

COLOR PLATE IIH.   Diffuse large-cell lymphoma involving stomach. (Original magnification, × 100.) (See page 411.)

CONTENTS

III SPECIFIC INFECTIONS AND MALIGNANT CONDITIONS

IV SPECIAL ASPECTS OF AIDS

I

THE VIRUS:
Its Transmission and Infection

1

ACQUISITION AND TRANSMISSION OF HIV

THOMAS R. O'BRIEN, MD, MPH
NATHAN SHAFFER, MD
HAROLD W. JAFFE, MD

The major transmission routes of human immunodeficiency virus type 1 (HIV-1)—sexual contact, parenteral exposure to blood and blood products, and perinatal transmission—were all described in the early 1980s. More recent information indicates that human immunodeficiency virus type 2 (HIV-2) has the same transmission routes as HIV-1 but may be transmitted at a lower rate. However, the rates of and risk factors for HIV transmission by these routes remain incompletely understood. In addition, unusual cases of HIV transmission are still reported. In this chapter recent information about the sexual and perinatal transmission of HIV-1 and HIV-2 is reviewed, and a recent case of apparent HIV-1 transmission from a dentist with acquired immunodeficiency syndrome (AIDS) to his patients is described.

SEXUAL TRANSMISSION

Homosexual Men

Early in the AIDS epidemic, epidemiologic studies established that receptive rectal intercourse was the predominant mode of HIV acquisition by homosexual men.[21,29,50,70,99] Other practices that could traumatize the rectal mucosa (e.g., rectal douching) appeared to increase further the infection risk for the receptive partner.[21,70,99] Insertive rectal sex could also place a man at risk for HIV infection, although the insertive partner would be at lower risk than the receptive partner.[21,50] Appropriately, receptive and insertive rectal sex were labeled as "unsafe" sexual practices and were abandoned by many homosexual men or were practiced only with condoms.

From the Division of HIV/AIDS, National Center for Infectious Diseases, Centers for Disease Control, U.S. Public Health Service, Atlanta, GA 30333.

Additional reports now suggest that other sexual practices of homosexual men may also transmit HIV.[32,62,65,88] For example, one report described HIV seroconversion in two homosexual men who denied having rectal intercourse for at least 5 years but had been the receptive partners in multiple episodes of unprotected oral intercourse with ejaculation.[62] Both men had gingival recession, although the possible role of this common oral condition in the acquisition of HIV is not known. Another brief report suggested acquisition of HIV infection by the insertive partners in oral sex, but the lack of detail in this report makes the conclusion difficult to interpret.[88] Thus, although clearly safer than rectal sex, unprotected oral sex between men should not be considered entirely safe.

Heterosexual Couples

On a worldwide basis sex between men and women apparently is the most common mode of acquiring HIV infection.[101] In Africa, the continent with the highest rates of HIV infection, heterosexual transmission accounts for the vast majority of cases.[80] In the United States AIDS cases attributed to heterosexual transmission, although still a small percentage of the total number of reported cases, comprise the most rapidly growing category.[41] Therefore an understanding of the rate at which HIV is transmitted between heterosexual couples and of the factors that may impede or enhance heterosexual transmission is important in slowing the worldwide HIV epidemic.

Heterosexual Transmission Between Steady Sex Partners

Studies that assess the prevalence of HIV infection in the steady heterosexual partners of HIV-infected persons (Table 1–1) have been valuable in gaining insight into the efficiency of heterosexual transmission of HIV. Retrospective studies of HIV-infected hemophilic men and their female sex partners have been particularly valuable because investigators have been able to enroll relatively large numbers of sexually active couples in which the female partners generally had no other risks for becoming HIV infected. Published results of these studies suggest that approximately 10% of the regular female sex partners of infected hemophilic men have themselves become infected with HIV.[1,13,54,63] These results are consistent with those of Peterman et al.[79] who found that 10 of 55 (18%) transfusion-infected men had transmitted HIV to their female partners.

Although most male-to-female HIV transmission results from vaginal sex, the per-contact risk from rectal sex may be somewhat greater than for vaginal intercouse, since heterosexual couples who engage in rectal sex are at increased risk of transmitting HIV infection.[37,76] This may, in part, account for the higher prevalence of HIV infection among female partners of infected bisexual men compared to partners of infected hemophilic men or transfusion recipients (see Table 1–1).

Higher rates of male-to-female HIV transmission have been reported in some studies of female partners of injecting drug users.[91] It is unclear, however, whether these higher rates reflect a truly higher risk of heterosexual transmission from injecting drug users compared to other HIV-infected men or additional sources of HIV risk in the female partners of injecting drug users. For example, women who

Table 1–1. Prevalence of Antibody to HIV-1 Among Regular Female Sexual Partners of HIV-Infected Men by Risk Group and Study

RISK GROUP OF INFECTED MEN (REFERENCE)	PROPORTION OF INFECTED PARTNERS (%)	
Hemophilic Men		
Kreiss et al. (54)	2/21	(10)
Allain (1)	10/148	(7)
Centers for Disease Control (13)	77/772	(10)
Lusher et al. (63)	21/201	(10)
Transfusion Recipients		
Peterman et al. (79)	10/55	(18)
Bisexual Men		
Padian et al. (76)	12/55	(22)
European Study Group (37)	11/33	(33)

are the sex partners of injecting drug users may themselves be injecting drug users or may have other male sex partners who are HIV infected.

Because in the United States and Europe HIV infection is more common in men than women, studies of female-to-male transmission of HIV infection are both fewer and smaller than studies of male-to-female transmission. Available data suggest female-to-male transmission may be less efficient than male-to-female transmission. Peterman et al.[79] found that 2 of 25 (8%) male partners of transfusion-infected females were themselves infected. Padian et al.[77] have also reported a lower risk of female-to-male transmission.

Overall, these American and European studies suggest that heterosexual transmission from HIV-infected persons to their regular sex partners is relatively inefficient, especially female-to-male transmission. Furthermore, the risk of heterosexual transmission is not related simply to the number of episodes of sex with an HIV-infected person because some people have remained uninfected after hundreds of such contacts[76,79] whereas others have become infected after a single episode of intercourse.[20]

In contrast to the relatively low incidence of heterosexual transmission observed in steady sex partners in American and European studies, researchers in Africa have demonstrated a high incidence of heterosexual transmission, including female-to-male transmission. Cameron et al.[12] reported an incidence of female-to-male transmission of 8.2% among men who developed symptoms of another sexually transmitted disease (STD) after a single sexual contact with an infected prostitute. This heterogeneity of risk of heterosexual HIV transmission may, in part, reflect biologic factors that play an important role in modulating heterosexual HIV transmission.

Biologic Risk Factors for Heterosexual Transmission

Multiple factors probably influence the infectivity of an HIV-infected person or the susceptibility of an uninfected person to infection with HIV (Table 1–2). An understanding of these factors is potentially important for designing public health interventions that will decrease the incidence of heterosexual HIV transmission.

Table 1–2. Factors that may Influence Heterosexual Transmission of HIV*

Infectivity Factors
Advanced HIV infection
Early HIV infection
Genital ulcer disease
Other sexually transmitted diseases
Antiretroviral therapy (may decrease infectivity)
Susceptibility Factors
Genital ulcer disease
Other sexually transmitted diseases
Lack of circumcision (men)
Traumatic sex
Defloration
Cervical ectopy
Oral contraceptives

*All factors listed are postulated to increase susceptibility or infectivity unless otherwise noted.

A number of studies suggest that HIV infectivity is greater in persons with advanced HIV infection. Goedert et al.,[39] in a study of HIV-infected hemophilic men and their female sex partners, first reported that HIV transmission was more common in partners of men with advanced disease as measured by low CD4 + cell count, development of AIDS, or p24 antigenemia. In a prospective study of heterosexual HIV transmission sponsored by the European Community, investigators observed seroconversions more commonly in partners of persons with symptomatic HIV infection than in partners of those with less advanced disease.[34]

The association between stage of infection and infectivity has also been assessed indirectly by use of HIV culture and the polymerase chain reaction (PCR) technique. Anderson et al.[4] reported a strong association between a CD4 + cell count <200 and a positive HIV semen culture. Using RNA PCR, Mermin et al.[67] found cellfree HIV RNA more commonly in semen of men with CD4 + cell counts <400.

Infectivity may also be higher during early infection before the development of antibodies to HIV. Although there is no direct evidence of such an effect, it would be consistent with reports of transient high levels of viremia in patients with acute HIV-1 infection[26] and might help to explain the rapid spread of HIV infection in highly sexually active populations.

Additionally, genital ulcer diseases and other STDs may increase the infectivity of HIV-infected persons. In a prospective study in Kenya, Cameron et al.[12] demonstrated a high rate of incident HIV infection in men who developed genital ulcer disease after contact with a prostitute. In the same population of seropositive female prostitutes, Kreiss et al.[52] detected HIV by culture from 4 of 36 (11%) ulcers. These data demonstrate that HIV is present in some ulcers and suggest that ulcers may provide a route for HIV transmission. In Kenya chancroid is the most important cause of genital ulceration, but syphilis and herpes simplex virus type 2 infection may also increase HIV infectivity.

Antiretroviral therapy may decrease infectivity, but data available to date are inconsistent. Although Krieger et al.[56] found no association between zidovudine use and positive HIV semen cultures, O'Brien et al.[74] reported that detection of HIV by semen culture was much less common in men receiving zidovudine therapy.

Conditions that compromise the barrier of the vaginal mucosa or penile epithelium may increase susceptibility to HIV infection. Kreiss et al.[55] first suggested genital ulceration as an important risk factor in epidemic acquisition of HIV infection by female prostitutes in Kenya. In another study among this cohort of prostitutes, Plummer et al.[82] reported that seroconversion was more common in women who had a genital ulcer or *Chlamydia trachomatis* infection. Therefore STDs that cause inflammation of the genital tract (e.g., chlamydia, gonorrhea, and *Trichomonas vaginalis* infections) may also lead to increased susceptibility to HIV infection. Laga et al.[57] have suggested that because these inflammatory conditions are more prevalent than ulcerative STDs, they may play a more important public health role in acquisition of HIV. However, studies of the role of other STDs in the heterosexual acquisition of HIV should be interpreted with some caution because the association of HIV transmission with certain STDs may, at least in part, reflect a high rate of dual infection (HIV and another STD) in the sex partners of study subjects. Nonetheless, aggressive STD intervention programs should be implemented in areas of high incidence of heterosexually acquired HIV infection, and these programs should be evaluated for their impact on HIV transmission.

Uncircumcised men may have increased susceptibility to HIV infection. Cameron et al.[12] found that men who were uncircumcised had an eightfold increased risk of becoming infected and that uncircumcised men who had a genital ulcer had the highest risk of acquiring HIV infection. Ecologic studies have also shown a strong association between the prevalence of HIV infection in certain regions of Africa and the practice of circumcision.[10] However, to date these findings have not been confirmed in European or American studies. The reason for an association between an intact penile foreskin and susceptibility to HIV infection is unclear, but it may result from trauma to the thin preputial epithelium during intercourse.

Other factors that may disrupt genital tract integrity have also been implicated as risk factors for acquiring HIV infection. Traumatic sex has been postulated as a risk factor for acquisition of HIV, as has defloration.[11] Peterman et al.[79] found higher rates of male-to-female transmission of HIV infection among older women and suggested that this could be due to increased susceptibility to vaginal trauma. Moss et al.[71] have reported that among wives of HIV-infected men, women with cervical ectopy are more likely to be infected with HIV.

Plummer et al.[82] found that Nairobi prostitutes who had used oral contraceptives were more likely to have become infected with HIV, even when the number of sexual contacts and condom use were considered. However, other investigators found no association between oral contraceptive use and acquisition of HIV infection.[73]

Heterosexual Transmission of HIV-2

Data emerging from West Africa suggest that HIV-2 infection is spreading more slowly than HIV-1 infection, even in areas where HIV-2 is the more prevalent virus,[31] but the reason for this observation is not yet clear. As noted previously, among persons with chronic HIV-1 infection transmission is more effective in persons with advanced disease. Since the rate of disease progression appears slower in HIV-2–infected persons than in HIV-1–infected persons,[64] the proportion of all HIV-2–infected persons with advanced disease may be low, resulting in lower rates of transmission. Alternatively, HIV-2 could be inherently less transmissible than HIV-1.

PERINATAL TRANSMISSION (see Chapter 27)

Rate

Mother-to-infant transmission of HIV-1 apparently is relatively efficient; approximately one in four infants born to seropositive mothers is infected. With the rapid spread of infection to women of reproductive age, perinatal transmission is now a major consequence of the HIV epidemic. According to the World Health Organization (WHO), by the end of 1992 more than 1 million infected infants will have been born worldwide.[19]

The precise rate of perinatal transmission in a given setting has been difficult to define because of problems in early, definitive diagnosis of HIV infection in the infant and difficulties in maintaining long-term follow-up. Uninfected children born to seropositive mothers may retain passively acquired maternal antibody for 6 to 18 months. Exposed children may not be identified as infected because of nonspecific symptoms or death from causes unrelated to HIV. Ongoing, prospective cohort studies have reported transmission rates of 16% to 30% in the United States,[5,40,48,66] 13% to 33% in Europe,[9,36,49] 30% to 52% in Africa,[30,45,58,60,90] and 25% in the Caribbean[43] (Table 1–3).

Table 1–3. Estimated Rates of HIV-1 Infection in Infants Born to Infected Mothers

SITE (REFERENCE)	SIZE OF COHORT*	INFECTED (%)
United States		
New York City (40)	33	21
New Haven (5)	43	16
Miami (48)	82	30
New York City (66)	55	29
Europe		
Italy (49)	281	33
France (9)	117	27
Europe (36)	372	13
Africa		
Zaire (90)	475	39
Zambia (45)	109	39
Congo (58)	64	52
Kenya (30)	361	45
Rwanda (60)	218	30
Caribbean		
Haiti (43)	230	25

*Number of children born to infected mothers included by authors in the calculation of the transmission rate.

Transmission rates apparently are higher in Africa than in Europe and the United States, although some of this difference may be explained by differences in the classification of children who were lost to follow-up or who died before definitive laboratory diagnosis could be established. Additionally, in some studies transmission rates were calculated on the basis of special information available only on a subset of infants. Calculated transmission rates have remained relatively constant over the past several years or, as in the European cohort study,[36] have been revised downward.

Risk Factors and Mechanisms

The timing, mechanisms, and risk factors for perinatal transmission are not well understood. Potential risk factors are being investigated with the hope of better predicting when transmission might occur and guiding the development of effective interventions. These factors include maternal stage of disease, maternal antibody response to infection, viral titer, variations in viral genotype and phenotype, and obstetric factors such as preterm birth, mode of delivery, and maternal or placental coinfection.

Perinatal transmission may be more likely in mothers with advanced disease or in those with newly acquired infection. Several studies have documented higher rates of infection in infants born to women with symptomatic HIV illness or AIDS or to women with a lower number or percent of CD4 + lymphocytes.[42,90,93] This result may reflect an increase in circulating virus presumed to occur at later stages of disease[23,47] or other characteristics of the virus not yet understood. There is some unconfirmed evidence that maternal viral burden, as measured by quantitative PCR[53] or by p24 antigenemia,[28] is associated with increased perinatal transmission risk. Consistent with this hypothesis, mothers with recently acquired infection, particularly those that seroconvert during pregnancy, may be at higher risk of transmission,[81] perhaps also because of high levels of plasma viremia. It is not known whether specific genetic viral sequences or virulence characteristics facilitate transmission.

If some mothers generated an antibody response that protects against transmission, either by helping to control the mother's infection or by providing protection in the infant, this factor might serve as the basis for inducing protective immunity. Preliminary reports suggested that the presence of epitope-specific antibodies to the principal neutralizing domain of the V3 loop of gp120 might be protective.[33,87] However, subsequent studies have not confirmed this hypothesis, at least with regard to V3 loop antibodies.[2,44,78] In addition, maternal levels of neutralizing antibody do not appear to protect against transmission.[51]

In at least one study infection in preterm infants was more common than in fullterm infants.[40] However, it is unclear whether fetal HIV infection predisposes to prematurity or whether preterm infants are at higher risk of acquiring infection during the birth process. Furthermore, particularly in the United States and Europe, maternal drug use may confound analyses of prematurity.[49,66]

A variety of maternal and placental conditions and coinfections might facilitate vertical transmission of HIV. If proved, they might suggest additional intervention strategies. In Zaire chorioamnionitis[90,93] and maternal anemia[93] were associated with transmission. The causes of these conditions are being investigated. The potential of other infectious agents, including syphilis, cytomegalovirus, herspesvirus, hepatitis B and C, and human T lymphotropic virus types I and II (HTLV I and II), to act as cofactors for transmission is unclear and is also being investigated in ongoing studies.

Timing

Perinatal HIV transmission can occur both in utero or at birth. Several lines of evidence support the occurrence of antenatal transmission. Trophoblastic cells of human placenta tissue express CD4+ receptors and are susceptible to HIV infection.[3,95] Virus has been isolated from amniotic fluid[72] and has been identified in fetal abortus tissue by culture,[59] PCR,[24] and in situ hybridization.[61] However, other investigators have not found HIV in fetal tissue,[35] and it is difficult to exclude contamination of these tissues by maternal blood. Clinically, the fact that subsets of infected infants have detectable virus at birth, immunologic abnormalities in the neonatal period, and rapid progression to AIDS in the first few months of life suggests in utero transmission. The proportion of infants actually infected in utero and the time during gestation when this is most likely to occur, however, are not known.

Intrapartum transmission, analogous to the vertical transmission of hepatitis B, likely occurs through direct contact with maternal blood and secretions as the infant is delivered through the birth canal. HIV has been isolated from cervical secretions.[98] Also the virus might be able to pass directly through maternal-fetal transfusions, particularly during placental separation at birth. The fact that many infected children are born without detectable virus or immunologic abnormalities supports the likelihood that delivery represents a high risk for HIV transmission. Interestingly, there has not been strong evidence that delivery by cesarean section is protective.[9,36,49] However, a recent report based on an international twin registry suggests that being the first of two twins delivered and vaginal delivery are risk factors for infection in twin births.[38] This hypothesis and its relevance for singleton births warrant further study. Although it has not been shown that intrapartum fetal scalp monitoring facilitates transmission, avoiding invasive monitoring of the fetus, whenever possible, seems prudent.

Postpartum Transmission (Breast-feeding)

Postpartum perinatal transmission of HIV through breast-feeding has been reported.[46,75,92] Free virus has been found in the cellfree fraction of breast milk[94] and might directly penetrate the infant's gastrointestinal mucosa. However, data from several cohort studies suggest that the additional risk of postpartum transmission is low in pregnant mothers already infected with HIV.[43,89] These findings may result from low viral titers in breast milk of previously infected women, concomitant maternal IgA antibody,[8,96] or some other factor. In contrast, the risk of transmission through breast-feeding in women with primary HIV infection who seroconvert during pregnancy or postpartum may be significantly higher. In a cohort of breast-feeding mothers seronegative at the time of delivery, nine of 16 (56%) infants born to mothers who seroconverted postpartum also seroconverted and were confirmed as infected, including four of 10 (40%) infants whose mothers seroconverted more than 3 months' postpartum.[97] Although WHO continues to recommend breast-feeding regardless of serostatus in areas where safe alternatives are not available,[100] these data suggest a high risk of transmission via breast milk in populations with a high incidence of new infections and present an especially difficult dilemma in the counseling of high-risk, seronegative women with regard to breast-feeding.

Transmission from infected children to breast-feeding mothers has been reported in one unusual outbreak in the Union of Soviet Socialist Republics (U.S.S.R), in which infants infected through contaminated, multiply used syringes apparently transmitted infection by blood-borne contact to their mothers.[83] Risk factors for transmission were aphthous ulcers in the infants' mouths and cracked nipples in the mothers.

Perinatal HIV-2 Transmission

In contrast to HIV-1, perinatal transmission of HIV-2 is considered rare,[85,86] although several cases of perinatally acquired HIV-2 infection resulting in AIDS have been documented in west Africa.[69] An ongoing perinatal transmission study in the Ivory Coast is investigating the relative rates of transmission and associated morbidity in mothers with HIV-1, HIV-2, and dual infections.

Clinical Interventions to Prevent Perinatal Transmission

Clinical trials are beginning to test chemoprophylaxis and immunoprophylaxis as interventions to interrupt perinatal transmission. These investigations may in themselves provide more information about the timing of and risk factors for transmission. The AIDS Clinical Trials Group has a protocol to evaluate whether zidovudine treatment of mothers during pregnancy and of their postpartum infants will decrease transmission. There have been, however, several case reports of vertical HIV transmission from mothers receiving zidovudine.[7,25] Another protocol is being planned to evaluate the effect on transmission of hyperimmune anti-HIV intravenous immunoglobulin administered to pregnant mothers who are also receiving zidovudine. Although development of a transmission-blocking vaccine is not likely in the near future, it is hoped that candidate vaccines soon will be available to test for their potential to decrease mother-to-infant transmission.

TRANSMISSION FROM INFECTED HEALTH CARE WORKERS TO THEIR PATIENTS

The eventual occurrence of HIV transmission from an HIV-infected health care worker to his or her patients was anticipated for two reasons. First, many reports have described transmission of hepatitis B virus, a blood-borne pathogen with transmission routes similar to those of HIV, from infected health care workers to patients during invasive medical and dental procedures.[16] Second, transmission of HIV from infected patients to health care workers after percutaneous exposure to infected blood is well documented (see Chapter 4).

However, it was not until July 1990 that the first case of possible HIV transmission from an infected health care worker to a patient was reported.[15] The patient was a young woman who, 2 years before developing AIDS, had her third maxillary molars extracted by a dentist with AIDS. Subsequent investigation revealed four additional patients who apparently also were infected while receiving care from the dentist.[17,18] All five infected patients had the following characteristics: (1) none had other confirmed exposures to HIV; (2) all had undergone one or more invasive procedures performed by the dentist; and (3) their HIV strains were genetically similar to each other and to the strain infecting the dentist but distinct from other HIV strains found in persons from the same geographic area.

Although all five of these patients apparently were infected during their dental care, the precise route of transmission remains unknown. One possibility is that some or all of the patients were directly exposed to the dentist's blood while undergoing the invasive procedures. These procedures, which included extractions and root canal therapy, require the use of sharp instruments that could have caused percutaneous injuries to the dentist. Although the patients were not aware that the dentist had injured himself while caring for them, he would not necessarily have informed them if such injuries had occurred. Although he wore gloves while caring for four of the five patients, gloves do not prevent all injuries caused by sharp instruments.

A second possibility is that the patients were infected indirectly through the use of instruments previously contaminated with the dentist's blood or the blood of a patient he had previously infected (see Chapter 4). This route appears less likely than the direct route for several reasons. First, although the dentist did not always follow recommended infection control procedures, HIV does not survive for extended periods in the environment and is susceptible to heat and the germicides used in this dental practice. Second, patient-to-patient transmission would most likely require days when more than one of the infected patients were seen in the office. Although several of the patients did visit the office on the same day, neither the time nor order of their appointments is known. An analysis of the procedures done on these days indicates that it is unlikely that the same instruments were used on more than one of the infected patients. Given the multiple dental visits made by these patients, their shared visit days may simply have occurred by chance.

Although the risk of HIV transmission from health care worker to patient is not known precisely, it probably is very small. Five additional investigations of the former patients of HIV-infected health care workers have been reported (Table 1–4). Of the 1235 patients tested for HIV antibody, only one was positive. This patient was a known injecting drug user whose clinical history suggested that he was infected before he had surgery. The Centers for Disease Control (CDC) is aware of a number of other "look-back" investigations that are still in progress. Although HIV-infected patients have been detected in several of these investigations, it is too early to know if any of these patients were infected during their surgical or dental care.

The CDC first published guidelines for the management of HIV-infected health care workers in 1987[14] and revised these guidelines in 1991.[16] Nonetheless, the subject of HIV transmission from infected health care workers to patients and the need for guidelines have been the subject of intense professional and public debate. This debate is likely to continue until more information can be obtained from the ongoing look-back studies.

Table 1–4.   HIV Testing of Patients of Infected Health Care Workers*

OCCUPATION OF WORKER	NO. PATIENTS TESTED	NO. POSITIVE	REFERENCE
General surgeon	616	1	68
General surgeon	76	0	84
General surgeon	75	0	6
Dental student	143	0	22
Family physician	325	0	27

*Excludes dental patients described in text.

CONCLUSION

During the first decade of the AIDS epidemic, much was learned about the routes of HIV transmission. Nonetheless, much remains to be learned about the specific determinants of transmission through these routes. Knowledge of these determinants is vital for the development of more effective behavioral and biologic interventions to prevent further transmission. In addition, the AIDS epidemic is far enough along that unusual cases of HIV transmission will occur. It is important that these unusual cases are recognized, that the circumstances that caused them are understood, and that appropriate action is undertaken to prevent them in the future.

REFERENCES

1. Allain J-P: Prevalence of HTLV-III/LAV antibodies in patients with hemophilia and in their sexual partners in France. N Engl J Med 315:517, 1986
2. Allain J-P, Matthews T, Coombs R, et al: Antibody to V3 loop peptide does not predict vertical transmission of HIV. In Abstracts of the Seventh International Conference on AIDS (Abstract W.C.3263). Florence, 1991
3. Amirhessami-Aghili N, Spector SA: Human immunodeficiency virus type 1 infection of human placenta: Potential route for fetal infection. J Virol 65:2231, 1991
4. Anderson D, Politch JA, Martinez A, et al: Prevalance and temporal variation of HIV-1 in semen. In Abstracts of the Sixth International Conference on AIDS (Abstract Th.C.553). San Francisco, 1990
5. Andiman WA, Simpson J, Olson B, et al: Rate of transmission of human immunodeficiency virus type 1 infection from mother to child and short-term outcome of neonatal infection. Am J Dis Child 144:758, 1990
6. Armstrong FP, Miner JC, Wolfe WH: Investigation of a health care worker with symptomatic human immunodeficiency virus infection: An epidemiologic approach. Milit Med 152:414, 1987
7. Barzilai A, Sperling RS, Hyatt AC, et al: Mother to child transmission of human immunodeficiency virus 1 infection despite zidovudine therapy from 18 weeks of gestation. Pediatr Infect Dis J 9:931, 1990
8. Belec L, Bouquety JC, Georges AJ, et al: Antibodies to human immunodeficiency virus in the breast milk of healthy, seropositive women. Pediatrics 85:1022, 1990
9. Blanche S, Rouzioux C, Moscato MLG, et al: A prospective study of infants born to women seropositive for human immunodeficiency virus type 1. N Engl J Med 320:1643, 1989

10. Bongaarts J, Reining P, Way P, et al: The relationship between male circumcision and HIV infection in African populations. AIDS 3:373, 1989

11. Bouvet E, De Vincenzi I, Ancelle R, et al: Defloration as risk factor for heterosexual HIV transmission. Lancet 1:615, 1989

12. Cameron DW, Simonsen JN, D'Costa LJ, et al: Female-to-male transmission of human immunodeficiency virus type 1: Risk factors for seroconversion in men. Lancet 2:403, 1989

13. Centers for Disease Control: HIV infection and pregnancies in sexual partners of HIV-seropositive hemophilic men—United States. MMWR 36:593, 1987

14. Centers for Disease Control: Recommendations for prevention of HIV transmission in health-care settings. MMWR 36(Suppl 2S):1, 1987

15. Centers for Disease Control: Possible transmission of human immunodeficiency virus to a patient during an invasive dental procedure. MMWR 39:489, 1990

16. Centers for Disease Control: Recommendations for preventing transmission of human immunodeficiency virus and hepatitis B virus to patients during exposure-prone invasive procedures. MMWR 40. (RR-8):1, 1991

17. Centers for Disease Control: Update: Transmission of HIV infection during an invasive dental procedure—Florida. MMWR 40:21, 1991

18. Centers for Disease Control: Update: Transmission of HIV infection during invasive dental procedures—Florida. MMWR 40:377, 1991

19. Chin J: Current and future dimensions of the HIV/AIDS pandemic in women and children. Lancet 336:221, 1990

20. Clumeck N, Taelman H, Hermans P, et al: A cluster of HIV infection among heterosexual people without apparent risk factors. N Engl J Med 321:1460, 1989

21. Coates RA, Calzavara LM, Read SE, et al: Risk factors for HIV infection in male sexual contacts of men with AIDS or an AIDS-related condition. Am J Epidemiol 128:729, 1988

22. Comer RW, Myers DR, Steadman CD, et al: Management considerations for an HIV positive dental student. J Dent Educ 55:187, 1991

23. Coombs RW, Collier AC, Allain J-P, et al: Plasma viremia in human immunodeficiency virus infections. N Engl J Med 321:1626, 1989

24. Courgnaud V, Laure F, Brossard A, et al: Frequent and early in utero HIV-1 infection. AIDS Res Hum Retroviruses 7:337, 1991

25. Crombleholme W, Wara D, Gambertoglio J, et al: Perinatal HIV transmission despite maternal/infant AZT therapy. In Abstracts of the Sixth International Conference on AIDS (Abstract Th.C.605). San Francisco, 1990

26. Daar ES, Moudgil T, Meyer RD, et al: Transient high levels of viremia in patients with primary human immunodeficiency virus type 1 infection. N Engl J Med 324:961, 1991

27. Danila RN, MacDonald KL, Rhame FS, et al: A look-back investigation of patients of an HIV-infected physician. Public health implications. N Engl J Med 325:1406, 1991

28. D'Arminio MA, Ravizza M, Muggiasca ML, et al: HIV infected pregnant women: Possible predictors of vertical transmission. In Abstracts of the Seventh International Conference on AIDS (Abstract W.C.49). Florence, 1991

29. Darrow WW, Echenberg DF, Jaffe HW, et al: Risk factors for human immunodeficiency virus (HIV) infections in homosexual men. Am J Public Health 77:479, 1987

30. Datta P, Embree J, Ndinya-Achola J, et al: Perinatal HIV-1 transmission in Nairobi, Kenya: 5 year followup. In Abstracts of the Seventh International Conference on AIDS (Abstract M.C.3). Florence, 1991

31. DeCock KM, Brun-Vezinet F, Soro B: HIV-1 and HIV-2 infections and AIDS in West Africa. AIDS 5[suppl 1]:S21-S28, 1991

32. Detels R, English P, Visscher BR, et al: Seroconversion, sexual activity, and condom use among 2915 HIV seronegative men followed for up to 2 years. J AIDS 2:77, 1989

33. Devash Y, Calvelli TA, Wood DG, et al: Vertical transmission of human immunodefiency virus is correlated with the absence of high-affinity/avidity maternal antibodies to the gp120 principal neutralizing domain. Proc Natl Acad Sci U S A 87:3445, 1990

34. DeVincenzi I, Ancelle-Park R: Heterosexual transmission of HIV: Follow-up of a European cohort of couples. In Abstracts of the Seventh International Conference on AIDS (Abstract M.C. 3028). Florence, 1991

35. Ehrnst A, Lindgren S, Dictor M, et al: HIV in pregnant women and their offspring: Evidence for late transmission. Lancet 338:203, 1991

36. European Collaborative Study: Children born to women with HIV-1 infection: Natural history and risk of transmission. Lancet 337:253, 1991

37. European Study Group: Risk factors for male to female transmission of HIV. Br Med J 298:411, 1989
38. Goedert JJ, Duliege A-M, Amos CI, et al: High risk of HIV-1 infection for first-born twins. Lancet 338:1471, 1991
39. Goedert JJ, Eyster ME, Biggar RJ, et al: Heterosexual transmission of human immunodeficiency virus: Association with severe depletion of T-helper lymphocytes in men with hemophilia. AIDS Res Hum Retroviruses 3:355, 1987
40. Goedert JJ, Mendez H, Drummond JE, et al: Mother-to-infant transmission of human immunodeficiency virus type 1: Association with prematurity or low anti-gp120. Lancet 2:1351, 1989
41. Greenspan A, Castro KG: Heterosexual transmission of HIV infection. Siecus Rep 19:1, 1990
42. Hague RA, Mok JYQ, MacCallum L, et al: Do maternal factors influence the risk of vertical transmission of HIV? In Abstracts of the Seventh International Conference on AIDS (Abstract W.C.3237). Florence, 1991
43. Halsey NA, Boulos R, Holt E, et al: Transmission of HIV-1 infections from mothers to infants in Haiti. JAMA 64:2088, 1990
44. Halsey NA, Markham R, Rossi P, et al: V3 loop peptide antibodies in Haitian women and infant HIV-1 infections. In Abstracts of the Seventh International Conference on AIDS (Abstract W.A.1311). Florence, 1991
45. Hira SK, Kamanga J, Phat GJ, et al: Perinatal transmission of HIV-1 in Zambia. Br Med J 299:1250, 1989
46. Hira SK, Mangrola G, Mwale C, et al: Apparent vertical transmission of human immunodeficiency virus type 1 by breast-feeding in Zambia. J Pediatr 117:421, 1990
47. Ho DD, Moudgil T, Alam M: Quantitation of human immunodeficiency virus type 1 in the blood of infected person. N Engl J Med 321:1621, 1989
48. Hutto C, Parks W, Lai S, et al: A hospital-based prospective study of perinatal infection with human immunodeficiency virus type 1. J Pediatr 118:347, 1991
49. Italian Multicentre Study: Epidemiology, clinical features, and prognostic factors of paediatric HIV infection. Lancet 2:1043, 1988
50. Kingsley LA, Detels R, Kaslow R, et al: Risk factors for seroconversion to human immunodeficiency virus among male homosexuals. Lancet 1:345, 1987
51. Krasinski K, Cao YZ, Friedman-Kien A, et al: Elevated maternal total and neutralizing anti-HIV1 antibody does not prevent perinatal HIV1. In Abstracts of the Sixth International Conference on AIDS (Abstract No. Th.C.45). San Francisco, 1990
52. Kreiss JK, Coombs R, Plummer F, et al: Isolation of human immunodeficiency virus from genital ulcers in Nairobi prostitutes. J Infect Dis 160:380, 1989
53. Kreiss J, Datta P, Willerford D, et al: Vertical transmission of HIV in Nairobi: Correlation with maternal viral burden. In Abstracts of the Seventh International Conference on AIDS (Abstract M.C.3062). Florence, 1991
54. Kreiss JK, Kitchen LW, Prince HE, et al: Antibody to human T-lymphotropic virus type III in wives of hemophiliacs: Evidence for heterosexual transmission. Ann Intern Med 102:623, 1985
55. Kreiss JK, Koech D, Plummer FA, et al: AIDS virus infection in Nairobi prostitutes. Spread of the epidemic to East Africa. N Engl J Med 314:414, 1986
56. Krieger JN, Coombs RW, Collier AC, et al: Recovery of human immunodeficiency virus type 1 from semen: Minimal impact of stage of infection and current antiviral chemotherapy. J Infect Dis 163:386, 1991
57. Laga M, Nzila N, Manoka AT, et al: Non ulcerative sexually transmitted disease as risk factors for HIV infection. In Abstracts of the Sixth International Conference on AIDS (Abstract Th.C.97). San Francisco, 1990
58. Lallemont M, Lallemant-Le Coeur S, Cheynier D, et al: Mother-child transmission of HIV-1 and infant survival in Brazzaville, Congo. AIDS 3:643, 1989
59. Lapointe N, Michaud J, Pekovic D, et al: Transplacental transmission of HTLV-III virus. N Engl J Med 312:1325, 1985
60. Lepage P, Van de Perre P, Msellati P, et al: Natural history of HIV-1 infection in children in Rwanda. A prospective cohort study. In Abstracts of the Seventh International Conference on AIDS (Abstract W.C.46). Florence, 1991
61. Lewis SH, Reynolds-Kohler C, Fox E, et al: HIV-1 in trophoblastic and villous Hofbauer cells, and haematological precursors in eight-week fetuses. Lancet 335:565, 1990
62. Lifson AR, O'Malley PM, Hessol NA, et al: HIV seroconversion in two homosexual men after receptive oral intercourse with ejaculation: Implications for counselling concerning safe sexual practices. Am J Public Health 80:1509, 1990

63. Lusher JM, Operskalski EA, Aledort LM, et al: Risk of human immunodeficiency virus type 1 infection among sexual and nonsexual household contacts of persons with congenital clotting disorders. Pediatrics 88:242, 1991
64. Marlink R, Thior I, Dia MC, et al: Prospective study of the natural history of HIV-2. In Abstracts of the Seventh International Conference on AIDS (Abstract Tu.C.104). Florence, 1991
65. Mayer KH, DeGruttola V: Human immunodeficiency virus and oral intercourse. Ann Intern Med 107:428, 1987
66. Mayers MM, Davenny K, Schoenbaum EE, et al: A prospective study of infants of human immunodeficiency virus seropositive and seronegative women with a history of intravenous drug use or of intravenous drug-using sex partners, in the Bronx, New York City. Pediatrics 88:1248, 1991
67. Mermin JH, Holodniy M, Katzenstein DA, et al: Detection of human immunodeficiency virus DNA and RNA in semen by the polymerase chain reaction. J Infect Dis 164:769, 1991
68. Mishu B, Schaffner W, Horan J, et al: A surgeon with AIDS. Lack of evidence of transmission to patients. JAMA 264:467, 1990
69. Morgan G, Wilkins HA, Pepin J, et al: AIDS following mother-to-child transmission of HIV-2. AIDS 4:879, 1990
70. Moss AR, Osmond D, Bacchetti P, et al: Risk factors for AIDS and HIV seropositivity in homosexual men. Am J Epidemiol 125:1035, 1987
71. Moss GB, Clemetson D, D'Costa L, et al: Association of cervical ectopy with heterosexual transmission of human immunodeficiency virus: Results of a study of couples in Nairobi, Kenya. J Infect Dis 164:588, 1991
72. Mundy DC, Schinazi RF, Gerber AR, et al: Human immunodeficiency virus isolated from amniotic fluid. Lancet 2:459, 1987
73. Musicco M, Sarraco A, Nicolosi A, et al: Incidence and risk factors of man to woman sexual HIV transmission: Longitudinal study on 171 women steady partners of infected men. In Abstracts of the Seventh International Conference on AIDS (Abstract M.C.4). Florence, 1991
74. O'Brien TR, Anderson DJ, Seage GR III, et al: Inverse association between zidovudine therapy and the prevalence of HIV in semen. In Abstracts of the Seventh International Conference on AIDS (Abstract M.C. 3092). Florence, 1991
75. Oxtoby MJ: Human immunodeficiency virus and other viruses in human milk: Placing the issues in broader perspective. Pediatr Infect Dis J 7:825, 1988
76. Padian N, Marquis L, Francis DP, et al: Male-to-female transmission of human immunodeficiency virus. JAMA 258:788, 1987
77. Padian NS, Shiboski SC, Jewell NP: Female-to-male transmission of human immunodeficiency virus. JAMA 266:1664, 1991
78. Parekh BS, Shaffer N, Pau C-P, et al: Lack of correlation between maternal antibodies to V3 loop peptides of gp120 and perinatal HIV-1 transmission. AIDS 5:1179, 1991
79. Peterman TA, Stoneburner RL, Allen JR, et al: Risk of human immunodeficiency virus transmission from heterosexual adults with transfusion-associated infections. JAMA 259:55, 1988
80. Piot P, Plummer FA, Mhalu FS, et al: AIDS: An international perspective. Science 239:573, 1988
81. Pizzo PA, Butler KM: In the vertical transmission of HIV, timing may be everything. (Editorial.) N Engl J Med 325:652, 1991
82. Plummer FA, Simonsen N, Cameron DW, et al: Cofactors in male-female sexual transmission of human immunodeficiency virus type 1. J Infect Dis 163:233, 1991
83. Pokrovsky VV, Kuznetsova I, Eramova I: Transmission of HIV-infection from an infected infant to his mother by breast-feeding. In Abstracts of the Sixth International Conference on AIDS (Abstract Th.C.48). San Francisco, 1990
84. Porter JD, Cruickshank JG, Gentle PH, et al: Management of patients treated by a surgeon with HIV infection. Lancet 335:113, 1990
85. Poulsen A-G, Kvinesdal B, Aaby P, et al: No evidence of vertical transmission of HIV-2 in Bissau. In Abstracts of the Fifth International Conference on AIDS (Abstract T.G.P.31). Montreal, 1989
86. Poulsen A-G, Kvinesdal B, Aaby P, et al: Prevalence of and mortality from human immunodeficiency virus type 2 in Bissau, West Africa. Lancet 1:827, 1989
87. Rossi P, Moschese V, Broliden P, et al: Presence of maternal antibodies to human immunodeficiency virus 1 envelope glycoprotein gp120 epitopes correlates with the uninfected status of children born to seropositive mothers. Proc Natl Acad Sci U S A 86:8055, 1989

88. Rozenbaum W, Gharakhanian S, Cardon B, et al: HIV transmission by oral sex. Lancet 1:1395, 1988
89. Ryder RW, Manzila T, Baende E, et al: Evidence from Zaire that breast-feeding by HIV-1–seropositive mothers is not a major route for perinatal HIV-1 transmission but does decrease morbidity. AIDS 5:709, 1991
90. Ryder RW, Wato N, Hassig SE, et al: Perinatal transmission of the human immunodeficiency virus type 1 to infants of seropositive women in Zaire. N Engl J Med 320:1637, 1989
91. Stiegbiegal NH, Maude DW, Feiner CJ, et al: Heterosexual transmission of HIV infection. In Abstracts of the Fourth International Conference on AIDS (Abstract 4057). Stockholm, 1988
92. Stiehm RE, Vink P: Transmission of human immunodeficiency virus infection by breast-feeding. J Pediatr 118:410, 1991
93. St. Louis ME, Kabagabo U, Brown C, et al: Maternal factors associated with perinatal HIV transmission. In Abstracts of the Seventh International Conference on AIDS (Abstract M.C.3027). Florence, 1991
94. Thiry L, Sprecher-Goldbrecher S, Jonckheer T, et al: Isolation of AIDS virus from cell-free breast milk of three healthy virus carriers. Lancet 2:891, 1985
95. Valente P, Main EK: Role of the placenta in perinatal transmission of HIV. Obstet Gynecol Clin North Am 17:607, 1990
96. Van de Perre P, Hitimana DG, Lepage P: Human immunodeficiency virus antibodies of IgG, IgA, and IgM subclasses in milk of seropositive mothers. J Pediatr 113:1039, 1988
97. Van de Perre P, Simonon A, Msellati P, et al: Postnatal transmission of human immunodeficiency virus type 1 from mother to infant. N Engl J Med 325:593, 1991
98. Vogt MW, Witt DJ, Craven DE, et al: Isolation of HTLV-III/LAV from cervical secretions of women at risk for AIDS. Lancet 1:525, 1986
99. Winkelstein W Jr, Lyman DM, Padian N, et al: Sexual practices and risk of infection by the human immunodeficiency virus, The San Francisco Men's Health Study. JAMA 257:321, 1987
100. World Health Organization: Breast feeding/breastmilk and human immunodeficiency virus (HIV). Wkly Epidemiol Rec 62:245, 1987
101. World Health Organization: Current and future dimensions of the HIV/AIDS pandemic: A capsule summary. September 1990. WHO/GPA/SFI/90.2

2

VIRAL AND IMMUNOLOGIC FACTORS IN HIV INFECTION

JAY A. LEVY, MD

HIV initially was isolated in 1983 from patients with AIDS and the AIDS-related complex (ARC). The virus was called lymphadenopathy-associated virus (LAV), human T cell lymphotropic virus type III (HTLV-III), and the AIDS-associated retrovirus (ARV).[5,23,54] An international committee on taxonomy of viruses recommended in 1986 a new term, *HIV (human immunodeficiency virus)*, to distinguish this virus as a newly recognized human pathogen.[16] In following that recommendation, we at the University of California, San Francisco, have renamed our isolates of HIV type 1, HIV-1$_{San Francisco}$ (HIV-1$_{SF}$). The second subtype of HIV, HIV-2, discussed below, is identified in our laboratory with the University of California subscript (HIV-2$_{UC}$). In this chapter we primarily refer to studies of HIV-1, designated in the text as HIV.

Studies by several groups indicated that HIV was associated with AIDS and the diseases linked to this syndrome.[5,23,54,57,76] Moreover, antibodies to the virus were found in individuals with disease or belonging to one of the groups known as at risk for AIDS.[23,41,42,54,78,79] These groups included homosexual or bisexual men, intravenous drug users, newborn children of seropositive mothers, transfusion and blood product recipients (hemophiliacs), and heterosexual contacts of virus-positive individuals. Moreover, individuals from Haiti and Africa had a high prevalence of HIV infection.[46,67,87] The source of infection in Haitians and Africans apparently was heterosexual activity, but transfusions and reuse of needles could also be factors. These epidemiologic and virologic studies indicated that the major route of HIV infection was by blood and intimate sexual contact. These sources of transmission have not changed.[6] All these early studies conclusively showed that HIV was the etiologic agent of this newly recognized human disease.

Research conducted by several laboratories has demonstrated that HIV is a member of the lentivirus subfamily of human retroviruses.[56,72] Other subfamilies include the Oncovirinae and the Spumavirinae, characterized by human T-cell leukemia

My work and that of my collegues cited in this paper were supported by grants from the American Foundation for AIDS Research, the California State University-Wide Task Force on AIDS, and the National Institutes of Health (grant numbers RO1-AI-24499 and PO1-AI-24286).

Table 2–1.   Characteristics of HIV That Resemble a Lentivirus

Clinical
1. Association with a disease with a long incubation period
2. Involvement of hematopoietic system
3. Involvement of the central nervous system
4. Association with immune suppression
Biologic
1. Cytopathic effect in certain infected cells (e.g., helper T cells) (fusion; multinucleated cells)
2. Infection of macrophages
3. Accumulation of unintegrated circular and linear forms of proviral DNA in infected cells
4. Latent infection in some infected cells
5. Morphology of viral particle by electron microscopy: cone-shaped nucleoid
Molecular
1. Large provirus size (9.7 kb)
2. Primer binding site, tRNA^{Lys}
3. Truncated *gag* gene: several processed *gag* proteins
4. Similar genomic base composition
5. Polymorphism, particularly in the envelope region
6. Novel central open reading frame in the viral genome that separates the *pol* and *env* regions
7. Presence of regulatory and accessory genes

virus, type 1, and the human foamy virus, respectively. All these viruses, as retroviruses, code for an enzyme, RNA-dependent DNA polymerase or reverse transcriptase, that permits transcription of the viral RNA into a DNA copy (cDNA).[49] In this form it can integrate into the celluar genome and replicate via the proviral DNA (see later discussion). The characteristics the AIDS virus shares with lentiviruses include its long genome (9.7 kilobases [kb]), its highly variable envelope genes (as demonstrated by selective serologic studies), its induction of a slow disease, and its cytopathic properties in cell culture. Moreover, like the animal lentiviruses, it infects the brain (Table 2–1).[29,35,55]

The major HIV proteins have been located in the virion by immunoelectron microscopy.[25] As demonstrated in Figure 2–1, the external envelope protein (gp120) is associated with small protrusions or spikes on the surface of the virion and attached to the viral capsid via the transmembrane protein, gp41. The *gag* proteins make up the core and the phosphoproteins that are found inside this nucleoid. The major *gag* protein has a molecular weight of 25,000 and is called *p25* (or *p24*); it forms the core shell. The *gag* protein p17 is located outside the core, right below the virion outer membrane (see Fig. 2–1). This location may explain the ability of some sera with antibodies to p17 to neutralize HIV.[68,77] Part of p17 may protrude through the viral capsid. Finally, reverse transcriptase (RT) is present in the core, intimately associated with the two strands of viral RNA, which are exact copies of each other. This diploid state is characteristic of all retroviruses and is important for their replicative cycle (for review, see Levy[49]).

WHAT CELLS ARE INFECTED BY HIV?

The initial studies of the AIDS virus revealed its presence in peripheral blood mononuclear cells (PMCs), particularly T-helper lymphocytes.[5,23,54] Subsequently,

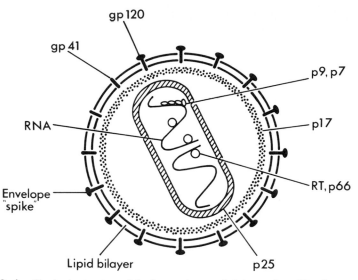

FIGURE 2–1. The basic structure of the human immunodeficiency virus. The diagram shows the location of the major structural proteins of the virion. (From Levy JA: Human immunodeficiency viruses and the pathogenesis of AIDS. JAMA 261:2997, 1989. Copyright 1989, American Medical Association.)

HIV was recovered from macrophages and was shown to infect a variety of other human cells, including B lymphocytes, promyelocytes, fibroblasts, and perhaps epidermal Langerhans cells.[56,58,85,86] The virus has been recovered from lymph nodes, bowel epithelium, and brain (see later discussion).

Integrated viral DNA has been detected in brain tissue,[81] and infectious virus has been isolated from all regions of the brain and cerebrospinal fluid (CSF).[35,37,55] The detection of infectious virus in CSF does not necessarily correlate with neurologic findings since individuals with fever or headaches alone have been found to have virus in this body fluid.[37] In situ hybridization studies have demonstrated HIV RNA primarily in brain macrophages but also in capillary endothelial cells and possibly glial cells in the brain, including oligodendrocytes.[47,52,92] Moreover, tissue culture studies have indicated the susceptibility of brain astrocytes to infection by the virus.[12]

HIV has been detected in the renal epithlium[17] and in the bowel epithelium, particularly in crypt cells and enterochromaffin cells.[64] This observation may explain the malabsorption and chronic diarrhea observed in some infected individuals and the syndrome of "slim disease" first described in Uganda.[80] The enterchromaffin cells have endocrine functions that control motility and digestive functions of the bowel. Thus, when infected, they could be responsible for the diarrhea. All these studies indicate the wide host cell range of the AIDS virus (Table 2–2).

Besides being found in several body tissues, HIV can be recovered from many body fluids (Table 2–3). In initial studies we found infectious virus in 30% of plasma or serum samples of infected individuals.[63] The estimated quantity was 10 to 50 infectious particles (IP)/ml. One individual had a titer as high as 25,000 IP/ml.[56] Subsequent reports have found HIV in most plasma samples of infected individuals, with the highest levels ($>10^4$ IP/ml) in patients with AIDS.[17a,34] We have confirmed this observation by assaying the plasma shortly after venipuncture

Table 2–2. Cells Susceptible to HIV

Hematopoietic	**Skin**
T lymphocytes	Langerhans cells
B lymphocytes	Fibroblasts
Macrophages	**Other**
Promyelocytes	Colon carcinoma cells
Dendritic cells	Bowel epithelium
Brain	Renal epithelium
Astrocytes	
Oligodendrocytes	
Capillary endothelium	
Macrophages	

and revising our cell culture procedures to detect virus production by the p25 antigen enzyme-linked immunosorbent assay (ELISA), a more sensitive assay than RT. Nevertheless, the relatively small amount of freely circulating virus in the blood could explain the low risk of infection following needle-stick injuries[26] compared with that of hepatitis B, which can be present in the blood of infected individuals at 10^8 IPs/ml. Other body fluids such as tears, saliva, and ear secretions contain at least one tenth to one hundredth the amount of virus in the blood and plasma and at less frequency.[56] Thus they essentially present no source of contagion. Genital secretions (vaginal or cervical and seminal fluids) vary in viral quantities but generally contain much less than blood.[56,88,93] CSF appears to yield high levels of virus (up to 1000 IPs/ml), reflecting good replication of HIV in certain brain cells. However, this body fluid would not be a natural source of infection.

Because of the relatively low level of infectious HIV particles present in body fluids, transmission of the virus in a free state seems less likely than transmission

Table 2–3. Isolation of HIV From Body Fluids

	VIRAL ISOLATION	ESTIMATED QUANTITY OF HIV
Cell Free Fluid		
Plasma	31/31	1-500
Tears	2/5	<1
Ear secretions	1/8	5-10
Saliva	3/55	<1
Urine	1/5	<1
Vaginal/cervical secretions	5/16	<1
Semen	5/15	10-50
Milk	1/5	<1
Cerebrospinal fluid	21/40	10-1000
Infected Cells		
Peripheral mononuclear cell	89/92	0.001%-01%
Saliva	4/11	<0.01%
Bronchial fluid	3/24	NK
Vaginal/cervical fluid	7/16	NK
Semen	11/28	0.01%-5%

NK, not known.

Results reflect number of specimens that contained HIV as determined by standard virologic procedures.[51,56,57]

by the infected cells also present.[32,50] Certain body fluids, particularly genital secretions, can contain substantial numbers of virus-infected cells.[50] In studies conducted in our laboratory, we found variations in the number of infected cells in these fluids among seropositive individuals. Up to 5% of white cells in seminal fluid can be HIV infected.[50] Since approximately 10^6 mononuclear cells are found in the ejaculate, this number of infected cells could be a major source of transmission. We believe this factor relates directly to the ability to transfer the virus to others. It can explain why several partners of some seropositive individuals do not get infected[65]; the genital fluids do not contain a large number of infected cells. In Africa sexually transmitted diseases are clearly a cofactor in the transmission of HIV, particularly in the case of genital ulcers caused by *Haemophilus ducreyi* or herpesvirus.[7,71,82] These infections produce open lesions that would permit contact of virus-infected cells with susceptible host cells. Moreover, venereal disease could bring copious amounts of inflammatory cells into the genital fluids, and many of them would be virus infected. This emphasis on the virus-infected cell as the major source of infection cannot be overstated. These cells pose a major problem in attempts at antiviral therapy and development of a vaccine. Probably only mechanisms that destroy HIV-carrying cells will lead to prevention and elimination of this viral infection.

HOW DOES HIV INFECT CELLS?

Retroviruses from all animal species require a cell surface receptor for attachment and penetration of the cell. It is generally accepted that HIV binds to the cell membrane primarily via the CD4 antigen complex. This protein was first recognized as a surface marker on helper T cells. It also has been found on a variety of hematopoietic cells, including B lymphocytes, macrophages, and some brain cells. The presence of the CD4 antigen appears to explain the susceptibility of many cells to HIV. However, as noted later, the virus also infects some cells lacking CD4 protein expression.

A direct interaction of viral gp120 with the CD4 molecule has been demonstrated by showing that both proteins are required for infection.[18,40,45,62] Monoclonal antibodies to specific epitopes on the CD4 protein block HIV infection, and antibodies to either CD4 or viral gp120 precipitate both proteins in a complex.[40,62] Nevertheless, work in our laboratory with cultured human fibroblasts,[85] and certain brain cells has indicated that CD4 is not the only receptor for HIV; these cells lack any evidence of CD4 protein or mRNA expression but can be infected by the virus.[12,85] Moreover, even CD8+ lymphocytes lacking the CD4 molecule can be infected if they are coinfected by another retrovirus such as HTLV-I[19] (C.Walker and J.A. Levy, unpublished observations). Clearly, other mechanisms for HIV entrance into a cell are involved.

Evidence from some laboratories has shown that antibodies to gp41, the transmembrane protein of HIV, can prevent virus infection.[36] This observation suggests that the virus may interact with the cell surface at two sites. The HIV envelope gp120 appears to attach to the CD4 protein, whereas gp41 could act as a fusion protein and interact with a separate cellular receptor (Figure 2–2).[22a] Thus both proteins working in concert permit the most efficient entrance of HIV into a cell.

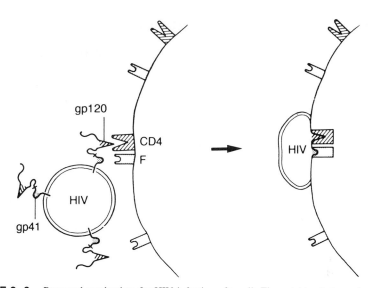

FIGURE 2–2. Proposed mechanism for HIV infection of a cell. The outside viral envelope protein, gp120, attaches to a cell surface receptor, most likely the CD4 antigen. The external portion of the transmembrane protein, gp41, attaches to a proposed specific fusion receptor (F) on the cell surface. Either receptor may permit viral entry into the cell, but both together would make this event more efficient.

A similar mechanism of infection has been shown for the paramyxoviruses.[70] Most recently, a potentially new virus receptor, galactosyl ceramide, has been found on brain-derived glial cells in culture.[31] Antibodies to this molecule block HIV infection of these CD4 − cells. This brain cell–specific glycolipid, however, is not present on all CD4-lacking cells such as fibroblasts. Thus still other receptors exist, or these CD4 − cells are infected via the gp41 receptor: fusion mechanism.

Once the virus enters the cell, its RNA, inside the central core, begins the process of reverse transcription that produces double-stranded DNA that circularizes and goes to the nucleus. This cDNA integrates into the host chromosome where it exists as a proviral DNA. The infected cell can remain in this latent state in which it makes little or no viral RNA or proteins. The cell can thus elude the host immune system possibly for years—a potential reason for long incubation periods.

Alternatively, the infected cell enters active virus production in which the proviral DNA makes the viral RNA and proteins, leading to release of infectious progeny. These infected cells can then spread the virus through production of infectious progeny or by fusion with uninfected cells.[59] This latter cell-to-cell interaction is important because it permits the transfer of viral information into an uninfected cell by a mechanism unaffected by neutralizing antibodies. The hypothetic fusion mechanism for virus entry that probably occurs between HIV gp41 and a cell receptor (see Fig. 2–2) might also mediate cell-to-cell contact. Both viral envelope proteins (gp41, gp120) are found on the surface of HIV-infected cells.[25] Finally, the cell latently infected by HIV may later become activated in the host by still undefined factors and enter into a virus-productive state.

ARE ALL HIV STRAINS THE SAME?

Soon after the identification of the three prototypes of HIV, it became clear, based on molecular studies, that a heterogeneity of HIV strains existed. Whereas LAV and HTLV-III were very similar, ARV and two other San Francisco isolates studied (ARV-3 and ARV-4) were quite distinct.[61,72] The genome of ARV versus LAV/HTLV-III differed by at least 6%; the predicted amino acid differences could be as high as 27%. Each HIV isolate has its own distinct restriction enzyme pattern and sequence identity. The major modifications in HIV occur in the envelope region[83] and in the regulatory proteins (e.g., *nef, tat*) for reasons that are unknown. Perhaps the accumulation of unintegrated proviral DNA copies of HIV in the cells during acute viral infection[56] permits genomic alterations because mutations and recombinations could occur more easily than if the virus were in an integrated state. This possibility is now under study.

HIV isolates can be distinguished not only by molecular but also by biologic features. They can differ in their ability to replicate in established T, B, and macrophage cell lines as well as PMCs and primary macrophages.[2,3,20,24,52,53,58] Moreover, the ability of HIV isolates to induce plaques in the MT4 T-cell line appears to correlate with differences in their cytopathic properties and replicating abilities in established T cell lines.[84] Those viruses that cause typical cytopathic effects, including formation of multinucleated cells and balloon degeneration leading to cell death (Figure 2–3), and that replicate best in T-cell lines readily induce plaques in the MT4 cells.[84]

By performing a variety of tissue culture studies in the laboratory, we have been able to identify specific biologic properties of HIV that distinguish the strains

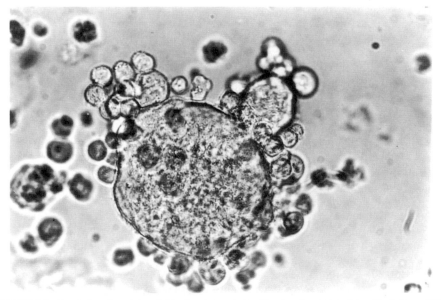

FIGURE 2–3.   Infected peripheral blood mononuclear cells showing cytopathic effects from HIV. Note the multinucleated cell caused by cell fusion and the large balloon forms ($\times$40).

Table 2–4. Biologic and Serologic Features of HIV-1 Strains Recovered From Different Tissues

CHARACTERISTICS	SOURCE OF VIRUS		
	PERIPHERAL BLOOD	BRAIN	BOWEL
Growth in CD4 + lymphocytes	+ +	+ +	+ +
Growth in established cell lines	+ +	–	±
Growth in macrophages	±	+ +	+
Modulation of CD4 antigen	+ +	–	+
Cell killing	+	–	+
Serum neutralization	+ +	–	+

associated with neurologic findings from those linked to immune suppression.[10] Those recovered from the brain do not replicate well in T cells but prefer primary macrophages. They are not neutralized efficiently by sera from HIV-infected individuals, and they are not very cytopathic in T cells and thus do not induce plaques in MT4 cells. Moreover, the evaluation of HIV isolates recovered from the bowel suggest that they may also have distinguishing biologic and serologic features.[4] Most notably, the bowel-derived isolates grow well in macrophages, but they do not grow readily in established T-cell lines. They are neutralized by serum antibodies. When bowel and blood isolates from the same individual are studied, these differences become most noteworthy[4] (Table 2–4). These initial studies suggest that other HIV strains may be found that will selectively grow in certain cells. Their disease-causing properties could be determined by their specific host range and biologic features and may differ from the initially recognized T-cell–tropic virus subtypes.

We have also demonstrated that the biologic properties of HIV can change in viruses recovered at different times from the same individual.[13] For example, one HIV isolate obtained from a patient with oral candidiasis was compared with an isolate recovered 5 months later from the same infected individual, who by that time had Kaposi's sarcoma and *Pneumocystis carinii* pneumonia. The second isolate showed greater replicating ability, a wider host range in cell culture, and more cytopathic changes, including the induction of MT4 cell plaques, than the initial HIV recovered. Yet both viral isolates were sensitive to neutralization by the same sera. Moreover, molecular studies strongly suggested that the genomes of these HIV were related since few differences were observed in restriction enzyme analyses and the genetic sequences.[13,14] These results and others with sequential HIV isolates emphasize the possibility that disease progression may occur with the emergence of more virulent strains of HIV in the individual (Table 2–5).

Most recent studies have been directed at identifying the "virulence" gene of HIV. These experiments have demonstrated that the viral envelope contains many of the regions necessary for virus infection of selected cell types, CD4 down modulation, cytopathology, and serum neutralization.[11] The regulatory regions of the virus (e.g., *tat, rev*) apparently are important for controlling intracellular replication of virus. Further studies have narrowed substantially the number of amino acid changes that may determine the replicative and cytopathic properties of

**Table 2–5. HIV Characteristics
Associated with Virulence
in the Host**

Enhanced cellular host range
Rapid kinetics of replication
High titers of viral production
Disruption or alteration in cell membrane permeability
Efficient cell killing

the virus.[14] These observations could eventually provide approaches for antiviral therapy.

Another subtype of HIV has been recovered from AIDS patients in West Africa. Existence of this virus, HIV-2, was suspected because antibodies to it, unlike those against HIV-1, cross-react with the simian immunodeficiency virus (SIV).[15,43] Molecular studies have indicated that its sequence differs from HIV-1 by 55%, with changes noted primarily in the envelope region.[28] Antibodies to HIV-2 have been found primarily in West Africa and in some individuals in Europe and South America. The virus has also been detected in the United States. Most tests for antibodies to HIV-1 can detect antibodies to HIV-2 unless only antibodies to HIV-2 envelope proteins are present in the serum. For this reason, screening tests for infection by an HIV should include the envelope protein of HIV-2 to detect exposure to either of these HIV subtypes. In our laboratory Evans et al.[21] have evaluated patients from the Ivory Coast. They have isolated several strains of HIV-2 and have identified individuals in Abidjan with antibodies to both HIV-1 and HIV-2.[21] In one individual studied, both HIV-1 and HIV-2 subtypes were recovered from the blood.[22] These results indicate that some individuals may be infected by both types of HIV.

We have characterized eight strains of HIV-2 recovered from patients infected in the Ivory Coast. The same kind of heterogeneity observed with HIV-1 strains, particularly in terms of cellular tropism and cytopathologic characteristics was observed.[8] One of the isolates, HIV-2$_{UC1}$, is noncytopathic in cell culture. It does not kill cells or induce cell fusion when infected cells are mixed with uninfected white blood cells from seronegative individuals.[21] Nevertheless, this HIV-2 strain was recovered from an individual who subsequently died of AIDS. This finding indicates that a noncytopathic HIV strain (perhaps attenuated) may be emerging in some parts of the world. Whether the individual at death had a more virulent form of this HIV-2 strain, as we have noted in HIV-1–infected individuals in whom AIDS later developed,[13] could not be determined.

HOW DOES THE HOST RESPOND TO HIV?

The outcome of any viral infection depends not only on the virulence of the virus, but also on the relative strength of the host's antiviral immune response. Because HIV attacks immune cells, its control poses an even greater challenge to an intact immune system.

The defense mechanism used by the host against viral infections consists of both humoral and cellular immune responses. B lymphocytes form the major arm of the humoral response. Through their interactions with macrophages and helper T lymphocytes, they make antibodies to foreign proteins, including invading organisms. For HIV, these include antibodies to the major structural and functional proteins of the virus that can be detected by standard immunoblot procedures.[66] Some of these antibodies can neutralize the virus; the titer depends on the specific B-cell response of the infected individual. We have demonstrated wide differences in serum levels of neutralizing antibodies among individuals.[9] Some investigators suggest that this antibody response decreases as the clinical state worsens.[73] This finding was not made, however, in longitudinal studies of infected individuals in our laboratory. In any case, neutralizing antibodies apparently are not protective once the viral infection has taken place. Thus vaccines made to induce these antibodies may help block initial infection by free virus but probably could not change the disease course after infection is established. Most important, because the virus-infected cell is a major source of transmission,[50] neutralizing antibodies in this situation would not protect an individual from infection.

Homsy in our laboratory has detected the presence of antibodies to HIV that enhance virus infection.[38,39] They were first noted in guinea pigs immunized with selected HIV-1 strains in attempts to induce type-specific neutralizing antibodies. Instead, antibodies that increased the ability of the virus to infect macrophages, T cells, and even fibroblasts were found. Subsequent studies indicated the presence of these antibodies in infected chimpanzees and in naturally infected human subjects. Enhancing antibodies have been demonstrated with infections by the flaviviruses, togaviruses, and other viral families,[30] but this is the first time such antibodies have been demonstrated for lentiviruses. The observation is important because vaccination with viral proteins must take into consideration the potential for inducing enhancing, not protective neutralizing, antibodies. These enhancing antibodies would not only increase the ability of the virus to infect T cells but might also change a lymphotropic virus into a macrophage-tropic virus. Our laboratory studies have further indicated that the mechanism for HIV entry into the macrophages and T cells after mixing with serum is the Fc receptor and does not depend on the CD4 molecule.[39] Thus enhancement is another mechanism by which HIV can enter cells without using the CD4 receptor (see the preceding). Robinson, Montefiori, and Mitchell[75] noted this enhancement of HIV infection in studies with complement-reconstituted serum and suggested that another mechanism for this phenomenon is through the complement receptor. The most recent studies suggest that the complement-mediated enhancement involves an interaction with the gp41 region of the viral envelope[74]; the Fc-mediated enhancement involves regions of gp120, particularly the third variable domain (V3 loop) (S. Kliks and J.A. Levy, unpublished observations), which has been linked to viral neutralization.[48]

The other major arm of the immune system, the cellular immune response, is often the most important defense against viral infections; with HIV this is also the case. This immune response is mediated primarily by T lymphocytes, macrophages, and natural killer (NK) cells. The T lymphocytes can be divided phenotypically into two major subgroups, helper T (CD4 +) and suppressor or cytotoxic (CD8 +) T cells. As noted earlier, the helper T lymphocytes are a major target for HIV, and suppressor T cells are rarely if ever infected by the virus. Macrophages are susceptible to HIV[24,56,58]; whether NK cells can be infected is not yet clear. The suppressor or cytotoxic T cells and the macrophages can function either by sup-

Table 2–6.   Autoantibodies in HIV Infection

TARGET	CLINICAL SIGN
Platelet	Immune thrombocytopenic purpura
Red blood cell	Anemia
Neutrophil	Neutropenia
Peripheral nerve	Neuropathy
Lymphocyte	Immune deficiency
Lupus anticoagulant (phospholipid)	? Neurologic disease; thrombosis
Nucleus (antinuclear antibody)	Autoimmunity

pressing viral replication or by killing the infected cell. In several laboratories cytotoxic responses have been observed with cells of infected individuals.[69,89] However, these studies have used systems in the laboratory that may not mimic the natural state. Thus we cannot yet be certain that HIV infection induces a protective cytotoxic response in the host.

Studies in our laboratory have indicated that in some individuals replication of HIV in PMCs can be suppressed by CD8+ T cells.[90] This suppression does not involve cell killing but is mediated in part by a diffusible factor (or cytokine) released by the CD8+ cells.[91] In comparing asymptomatic individuals with those who have active disease, we have found that the suppression by CD8+ cells can be observed best in the healthy individuals. In one case, that of an AIDS patient whose Kaposi's sarcoma lesions had gone into remission, this antiviral reaction was also noted.[90] We are attempting to identify the cytokine produced by the CD8+ cells and develop methods to sustain CD8+ cell control of HIV replication. Most recent studies suggest that the cytokine is not interferon, tumor necrosis factor, or any of the known lymphokines; it apparently is a novel product of CD8+ cells that awaits identification.

Although the immune system may limit viral replication either through neutralizing antibodies or through suppressor or cytotoxic T cells, viral infection often leads to other types of disarray in immune function. For instance, infection with many herpesviruses (e.g., Epstein-Barr) leads to activation of B cells, with resulting hypergammaglobulinemia and production of antibodies to a variety of cellular antigens.[33] In many individuals infected with HIV, a similar response can be seen with proliferation of B cells and production of antibodies. This feature is found particularly in newborn infants and young children.[1] In some individuals the antibodies are directed against normal cellular proteins and induce an autoimmune state. A variety of autoimmune syndromes have been observed in AIDS patients (Table 2–6). Each of them has been linked to an antibody to a normal protein present on the target cell.[44,51] Production of these autoantibodies may result from B-cell proliferation, carrier-hapten mechanism,[60] or from viral properties shared either by sequence or antigenic nature with a cellular protein. An example of this latter phenomenon of "molecular mimicry" is the cross-reactivity of certain viral envelope epitopes with human leukocyte antigens (HLAs).[27] Antibodies to the envelope may induce these anti-HLA antibodies that could play a role in destroying lymphocytes in the host. These possibilities are under study. Thus HIV infection might lead to the production of autoantibodies that further compromise the immune system and contribute to the progression to disease.

SUMMARY

This chapter reviews briefly the important characteristics of the AIDS virus, the parameters of HIV infection, and the fact that this virus, after infection of the host, can spread to many body tissues. Its major mode of transmission apparently is via virus-infected cells that must be destroyed or controlled by a strong immune system. The ultimate outcome of the infection depends on the host's immune reaction to the virus either through suppression of HIV replication or through killing of the infected cell. In some individuals an active immune system has prevented development of the disease for more than 10 years (J.A. Levy, unpublished observations). The factors important in maintaining this immune response are not yet known and merit close attention. In some individuals, for example, the immune system appears to make enhancing antibodies to HIV, and this phenomenon occurs particularly with progression of disease.[38] It is related to changes in the antibodies made and in some cases to modifications in the virus so that it is more sensitive to enhancing antibodies.[38] Moreover, the immune system can hyperreact, with production of auto-antibodies that might also hasten the development of disease. Clearly changes in the virus and the immune response of the host play important roles in the ultimate steps leading to AIDS.

We have come a long way in understanding AIDS and its causative agent, HIV. Only through continued studies of its biologic, serologic, and molecular properties can we hope to learn the approaches that will eventually lead to effective antiviral therapy and a vaccine.

REFERENCES

1. Ammann A, Levy JA: Laboratory investigation of pediatric acquired immunodeficiency syndrome, Clin Immunol Immunopathol 40:122, 1986
2. Anand R. Reed C, Forlenza S, et al: Non-cytocidal natural variants of human immunodeficiency virus isolated from AIDS patients with neurological disorder. Lancet 2:234, 1987
3. Asjo B, Albert J, Karlsson A, et al: Replicative capacity of human immunodeficiency virus from patiens with varying severity of HIV infection. Lancet 2:660, 1986
4. Barnett S, Barboza A, Wilcox CM, et al: Characterization of human immunodeficiency virus type 1 strains recovered from the bowel of infected individuals. Virology 182:802, 1991
5. Barre-Sinoussi F, Nugeyre M, Dauguet C, et al: Isolation of a T-lymphotropic retrovirus from a patient at risk for acquired immune deficiency syndrome. Science 220:868, 1986
6. Brookmeyer R: Reconstruction and future trends of the AIDS epidemic in the United States. Science 253:37, 1991
7. Cameron DW, Simonsen JN, D'Costa LJ, et al: Female to male transmission of human immunodeficiency virus type 1: Risk factors for seroconversion in men. Lancet 2:403, 1989
8. Castro BA, Barnett SW, Evans LA, et al: Biologic heterogeneity of human immunodeficiency virus type 2 (HIV-2). Virology 178:527, 1990
9. Cheng-Mayer C, Homsy J, Evans LA, et al: Identification of HIV subtypes with distinct patterns of sensitivity to serum neutralization. Proc Natl Acad Sci U S A 85:2815, 1988
10. Cheng-Mayer C, Levy JA: Distinct biologic and serologic properties of HIV isolates from the brain. Ann Neurol 23:S58, 1988
11. Cheng-Mayer C, Quiroga M, Tung JW, et al: Viral determinants of HIV-1 T-cell/macrophage tropism, cytopathicity, and CD4 antigen modulation. J Virol 64:4390, 1990
12. Cheng-Mayer C, Rutka JT, Rosenblum ML, et al: The human immunodeficiency virus (HIV) can productively infect cultured human glial cells. Proc Natl Acad Sci U S A 84:3526, 1987
13. Cheng-Mayer C, Seto D, Levy JA: Biologic features of HIV that correlate with virulence in the host. Science 240:80, 1988
14. Cheng-Mayer C, Shioda T, Levy JA: Host range, replicative, and cytopathic properties of human

immunodeficiency virus type 1 are determined by very few amino acid changes in *tat* and gp120. J Virol 65:6931, 1991

15. Clavel F, Guetard D, Brun-Vezinet F, et al: Isolation of a new human retrovirus from West African patients with AIDS. Science 233:343, 1986

16. Coffin J, Haase A, Levy JA, et al: Human immunodeficiency viruses. Science 232:697, 1986

17. Cohen AH, Sun NCJ, Shapshak P, et al: Demonstration of human immunodeficiency virus in renal epithelium in HIV-associated nephropathy. Mod Pathol 2:125, 1989

17a. Coombs RW, Collier AC, Allain JP, et al: Plasma viremia in human immunodeficiency virus infection. N Engl J Med 321:1626, 1989

18. Dalgleish A, Beverly P, Clapham P, et al: The CD4 (T4) antigen is an essential component of the receptor for the AIDS retrovirus. Nature 312:763, 1984

19. de Rossi A, Franchini G, Alsovini A, et al: Differential response to the cytopathic effects of human T cell lymphotropic virus type III (HTLV-III) superinfection in T4+ (helper) and T8+ (suppressor) T-cell clones transformed by HTLV-I. Proc Natl Acad Sci U S A 83:4297, 1986

20. Evans LA, McHugh TM, Stites DP, et al: Differential ability of human immunodeficiency virus isolates to productively infect human cells. J Immunol 138:3415, 1987

21. Evans LA, Moreau J, Odehouri K, et al: Characterization of a noncytopathic HIV-2 strain with unusual effects on CD4 expression. Science 240:1522, 1988

22. Evans LA, Moreau J, Odehouri K, et al: Simultaneous isolation of HIV-1 and HIV-2 from an AIDS patient. Lancet 2:1389, 1988

22a. Gallaher WR: Detection of a fusion peptide sequence in the transmembrane protein of human immunodeficiency virus. Cell 50:327, 1987

23. Gallo R, Salahuddin S, Popovic M, et al: Frequent detection and isolation of cytopathic retrovirus (HTVL-III) from patients with AIDS and at risk for AIDS. Science 224:500, 1984

24. Gartner S, Markovits P, Markovitz DM, et al: The role of mononuclear phagocytes in HTLV-III/LAV infection. Science 233:215, 1986

25. Gelderblom HR, Hausmann EHS, Ozel M, et al: Fine structure of human immunodeficiency virus (HIV) and immunolocalization of structural proteins. Virology 156:171, 1987

26. Gerberding JL, Bryant-LeBlanc CE, Nelson K, et al: Risk of human immunodeficiency virus, cytomegalovirus, and hepatitis B virus transmission to health care workers exposed to patients with acquired immunodeficiency syndrome (AIDS) and AIDS-related conditions. J Infect Dis 156:1, 1987

27. Golding H, Robey FA, Gates FT III, et al: Identification of homologous regions in human immunodeficiency virus 1 gp41 and human MHC Class II beta 1 domain. J Exp Med 167:914, 1988

28. Guyader M, Emerman M, Sonigo P, et al: Genome organization and transactivation of the human immunodeficiency virus type 2. Nature 326:662, 1987

29. Haase A: The slow infection caused by visna virus. Curr Top Microbiol Immunol 72:101, 1975

30. Halstead SB, O'Rourke EJ: Dengue viruses and mononuclear phagocytes. J Exp Med 146:201, 1977

31. Harouse JM, Bhat S, Spitalnik SL, et al: Inhibition of entry of HIV-1 in neural cell lines by antibodies against galactosyl ceramide. Science 253:320, 1991

32. Harper ME, Marselle LM, Gallo RC, et al: Detection of lymphocytes expressing human T-lymphotropic virus type III in lymph nodes and peripheral blood from infected individuals by in situ hybridization. Proc Natl Acad Sci U S A 83:772, 1986

33. Henle G, Henle W: Immunology of Epstein-Barr virus. In Roizman B (ed): The Herpesviruses. New York, Plenum Press, 1982, p 209

34. Ho DD, Moudgil T, Alam M: Quantitation of human immunodeficiency virus type 1 in the blood of infected persons. N Engl J Med 321:1621, 1989

35. Ho DD, Rota T, Schooley R, et al: Isolation of HTLV-III from cerobrospinal fluid and neural tissues of patients with neurologic syndromes related to the acquired immunodeficiency syndrome. N Engl J Med 313:1493, 1985

36. Ho DD, Sarngadharan MG, Hirsch MS, et al: Human immunodeficiency virus neutralizing antibodies recognize several conserved domains on the envelope glycoproteins. J Virol 61:2024, 1987

37. Hollander H, Levy JA: Neurologic abnormalities and human immunodeficiency virus recovery from cerebrospinal fluid. Ann Intern Med 106:692, 1987

38. Homsy J, Meyer M, Levy JA: Serum enhancement of HIV infection correlates with disease in HIV-infected individuals. J Virol 64:1437, 1990

39. Homsy J, Meyer M, Tateno M, et al: The Fc and not the CD4 receptor mediates antibody enhancement of HIV infection in human cells. Science 244:1357, 1989
40. Hoxie JA, Alpers JD, Rackowski JL, et al: Alterations in T4 (CD4) protein and mRNA synthesis in cells infected with HIV. Science 234:1123, 1986
41. Kalyanaraman VS, Cabradilla CD, Getchell JP, et al: Antibodies to the core protein of lymphadenopathy-associated virus (LAV) in patients with AIDS. Science 225:321, 1984
42. Kaminsky LS, McHugh T, Stites D, et al: High prevalence of antibodies to AIDS-associated retroviruses (ARV) in acquired immune deficiency syndrome and related conditions and not in other disease states. Proc Natl Acad Sci U S A 82:5535, 1985
43. Kanki PJ, Barin F, M'Boup S, et al: New human T-lymphotropic retrovirus related to simian T-lymphotropic virus type III (STLV-III$_{agm}$). Science 232:238, 1986
44. Kiprov DD, Anderson RE, Morand PR, et al: Antilymphocyte antibodies and seropositivity for retroviruses in groups at high risk for AIDS. N Engl J Med 312:1517, 1985
45. Klatzmann D, Champagne E, Chamaret S, et al: T-lymphocyte T4 molecule behaves as receptor for human retrovirus LAV. Nature 312:767, 1984
46. Koenig RE, Pittluga J, Bogart M, et al: Differences in prevalence of antibodies to the human immunodeficiency virus (HIV) in Dominicans and Haitians in the Dominican Republic. JAMA 257:631, 1987
47. Koenig S, Gendelman HE, Orenstein JM, et al: Detection of AIDS virus in macrophages in brain tissue from AIDS patients with encephalopathy. Science 233:1089, 1986
48. LaRosa GJ, Davide JP, Weinhold K, et al: Conserved sequence and structural elements in the HIV-1 principal neutralizing determinant. Science 249:932, 1990
49. Levy JA: The multifaceted retrovirus. Cancer Res 46:5457, 1986
50. Levy JA: The transmission of AIDS: The case of the infected cell. JAMA 259:3037, 1988
51. Levy JA: Human immunodeficiency viruses and the pathogenesis of AIDS. JAMA 261:2997, 1989
52. Levy JA, Evans LA, Cheng-Mayer C, et al: The biologic and molecular properties of the AIDS-associated retrovirus that affect antiviral therapy. Ann Inst Pasteur 138:101, 1987
53. Levy JA, Evans LA, Pan L-Z, et al: The biologic heterogeneity of HIV and host immune response during HIV infection. In Ginsburg H, Lerner R, Chanock R (eds): Vaccines 1987. Cold Spring Harbor, Cold Spring Harbor Laboratories, 1987, p 168
54. Levy JA, Hoffman AD, Kramer SM, et al: Isolation of lymphocytopathic retroviruses from San Francisco patients with AIDS. Science 225:840, 1984
55. Levy JA, Hollander H, Shimabukuro J, et al: Isolation of AIDS-associated retroviruses from cerebrospinal fluid and brain of patients with neurological symptoms. Lancet 2:586, 1985
56. Levy JA, Kaminsky LS, Morrow WJW, et al: Infection by the retrovirus associated with the acquired immunodeficiency syndrome. Ann Intern Med 103:694, 1985
57. Levy JA, Shimabukuro J: Recovery of AIDS-associated retroviruses from patients with AIDS, related conditions and clinically healthy individuals. J Infect Dis 152:734, 1985
58. Levy JA, Shimabukuro J, McHugh T, et al: AIDS-associated retroviruses (ARV) can productively infect other cells besides human T helper cells. Virology 147:441, 1985
59. Lifson JD, Feinberg MB, Reyes GR, et al: Induction of CD4-dependent cell fusion by the HTLV-III/LAV envelope glycoprotein. Nature 323:725, 1986
60. Lindenmann J: Viruses as immunological adjuvants in cancer. Biochem Biophys Acta 49:355, 1974
61. Luciw PA, Potter SJ, Steimer K, et al: Molecular cloning of AIDS-associated retrovirus. Nature 312:760, 1984
62. McDougal J, Kennedy M, Sligh J, et al: The binding of HTLV-III/LAV to T4+ T cells by a complex of the 110 kD viral protein (gp110) and the T4 molecule. Science 231:382, 1986
63. Michaelis B, Levy JA: Recovery of human immunodeficiency virus from serum. JAMA 257:1327, 1987
64. Nelson JA, Wiley CA, Reynolds-Kohler C, et al: Human immunodeficiency virus detected in bowel epithelium from patients with gastrointestinal symptoms. Lancet 1:259, 1988
65. Padian NS, Shiboski S, Jewell NP: Female-to-male transmission of human immunodeficiency virus. JAMA 266:1664, 1991
66. Pan L-Z, Cheng-Mayer C, Levy JA: Patterns of antibody response in individuals infected with the human immunodeficiency virus. J Infect Dis 155:626, 1987
67. Pape JW, Liautaud B, Thomas F, et al: The acquired immunodeficiency syndrome in Haiti. Ann Intern Med 103:674, 1985

68. Papsidero LD, Sheu M, Ruscetti FW: Human immunodeficiency virus type 1–neutralizing mono-clonal antibodies which react with p17 core protein: Characterization and epitope mapping. J Virol 63:267, 1989

69. Plata F, Autran B, Martins LP, et al: AIDS virus-specific cytotoxic T lymphocytes in lung disorders. Nature 328:348, 1987

70. Protner A, Scroggs RA, Naeve CW: The fusion glycoprotein of Sendai virus: Sequence analysis of an epitope involved in fusion and virus neutralization. Virology 157:556, 1987

71. Quinn TC, Mann JM, Curran JW, et al: AIDS in Africa: An epidemiologic paradigm. Science 234:955, 1986

72. Rabson A, Martin M: Molecular organization of the AIDS retrovirus. Cell 40:477, 1985

73. Robert-Guroff M, Giardina PJ, Robey WG, et al: HTLV-III neutralizing antibody development in transfusion-dependent seropositive patients with B-thalassemia. J Immunol 138:3731, 1987

74. Robinson WE Jr, Kawamura T, Gorny MK, et al: Human monoclonal antibodies to the human immunodeficiency virus type 1 (HIV-1) transmembrane glycoprotein gp41 enhance HIV-1 infection in vitro. Proc Natl Acad Sci U S A 87:3185, 1990

75. Robinson WE Jr, Montefiori DC, Mitchell WM: Antibody-dependent enhancement of human immunodeficiency virus type 1 infection. Lancet 1:790, 1988

76. Salahuddin SZ, Markham PD, Popovic M, et al: Isolation of infectious human T-cell leukemia/lymphotropic virus type III (HTLV-III) from patients with acquired immunodeficiency syndrome (AIDS) or AIDS-related complex (ARC) and from healthy carriers: A study of risk groups and tissue sources. Proc Natl Acad Sci U S A 82:5530, 1985

77. Sarin PS, Sun DK, Thornton AH, et al: Neutralization of HTLV-III/LAV replication by antiserum to thymosin alpha-1. Science 232:1135, 1986

78. Sarngadharan MG, Popovic M, Bruch L, et al: Antibodies reactive with human T-lymphotropic retroviruses (HTLV-III) in the serum of patients with AIDS. Science 224:506, 1984

79. Schupbach J, Haller O, Vogt M, et al: Antibodies to HTLV-III in Swiss patients with AIDS and pre-AIDS and in groups at risk for AIDS. N Engl J Med 312:265, 1985

80. Serwadda D, Mugerwa RD, Sewandambo NK: Slim disease: A new disease in Uganda and its association with HTLV-III infection. Lancet 2:849, 1985

81. Shaw G, Harper M, Hahn B, et al: HTLV-III infection in brains of children and adults with AIDS encephalopathy. Science 227:177, 1985

82. Simonsen JN, Cameron DW, Gaknya MN, et al: Human immunodeficiency virus infection among men with sexually transmitted diseases. N Engl J Med 319:274, 1988

83. Starcich BR, Hahn BH, Shaw GM, et al: Identification and characterization of conserved and variable regions in the envelope gene of HTLV-III/LAV, the retrovirus of AIDS. Cell 45:637, 1986

84. Tateno M, Cheng-Mayer C, Levy JA: MT-4 plaque formation can distinguish cytopathic subtypes of the human immunodeficiency virus (HIV). Virology 167:299, 1988

85. Tateno M, Gonzalez-Scarano F, Levy JA: The human immunodeficiency virus can infect CD4-negative human fibroblastoid cells. Proc Natl Acad Sci U S A 86:4287, 1989

86. Tschachler E, Groh V, Popovic M, et al: Epidermal Langerhans cells: A target for HTLV-III/LAV infection. J Invest Dermatol 88:233, 1987

87. Van de Perre P, Lepage P, Kestelyn P, et al: Acquired immunodeficiency syndrome in Rwanda. Lancet 2:62, 1984

88. Vogt M, Craven D, Crawford D, et al: Isolation of HTLV-III/LAV from cervical secretions of women at risk for AIDS. Lancet 1:525, 1986

89. Walker B, Chakrabarti S, Moss B, et al: HIV-specific cytotoxic T lymphocytes in seropositive individuals. Nature 328:345, 1987

90. Walker C, Moody D, Stites DP, et al: CD8+ lymphocytes can control HIV infection in vitro by suppressing virus replication. Science 234:1563, 1986

91. Walker CM, Levy JA: A diffusible lymphokine produced by CD8+ T lymphocytes suppresses HIV replication. Immunology 66:628, 1989

92. Wiley CA, Schrier RD, Nelson JA, et al: Cellular localization of the AIDS retrovirus infection within the brains of acquired immune deficiency syndrome patients. Proc Natl Acad Sci U S A 83:7089, 1986

93. Wofsy CB, Cohen JB, Hauer LB, et al: Isolation of the AIDS-associated retrovirus from genital secretions from women with antibodies to the virus. Lancet 1:527, 1986

3

AIDS TESTING
Now and in the Future

MICHAEL S. SAAG, MD

When considering what is the optimum "AIDS test," AIDS testing must be placed into appropriate historical context. AIDS was first described as a syndrome, a collection of clinical features that were the result of a weakened immune sytem. It was not until the causative agent of AIDS, human immunodeficiency virus type 1 (HIV-1), was discovered in 1984 that "tests for AIDS" became available. However, since AIDS is a clinical syndrome, there is no such thing as a laboratory test for AIDS per se; rather, all "AIDS tests" are designed to detect, either directly or indirectly, the presence of underlying HIV-1 infection.

The first test developed to detect HIV-1 infection was isolation of the virus through tissue culture. This was the technique used originally to establish HIV-1 as the causative agent of AIDS. Unfortunately, although sensitive for viral isolation, the tissue culture procedure is expensive, time consuming, and labor intensive. As a result, soon after the initial discovery of HIV-1, several tests were developed using protein products of the newly discovered virus to detect antibodies produced by the infected host. Through these newer techniques, the immunologic "footprints" (i.e., antibodies) to the viral infection are detected rather than the virus itself.

The two antibody tests used most commonly are the enzyme-linked immuno-sorbent assay (ELISA) and the Western blot. In addition to being less expensive, faster, and easier to perform than viral culture, the ELISA and the Western blot test do not require working with live virus and therefore are safer. Nonetheless, no test is perfect, and the HIV-1 antibody tests are limited by their reliance on the production of antibody by the host and the absence of cross-reacting antibodies.

Over the last 3 to 4 years, several novel techniques have been developed that directly detect viral protein products or amplify minute fragments of viral RNA and DNA to avoid the pitfalls of antibody testing and the dangers and expense of live virus culture.[23,71] Yet these tests have their own limitations, not the least of which is the interpretation of the results by the clinician ordering the test.

This work was supported in part by the University of Alabama at Birmingham General Clinical Research Center (RR00032), the University of Alabama at Birmingham Aids Center (AI27767), and the Birmingham Veterans Affairs Medical Center.

The best way to minimize errors in interpretation of laboratory findings is to understand the methodology of the test, the advantages and limitations of the testing technology, and the application of the test in the context of what is known about the epidemiology and pathogenesis of the underlying disease. This chapter reviews the methodologies of currently available tests for HIV-1, examines their appropriate use and limitations, and discusses the role of each test in the context of diagnosis and as measurements of response to antiretroviral therapy.

METHODOLOGIES

HIV-1 tests can be divided into several groups: virus culture techniques, antibody detection tests, antigen detection tests, viral genome amplification tests, and immune function tests.

Virus Culture Techniques

PBMC Coculture for HIV-1 Isolation

This technique was used initially to establish HIV-1 as the causative agent of AIDS.[7,61] Viable peripheral blood mononuclear cells (PBMCs) from HIV-1–infected patients are obtained via centrifugation of anticoagulated whole blood (collected in either acid citrate dextran [ACD] tubes or syringes containing preservative-free heparin) over ficoll-hypaque lymphocyte separation medium. Infected PBMCs then are cocultured with PBMCs derived from an uninfected human donor that have been stimulated previously for 24 to 48 hours with phytohemagglutinin (PHA). Growth of the cells in tissue culture is supported by special media (RPMI-1640) that has been supplemented with L-glutamine, fetal bovine serum, gentamicin, and interleukin-2 (to stimulate expression of CD4 receptors for enhanced viral replication and proliferation of lymphocytes). The cultures are observed for evidence of syncytial formation (i.e., multinucleated giant cell formation) as a sign of viral infection in vitro and for the presence of either HIV-1 reverse transcriptase (RT) activity or HIV-1 p24 antigen production in the culture supernatant. Cultures are declared "positive" when at least two consecutive assays detect the presence of RT or p24 antigen in increasing magnitude above a predetermined cut-off value. When performed properly, HIV-1 isolation by PBMC coculture is positive in 95% to 99% of HIV-1–infected patients.[23,71]

Quantitative Cell Culture

Quantitative cell culture is a technique that measures the relative amount of viral load within cells. The cell culture technique is the same as described previously; however, in addition to cocultivating 10^6 patient cells with 10^6 donor cells, serial dilutions of patient cells are also set in culture in decreasing amounts (e.g., 10^6, 10^5, 10^4, 10^3) with 10^6 donor cells[38] (Figure 3–1A). In this way fewer patient cells are introduced into the coculture system, thereby allowing measurement of relative viral burden. The last positive culture with the fewest number of patient cells represents the end point. The reciprocal of the end-point dilution indicates the

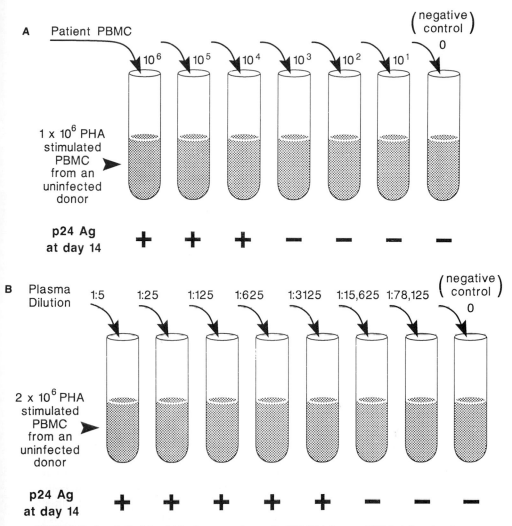

FIGURE 3–1. *A*, Peripheral blood mononuclear cells (PBMCs) from an HIV-1–infected patient are added in tenfold serial dilutions to a standard amount (e.g., 1×10^6) of phytohemagglutin (PHA)-stimulated PBMC from an uninfected donor. The lowest dilution yielding a positive result, as determined by p24 antigen (p24 Ag) positivity in the culture supernatant, represents the end point. In this example, the end-point dilution is 1×10^4 cells/mm³. *B*, Serial fivefold dilutions of plasma from an HIV-1–infected patient are cocultivated with a standard amount (e.g., 2×10^6) of peripheral blood mononuclear cells from an uninfected donor. As in the quantitative cell dilution assay, the least amount of plasma required to yield a positive culture result represents the end point. In the example above, the end-point titer is 1:3125.

relative number of infected cells in the patient. For example, if the last positive titer is 1×10^4 (10,000), the relative burden signifies one out of every 10,000 patient cells is infected. If the end-point titer is 1×10^3 (1000), approximately one out of 1000 cells is infected. This procedure can be improved further by using serial dilutions on a 1:3 basis rather than a 1:10 basis.

Quantitative Plasma Culture

Another means of measuring viral load is through the measurement of free infectious virus in the plasma.[17,19,38,68] This is accomplished through quantitative plasma culture techniques (Figure 3–1*B*). Serial dilutions of plasma are prepared by mixing 0.6 ml of plasma with 2.4 ml of culture media consisiting of RPMI-1640, supplemented with L-glutamine, gentamicin, fetal bovine serum, and inter-leukin-2. One milliliter of each of the dilutions is added to 2×10^6 PHA-stimulated PBMC from an uninfected donor in a microtiter, 96-well tissue culture plate. Culture supernatants are monitored for viral replication at days 7 and 14 after cultivation by an HIV-1 p24 antigen test (see below). The end-point dilution is defined as the smallest volume of plasma that yields a positive culture result. The reciprocal of the smallest volume of plasma indicates the titer expressed as the tissue culture infectious doses per milliliter of plasma. As shown in Figure 3–1*B*, a positive dilution of 1:3125 implies that there are more than 3000 free infectious virions per milliliter of plasma in that patient. To ensure accuracy, these tests are usually performed in duplicate and, under special circumstances, in quadruplicate.

HIV Antibody Tests

ELISA

The technology to perform the ELISA was available before the discovery of HIV in 1983 and 1984. This technology was applied rapidly for use as an HIV-1 diagnostic test and was in widespread use by the summer of 1985.[15] As shown in Figure 3–2, this test uses HIV antigens (proteins) produced in a tissue culture system. After the virus has been grown to high titers, the cell culture is lysed. The soluble antigens are then coated onto the wells of a microtiter plate. The test is initiated by adding patient serum to the antigen-coated wells. Anti–HIV-1-specific antibody present in the patient's serum will bind very tightly and specifically with the HIV-1 antigens in the plate. After a washing procedure to remove unbound materials, the specific anti–HIV-1 antibodies that have bound to the coated antigen are detected through the addition of a goat anti-human antibody that binds very tightly and specifically to any anti–HIV-1 human antibody bound to HIV-1 antigens on the plate. The goat anti–human antibody has been conjugated to an enzyme that specifically cleaves a colorless substrate and into a product with color (usually yellow). After a washing procedure, the substrate for the enzyme is added. The amount of color present in the well is proportional to the amount of conjugated enzyme bound to the human antibody present. By spectrophotometrically measuring the optical density in the sample well versus that in the negative control well, the amount of HIV-1 antibody can be determined quantitatively.

Through examination of large panels of known HIV-positive sera and comparison of their optical densities with those of known seronegative controls, a cutoff optical density measurement can be determined that distinguishes between a positive and negative result. To make the test more sensitive, the optical density cutoff is established at a lower value; conversely, to improve specificity the cutoff can be established at a higher value.

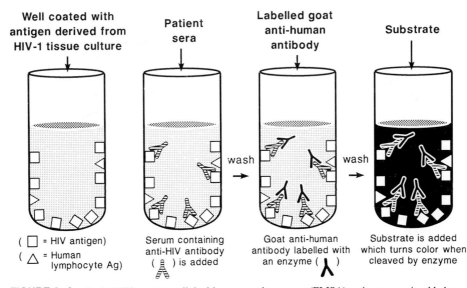

| Well coated with antigen derived from HIV-1 tissue culture | Patient sera | Labelled goat anti-human antibody | Substrate |

(☐ = HIV antigen)
(△ = Human lymphocyte Ag)

Serum containing anti-HIV antibody (⚥) is added

Goat anti-human antibody labelled with an enzyme (⅄)

Substrate is added which turns color when cleaved by enzyme

FIGURE 3–2. In the HIV-1 enzyme-linked immunosorbent assay (ELISA) patient serum is added to a microwell plate that has been coated with antigens derived from an HIV-1 tissue culture lysate. Bound anti-HIV antibody from the infected patient is detected via a goat anti-human antibody that has been labeled with an enzyme designed to react with a specific substrate. The cleaved substrate product yields a color that can be measured photometrically. Because the HIV-1 antigens are derived from tissue culture, some human lymphocyte antigens (Ag) may also be present in the well, potentially yielding a false-positive test result (see text for details).

Western Blot Test

The Western blot test is also designed to detect the presence of anti-HIV-1 antibodies; however, in addition to identifying the presence of such antibodies, the Western blot test allows determination of the specific antigen against which the antibody is directed. As shown in Figure 3–3A, HIV-1 antigens are prepared from a lysate of HIV-1–infected cells and are separated electrophoretically in a poly-acrylamide gel. The electrophoretic procedure separates the antigens according to their size: the larger fragments remain toward the top of the gel, and the smaller fragments migrate further down the gel, thereby creating a gradient of antigen by size within the gel. The proteins within the gel are then transferred (blotted) onto nitrocellulose filter paper, which holds the antigens in place for further testing. The nitrocellulose filter is cut into strips that can be incubated with the patient's serum. Anti–HIV-1 antibodies present in this serum bind tightly and specifically to the antigens on the nitrocellulose paper at the point where the antigens migrated. The anti–HIV-1 antibodies can then be detected by goat anti-human antibody, which is conjugated to either an enzyme or a radioactive probe. Once processed, bands appear at the location where the antibody has bound to antigen. Through the use of reference bands produced as a positive control, the reactivity of the antibodies against specific antigens can be determined (Figure 3–3B).

The precise criteria for what constitutes a positive Western blot test remain controversial.[6,14,18,56] In general, positive bands from two of the three major antigen

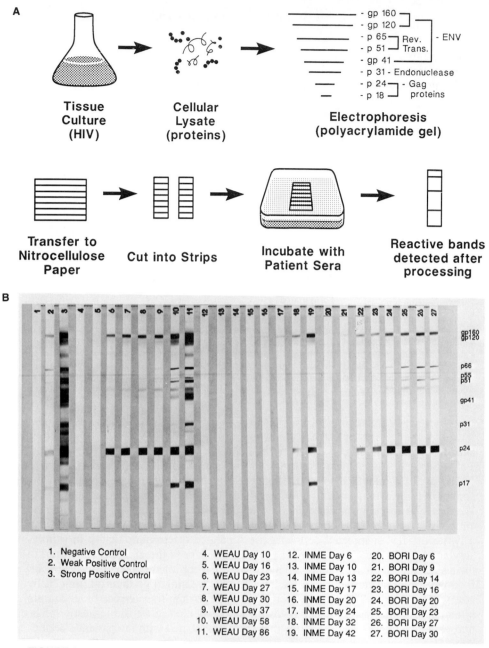

FIGURE 3-3. *A,* Western blot test is performed by separating tissue culture–derived HIV-1 proteins (p) and glycoproteins (gp) via polyacrylamide gel electrophoresis, transferring (blotting) the separated proteins onto nitrocellulose paper, incubating the cut strips of nitrocellulose paper with patient serum, and detecting anti–HIV antibodies that have bound to the HIV-1–associated proteins at the precise point at which they migrated in the gel. Through this procedure the antibody reactivity against specific antigens can be determined (e.g., anti-*gag,* anti-*env,* or anti-endonuclease antibodies). *B,* Examples of Western blot tests from three patients (WEAU, BORI, and INME) identified at the time of acute HIV-1 infection (seroconversion). Each lane represents a time point (in days) from the time of presentation with symptomatic acute HIV-1 disease or a positive or negative control (lanes 1 to 3).

groups, the *gag, pol,* and *env* regions of the virus, are required for a positive test. The *gag* proteins consist of p55, p24 and p18 proteins (*p* stands for protein); the *pol* region codes for reverse transcriptase (p66 and p51) and an endonuclease (p31); and the *env* region codes for the envelope glycoprotein gp160 (the precursor product) and its two major subunits, gp120 and gp41 (*gp* stands for glycoprotein). Recent analyses suggest the use of criteria developed by the Centers for Disease Control and the Association of State, Territorial, and Public Health Laboratory Directors (CDC/ASTPHLD) as the most appropriate for judging results of the Western blot tests.[78] The CDC/ASTPHLD criteria require the presence of at least two of the following bands—p24, gp41, or gp160/120—for a positive result; the presence of no bands for a negative result; and the presence of any HIV-1–related (or non-HIV-1–related) band(s) not meeting the criteria for a positive result as an indeterminate result.[56]

Radioimmunoprecipitation Assay

The radioimmunoprecipitation assay (RIPA) is a more time consuming and labor intensive test than the Western blot, yet it provides much finer resolution of the high-molecular-weight envelope proteins than the Western blot test.[12] The RIPA requires ongoing cell culture of HIV-1 to provide the appropriate substrate for the assay. HIV-1 replication in lymphocytic cell lines occurs in the presence of radiolabeled amino acids (e.g., ^{35}S-methionine or ^{35}S-cysteine). The radiolabeled amino acids are incorporated into viral proteins during viral replication. A cell lysate is prepared via homogenization of infected cells, and the lysate is then incubated in the presence of patient serum. Anti–HIV-1 antibodies present in the serum react with the radiolabeled antigens and form immune complexes. These complexes are removed by incubating the reaction mixture with protein-A–coated Sepharose beads, which bind the Fc portion of immunoglobulin molecules. The beads are separated from the reaction mixture through centrifugation, and the antibody-antigen complexes are eluted from the separated beads by adding a detergent and heating. The immunoprecipitants are then run through an electrophoretic gel, which separates them according to their molecular weight (as in the Western blot procedure). An audioradiograph of the gel yields a banding pattern very similar to that of the Western blot test.

The RIPA is considered more sensitive and specific than the Western blot test[12,16,32,36]; however, the time, expense, and need for active cell lines and radioactive materials make the RIPA a poor choice for routine testing in commercial laboratories. Rather, its use is best reserved for difficult-to-diagnose cases.

Indirect Immunofluorescence Assay

Like the RIPA, the indirect immunofluorescence assay (IFA) requires preparation of HIV-1 antigens that are expressed on infected cells and are stained subsequently.[23] Infected cells are placed on glass slides in a fixed monolayer and are incubated with patient serum. Anti–HIV-1 antibodies present within the serum bind to antigens expressed on the surface of cells, and these bound antibodies are then detected with anti-human antibody that has been labeled with fluorescein isothiocyanate (FITC), an ultraviolet-activated dye compound. After appropriate processing, the slide is viewed under a fluorescent microscope, and the number of cells, the intensity of staining, and the staining pattern are assessed. IFA can detect the earliest serologic response against the virus (lgM antibodies) during acute infection[21]; however, the time, expense, and expertise required for the IFA procedure makes its routine use in a commercial laboratory impractical.

Other Anti–HIV-1 Antibody Tests

A number of rapid screening tests have been developed that may be useful in evaluation of field isolates when large numbers of samples must be screened. The rapid latex agglutination assay uses polystyrene beads that have been coated with recombinant HIV-1 proteins.[66] In the presence of antibodies against these proteins, the beads agglutinate. This test apparently is quite accurate when used by experienced personnel in areas where HIV infection is endemic.[23,64] However, further testing is required to establish its usefulness among populations with lower rates of infection.

An autologous red cell agglutination assay has been developed.[43] In this test a mouse monoclonal antibody directed against human red cells is conjugated with synthetic gp41 envelope protein from HIV. When added to whole blood from the patient, the antibody-gp41 complex binds to the human red cells, and if anti-gp41 antibodies are present in the plasma, agglutination of the red cells occurs rapidly (within a few minutes). Further testing is required to establish the sensitivity and specificity of this assay in large populations.

p24 ANTIGEN ASSAYS

HIV p24 Antigen Test

This assay measures the amount of free viral protein (p24) present in the plasma or tissue culture supernatant.[2] Although this protein may be present in the plasma of patients at all stages of HIV infection, p24 antigenemia is most prevalent during the time of initial seroconversion and again later in the course of more advanced HIV disease.[3,17,34,59,68] The test uses an ELISA sandwich technique in which antibodies to p24 are bound to the bottom of a microtiter well or onto polystyrene beads (Figure 3–4). The bound antibodies are incubated with patient serum or plasma. If free p24 antigen is present in the serum, the antigen is bound tightly and specifically to the "capture" anti-p24 antibody. After a washing procedure, a second "detector" anti-p24 antibody is added, followed by addition of an enzyme-linked immunoglobulin, which is directed against the second p24 antibody. With the addition of substrate, the conjugated enzyme cleaves the substrate into a color-generating product that can be measured spectrophotometrically (as in the ELISA anti-HIV antibody procedure). This test was originally developed with the second anti-p24 antibody's having a polyclonal nature. More recently, the use of monoclonal anti-p24 antibodies has increased the sensitivity of the assay substantially. With the more advanced test, p24 antigen levels as low as 7 to 10 pg/ml can be detected reliably.

Well with anti-HIV capture antibody	→ Add sera containing HIV antigen (p 24)	→ Add rabbit anti-HIV detection antibody	→ Add goat anti-rabbit antibody (labeled)	→ Add substrate; measure color photometrically

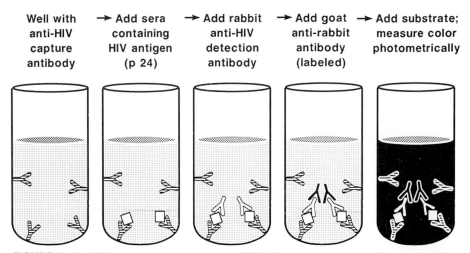

FIGURE 3–4. HIV-1 antigen capture assay is an ELISA-based test that detects the presense of free HIV-1 p24 antigen in patient serum. Free antigen is bound (captured) by specific anti-p24 "capture" antibodies that have been coated onto a microwell. Bound antigen is detected by specially designed rabbit anti-HIV p24 (detection antibodies), which, in turn, are detected by goat anti-rabbit antibodies. The goat antibodies have been conjugated with an enzyme that cleaves a specific substrate, yielding a colored product. By photometrically measuring the degree of color in the well, the amount of HIV-1 p24 antigen can be determined quantitatively.

Acidified p24 Antigen Procedure

Very recently a modification of the p24 antigen test was introduced that further increases its sensitivity. This modification is based on the concept that p24 antigen, when produced in the presence of significant amounts of anti-p24 antibody, forms antigen-antibody complexes that bind free antigen and prevent detection. Through acidification of plasma, the antigen-antibody complexes can be disrupted, releasing free antigen for detection by the antigen assay.[44,55,62]

The procedure is performed by pretreating patient plasma (or serum) with glycine and incubating it for 1 hour at 37° C. After stabilization of the plasma, the plasma is analyzed for the presence of p24 antigen as described previously. Studies are currently underway to assess the degree of increased sensitivity through this technique. Preliminary results indicate that it may be especially helpful in detecting p24 antigen in HIV-1–infected infants in the perinatal period. The acidified p24 antigen assay may also be useful in following patient responses to antiretroviral therapy in clinical trials.

Polyethylene Glycol Precipitation

Another approach to enhancing p24 antigen sensitivity is through polyethylene glycol precipitation of antibody-antigen complexes before p24 antigen testing. In one study the sensitivity increased from 38% to 59% after polyethylene glycol precipitation of the complexes.[29] This technique is still under investigation.

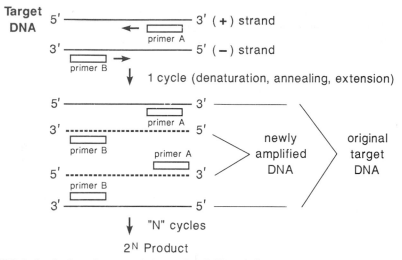

FIGURE 3–5. In the polymerase chain reaction (PCR) technique, target DNA is amplified through a series of cycles, each consisting of (1) denaturation of the double-stranded target DNA, (2) annealing of specially designed complementary primers (A and B) to the target DNA, and (3) extension of the primers into complementary new strands of DNA through the use of a unique heat-stable DNA polymerase (Taq polymerase). By repeating the cycles "N" times, the amount of original target DNA is amplified exponentially, 2^N (see text for details).

Polymerase Chain Reaction Techniques

Polymerase chain reaction (PCR) technique, introduced in the late 1980s, represents a major advance in the diagnosis of many disorders, including HIV infection.[58,69] This powerful technique can amplify target DNA existing in very small quantities (as few as one copy of HIV per 100,000 cells) through a series of binary replicative cycles (Figure 3–5).[58,69] Oligonucleotide primers, approximately 25 to 30 bp in length, are carefully designed to bind to a known sequence of the target DNA. These complementary primers bind to highly conserved regions of the genome, usually spaced 150 to 600 bp apart.

Each PCR cycle consists of a period of denaturation (during which the temperatures reach 95° C), followed by an annealing period during which the primers bind to the target DNA (typically with temperatures of 55° to 60° C) and finally by an extension period during which complementary sequences are generated (temperature, 72° C). The key to the entire reaction is the Taq polymerase, a unique DNA polymerase derived from the bacteria *Thermus aquaticus,* that maintains its activity at high temperatures (72° C). In addition to the Taq polymerase enzyme and primers, the reaction mixture contains the necessary phosphorylated nucleotide products (dATP, dGTP, dCTP, and dTTP), appropriate concentrations of divalent cations (e.g., magnesium), buffers, and the target DNA to allow optimum amplification to occur.

The duration of each portion of the cycle is generally 1 to 3 minutes. At the end of each completed cycle the amount of DNA in the region of interest is doubled. After a total of a specified number (*N*) of cycles, the amplified region of DNA exists at 2^N power (usually 20 to 30 cycles are used). Therefore, even if the target DNA initially exists in only a small copy number, the PCR reaction magnifies it several hundred millionfold (e.g., 2^{30} after 30 cycles). The amount of amplified product is easily detected on agarose gel electrophoresis.

The PCR procedure can also be applied to RNA.[35,37,39] In such an instance RNA is reverse transcribed into cDNA with an animal retrovirus reverse transcriptase (e.g., murine leukemia virus RT), and the cDNA product is then amplified as described above. In the case of HIV, proviral HIV-1 DNA, genomic RNA, and mRNA have all been successfully amplified.

The major problem with PCR amplification, ironically, is also its greatest strength, that is, its incredible sensitivity. When performed properly, there is probably no more powerful molecular biologic technique. Unfortunately, inadvertent contamination of reagents and/or target DNA can lead to false-positive results even in laboratories with the most experienced personnel.[49] The problem with contamination is the limiting obstacle to the widespread use of the PCR technique in clinical practice. Nonetheless, when used properly in laboratories with experienced personnel, this technique allows early detection of infection before the development of a serologic response.[22,78]

Quantitative PCR

Although not perfected or standardized to date, many laboratories have established techniques to quantitate the amount of HIV proviral DNA and genomic RNA as relative measures of viral load.[1,8,22,24,39,57] The usual approach is to create serial dilutions of the target DNA (or cDNA) and then PCR-amplify the desired products under standard conditions. Co-amplification of a highly conserved sequence of host genomic DNA such as the β-globin gene serves as a positive control. Because of the difficulties with potential contamination of DNA, inefficient RNA extraction, and problems with DNAse or RNAse contamination, quantitative PCR has not yet been applied on a widespread basis. However, it does hold much promise for future use.

EVALUATION OF IMMUNOLOGIC STATUS

CD4 Cell Count

The pool of human lymphocytes possesses specific glycoproteins on their surface that play an important role in the cell's activity and function. Although many surface glycoproteins have been identified, the CD3, CD4, and CD8 cell-surface markers are used most often in the context of HIV infection.[47] The CD3 (T3) cell marker is present on all adult human lymphocytes. The CD8 (T8) cell marker is present on the subset of suppressor or cytotoxic lymphocytes that control or suppress specific ongoing immunologic activity. In contrast, the lymphocytes bearing the CD4 (T4) cell surface marker help or induce immunologic reactions.

CD4 cells respond to the class II major histocompatibility complex (MHC) antigens and release cytokines that activate and augment the immunologic response. CD4-positive lymphocytes are the primary targets of HIV infection, and the CD4 receptor is the primary binding site of HIV-1. Throughout the course of chronic HIV-1 infection, the number of CD4 lymphocytes is depleted, and the loss of these cells is associated with development of the characteristic opportunistic infections and malignancies of AIDS.[23,26,27,33,53,60,65] Thus the measurement of CD4-positive lymphocytes is one of the most important determinates for clinically staging the disease status of HIV-1–infected patients.

The numbers of CD4 and CD8 cells are measured through the use of specific monoclonal antibodies directed against the surface glycoprotein. These monoclonals are labeled with fluorescent markers, which can be detected when light is passed through the sample. Specialized fluorescent antibody cell sorting (FACS) machines have been developed that automatically count the number of cells labeled with the monoclonal antibody. Using this flow cytometric technique, the percentage of cells bearing the CD4 or CD8 cell-surface markers can be determined.

The FACS analysis yields the percentage of cells carrying a certain surface marker. The absolute CD4 count cannot be measured directly but is calculated by the following formula:

$$\text{Absolute CD4 count} =$$
$$\text{Total white blood count} \times \text{Percent lymphocytes} \times \text{Percent CD4 cells}$$

Clinical staging can be based on either the CD4 percent or the absolute CD4 count; however, most clinical studies have used the absolute CD4 count, even though the percentage value is less subject to fluctuations.[50,74]

Variability in the CD4 percent and the absolute CD4 cell count can be a significant problem both over time and with repeated determinations. CD4 counts normally undergo diurnal variation, with fluctuations of as much as a 150- to 300-cells/mm^3 difference between morning and evening values in normal hosts.[50] Additionally, the longer samples set before processing, the more likely CD4 count values will be artificially elevated. Refrigeration also dramatically increases CD4 cell count values. Such variation has posed difficulties both in clinically staging patients and in following response to therapy in clinical trials.

Another means of clinically following patients is to use the CD4:CD8 ratio.[74] It is determined by dividing the number of CD4 cells by the number of CD8 cells. In uninfected controls normal values for the CD4:CD8 ratio are 0.5 to 2.0. Normal values for CD4 percent are 40% to 70%, and CD4 counts are generally 500 to 1600 cell/mm^3 in adults.

β₂-Microglobulin

β_2-microglobulin is a protein present on the surface of all nucleated cells and serves as the light chain of the class 1 MHC complex.[23] Measurable levels of β_2-microglobulin are increased whenever mononuclear cell activation or cell destruction occurs, as is the case with HIV-1 infection. Serum levels of β_2-microglobulin are determined through radioimmunoassay determination or through an enzyme immunoassay. Several clinical studies have shown that levels >3 mg/L are associated with increased risk of progression to AIDS among HIV-infected patients.[11,45,48,73] When levels are >5 mg/L, the likelihood of occurrence of new opportunistic diseases or death increases further.[5,52] Some investigators have proposed following

β_2-microglobulin levels as a useful means of assessing the effectiveness of anti-retroviral drugs.[42] However, more data are needed to assess fully the best application of this test.

Serum Neopterin

Neopterin is produced during guanosine triphosphate metabolism and is increased during periods of cellular activation. The primary source of neopterin apparently is cells of the monocyte-macrophage lineage that release increased amounts of neopterin after stimulation with interferon-γ. Neopterin levels can be determined through high-pressure liquid chromatography or by competitive radioimmunoassay and can be detected in both serum and urine.

Like β_2-microglobulin, elevated levels of neopterin have been correlated to advancing clinical HIV disease.[28,30,31] Levels >15 ng/ml are noted in patients with AIDS as compared to levels in the 3 to 5 ng/ml range for asymptomatic seropositive patients.[64] In some studies the prognostic value of combining serum neopterin levels and CD4 counts was greater than that of either test used alone.[28] The relative value of neopterin levels in clinical trials has not been fully elucidated.

TEST INTERPRETATION

To interpret results of any HIV-related test appropriately, the natural history of HIV infection and the host immune response must be understood. After initial primary infection with HIV there is an immunologically silent-window period before the development of detectable antibody (Figure 3–6). The median time from initial

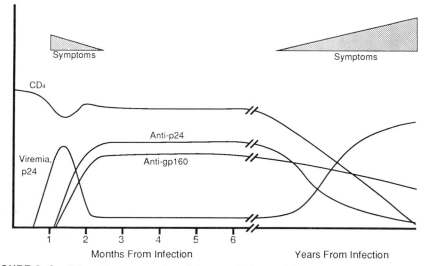

FIGURE 3–6.   Schematic representation of the natural history of HIV-1 infection. (From Clark SJ, Saag MS, Decker WD, et al: High titers of cytopathic virus in plasma of patients with symptomatic primary HIV-1 infection. Reprinted by permission of N Engl J Med 324(14):959, 1991.)

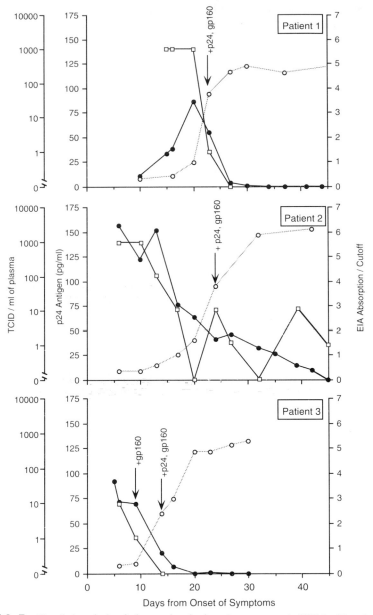

FIGURE 3–7. Detailed analysis of plasma viremia titers (*open squares*), HIV-1 p24 antigen levels (*closed circles*), and anti-p24 antibody levels (*open circles*) in three patients with acute primary HIV-1 infection. The arrows indicate the time of first detection of both gp160 and p24 antibodies by Western blot technique (see Figure 3–3B; From Clark SJ, Saag MS, Decker WD, et al: High titers of cytopathic virus in plasma of patients with symptomatic primary HIV-1 infection. Reprinted by permission of N Engl J Med 324(14):956, 1991.)

infection to the development of detectable antibody is 2.1 months, with 95% of individuals developing antibody within 5.8 months of initial infection.[40] Although the majority of individuals notice very few, if any, symptoms associated with seroconversion, an estimated 40% to 60% of individuals will develop symptoms of an acute mononucleosis-like syndrome, consisting of sore throat, headache, fever, myalgias, lymphadenopathy, and skin rash.[17,20,41,75,76] When such symptomatic patients have been studied carefully, p24 antigen levels are typically quite high, and free virus is present in the plasma at high titer[17,22] (Figure 3–7). Within 14 to 21 days after the onset of symptoms, anti–HIV-1 antibodies become detectable, and titers rise very rapidly against both the envelope glycoproteins and p24. Once a patient develops a mature antibody response, it usually remains detectable for life. The rise in detectable antibody response is associated with a rapid decline in both the p24 antigenemia and plasma viremia, usually to undetectable levels within weeks. The p24 antigenemia and plasma viremia generally return to detectable levels as the patient approaches more advanced disease.[19,38,68]

The CD4 count generally decreases during the acute viral-like illness of acute seroconversion (as CD4 counts do with most acute viral syndromes) but usually returns toward normal levels as a healthy immune response is established. Over a period of many years the CD4 count declines. As the cell count drops below 500 cells/mm³, antiretroviral therapy is usually initiated.[54] The risk of serious opportunistic infections and death increases substantially as CD4 counts drop below 200 cells/mm³.[26,27,33,53,60,65] Prophylactic therapy against the development of *Pneumocystis carinii* pneumonia is indicated when the CD4 cell count approaches 200 cells/mm³.[54] Much controversy still exists about routine prophylaxis of other opportunistic diseases when CD4 counts drop below 50 cells/mm³ (see Chapter 6).

SENSITIVITY, SPECIFICITY, AND MISLEADING TEST RESULTS

Any discussion of HIV testing must address the questions of sensitivity, specificity, positive predictive value, and negative predictive value (Table 3–1). By definition, sensitivity refers to the ability to detect accurately an individual with a particular disorder among those individuals who truly have the disorder. In contrast, specificity is the ability to identify accurately all those individuals who truly do not have the disorder out of all of those individuals within a population who are unaffected. The sensitivity and specificity of a given test are **test specific** and are not dependent on the population being tested. Positive and negative predictive values, on the other hand, refer to the test's ability to **predict** accurately who does or does not have a particular disorder and are critically related to the prevalence of the disorder within the population being tested.

False-negative antibody test results can occur any time an individual is within that 2- to 3-month seronegative window period between the time of initial infection and the development of a detectable immune response. Fortunately, this time period is short and, based on blood-bank transfusion data, the number of false-negative results among low-risk populations is approximately one in 40,000 to one in 150,000.[77] Other causes of false-negative ELISA reactions to HIV-1 include replacement transfusions, bone marrow transplantation, and commercially available

Table 3–1. HIV Testing Results

		HIV	INFECTION
		Present	**Absent**
TEST RESULT	**Positive**	True positive (A)	False positive (B)
	Negative	False negative (C)	True negative (D)

$$\text{Sensitivity (\%)} = \frac{A}{A + C} \, (\times \, 100). \qquad \text{Positive predictive value (\%)} = \frac{A}{A + B} \, (\times \, 100).$$

$$\text{Specificity (\%)} = \frac{D}{D + B} \, (\times \, 100). \qquad \text{Negative predictive value (\%)} = \frac{D}{D + C} \, (\times \, 100).$$

test kits that detect antibody to p24 only (e.g., the ELISA test using recombinant p24 antigen).

False-positive ELISA reactions generally result from cross-reacting antibodies such as those against class II human leukocyte antigens (HLA-DR-4 and DQw-3).[4,10,46] Such antibodies are most often observed in multiparous women and in individuals who have received multiple transfused units of blood. Other autoantibodies (e.g., those against smooth muscle or parietal cells; anti-mitochondrial antibodies; antinuclear antibodies; and anti–T-cell antibodies) can lead to false-positive results.[9,67,70,72]

A common misconception is that a false-positive ELISA will always be corrected by the confirmatory Western blot test. In fact, false-positive Western blot results do occur, although the frequency of false-positive Western blot results is generally less common than with ELISA results.[70] Antibodies against HLA class I antigens may lead to false-positive gp41 bands, whereas antibodies to class II HLA antigens cause false-positive bands at p31. Other autoantibodies (e.g., antimitochondrial, antinuclear, anti–T-cell, and antileukocyte antibodies) that react with proteins present in the T-lymphocyte cell line that propagated the virus used in the Western blot test may also lead to false-positive test results.[67,70]

The most important parameter when interpreting HIV tests is the positive predictive value. The probability of a positive test result's occurring in a truly infected individual is critically dependent on the prevalence of HIV infection of the population tested.[51] As an example, assuming tests (ELISA and Western blot) of 100% sensitivity and a joint false-positive rate of 0.01%, the rates of truly infected patients among those with positive ELISA and Western blot results vary dramatically, depending on who is tested. In testing intravenous drug users from a major U.S. metropolitan center in which the seroprevalence is 50%, the positive predictive value would approach 100%. Conversely, in screening female school teachers from a rural area in the United States where the prevalence of HIV infection is 0.01%, 50% of the women testing positive would have false-positive test results. If the joint false-positive rate increases to 0.1%, 90% of the women with positive ELISA and Western blot results would be falsely labeled as HIV infected[51] (Figure 3–8).

Although test specificity has improved over the last 3 to 5 years, the specificities

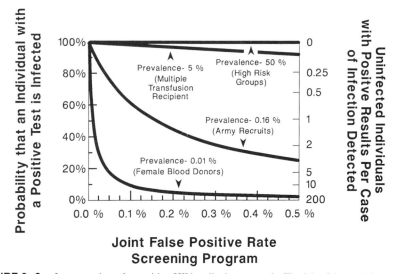

Joint False Positive Rate
Screening Program

FIGURE 3–8.   Interpretation of a positive HIV antibody test result. The joint false-positive rate from the ELISA and Western blot tests is shown on the horizontal axis. The left verticle axis demonstrates the probability that a person with a positive test result is truly infected with HIV. The right verticle scale shows the number of uninfected individuals falsely identified as infected for every infected person correctly identified. The four bold lines represent four populations that might be screened (high-risk groups, transfusion recipients, army recruits, and female blood donors), each of which has a different prevalence of HIV infection (listed accordingly). (From Meyer KB, Pauker SG: Sounding Board, Screening for HIV: Can we afford the false positive rate? Reprinted by permission of N Engl J Med 317(4):240, 1987.)

do not equal 100% and in some instances, depending on the experience of the laboratory personnel, may be 99.9% (false-positive rate, 0.1%). For most other tests this is an acceptable false-positive rate; however, when considering the difficulties in counseling an individual who has a low risk of HIV infection who has just been diagnosed as HIV positive, it becomes quite difficult to know what precisely to tell the patient. In such instances in which the test result does not match the clinical presentation, it is best initially to repeat both the ELISA and the Western blot test at a different laboratory. If the results do not change or are indeterminate, testing at specialized laboratories using either RIPA, IFA, HIV-1 isolation by cell culture, or PCR techniques may be of some benefit.

Another difficult problem in antibody test interpretation is how to deal with an indeterminate Western blot result. As described earlier, this situation is created when bands are present on the Western blot that do not meet criteria of a truly positive test. Several algorithms have been proposed in the literature for dealing with indeterminate Western blots; however, the applied concepts of assessing the risk to the patient combined with repeat testing in another laboratory is a common theme throughout these algorithms.[13,25] When retesting a patient who has had an indeterminate result at more than one laboratory, it is recommended that the individual be retested at 3 and 6 months to determine whether he or she was in the process of seroconverting at the original time of testing.

The use of PCR as a routine diagnostic test should be discouraged. The rate of false positivity in laboratories with inexperienced personnel can be quite substantial.

Even in the best laboratories using appropriate controls and sterile technique, contamination can and does occur.

Use of Markers in Clinical Trials

Since the discovery of zidovudine (AZT) as an effective antiretroviral agent, it is no longer ethically appropriate to have untreated placebo groups in patients with advanced HIV infection; neither is it appropriate to rely on gross measurements of antiviral efficacy such as advancing morbidity or mortality as a means of assessing relative antiviral activity of one compound versus another. As a result, surrogate markers of viral replication such as p24 antigenemia, plasma viremia, quantitative cell culture, quantitative PCR, CD4 counts, β_2-microglobulin, and neopterin levels are being used in various combinations to assess the relative antiretroviral **activity** of one compound versus another. Although the definitions of how to use each test most appropriately are still being clarified, many of these surrogate markers will be used with increasing frequency in the assessment of the antiretroviral effect of drugs in clinical trials.

From a clinical standpoint, however, it is important to separate the goals of experimental therapeutics and the goals of optimum patient care. In fact, outside of clinically staging patients with CD4 counts, the use of these other techniques remains controversial. The use of plasma viremia, quantitative cell markers, and quantitative PCR is not indicated in routine clinical practice. The use of p24 antigenemia, neopterin, and/or β_2-microglobulin levels may become more important as more antiretroviral drugs and combinations of drugs become commercially available and the role of surrogate markers is better defined.

In essence, clinicians should ask themselves, "How will this test result change the care I am providing for my patient?" The answer to that question will dictate which tests are indicated, although most often the only test for clinical use will be the CD4 lymphocyte count. Nonetheless, since the treatment of HIV infection is constantly in a state of flux, some of these other tests may become more reliable, readily available, and useful in therapeutic decision making over the next several years.

ACKNOWLEDGMENT

Thanks to Ms. Jane Garrison for her expert assistance in the preparation of this manuscript, to Katharine Coleman for preparation of the figures, and to Dr. Victoria Johnson for her critical review.

REFERENCES

1. Abbott MA, Poiesz BJ, Byrne BC, et al: Enzymatic gene amplification: Qualitative and quantitative methods for detecting proviral DNA amplified in vitro. J Infect Dis 158(6);1158-1169, 1988
2. Allain J-P, Laurian Y, Paul DA, et al: Long-term evaluation of HIV antigen and antibodies to p24 and gp41 in patients with hemophilia. N Engl J Med 317:1114-1121, 1987
3. Allain J-P, Laurian Y, Paul DA, et al: Serological markers in early stages of human immunodeficiency virus infection in hemophiliacs. Lancet 2:1233-1236, 1986

4. Ameglio F, Dolei A, Benedetto A, et al: Antibodies reactive with nonpolymorphic epitopes on HLA molecules interfere in screening tests for the human immunodeficiency virus. J Infect Dis 156(6):1034-1035, 1987
5. Anderson RE, Lang W, Shiboski S, et al: Use of β_2-microglobulin level and CD4 lymphocyte count to predict development of acquired immunodeficiency syndrome in persons with human immunodeficiency virus infection. Arch Intern Med 150:73-77, 1990
6. Barnes DM: New questions about AIDS test accuracy. Science 238:884-885, 1987
7. Barre-Sinoussi F, Chermann JC, Rey F, et al: Isolation of a T-lymphotropic retrovirus from a patient at risk for acquired immune deficiency syndrome (AIDS). Science 220:868-871, 1983
8. Becker-Andre M, Hahlbrock K: Absolute mRNA quantification using the polymerase chain reaction (PCR). A novel approach by a PCR aided transcript titration assay (PATTY). Nucleic Acids Res 17:9437-9446, 1989
9. Biberfeld G, Bredberg-Raden U, Bottinger B, el al: Blood donor sera with false-positive Western blot reactions to human immunodeficiency virus. Lancet 2:289-290, 1986
10. Blanton M, Balakrishnan K, Dumaswala U, et al: HLA antibodies in blood donors with reactive screening tests for antibody to the immunodeficiency virus. Transfusion 27:118, 1987
11. Calabrese LH, Proffitt MR, Gupta MK, et al: Serum β_2-microglobulin and interferon in homosexual males: Relationship to clinical findings and serologic status to the human T lymphotropic virus (HTLV-III). AIDS Res 1:423-438, 1984
12. Carlson JR, Yee J, Hinrichs SH, et al: Comparison of indirect immunofluorescence and Western blot for detection of antihuman immunodeficiency virus antibodies. J Clin Microbiol 25:494-497, 1987
13. Celum CL, Coombs RW, Lafferty W, et al: Indeterminate human immunodeficiency virus type 1 Western blots: Seroconversion risk, specificity of supplemental tests, and an algorithm for evaluation. J Infect Dis 164:656-664, 1991
14. Centers for Disease Control: Interpretation and use of the Western blot assay for serodiagnosis of human immunodeficiency virus type 1 infections. MMWR 38:1-7, 1989
15. Centers for Disease Control: Update: Serologic testing for antibody to human immunodeficiency virus. MMWR 36:833-840, 1988
16. Chiodi F, Bredberg-Raden U, Biberfeld G, et al: Radioimmunoprecipitation and Western blotting with sera of human immunodeficiency virus infected patients: A comparative study. AIDS Res Hum Retroviruses 3:165-176, 1987
17. Clark SJ, Saag MS, Decker WD, et al: High titers of cytopathic virus in plasma of patients with symptomatic primary HIV-1 infection. N Engl J Med 324:954-960, 1991
18. Consortium for Retrovirus Serology Standardization: Serological diagnosis of human immuno-deficiency virus infection by Western blot testing. JAMA 260:674-679, 1988
19. Coombs RW, Collier AC, Allain J-P, et al: Plasma viremia in human immunodeficiency virus infection. N Engl J Med 321:1626-1631, 1989
20. Cooper DA, Gold J, Maclean P, et al: Acute AIDS retrovirus infection. Lancet 1:537-540, 1985
21. Cooper DA, Imrie AA, Penny R: Antibody response to human immunodeficiency virus after primary infection. J Infect Dis 155:1113-1118, 1987
22. Daar ES, Moudgil T, Meyer RD, et al: Transient high levels of viremia in patients with primary immunodeficiency type 1 infection. N Engl J Med 324:961-964, 1991
23. Davey RT Jr, Lane HC: Laboratory methods in the diagnosis and prognostic staging of infection with human immunodeficiency virus Type 1. Rev Infect Dis 12(5):912-930, 1990
24. Dickover RE, Donovan RM, Goldstein E, et al: Quantitation of human immunodeficiency virus DNA by using the polymerase chain reaction. J Clin Microbiol 28:2130-2133, 1990
25. Dock NL, Kleinman SH, Rayfield MA, et al: Human immunodeficiency virus infection and indeterminate Western blot patterns. Arch Intern Med 151:525-530, 1991
26. El-Sadr W, Marmor M, Zolla-Pazner S, et al: Four year prospective study on homosexual men: Correlation of immunologic abnormalities, clinical status and serology to human immunodefi-ciency virus. J Infect Dis 155:789-793, 1987
27. Eyster ME, Gail MH, Ballard JO, et al: Natural history of human immunodeficiency virus infection in hemophiliacs: Effects of T-cell subsets, platelet counts, and age. Ann Intern Med 107:1-6, 1987
28. Fahey JL, Taylor JMG, Detels R, et al: The prognostic value of cellular and serologic markers in infection with human immunodeficiency virus type 1. N Engl J Med 322:166-172, 1990
29. Fiscus SA, Wallmark EB, Folds JD, et al: Detection of infectious immune complexes in human immunodeficiency virus type 1 (HIV-1) infections: Correlation with plasma viremia and CD4 cell counts. J Infect Dis 164:765-769, 1991

30. Fuchs D, Hausen A, Reibnegger G, et al: Neopterin as a marker for activated cell-mediated immunity: Application in HIV infection. Immunol Today 9:150-155, 1988
31. Fuchs D, Spira TJ, Hausen A, et al: Neopterin as a predictive marker for disease progression in human immunodeficiency virus type 1 infection. Clin Chem 35:1746-1749, 1989
32. Gallo D, Diggs JL, Shell GR, et al: Comparison of detection of antibody to the acquired immune deficiency syndrome virus by enzyme immunoassay, immunofluorescence, and Western blot methods. J Clin Microbiol 23:1049-1051, 1986
33. Goedert JJ, Biggar RJ, Melbye M, et al: Effect of T4 count and cofactors on the incidence of AIDS in homosexual men infected with human immunodeficiency virus. JAMA 257:331-334, 1987
34. Goudsmit J, DeWolf F, Paul DA, et al: Expression of human immunodeficiency virus antigen (HIV-Ag) in serum and cerebrospinal fluid during acute and chronic infection. Lancet 2:177-180, 1986
35. Hart C, Schochetman G, Spira T, et al: Direct detection of HIV RNA expression in seropositive subjects. Lancet 2:596-599, 1988
36. Hedenskog M, Dewhurst S, Ludvigsen C, et al: Testing for antibodies to AIDS-associated retrovirus (HLTV-III/LAV) by indirect fixed cell immunofluorescence: Specificity, sensitivity, and applications. J Med Virol 19:325-334, 1986
37. Hewlett IK, Gregg RA, Ou CY, et al: Detection in plasma of HIV-1 specific DNA and RNA by polymerase chain reaction before and after seroconversion. J Clin Immunoassay 11:161-164, 1988
38. Ho DH, Moudgil T, Alam M: Quantitation of human immunodeficiency virus type 1 in the blood of infected persons. N Engl J Med 321:1621-1625, 1989
39. Holodniy M, Katzenstein DA, Sengupta S, et al: Detection and quantification of human immunodeficiency virus RNA in patient serum by use of the polymerase chain reaction. J Infect Dis 163:862-866, 1991
40. Horsburgh CR Jr, Ou CY, Jason J, et al: Duration of human immunodeficiency virus infection before detection of antibody. Lancet 2:637-639, 1989
41. Isaksson B, Albert J, Chiodi F, et al: AIDS two months after primary human immunodeficiency virus infection. J Infect Dis 158:866-868, 1988
42. Jacobson MA, Abrams DI, Volberding PA, et al: Serum β_2-microglobulin decreases in patients with AIDS or ARC treated with azidothymidine. J Infect Dis 159:1029-1036, 1989
43. Kemp BE, Rylatt DB, Bundesen PG, et al: Autologous red cell agglutination assay for HIV-1 antibodies: Simplified test with whole blood. Science 241:1352-1354, 1988
44. Kestens L, Goofd G, Gigase PL, et al: HIV antigen detection in circulating immune complexes. J Virol Methods 31:67-76, 1991
45. Klein E, Gindi EJ, Brown DK, et al: Cross-sectional study of immunologic abnormalities in intravenous drug abusers on methadone maintenance in New York City. AIDS 3:235-237, 1989
46. Kuhnl P, Seidl S, Holzberger G: HLA DR4 antibodies cause positive HTLV-III antibody ELISA results. Lancet 1:1222-1223, 1985
47. Lane HC, Fauci AS: Immunologic abnormalities in the acquired immunodeficiency syndrome. Annu Rev Immunol 3:477-500, 1985
48. Lazzarin A: Raised serum β_2-microglobulin levels in different stages of human immunodeficiency virus infection. J Clin Lab Immunol 27:133-137, 1988
49. Lifson AR, Stanley M, Pane J, et al: Detection of human immunodeficiency virus DNA using the polymerase chain reaction in a well-characterized group of homosexual and bisexual men. J Infect Dis 161:436-439, 1990
50. Malone JL, Simms TE, Gray GC, et al: Sources of variability in repeated T-helper lymphocyte counts from human immunodeficiency virus type 1–infected patients: Total lymphocyte count fluctuations and diurnal cycle are important. J Acquir Immune Defic Syndr 3:144-151, 1990
51. Meyer KB, Pauker SG: Sounding Board: Screening for HIV: Can we afford the false positive rate? N Engl J Med 317(4):238-241, 1987
52. Moss AR, Bacchetti P: Natural history of HIV infection. AIDS 3:550-561, 1989
53. Moss AR, Bacchetti P, Osmond D, et al: Seropositivity for HIV and the development of AIDS or AIDS related condition: Three year follow-up of the San Francisco General Hospital cohort. BMJ 296:745-750, 1988
54. NIH State-of-the-Art Conference: State-of-the-Art conference on azidothymidine therapy for early HIV infection. Am J Med 89:335-344, 1990
55. Nishanian P, Huskins KR, Stehn S, et al: A simple method for improved assay demonstrates that

HIV p24 antigen is present as immune complexes in most sera from HIV-infected individuals. J Infect Dis 162:21-28, 1990

56. O'Gorman MRG, Weber D, Landis SE, et al: Interpretive criteria of the Western blot assay for serodiagnosis of human immunodeficiency virus type 1 infection. Arch Pathol Lab Med 115:26-30, 1991

57. Oka S, Urayama K, Hirabayashi Y, et al: Quantitative analysis of human immunodeficiency virus type 1 in asymptomatic carriers using the polymerase chain reaction. Biochem Biophys Res Commun 167:1-8, 1990

58. Ou CY, Kwok S, Mitchell SW, et al: DNA amplification for direct detection of HIV-1 DNA of peripheral blood mononuclear cells. Science 239:295-297, 1988

59. Paul DA, Falk LA, Kessler HA, et al: Correlation of serum HIV antigen and antibody with clinical status in HIV-infected patients. J Med Virol 22:257-363, 1987

60. Polk BF, Fox R, Brookmeyer R, et al: Predictors of the acquired immunodeficiency syndrome developing in a cohort of seropositive homosexual men. N Engl J Med 316:61-66, 1988

61. Popovic M, Sarngadharan MG, Read E, et al: Detection, isolation, and continuous production of cytopathic retroviruses (HTLV-III) from patients with AIDS and pre-AIDS. Science 224:497-500, 1984

62. Portera M, Vitale F, La Licata R, et al: Free and antibody-complexed antigen and antibody profile in apparently healthy HIV seropositive individuals and in AIDS patients. J Med Virol 30:30-35, 1990

63. Quinn TC, Riggin CH, Kline RL, et al: Rapid latex agglutination assay using recombinant envelope polypeptide for the detection of antibody to the HIV. JAMA 260:510-513, 1988

64. Reddy MM, Grieco MH: Neopterin and alpha and beta interleukin-1 levels in sera of patients with human immunodeficiency virus infection. J Clin Microbiol 27:1919-1923, 1989

65. Redfield RR, Wright DC, Tramont EC: The Walter Reed staging classification for HTLV-III/LAV infection. N Engl J Med 314:131-132, 1986

66. Riggin CH, Beltz GA, Hung C-H, et al: Detection of antibodies to human immunodeficiency virus by latex agglutination with recombinant antigen. J Clin Microbiol 25:1772-1773, 1987

67. Saag MS, Britz J: Asymptomatic blood donor with a false positive HTLV-III Western blot. N Engl J Med 314(2):118, 1986

68. Saag MS, Crain MJ, Decker WD, et al: High-level viremia in adults and children infected with human immunodeficiency virus: Relation to disease stage and CD4+ lymphocyte levels. J Infect Dis 164:72-80, 1991

69. Saiki RK, Gelfand DH, Stoffel S, et al: Primer-directed enzymatic amplification of DNA with a thermostable DNA polymerase. Science 239:487-491, 1988

70. Schleupner CJ: Diagnostic tests for HIV-1 infection. In Mandell, Douglas, and Bennet (eds): Principles and Practice of Infectious Diseases, Update 1. New York, Churchill Livingstone, 1989, p 3

71. Sloand EM, Pitt E, Chiarello RJ: HIV testing—State of the art. JAMA 266(20):2861-2866, 1991

72. Smith DM, Dewhurst S, Shepherd S, et al: False-positive enzyme-linked immunosorbent assay reactions for antibody to human immunodeficiency virus in a population of Midwestern patients with congenital bleeding disorders. Transfusion 127:112, 1987

73. Taylor CR, Krailo MD, Levine AM: Serum beta-2 microglobulin levels in homosexual men with AIDS and with persistent, generalized lymphadenopathy. Cancer 57:2190-2192, 1986

74. Taylor JMG, Fahey JL, Detels R, et al: CD4 percentage, CD4 number, and CD4:CD8 ratio in HIV infection: Which to choose and how to use. J Acquir Immune Defic Syndr 2:114-124, 1989

75. Tindall B, Barker S, Donovan E, et al: Characterization of the acute clinical illness associated with human immunodeficiency virus infection. Arch Intern Med 148:945-949, 1988

76. Ward JW, Bush TJ, Perkins HA, et al: The natural history of transfusion-associated infection with human immunodeficiency virus: Factors influencing the rate of progression to disease. N Engl J Med 321(14):947-952, 1989

77. Ward JW, Holmberg SD, Allen JR, et al: Transmission of human immunodeficiency virus (HIV) by blood transfusions screened as negative for HIV antibody. N Engl J Med 318(8):473-478, 1988

78. Wolinsky SM, Rinaldo CR, Kwok S, et al: Human immunodeficiency virus type 1 (HIV-1) infection a median of 18 months before a diagnostic Western blot. Ann Intern Med 111:961-972, 1989

4

HIV TRANSMISSION TO PROVIDERS AND THEIR PATIENTS

JULIE LOUISE GERBERDING, MD, MPH

Health care providers exposed to blood and other body fluids risk infection with human immunodeficiency virus (HIV). Defining the risks of occupational HIV transmission and developing policies for protecting health care providers are important concerns in the AIDS era. HIV transmission from infected providers to patients is also an important issue that gained visibility after reports linked HIV transmission in five patients to an infected dentist. This chapter provides an update of the current status of risk assessment and risk reduction strategies for preventing HIV infection among providers and their patients.

RISK ASSESSMENT

The risk from occupational exposure to HIV has been prospectively evaluated in cohorts of intensively exposed health care providers at several medical centers around the world. Since both the numerator (number of infections) and the denominator (number of exposures) are known, these studies allow estimation of the rate of transmission following various types of exposure. More than 4000 health care providers from a variety of occupational categories, including more than 2000 with a history of accidental parenteral inoculation with HIV-infected materials, have been enrolled in such studies and periodically tested for HIV antibody.[4,9,14,16,17,20,22,27,30,38]

After 5 years of observation, direct inoculation of infected material during accidental needle-stick or similar parenteral injury is the only mechanism of transmission observed among study patients. The rate of nosocomial HIV transmission following parenteral exposure is approximately 0.32% (six infections in more than 2008 needle sticks involving HIV-infected blood).[4,6,9,14,16,17,20,22,27,30,38] The risk from mucous membrane contact or inoculation of nonintact skin with HIV-infected blood or body fluids is too low for quantification in these studies to date, despite the fact that at least 1000 exposures of this type have been assessed.

More than 40 documented cases of occupational HIV transmission (including the six mentioned previously) have been reported in the world's medical literature since 1981. In the majority of these cases occupational transmission was proved by demonstrating seroconversion temporally related to a discrete accidental HIV exposure event.[1,6,11,16,21,27,31-33,38,43,45,46,48] Needle-stick exposure or lacerations contaminated by infected blood produced infection in the majority. Inapparent parenteral exposure to blood through breaks in the skin or mucous membrane inoculation with blood was the most likely route of transmission in a small number of cases.[11,46] At least two workers were infected via exposure to virus concentrate (parenteral and nonintact skin contamination) in research laboratories.[48] In several cases occupational transmission was considered possible but was not proved by demonstrating seroconversion.[13,27,36,49] These published anecdotes most certainly do not include all cases of occupational infection because in many states occupational infection is not a reportable condition until AIDS develops, and some cases may not yet be recognized or reported. Efforts to coordinate surveillance and reporting of occupationally acquired HIV infection are in progress by the Centers for Disease Control (CDC) so that a more complete assessment of the frequency of such events will be possible.

The risk of transmission may be influenced by a variety of factors that are as yet poorly defined. Most authorities believe that the volume of the inoculum and/or quantity of virus involved in the exposure influences the degree of risk. Deep (intramuscular) penetrations, large-bore hollow needles, and injections of blood are factors associated with most of the reported needle-stick accidents causing occupational infections. Large volumes of blood, prolonged duration of contact, and a portal of entry are common denominators in the reported mucocutaneous cases. The stage of infection in the source patient also may be linked to the probability of transmission. Circulating titers of HIV are believed highest at the time of seroconversion and during advanced stages of symptomatic infection, but the relationship of this observation to the probability of occupational transmission remains speculative.[18] The efficiency of transmission could also be affected by the presence of intracellular (as opposed to cellfree) virus in the inoculum. Finally, the immunologic status of the recipient health care provider could influence the probability of successful infection.

The use of gloves may reduce the risk of transmission during needle-stick injuries to the hands. In a laboratory model needles passed through glove material transferred at least 50% less blood than when glove material was not present. This effect was apparent regardless of the specific type of glove material tested, and no advantage of latex over vinyl material was detected.[28]

Blood has been implicated as the source of the exposure in all infections occurring in clinicians. Other body fluids, including saliva, tears, and urine, may contain the virus, but the titer of HIV in these fluids is usually much lower than the titer found in blood and semen. Although HIV transmission therefore is unlikely following exposure to most nonbloody body fluids, these other body fluids could contain other viruses or pathogens and should be considered potentially infectious when planning infection control interventions.

Cutaneous exposure to blood involving normal skin has not been linked to HIV infection in any setting. Although Langerhans' cells and other subcutaneous cells possess CD4 receptors and contain HIV in most infected patients, these cells are protected from primary infection by an intact integument. However, transcutaneous inoculation during parenteral needle-stick injury or contamination of skin lesions has been hypothesized to promote primary infection of subcutaneous target cells. No risk from close personal contact with patients, exposure to airborne droplets or aerosols, or contact with contaminated environmental surfaces or fomites has been observed.

Aerosols of infected blood or saliva can occur in dental, pathology, laboratory, and surgical environments. Because masks do not prevent exposure to a aerosolized particle smaller than the pore diameter of the mask material, concern about the possibility of aerosolized HIV transmission has alarmed some health care providers. Hepatitis B virus, which is present in much higher titers than HIV among infected patients, has not been recovered from aerosols during experiments performed in dental operatories and dialysis units.[34,35] The absence of HIV seroconversion in prospective studies of dentists practicing in areas where HIV is highly prevalent strongly suggests that aerosol transmission is unlikely to confer a measurable occupational hazard.[9] In fact, aerosols have not been associated with HIV infection in any setting to date. Even if aerosols contain viable HIV, the magnitude of risk is unlikely to be greater than the risk from mucous membrane splashes (see above).

The cumulative professional risk from repeated exposure to HIV has not been adequately assessed. The overall risk to a given health care provider depends on the risk from discreet exposure events, the frequency of exposure to body fluids, and the prevalence of HIV in the workplace. Health care providers such as nurses, dentists, surgeons, emergency care providers, and labor and delivery personnel are at highest risk for acquiring HBV and also may be at higher risk for HIV infection over a lifetime of practice, particularly when practicing in areas with a high prevalence of HIV.[12,50] Large prospective studies of these individuals are needed to define the true magnitude of risk among various professionals. One such study of more than 3400 orthopedic surgeons documented two cases of nonoccupational infection, but no cases attributable to occupational exposure.[37]

Transmission of HIV to patients could occur directly by inoculation of blood or other infected body fluids or indirectly through the use of contaminated instruments. Direct inoculation is possible when an infected provider is injured and then bleeds into the patient or when the contaminated instrument causing injury recontacts the patient's tissue. The frequency of injuries severe enough to cause bleeding into the wounds or tissues of patients undergoing invasive procedures is unknown but probably is extremely rare. The frequency of recontact exposures such as occur when a suture needle injuring the provider is passed back through the tissue of the patient may be more common, but the transmission risk associated with these exposures is unknown. To date, no infections linked to recontacts during surgical procedures have been detected in any setting.

Instruments contaminated with blood from infected patients or providers could transmit HIV to patients if proper disinfection procedures are not followed. Even though HIV is a relatively fragile virus, survival in clots of blood or tissue, especially when environmental conditions such as warmth or moisture are present, is possible. Indeed, many experts suspect that the nosocomial transmission to the Florida dental patients occurred during procedures performed with contaminated instruments previously used in the mouth of the HIV-infected dentist.[39] The fact that disinfection procedures in this practice were lax adds credence to this view and has implications for infection control policy formation. If disinfection protocols are not rigorously followed, nosocomial transmission from patient to patient is potentially a much more common event than transmission from provider to patient.

Allaying Fears

Fear of AIDS may be masked by denial. Beliefs that HIV-infected patients are not present, that infected patients can be identified and avoided, or that transmission is impossible are often perpetuated until the reality of occupational risk becomes apparent. The first experience with occupational exposure or infection may precipitate a crisis. Intense anger, depression, surprise, and aggressiveness are reactions frequently described in this setting. Although creating a "zero risk" of infection is not a realistic possibility, a demand for excessive or unreasonable infection control measures often follows the initial crisis. Recognition that some degree of risk is unavoidable and that all care providers are at shared risk should be made. On the other hand, providers should be reassured that occupational infection is less likely when infection control procedures are implemented. Involving workers at risk for exposure in the development of infection control precautions can help channel concerns into constructive outlets.

Fear of acquiring HIV among clinicians who recognize their risk for exposure is not irrational when the degree of fear is appropriate for the degree of risk present. Lack of knowledge about the magnitude of risk or routes of transmission, the epidemic nature of the disease, the high mortality rate, and the lack of effective treatment can amplify the perceived risk and should be addressed. In addition, the anxiety aroused by confronting the complex psychologic issues related to homosexuality, morality, and mortality evoked by AIDS patients may be communicated as fear of infection. For some health care professionals, it is easier to avoid the AIDS patient altogether than to deal with the emotional conflicts encountered while providing care; fear of contagion provides a convenient and more publicly acceptable excuse. Constructive methods to acknowledge openly the stresses inherent in dealing with AIDS patients should be included in clinical training curricula and staff development programs.

The publicity surrounding the reports of five patients infected in the office of the Florida dentist with AIDS has alarmed the public. The uncertainty surrounding the modes of transmission to these patients has added to the confusion, exaggerated perceptions of risk, and stymied efforts to implement sensible infection control interventions. Health care workers, especially those who perform invasive procedures, should be alert to the concerns patients may experience and openly address these issues. Frank communication about transmission risks and infection control practices will help establish mutual trust between providers and patients and alleviate fear. Providers should also be prepared to answer queries about HIV status honestly (e.g., "I've not been tested," "I am/am not infected," or "I do not choose to discuss my HIV testing status with my patients").

RISK REDUCTION: INFECTION CONTROL

Avoiding contact with potentially infected body fluids and tissues is an essential component of risk reduction for health care providers.[6,10,26,40,47] Preventing needlestick injuries and other parenteral exposures is likely to have the biggest impact on reducing HIV transmission in most health care settings.[19,40] Athough blood is the only body fluid associated with occupational HIV transmission to date, common sense and concern for preventing transmission of other nosocomial pathogens would dictate that other body fluids also should be considered potentially infectious.

Universal precautions are recommended by the CDC for all patients, regardless of diagnosis, for preventing transmission of blood-borne pathogens.[40] Use of additional isolation precautions is advised for patients with infections transmitted by other routes. The universal precautions include the use of gloves for procedures in which contact with blood, bloody body fluids, and certain other fluids (amniotic fluid, semen, vaginal fluid, cerebrospinal fluid, serosal transudates and exudates, and inflammatory exudates) might occur, the use of masks and protective eyewear when splatter of such body fluids is anticipated, and the use of gowns or other protective garments when soilage of clothing is likely.[40]

Body substance precautions (BSP), or body substance isolation (BSI), is an alternative system of infection control practiced by an increasing number of institutions.[26,28] A single standard of precautions, based on the anticipated degree of exposure with **all** body fluids and tissues, regardless of the infectious disease diagnosed or suspected, is implemented at the moment of initial contact with the patient.[26,28] The main difference between these two infection control systems is that the CDC isolation system considers the type of infection suspected, whereas BSP is based on the degree of contact anticipated. However, both universal precautions and BSP emphasize prevention of needle-stick injury and barrier protection for avoiding exposure to potentially infectious materials, and neither requires the use of labeling of patients or specimens for implementation. Compliance with either policy is likely to reduce exposure to blood-borne pathogens and should be encouraged in all health care settings.

Nosocomial transmission to patients is avoidable if proper disinfection and needle-stick safety protocols are followed. Sterilization or disinfection cannot be accomplished if instruments are not properly cleaned to remove blood, tissue, or other debris before processing. Liquid disinfectants lose their potency if solutions age or are diluted below their effective strength. Timing of the disinfection process is also important, and careful monitoring of the duration of exposure to the agent is essential.

Techniques involving needles and other sharp instruments during invasive procedures are undergoing scrutiny to prevent injuries that could expose the patient to provider's blood. Using the index finger of the nondominant hand to retract tissue or to palpate the needle tip during suturing accounts for a large proportion of intraoperative injuries. Substituting instruments for manual manipulations or use of special protective coverings is advocated to ameliorate this problem. Gloves constructed of monofilament polymers resistant to laceration recently have become available for use when manipulation of bone fragments or suture wires is needed. Efforts are underway to identify other changes that may affect intraoperative injury risk rates favorably. Health care providers with open sores, exudates, or other skin lesions should never provide direct care to patients, regardless of HIV status. Although transmission by this route is unlikely, some degree of risk is present, and gloves are not adequate to prevent exposure.

HIV Testing for Infection Control

The list of valid indications for considering HIV testing continues to expand, especially since the advent of effective antiretroviral therapy and prophylaxis for pneumocystic pneumonia. Unlike most other laboratory tests, testing for HIV can incur special risks to the patient. Because effective antidiscrimination legislation has not yet been passed in most areas, many HIV-infected persons risk employment, housing, insurance, and even medical discrimination. Most states have recognized both the benefits and risks associated with HIV testing and require informed consent before the test is performed.

Testing for HIV to implement infection control procedures remains controversial. Some health care providers believe that testing and labeling infected patients will improve compliance with infection control procedures or that safer surgical techniques should be selectively used for those with diagnosed HIV infection. In some hospitals such as San Francisco General surgeons can opt to test patients preoperatively (after informed consent is obtained) and adjust infection control practices accordingly. Other institutions prohibit HIV testing unless a medical indication is present, and some routinely test all patients. Currently no evidence supports the validity of any of these approaches. Clearly more research is warranted to determine if benefit (reduced exposure) at minimum risk to the patient (good surgical outcome, confidentiality) and cost to the institution (excessive expenditures) can be achieved through identifying infected patients preoperatively.

Managing Exposures to HIV

The CDC has published guidelines for managing health care workers who sustain accidental exposures to HIV.[2] Determining whether or not exposure has actually occurred is rarely simple. Health care workers may not report exposures for a variety of reasons and may underestimate or overestimate the severity of the exposure. Obtaining a careful history will usually permit categorization of the exposure route into one of the following broad categories: (1) needle stick (or similar injury resulting in direct transcutaneous exposure); (2) mucous membrane inoculation; (3) contamination of open skin wound or lesion; or (4) contamination of nonintact skin. Needle sticks and other percutaneous accidents should be characterized further by the size and type of needle or instrument involved (e.g., suture, hollow, scalpel), approximate depth of penetration, volume of blood injected (if any), site, wound appearance, amount of bleeding produced, and how long the contaminating fluid was ex vivo before the exposure occurred. The type, volume, and duration of contact should be estimated for mucous membrane and skin wound contacts.

A system for estimating exposure severity developed at San Francisco General Hospital classifies exposures as "massive" (transfusions, parenteral exposure to HIV concentrates), "definite parenteral" (intramuscular parenteral inoculations or injections of blood or bloody fluids), "possible parenteral" (subcutaneous or superficial percutaneous exposures, mucous membrane splashes, contamination of open wounds), "doubtful parenteral" (exposures involving nonbloody body fluids such as saliva, urine, tears), and "nonparenteral" (contamination of normal skin) (Table 4–1).[15] Although the relationship of these designations to the actual risk of transmission remains unproved, clinicians have found the classification scheme useful in counseling exposed workers and planning follow-up interventions (see below).

Establishing the presence of infection in the source patient is often difficult but can help clarify the degree of risk induced by the exposure event. HIV infection can be assumed when patients are diagnosed with AIDS or are known to be HIV infected. Institutions vary in testing policies for source patients whose HIV status

Table 4–1. Zidovudine Prophylaxis for Occupationally Exposed Health Care Providers* (zidovudine, 200 mg q4h × 72h, then 200 mg q4h five times per day for 25 days)

EXPOSURE	TREATMENT
Massive (transfusion)	Recommended
Definite parenteral (intramuscular injection)	Endorsed
Possible parenteral (subcutaneous or mucosal)	Not encouraged
Doubtful parenteral (nonbloody)	Discouraged
Nonparenteral (cutaneous)	Not provided

Modified from Henderson DK, Gerberding JL: Prophylactic zidovudine after occupational exposure to the human immunodeficiency virus: An interim analysis. J Infect Dis 160:321, 1989.
  *Interim protocol, 1991.
  †Treatment ideally started within 1 hour of exposure.

is less clear. In most the probability of HIV infection is assessed by clinical and epidemiologic criteria. Patients perceived at risk are then counseled and asked to consent to testing. Routine testing of all source patients is gaining acceptance, although mandatory source patient testing (without informed consent) is not yet widespread. Regardless of the testing strategy used, every effort must be made to protect the confidentiality of the source patient.

The exposed health care worker should be encouraged to undergo baseline HIV testing or at least serum banking as soon as possible after exposure has occurred. Without a negative baseline HIV test, proving that infection was temporally related to the exposure event is extremely difficult. Consequently, the worker's ability to claim workers' compensation and other benefits may be seriously jeopardized. Subsequent HIV testing, usually performed 6 weeks, 3 months, and 6 months after exposure, is recommended when HIV is present or potentially present in the exposure source. Sequential testing is extremely useful in allaying fears, documenting seronegativity, and rarely, diagnosing HIV infection.

Because symptoms of acute retroviral infection (fever, lymphadenopathy, rash, headache, profound fatigue) are associated with the majority of reported occupational infections, persons sustaining exposures should be advised to return for evaluation if a compatible illness occurs. Enzyme-linked immunosorbent assay (ELISA) HIV antibody tests may be negative or indeterminant during the early phases of seroconversion illness. Western blot, viral culture, or HIV p24 antigen tests may be more sensitive methods for detecting early infection. The value of gene amplification technology (polymerase chain reaction [PCR]) in identifying infection in seronegative health care workers remains unproved, but preliminary studies suggest that latent infections detected by PCR rarely, if ever, are detected in seronegative health care workers.[7]

Postexposure counseling by experienced care providers familiar with the special medical and psychologic needs of exposed health care providers is essential. Counseling should provide information about the degree of risk present, options for follow-up care, a description of the confidentiality procedures in place, and infection control procedures to prevent similar occurrences in the future. Counselors should be alert to the concerns of the sexual partners, coworkers, family, and friends of the exposed worker.

The CDC recommends "safer" sexual practices and other behavior changes to minimize the potential for transmission until infection has been ruled out by a negative antibody test 6 months after the exposure.[2] Unfortunately, offering this advice frequently produces confusion and anxiety in the exposed person. Counselors are faced with the difficult task of communicating a "mixed message" about the risk of infection: reassurance that occupational transmission is statistically unlikely and, on the other hand, advocacy of behaviors to prevent exchange of body fluids, to avoid pregnancy, and to defer blood donation until infection has been ruled out. In some centers advice is individualized to the specific situation. For example, persons sustaining trivial punctures with small-bore nonhollow needles minimally contaminated by blood from a low-risk untested source patient may decide to return for follow-up HIV testing for 6 months but to comply with safer sex guidelines for a shorter interval of time. Likewise recipients of deep intramuscular injections of infected blood may be cautioned to follow guidelines for preventing transmission compulsively for more than 6 months and to continue follow-up for 12 months.

Patients exposed to provider's blood should be managed with the same standard of care applied to occupational exposures. A system for confidential reporting of such exposures should be developed and communicated to hospital staff. It is the ethical and professional responsibility of the involved provider to undergo testing for blood-borne pathogens and to communicate test results to the clinician responsible for the patient's postexposure care.

POSTEXPOSURE CHEMOPROPHYLAXIS

Interest in postexposure chemoprophylaxis for occupationally exposed health care workers has increased since zidovudine was licensed for palliating HIV infection in persons with advanced disease. Theoretically zidovudine or other nucleoside analogs could prevent successful HIV infection when administered soon after exposure by preventing HIV replication in the initial target cells.

The relevance of animal models of retrovirus infection to human infection with HIV has not been established. Experiments using murine, feline, and human retroviruses in animals inoculated with high titers of virus indicate that zidovudine can prevent viremia and illness under some conditions.[41,42,44] Protection is most apparent when treatment is started within 24 hours of exposure. However, the efficacy of zidovudine in preventing the establishment of asymptomatic latent infection has not been proved in any primate models.[8,25,29]

Failure of postexposure zidovudine chemoprophylaxis in at least three patients has been documented.[3,23,24] In one treatment was delayed for 6 hours and may have involved a zidovudine-resistant strain of virus. In the other two exposure to unusually large inocula of blood occurred, and in one of them blood was injected intravenously. These cases indicate that zidovudine chemoprophylaxis is not 100% effective, but its value in more typical situations remains unknown. Ultimately, the efficacy of zidovudine or other antiretroviral therapies in preventing latent infection in exposed health care workers will be difficult to assess because the low rate of seroconversion mandates an extremely large sample size. Furthermore, detecting infection in treated individuals may be complicated by delayed seroconversion related to drug-induced inhibition of viral replication. Anecdotal experience with zidovudine use for short intervals in healthy health care workers indicates that reversible hematologic toxicity rarely occurs but that less serious intolerances, including subjective symptoms of fatigue, insomnia, and flulike symptoms, are common.[5]

Collaborative efforts to evaluate the safety of prophylactic zidovudine by investigators at the National Institutes of Health (NIH) and San Francisco General Hospital are in progress. In the meantime, some institutions (including the NIH and San Francisco General Hospital) have developed protocols for offering prophylactic zidovudine to selected health care workers exposed to HIV.[5] Until more information is available, protocols for prophylactic treatment should be considered experimental therapy, with written informed consent required from the health care worker electing treatment.

At San Francisco General Hospital and the NIH the option of taking zidovudine is discussed with all exposed health care providers, and expert consultation is readily available. Although the decision to take zidovudine is ultimately left to the health care worker, the advice given at San Francisco General Hospital is highly influenced by the severity of exposure (see Table 4–1). This approach assumes that exposure severity is a major predictor of infection risk and that the benefit from prophylactic zidovudine will be most evident for high-risk exposures.

Most authorities believe that prophylactic zidovudine treatment should be started as soon as possible (minutes to hours) after the exposure to maximize the chance of efficacy. The optimum dose and duration for chemoprophylaxis have not been established, but most protocols use 1 to 1.2 grams/day for 2 to 6 weeks. Treatment of pregnant women or persons not practicing effective contraception is discouraged. Close monitoring for hematologic, hepatic, renal, and neurologic dysfunction is essential. Adverse reactions should be reported to the Food and Drug Administration.

Clearly further in vitro and animal research on chemoprophylaxis with zidovudine and other antiretroviral agents is warranted. Until efficacy and toxicity of any agent are established, chemoprophylaxis will remain a promising but unproved strategy for preventing HIV infection in health care providers.

REFERENCES

1. Apparent transmission of human T-lymphotropic type III/lymphadenopathy–associated virus from a child to a mother providing health care. MMWR 35:76-79, 1986
2. Centers for Disease Control: Public health service statement on management of occupational exposure to human immunodeficiency virus, including considerations regarding zidovudine use. MMWR 39:1-14, 1990
3. Durand E, LeJuenne C, Hugues FC: Failure of prophylactic zidovudine after suicidal self-inoculation of HIV-infected blood. N Engl J Med 324:1062, 1991
4. Gerberding JL, Bryant-LeBlanc CE, Nelson KN, et al: Risk of transmitting the human immunodeficiency virus, cytomegalovirus, and hepatitis B virus to health care providers exposed to patients with AIDS and AIDS-related conditions (ARC). J Infect Dis 156:1-8, 1987
5. Gerberding JL, Fahrner R, Berkvam G, et al: Zidovudine post-exposure chemoprophylaxis for health care workers exposed to HIV at San Francisco General Hospital. Paper presented at the Thirty-first Interscience Congress on Antimicrobial Agents and Chemotherapy. Chicago, 1991.

6. Gerberding JL, Henderson DK: Design of rational infection control guidelines for human immunodeficiency virus infection. J Infect Dis 156:861-864, 1987
7. Gerberding JL, Littell C, Louie P: Gene amplification to detect latent HIV in health care workers at risk for low inoculum exposures. In Programs and Abstracts of the 29th Interscience Conference on Antimicrobial Agents and Chemotherapy. (Abstract No. 1171.) Washington, DC, American Society for Microbiology, 1989
8. Gerberding JL, Marx P, Gould R, et al: Simian model of retrovirus chemoprophylaxis with constant infusion zidovudine with or without interferon-alpha. Paper presented at the Thirty-first Interscience Congress on Antimicrobial Agents and Chemotherapy. Chicago, 1991
9. Gerberding JL, Nelson K, Greenspan D, et al: Risk to dentists from occupational exposure to human immunodeficiency virus (HIV): Followup. In Programs and Abstracts of the 27th Interscience Conference on Antimicrobial Agents and Chemotherapy. (Abstract No. 698.) Washington, DC, American Society for Microbiology, 1987
10. Gerberding JL, University of California, San Francisco Task Force on AIDS: Recommended infection-control policies for patients with human immunodeficiency virus infection: An update. N Engl J Med 315:1562-1564, 1986
11. Gioannini P, Sinicco A, Cariti G, et al: HIV infection acquired by a nurse. Eur J Epidemiol 4:119-120, 1988
12. Grady GF, Lee VA, Prince AM, et al: Hepatitis B immune globulin for accidental exposures among medical personnel: Final report of a multicenter controlled trial. J Infect Dis 138:625-638, 1978
13. Grint P, McEvoy M: Two associated cases of the acquired immunodeficiency syndrome (AIDS). PHLS Commun Dis Rep 42:4, 1985
14. Health and Welfare Canada: National surveillance program on occupational exposure to HIV among health care workers in Canada. Can Dis Wkly Rep 13(37):163-166, 1987
15. Henderson DH, Gerberding JL: Post-exposure zidovudine chemoprophylaxis for health care workers occupationally exposed to the human immunodeficiency virus: An interim analysis. J Infect Dis 1989
16. Henderson DK, Fahey, BS, Saah AJ, et al: Longitudinal assessment of the risk for occupational/nosocomial transmission of human immunodeficiency virus, type 1 in health care workers. In Programs and Abstracts of the 28th Interscience Conference on Antimicrobial Agents and Chemotherapy. (Abstract No. 634.) Washington, DC, American Society for Microbiology, 1988
17. Henderson DK, Saah AJ, Zak BJ, et al: Risk of nosocomial infection with human T-cell lymphotropic virus type III/lymphadenopathy–associated virus in a large cohort of intensively exposed health care providers. Ann Intern Med 104:644-647, 1986
18. Ho DD, Moudgil TM, Alam M: Quantitation of human immunodeficiency virus type-1 in the blood of infected persons. N Engl J Med 321:1621-1625, 1989
19. Jagger J, Hunt EH, Bland-Elnaggar J, Pearson RD: Rates of needlestick injury caused by various devices in a university hospital. N Engl J Med 319:284-288, 1988
20. Joline C, Wormser GP: Update on a prospective study of health care providers exposed to blood and body fluids of acquired immunodeficiency syndrome patients. Am J Infect Control 15:86, 1987
21. Klein RS, Phelan JA, Freeman K, et al: Low occupational risk of HIV infection among dental professionals. N Engl J Med 318:86-90, 1988
22. Kuhls TL, Viker S, Parris NB, et al: Occupational risk of HIV, HBV, and HSV-2 infections in health care personnel caring for AIDS patients. Am J Public Health 77:1306-1309, 1987
23. Lange JMA, Boucher CAB, Hollak CEM, et al: Failure of zidovudine prophylaxis after accidental exposure to HIV. N Engl J Med 322:1375-1377, 1990
24. Looke DFM, Grove DI: Failed prophylactic zidovudine after needlestick injury (letter). Lancet 335:1280, 1990
25. Lundgren B, Hedstrom KG, Norrby E, et al: Inhibition of early occurrence of antigen in SIV-infected macaques as a measurement of antiviral efficacy (abstract). Symposium on Non-human Primate Models for AIDS. November 1990
26. Lynch P, Jackson MM, Cummings MJ, Stamm WE: Rethinking the role of isolation practices in the prevention of nosocomial infections. Ann Intern Med 107:243-246, 1987
27. Marcus R, The Cooperative Needlestick Surveillance Group: Surveillance of health care workers exposed to blood from patients infected with the human immunodeficiency virus. N Engl J Med 319:1118-1123, 1988
28. Mast S, Gerberding JL: Factors predicting needlestick infectivity following exposure to HIV: An in vitro model. Clin Res 39(2):, 1991.

29. McClure HM, Anderson DC, Fultz P, et al: Prophylactic effects of AZT following exposure of macaques to an acutely lethal variant of SIV (SIV/SMM/PBj-14) (abstract). Fifth International Conference on AIDS. Montreal, June 4-9, 1989, p 522
30. McEvoy M, Porter K, Mortimer P, et al: Prospective study of clinical, laboratory, and ancillary staff with accidental exposures to blood or other body fluids from patients infected with HIV. Br Med J 294:1595-1597, 1987
31. Needlestick transmission of HTLV-III from a patient infected in Africa. Lancet 2:1376-1377, 1984
32. Neisson-Verant C, Arfi S, Mathez D, et al: Needlestick HIV seroconversion in a nurse. Lancet 2:814, 1986
33. Oskenhendler E, Harzic M, Le Roux JM, et al: HIV infection with seroconversion after a superficial needlestick injury to the finger. N Engl J Med 315:582, 1986
34. Petersen NJ: An assessment of the airborne route in hepatitis B transmission. Ann N Y Acad Sci 253:157-166, 1980
35. Petersen NJ, Bond WW, Favero MS: Air sampling technique for hepatitis B surface antigen in a dental operatory. J Am Dent Assoc 99:465-467, 1979
36. Ponce de Leon RS, Sanchez-Mejorada G, Zaidi-Jacobson M: AIDS in a blood bank technician in Mexico City (letter). Infect Control Hosp Epidemiol 9:101-102, 1988
37. Preliminary analysis: HIV serosurvey of orthopedic surgeons, 1991. MMWR 40:309-311, 1991
38. Ramsey KM, Smith EN, Reinarz JA: Prospective evaluation of 4 health care workers exposed to human immunodeficiency virus-1, with one seroconversion (abstract). Clin Res 36:22A, 1988
39. Recommendations for preventing transmission of human immunodeficiency virus and hepatitis B virus to patients during exposure-prone procedures. MMWR 40:1-9, 1991
40. Recommendations for prevention of HIV transmission in health-care settings. MMWR 36(suppl 2S), 1987
41. Ruprecht RM, O'Brien LG, Rossoni LD, Nusinoff-Lehrman S: Suppression of mouse viraemia and retroviral disease by 3'-azido-3'-deoxythymidine. Nature 323:467-469, 1986
42. Shih CC, Kaneshima H, Rabin L, et al: Post-exposure prophylaxis with zidovudine suppresses human immunodeficiency virus type-1 infection in SCID-hu mice in a time-dependent manner. J Infect Dis 163:625-627, 1991
43. Stricof RL, Morse DL: HTLV-III/LAV seroconversion following a deep intramuscular needlestick injury (letter). N Engl J Med 314:1115, 1986
44. Travares L, Roneker C, Johnston K, et al: 3'-Azido-3'-deoxythymidine in feline leukemia virus-infected cats: A model for therapy and prophylaxis of AIDS. Cancer Res 47:3190-3194, 1987
45. Update: Acquired immunodeficiency syndrome and human immunodeficiency virus infection among health care workers. MMWR 37:229-239, 1988
46. Update: Human immunodeficiency virus infections in health care workers exposed to blood from infected patients. MMWR 36:285-289, 1987
47. US Department of Labor, US Department of Health and Human Services: Joint Advisory Notice: Protection against occupational exposure to hepatitis B virus (HBV) and human immunodeficiency virus (HIV). Federal Register 52:41818-41824, 1987
48. Weiss SH, Goedert JJ, Gartner S, et al: Risk of human immunodeficiency virus (HIV-1) infection among laboratory workers. Science 239:68-71, 1988
49. Weiss SH, Saxinger WC, Rechtman D, et al: HTLV-III infection among health care workers: Association with needlestick injuries. JAMA 254:2089-2093, 1985
50. Werner BJ, Grady GF: Accidental hepatitis-B-surface antigen-positive inoculations: Use of e antigen to estimate infectivity. Ann Intern Med 97:367-369, 1982

II

MANAGEMENT OF HIV INFECTIONS AND ITS COMPLICATIONS

5

PRIMARY HIV INFECTION

BRETT TINDALL, BAppSc, MSc
ALLISON IMRIE, BSc
BASIL DONOVAN, MB, BS, FACVen, FAFPHM
RONALD PENNY, MD, DSc, FRACP, FRCPA
DAVID A. COOPER, BSc (Med), MD, FRACP, FRCPA,
FACVen, FAFPHM

The first encounter of HIV-1 with the human immune system provides valuable insights into the immunopathology of HIV-1 infection and the host response to HIV-1. The increasing recognition of this early stage of infection has allowed the definition and investigation of its characteristic clinical, serologic, and immunologic features.[109] Information about these early events could suggest approaches to arresting initial viral infection and spread. Moreover, the identification of patients at this stage of infection affords a rare opportunity to institute counseling to avoid further dissemination of HIV-1 infection in the community.

EPIDEMIOLOGY

Transmission Category

Symptomatic primary HIV-1 infection has been reported in persons from each of the major groups affected by HIV-1 infection: homosexual men, heterosexual men and women, injecting drug users, persons with hemophilia, recipients of contaminated blood, blood components, or organs, and health care workers in association with significant occupation injuries.

It is not yet clear whether the risk of developing symptomatic primary HIV-1 infection after inoculation is greater in any of these groups. If differences do exist, they might be attributable to factors such as differences in dose of inoculum associated with the various transmission routes and differences in the antecedent immunocompetence of the various groups.

Incidence

An acute clinical illness associated with seroconversion for HIV-1 has been reported in 53% to 93% of cases.[36,77,108] Although asymptomatic seroconversion does occur, a high index of clinical suspicion and prior experience with primary HIV-1 infection greatly increase the recognition rate.

Incubation Period and Duration

The time from exposure to HIV-1 until the onset of the acute clinical illness is typically 2 to 4 weeks,[24,30,36,84,112] although longer incubation periods have been reported.

The clinical illness is acute in onset[14,36,47,54,112] and lasts from 1 to 2 weeks.[14,30,47,54,99,112] It can be associated with an appreciable degree of morbidity, and patients may require hospitalization.[24,36,44,112] Most of the clinical manifestations of primary HIV-1 infection are self-limited and do not recur after resolution.

CLINICAL PRESENTATION

The main clinical features of primary HIV-1 infection reflect both the lymphocytopathic and neurologic tropism of HIV-1 (Table 5–1). Patients typically present with an illness of acute onset characterized by fever, lethargy, malaise, myalgias, headaches, retro-orbital pain, photophobia, sore throat, lymphadenopathy, and a maculopapular rash. Meningoencephalitis may also occur.

General Features

Fever is a consistent sign in patients with symptomatic primary HIV-1 infection and may or may not be associated with night sweats. Myalgia is also common[8,19,24,30,44,47,54,99] and may be associated with muscle weakness and an increased level of serum creatine kinase. Arthralgia may also occur.[24,47,54,99,102]

Lethargy and malaise are frequent, often severe, and may persist for several months after resolution of the other clinical manifestations of primary HIV-1 infection.[10,24,102]

Lymphocytopathic Features

Lymphadenopathy develops in approximately 70% of persons, generally in the second week of the illness and usually concomitant with the development of peripheral lymphocytosis.[108] The lymphadenopathy may be generalized,[99,102] but the axillary, occipital, and cervical nodes are most commonly involved.[14,19,24,54,102] The lymph node enlargement persists after the acute illness[24,30] but tends to decrease with time.

Table 5–1.   Clinical Manifestations of Primary HIV-1 Infection

General	Dermatologic
Fever	Erythematous maculopapular rash
Pharyngitis	Roseola-like rash
Lymphadenopathy	Diffuse urticaria
Arthralgia	Desquamation
Myalgia	Alopecia
Lethargy/malaise	Mucocutaneous ulceration
Anorexia/weight loss	**Gastrointestinal**
Neuropathic	Oral/oropharyngeal candidiasis
Headache/retro-orbital pain	Nausea/vomiting
Meningoencephalitis	Diarrhea
Peripheral neuropathy	
Radiculopathy	
Brachial neuritis	
Guillain-Barré syndrome	
Cognitive/affective impairment	

Splenomegaly has also been reported.[18,24,39,82,84,85,96,99,120] The mechanism for this splenomegaly is not apparent; it may be related to increased clearance of virally infected lymphocytes.

Dermatologic Features

The most frequently reported dermatologic evidence of primary HIV-1 infection is an erythematous, nonpruritic, maculopapular rash (color plate IA).[6,8,10,14,16,27,39,47,49,54,70,83,84,95,99] This rash is generally symmetric, with lesions 5 to 10 mm in diameter, and affects the face or trunk, but it can also affect the extremities, including the palms and soles,[14,30] or can be generalized.

Other skin lesions noted during primary HIV-1 infection include a roseola-like rash,[76] diffuse urticaria,[47] a vesicular, pustular exanthem and enanthem,[16] desquamation of the palms and soles,[27,71] and alopecia.[19,54]

Mucocutaneous Ulceration

Mucocutaneous ulceration is a distinctive feature of primary HIV-1 infection. Ulcers have been reported on the buccal mucosa, gingiva, or palate,[10,24,31,39,49,70,84,120] esophagus,[39,49,54,84] anus,[39] and penis.[10,39,49] They are generally round or oval and sharply demarcated, with surrounding mucosa that appears normal.

In one series seven (35%) of 20 subjects had mucocutaneous ulceration at the time of presentation, and a further five presented with retrosternal pain on swallowing that probably was caused by esophageal ulceration.[39] Rabeneck et al.[84] reported on a series of 16 homosexual men who presented with odynophagia during primary HIV-1 infection and in whom endoscopy demonstrated esophageal ulcers. Electron microscopy revealed viral particles that morphologically resembled human retroviruses in specimens of ulcer tissue obtained from eight patients, and HIV-1 was isolated from ulcer tissue in one patient.

Neurologic Features

The isolation of HIV-1 from cerebrospinal fluid (CSF) during primary HIV-1 infection[31,96] indicates that infection of the central nervous system (CNS) occurs soon after exposure (see Chapter 13). Elevated neopterin and β_2-microglobulin levels have also been found in CSF during primary HIV-1 infection, both in individuals with and without clinical meningitis,[101] suggesting that the cellular immune system in the CNS may be activated during this stage even without the development of overt neurologic symptoms or signs.

The most common neurologic symptoms are headaches,[8,18,19,24,44,84] retro-orbital pain (particularly during eye movement),[84] and photophobia.[47,84] Several cases of aseptic meningoencephalitis during primary HIV-1 infection have been reported.[10,17,44,46,47] Depression, irritability, and mood changes[17,108] suggest that early CNS involvement may also manifest as cognitive or affective impairment.

Other neurologic conditions that may be associated with primary HIV-1 infection include myelopathy,[31] peripheral neuropathy,[82] meningoradiculitis,[74] brachial neuritis,[15,16] facial palsy,[71,82,120] and Guillain-Barré syndrome.[43] The neurologic manifestations of primary HIV-1 infection are generally self-limited, but persistent neurologic deficit has been reported.[16]

Gastrointestinal Features

Sore throat and pharyngeal edema are common during primary HIV-1 infection.[10,14,24,112] Anorexia, nausea, vomiting, and diarrhea have also been reported.[10,19,24,30,99] Oral candidiasis may occur during primary HIV-1 infection, and several cases of esophageal candidiasis have also been reported.[26,76,83,111] In each of these cases of esophageal candidiasis there was an appreciable decline in the absolute number of peripheral CD4+ cells, reflecting that the development of this AIDS-defining condition occurred in the setting of transient but severe immunodeficiency.[111]

Respiratory Features

Respiratory presentations are not common, although some patients may have a dry cough. Several cases of acute pneumonitis with bilateral diffuse interstitial abnormalities revealed by chest roentgenogram and nonspecific inflammation revealed by fiberoptic bronchoscopy have been reported.[18,19]

Primary HIV-2 Infection

Two cases of symptomatic primary HIV-2 infection have been reported. In the first case a 19-year-old woman developed an acute clinical illness 3 weeks after her first sexual relationship (with an African man of unknown HIV-1 and HIV-2 antibody status).[9] The illness was characterized by painful cervical nodes, shivering, intense fatigue, and a maculopapular rash on the face and thorax. The illness resolved within a few days. A serum sample obtained 26 days after the presumed infection was negative for antibodies to HIV-2, but samples obtained 69, 84, 118, and 150 days after the presumed infection were positive for antibodies to HIV-2. In the second case a 50-year-old French male resident of the Ivory Coast presented with polyneuritis in association with seroconversion to HIV-2.[91]

LABORATORY FINDINGS

Hematology

After an initial and transient lymphopenia, lymphocytosis comprised mainly of CD8 + lymphocytes develops (generally in the second to third weeks of infection). The appearance of atypical lymphocytes concomitant with this CD8 + lymphocytosis has been noted in several case reports.[61,102] However, in a series of 20 patients with primary HIV-1 infection, atypical lymphocytes were detected in less than 50% of them.[39]

Mild thrombocytopenia is a common finding in the first 2 weeks of illness,[16,18,19,27,31,39,47,76,112,120] but there are no reports showing it is of clinical significance. Antiplatelet antibodies and reduced numbers of megakaryocytes on bone marrow examination have been demonstrated during primary HIV-1 infection,[61] suggesting that several viral-mediated or immune-mediated mechanisms are responsible for the thrombocytopenia. The presence of other autoantibodies have not been documented during primary HIV-1 infection.

The erythrocyte sedimentation rate (ESR) may be increased.[16,19,39,47] No characteristic alterations in hemoglobin levels have been reported.

The proportion of banded neutrophils increases during the first week of illness, and segmented neutrophils decrease during the third and fourth weeks of illness.[39] C-reactive protein is raised in approximately 50% of patients.[39]

Liver Function Tests

Elevated serum levels of alkaline phosphatase and aspartate transaminase have been noted[10,16,17,31,39,82,85,102] but are infrequently associated with clinical hepatitis.[99]

T-Lymphocyte Subset Enumeration

Primary HIV-1 infection is characterized by rapid changes in peripheral T-cell subsets[29,41,75,92]; therefore the values obtained at enumeration depend on the time after infection.

During the first 1 to 2 weeks after onset of primary HIV-1 infection there characteristically is lymphopenia that affects both CD4 + and CD8 + subsets. It may be profound, and the level of CD4 + cells may be as low as that of patients with advanced HIV-1 disease. This transient lymphopenia is followed 3 to 4 weeks after infection by peripheral lymphocytosis. Although both CD4 + and CD8 + cells contribute to this lymphocytosis, the increase in CD8 + cells is relatively greater, leading to an inversion of the CD4 + :CD8 + ratio. The level of CD8 + cells typically remains higher than that of the CD4 + cells, and there is sustained inversion of the CD4 + :CD8 + ratio.

Roos et al.[92] recently have found that the most marked increase in the absolute number of CD8 + lymphocytes (and activated CD8 + lymphocytes) was observed in individuals with the most pronounced clinical signs of primary HIV-1 infection.

Immune Function Studies

Severe lymphocytic hyporesponsiveness to both mitogens and antigens occurs during primary HIV-1 infection[29,75] and persists after resolution of the acute illness. Rapid and persistent impairment of B-cell function follows primary HIV-1 infection.[104,105] Terpstra et al.[105] found that inducible in vitro B-cell activity is impaired soon after seroconversion and remains impaired throughout the first year of infection. Teeuwsen et al.[104] found that there is impairment of mitogen and antigen responses in the 3 months after seroconversion.

Antibodies to Structural Proteins

Primary HIV-1 infection is confirmed serologically by the appearance of HIV-specific serum antibodies (see Chapter 3). The HIV-1 provirus codes for several major structural proteins, including *gag* (p55, p24, p18), *pol* (p68, p53, p34), and *env* (gp160, gp120, gp41). The rapid and early diagnosis of primary HIV-1 infection has been aided by the characterization of the timing and order in which antibodies to these proteins appear and the development of specific and sensitive tests for their detection.

In persons with symptomatic primary HIV-1 infection, specific HIV-1 antibodies are usually detectable within the first few weeks of onset of the acute illness.[28,40] Antibodies are generally detected first by immunofluorescent assay (IFA) or enzyme-linked immunosorbent assay (ELISA) for IgM antibody. IgG antibody is then detected, usually 2 to 6 weeks after the onset of illness.[28,40] Differences in the length of the window period according to the type of the ELISA screening tests emphasize the need for consistent use of sensitive screening tests. Immunoblotting usually first shows antibody to p24 or gp41.[28,40] Gaines et al.[40] found that all serum samples obtained 2 weeks or more after onset of symptomatic primary HIV-1 infection in 20 patients were seropositive by immunoblotting.

Antibodies to Regulatory Proteins

The HIV-1 provirus also codes for several proteins that control the expression of HIV-1 itself. Although these proteins are not used for routine diagnostic tests, they provide further information about the window period of HIV-1 seroconversion. The *nef* protein is involved in the down-regulation of viral expression and may participate in the establishment and maintenance of viral latency. Anti-*nef* antibodies are elicited early in infection, generally concomitant with, but in some cases before, *gag* and *env* seroconversion.[5,22,32,89] Antibodies to *tat* (a protein that accelerates the production of HIV), *rev* (a protein that positively regulates HIV-1 replication), and *vpu* and *vpr* (precise function not known) have also been found in a small proportion of cases up to 6 months before *gag* and *env* seroconversion.[88,90]

The significance of the presence of antibodies to regulatory proteins months before *gag* and *env* seroconversion is not clear. The demonstration of anti-*nef* antibodies in HIV-1 seronegative patients without risk factors for HIV-1 infection[86] suggests that there may be an immunologic cross-reaction between *nef* and some cellular protein.

IgM Antibody

The detection of HIV-specific IgM antibodies is a sign of recent infection. IgM antibodies to HIV-1 appear within 2 weeks of infection, precede the IgG response, reach peak titers at 2 to 5 weeks, and then decline to undetectable levels within approximately 3 months.[28,38,40] The first IgM antibodies to appear are directed against *gag* or *env* proteins.[38] However, IgM antibody is not always detected within the first few weeks of infection, and a negative result therefore is not conclusive.[57] Further, technical difficulties with IgM assays, including lack of specificity, reproducibility, and standardization, indicate a need for care in the interpretation of IgM results.

Seronegative HIV-1 Infection

Much controversy has surrounded the occurrence and prevalence of "silent" HIV-1 infection among persons who test negative for HIV-1–specific serum antibodies. The potential for silent HIV-1 infection has profound implications for the public health and also for understanding of HIV-1 immunopathogenesis.

Ranki et al.[87] first reported the detection of low titer antibodies to recombinant structural or accessory proteins or free HIV-1 antigen in serum from homosexual men 6 to 14 months before ELISA seroconversion. A subsequent study found an appreciable rate of HIV-1 isolation from homosexual men who remained seronegative for a long period.[50] However, results from other cohort studies did not support these findings,[48,60] and it was suggested that the use of relatively insensitive ELISAs in the first studies may have been responsible for misclassification of patients as HIV-1 seronegative in at least some instances.[97]

Several investigators have examined the prevalence of silent infection in high-risk seronegative persons further by using the polymerase chain reaction (PCR) method, viral isolation, and in situ hybridization. The results of these studies have been conflicting. Some have demonstrated an appreciable prevalence of seronegative infection,[25,35,50,59,63,80,81,121,122] whereas others have found no such evidence.[3,52,58-60,67]

It has been suggested that in some studies intermittent positive and low-intensity PCR readouts may be false-positive findings.[119] Sheppard et al.[98] have reported that a major weakness of many studies is that they fail to report the rate of positive PCR results in low-risk individuals. They found an identical frequency and distribution of equivocal PCR reactions in homosexual men who had been at risk for HIV-1 infection and in heterosexual men with presumed low levels of risk. Of all samples, 8.6% showed weak PCR reactivity with one or more primer sets; but all samples were negative with at least one primer, and no sample was conclusively positive. Their findings suggested that latent HIV-1 infection in seronegative homosexual men, if it occurred at all, was a rare phenomenon.

Of those studies that have reported patients with seronegative infection, none has determined the infectious potential of such patients. In our experience testing of the index cases from whom patients have acquired primary HIV-1 infection has always revealed positive ELISA and Western blot HIV serology. However, transmission of HIV-1 from infected persons who are themselves in the process of seroconverting has been reported,[21,118] emphasizing that a negative serologic result must always be interpreted in the context of the clinical presentation and the case history.

p24 Antigen

p24 antigen can be detected in serum and CSF in the period before *gag* and *env* seroconversion[4,16,37,51,54,67,103,115] and has been detected in serum as early as 24 hours after the onset of acute illness.[54,114] In one series antigen was detected in all of 13 patients for whom serum samples were available during the first 18 days after the onset of illness.[114]

The level of serum p24 antigen typically decreases as immune complexes develop,[99,114] and the level of serum HIV-1 antibodies increases.[42,51,54,114] Persistent antigenemia or the reappearance of antigenemia at a later time is associated with an increased risk for the development of severe HIV-1 disease.[33,78]

The isolation of HIV-1 from a range of host cells and tissues during primary HIV-1 infection indicates that the antigenemia of the acute period reflects a true viremia and that patients are potentially highly infectious during the period of primary HIV-1 infection.

Viral Isolation

HIV-1 has been isolated from peripheral blood mononuclear cells (PBMCs),[2,40,47,51,84,96] cellfree plasma,[2,37,40] CSF,[31,96] bone marrow cells,[96] and seminal fluid (B. Tindall, unpublished data) during primary HIV-1 infection.

Histopathology

Histopathologic examination of lymph nodes or skin may be required in some cases of primary HIV-1 infection.

Lymph node biopsies typically show a reduction of extrafollicular B cells, CD8 + cell follicular infiltration, and only little activation and proliferation of the germinal center cells.[99] The *env* proteins gp120 and gp160 have been found in interfollicular and follicular lymphocytes, endothelial cells, and interdigitating and dendritic reticulum cells.[99] The relative normality of the structure of the germinal centers during primary HIV-1 infection contrasts with the follicular hyperplasia associated with established HIV-1 infection.

Immunohistologic features of the typical erythematous rash generally reveal a normal epidermis and a sparse dermal, mainly perivascular, lymphocytic, and his-tiocytic infiltrate around vessels of the superficial plexus.[8,14,70] One report noted the infiltrate around the superficial vessels was composed of predominantly CD4+ cells and p24 antigen was detected in occasional cells (possibly Langerhans' cells) of the infiltrate.[70] These findings suggest that the rash of primary HIV-1 infection may be caused by a T-cell–mediated immunoreaction, possibly against Langerhans' cells.

DIFFERENTIAL DIAGNOSIS

Although originally described as "mononucleosis-like"[27] and still described as such in the Centers for Disease (CDC) classification system of HIV-1 disease,[20] symptomatic primary HIV-1 infection is a distinct and recognizable clinical syn-drome.

The diagnosis of primary HIV-1 infection should be considered in any person with known possible recent exposure to HIV-1 and who has a febrile illness of acute onset (Table 5–2). The major symptoms and signs that strengthen this di-agnosis include mucocutaneous ulceration, maculopapular rash, lymphadenopathy, and pharyngitis.

The skin rash associated with primary HIV-1 infection is a valuable diagnostic aid. Skin eruptions are rare in patients with Epstein-Barr virus (EBV) infection (unless antibiotics have been given), toxoplasmosis, and cytomegalovirus (CMV) infection and do not affect the palms and soles in patients with rubella. The rash of pityriasis rosea is typically scaly and may be pruritic; both these features are not found in the rash of a patient with primary HIV-1 infection. Further, constitutional symptoms are generally mild or absent in persons with pityriasis rosea. Histolog-ically, epidermal changes are absent with primary HIV-1 infection, excluding pit-yriasis rosea as the diagnosis. Mucocutaneous ulceration is a fairly distinctive finding because it is unusual in most of the other differential diagnoses.

The major differences between primary HIV-1 infection and EBV mononucleosis have been detailed by Gaines et al.[39] and are summarized in Table 5–3. Although serologic testing for HIV-1 and EBV usually provides the definitive diagnosis, clinicians should be aware that false-positive tests for heterophil antibodies may

Table 5–2.   Major Differential Diagnoses

Primary HIV-1 infection
Epstein-Barr virus mononucleosis
Cytomegalovirus mononucleosis
Toxoplasmosis
Rubella
Viral hepatitis
Secondary syphilis
Disseminated gonococcal infection
Primary herpes simplex virus infection
Other viral infection
Drug reaction

Table 5–3. Clinical Factors Differentiating Epstein-Barr Virus (EBV) Mononucleosis From Primary HIV-1 Infection

PRIMARY HIV-1 INFECTION	EBV MONONUCLEOSIS
Acute onset	Insidious onset
Little or no tonsillar hypertrophy	Marked tonsillar hypertrophy
Enanthema on hard palate	Enanthema on border of both hard and soft palates
Exudative pharyngitis uncommon	Exudative pharyngitis common
Mucocutaneous ulcers common	No mucocutaneous ulcers
Rash common	Rash rare
Jaundice rare	Jaundice (8%)
Diarrhea possible	No diarrhea

From Gaines H, von Sydow M, Pehrson PO, Lundbergh P: Br Med J 297:1363-1368, 1988.

occur during primary HIV-1 infection. Because HIV-1 remains predominantly a sexually transmitted disease (STD) and because the incubation period of primary HIV-1 infection is comparable to that of most common STDs, primary care physicians managing other STDs should be particularly alert to its clinical manifestations and include them in their differential diagnosis.

PROGNOSIS

After resolution of the acute clinical illness, most patients enter a stage of asymptomatic infection that lasts from many months to years. The development of severe HIV-1–related disease within the first 2 years after infection is unusual, although such cases have been reported.[51]

Other viral models have shown that the nature of the acute clinical response may have a role in subsequent disease progression. For example, in hepatitis B virus infection the person with sudden onset and deep jaundice usually recovers completely, and survivors of fulminant viral hepatitis rarely develop progressive disease. In such patients the severe acute clinical illness reflects an effective cytotoxic immunologic response.

Pedersen et al.[77] found that the 3-year progression rate to CDC group IV HIV-1 disease was eight times higher among patients who had a primary illness lasting longer than 14 days than in those with illnesses of shorter duration. Further, each of six patients who developed AIDS during this period had long-lasting illnesses. The 3-year progression rates to CD4+ cell counts of $<500 \times 10^6/L$ and to recurrence of HIV-1 antigenemia were also significantly higher for those patients who had long-lasting primary HIV-1 infection. These findings suggest that a severe primary illness could be related to an early and extensive spread of HIV-1 caused by a defective host immune response that could, in turn, adversely influence long-term prognosis.[77] Anecdotal case reports of fatal primary HIV-1 infection in immunosuppressed persons[7,96] and of rapid progression to AIDS in a person treated with prednisolone[79] support this notion.

In a further study it was found that persons with low p24 antibody titers and high gp120 antibody titers at seroconversion developed severe HIV-1 disease more rapidly than did those with high p24 and low gp120 antibody titers and were more likely to have developed p24 antigenemia.[23] Possibly higher quantities of infecting virus may lead to more rapid progression of disease and suppress production of p24 antibody by interfering with the cooperation of T cells with B cells to produce antibodies.[72]

Although these studies require validation, they suggest that there may be subgroups of patients who should be monitored more intensively and targeted for early intervention.

PREDISPOSING FACTORS

The factors that determine whether an infected person develops symptomatic primary HIV-1 infection or the severity of his or her clinical response, have not been elucidated fully. However, several factors seem, at least theoretically, plausible.

Susceptibility

HIV-1 itself may be an opportunistic infection in an immunocompromised host. In a group of persons with hemophilia, HIV-1 seroconversion after administration of HIV-infected factor VIII preparation was more likely in those who had a pre-existing low CD4 + cell count or CD4 + :CD8 + ratio.[65] However, in a large group of homosexual men no difference was found between the antecedent T-cell profiles of 45 seroconverters and 90 matched seronegative controls.[108] A further study supported these findings but found that anergy to dinitrochlorobenzene (DNCB), a novel antigen, was predictive of subsequent seroconversion and suggested that individuals who could not mount an adequate primary immune response to DNCB (or other novel antigens) were at increased risk of HIV-1 seroconversion.[66] In contrast, anergy to three recall antigens was not predictive of seroconversion.

Source of Infection

There is limited evidence that persons who acquire HIV-1 infection from an index case who has late stage HIV-1 disease may have a higher incidence of symptomatic primary HIV-1 infection than those who acquire infection from an index case who is at an earlier stage of infection. Ward et al.[117] found that symptomatic primary HIV-1 infection was more frequent in 31 patients who were infected by donors in whom AIDS developed within 29 months from the date of donation than in 31 subjects who were infected by donors who developed AIDS more than 29 months after donation (58% versus 23%). Individuals from the first group were also more likely to have developed AIDS 4 years after infection (49% versus 4%). Similarly, van Griensven et al.[113] have reported that history of sex with someone with AIDS is a risk factor for accelerated development of severe disease.

Although these studies have not been substantiated, they suggest that either the nature of the virus in persons with late-stage disease or the viral load from such persons may affect the expression of primary HIV-1 infection in the recipient. Ho, Moudgill, and Alam[45] have shown that titers of infectious virus are increased in persons with AIDS and infection from such persons with advanced disease may therefore contain a larger viral inoculum. Tersmette et al.[106,107] have shown that persons with severe HIV-1 disease have high replicating and syncytium-inducing (SI) HIV-1 variants, which apparently are more virulent in vitro. Roos et al.[92] recently examined the virus phenotype in 19 patients with primary HIV-1 infection who were reviewed for 1 year after infection. They found that the number of CD4 + cells remained relatively stable in 15 of 16 patients with primary HIV-1 infection who were infected with non–syncytium-inducing (NSI) variants but declined rapidly in each of three individuals infected with SI variants (one of whom was treated with zidovudine during primary HIV-1 infection).

Concurrent Viral Infections

The host's clinical and immunologic response to primary HIV-1 infection may, in theory, be influenced by concurrent infection with other potentially immuno-depressive viruses. If so, this may be particularly relevant in groups of persons such as homosexual men and blood component recipients with a high prevalence of infection with such viruses, including EBV and CMV.

Coinfection of T-cell or monocyte cell lines with CMV and HIV-1 has resulted in enhanced in vitro replication of HIV-1 as measured in a virus-yield assay or by radioimmunoassay for p24 antigen.[100] Further, on the molecular level products of genes of CMV and other herpesviruses are able to transactivate the long terminal repeat of HIV-1 in the presence of the *tat* gene.[73]

There are few clinical data on these factors. Three cases of simultaneous infection with CMV and HIV-1 have been reported. In two of them the severity of the acute clinical illness was reported as more severe and of greater duration than that which the authors had generally encountered in either infection alone.[12] In the third case p24 antigenemia and low absolute numbers of CD4 + cells developed within 18 months of primary HIV-1 infection, suggesting that simultaneous primary infection with CMV may have accelerated expression of HIV-1.[85]

PATHOGENESIS
Viral Burden During Primary HIV-1 Infection

The heterogeneous and widespread clinical manifestations of primary HIV-1 infection apparently are based on an immunologic response to rapid and widespread dissemination of HIV-1 after infection.

Several recent reports have attempted to quantitate the viral burden during primary HIV-1 infection. Clark et al.[24] found high titers of infectious HIV-1 (from 10 to 10^3 tissue-culture–infective doses [TCID] per milliliter of plasma) in three patients 6 to 15 days after onset of symptomatic primary HIV-1 infection. These titers fell by day 27, and this fall was associated with an improvement in clinical symptoms and an increase in levels of anti–HIV-1 antibodies. Sequential isolates of virus from plasma and PBMC obtained throughout the period of primary HIV-1 infection and virus derived from two molecular proviral clones were highly cytopathic for normal-donor PBMC and immortalized T cells. These high levels of infectious HIV-1 in plasma and PBMC were also reported in four other patients by Daar et al.[30]

It is not yet clear whether a clinical illness is necessarily related to a greater viral burden (or antigenemia). Lindhardt et al.[62] found that p24 antigenemia was significantly more common in seroconverters with symptomatic primary HIV-1 infection than in those who seroconverted asymptomatically (56% versus 19%). However, patients who were p24 antigenemic may have been more severely ill and therefore more likely to present clinically. Pedersen et al.[77] found no significant difference in the proportion of patients with a long-lasting illness and those without a long-lasting illness who were p24 antigenemic (50% and 41%, respectively).

Cytokines

Increased levels of interferon-α (IFN-α), tumor necrosis factor-α (TNF-α) neopterin, and β_2 microglobulin have been detected in blood and CSF during primary HIV-1 infection,[41,68,101,115] reflecting activation of the cellular immune system. High circulating levels of these cytokines are also presumably responsible for the pathogenesis of some of the major clinical manifestations of primary HIV-1 infection (e.g., the symptoms of primary HIV-1 infection such as fevers, chills, myalgia, headache, fatigue, leukopenia, and weight loss are very similar to those found in people receiving exogenous IFN-α).

The order of appearance of these markers in relation to HIV-1 seroconversion in humans remains unclear.

CONTROL OF VIREMIA

After HIV-1 infection there is a short and intense period of viral replication,[24,30] followed in the ensuing weeks by a rapid decline in viral load and resolution of the acute illness. This viral clearance might be due either to a progressive lack of susceptible target cells or, more likely, to the emergence of an effective host mechanism for viral clearance. The mechanisms of viral clearance during primary HIV-1 infection are not fully delineated, but humoral, cellular, and cytokine responses all apparently play a role.

Humoral Immune Responses

HIV-1 immune complexes appear in the blood during the period of declining concentrations of free antigen and increasing concentrations of IgM and IgG antibodies.[114] They can be detected before overt seroconversion.[56]

Neutralizing antibodies may also contribute to viral clearance. Albert et al.[1] found that isolate-specific neutralizing antibodies develop rapidly after primary HIV-1 infection. They also identified the subsequent emergence of viral variants with reduced sensitivity to neutralization by autologous but not heterologous sera. The emergence of such viral variants that the person fails to neutralize could contribute to disease progression. Boucher et al.[13] found that 17 (23%) of 75 men with *gag* and *env* seroconversion concomitantly developed antibodies to a synthetic peptide covering a lymphadenopathy-associated virus type 1 (LAV-1)/human T lymphotropic virus type IIIB (HTLV-IIIB) neutralization epitope. The temporal association indicates that these neutralizing antibodies are stimulated by either the inoculating strain or an early variant.

Antibodies that inhibit syncytium formation and antibodies that mediate antibody-dependent cellular cytotoxicity (ADCC) against virally infected target cells also develop soon after seroconversion.[11]

Cellular Immune Responses

CD8+ lymphocytosis has been reported in patients with primary HIV-1 infection,[27,29,41,75] generally beginning in the second week after onset of illness. CD8+ lymphocytosis is also characteristic of other primary viral infections and controls these infections through cytotoxic or suppressor mechanisms.

We have previously shown that the increase in the number of CD8+ cells during primary HIV-1 infection occurs concomitant with resolution of clinical symptoms and a decrease in the detectable levels of serum p24 antigen,[29] suggesting that the CD8+ cell response to primary HIV-1 infection has a role in controlling viral replication in vivo as it has been shown to have in vitro.[116]

Recently Roos et al.[92] reported that activated CD8+ cells were found in all patients with primary HIV-1 infection but were only transiently elevated in those patients with infection with SI variants of HIV. They hypothesised that, after primary HIV-1 infection, SI variants may be selectively cleared by the host immune response and that the isolation of SI variants from these patients may reflect the failure of the CD8+ response to clear the SI variants.

Cytokine Response

Primary HIV-1 infection is associated with an early, transient rise in IFN-α and TNF-α in some individuals. Von Sydow et al.[115] found that the IFN-α response was sufficiently high to induce suppression of HIV-1 replication. In accordance with this discovery, they found that p24 antigen concentrations rapidly declined to undetectable levels following the peak of the IFN-α response. They found the IFN-α response before the development of HIV-specific antibodies and before the rise in CD8+ cells, suggesting that it is a first line of defense against HIV-1 infection.

MANAGEMENT

The mainstays of treatment of primary HIV-1 infection are early recognition and symptomatic treatment. Recognition and early diagnosis of HIV-1 infection are important in order to institute appropriate counseling and prevent further spread of the virus. Moreover, early diagnosis obviates the need for further investigations or empiric therapy, which may not be appropriate. This is especially important in those cases in whom neurologic signs are present. Although not yet proved, it is possible that antiretroviral intervention during primary HIV-1 infection could prevent persistent HIV-1 infection or lessen the initial viral load and subsequently improve long-term prognosis.

Zidovudine

In some animal retroviral models zidovudine has prevented persistent infection or significantly altered disease progression if it was given soon after inoculation.[69,93,94] Although these studies suggest that zidovudine may have some role in the postexposure prophylaxis of retroviruses, including HIV-1, their direct applicability to humans is tenuous. However, based on these animal studies, zidovudine has been used by several investigators in the postexposure prophylaxis of HIV-1 in humans. In the absence of a controlled clinical trial format, it is not possible to evaluate the efficacy of the use of zidovudine in these studies. However, cases have been reported in which zidovudine clearly failed to prevent persistent HIV-1 infection when administration was begun 45 minutes to 6 hours after inoculation (see Chapter 4).[53,55,64]

If zidovudine is to have any role in the postexposure prophylaxis of HIV-1 infection, it would probably be most efficacious if it were administered during the initial replicative cycle. By the time symptomatic primary HIV-1 infection develops, widespread viral dissemination has already occurred, and it seems unlikely that treatment at this stage would prevent the establishment of persistent HIV-1 infection.

So far only one report has discussed the effect of treatment with zidovudine during symptomatic primary HIV-1 infection. In a joint Australian-Swedish study 11 patients with symptomatic primary HIV-1 infection were treated with 1 g of zidovudine daily for a median period of 56 days.[110] Compared with a group of historical controls, no clear evidence of any clinical benefit in terms of resolution of the clinical illness and no indication that the intervention would prevent development of persistent infection emerged. These patients are being monitored to determine long-term outcome. In addition to this seminal study, an international collaborative, double-blind, placebo-controlled clinical trial is presently in progress to examine the efficacy of zidovudine in the treatment of primary HIV-1 infection.

Other Potential Agents

Several other drugs, including nucleoside analogs, are being developed and tested in clinical trials for the treatment of established HIV infection, including didanosine (ddI) and zalcitabine (ddC). Some of them may be tested for the treatment of primary HIV-1 infection, either as sole agents or in combination, in the future.

Counseling

A diagnosis of HIV infection can be associated with profound psychosocial consequences. Specific factors that must be considered in counseling persons with primary HIV-1 infection include the acute physical distress that many persons experience, the tentative nature of the diagnosis before seroconversion occurs, self-reproach resulting from recent risk behavior, and the potential development of mood disorders during primary HIV-1 infection.[17,108]

The identification of a patient with primary HIV-1 infection necessarily implies the existence of a source case of infection. When possible, contact tracing should be implemented to identify this source case. If he or she is identified, counseling for the source person is also indicated. Such persons may be unaware of their infection, may be in the process of seroconverting themselves, or may be unaware of what constitutes safe sex or safe injecting practices. Counseling of such patients also must address their emotional reactions to having infected another individual.

Prevention

Prevention of primary HIV-1 infection remains the only proved intervention strategy. Most cases of primary HIV-1 infection occur as the result of intimate, consensual human activity, and spread of HIV-1 through these modes is totally preventable. The significant changes in sexual practices among homosexual men in urban areas demonstrate that sustained behavior change can be achieved.

REFERENCES

1. Albert J, Abrahamsson B, Nagy K, et al: Rapid development of isolate-specific neutralizing antibodies after primary HIV-1 infection and consequent emergence of virus variants which resist neutralization by autologous sera. AIDS 4:107-112, 1990
2. Albert J, Gaines H, Sonnerborg A, et al: Isolation of human immunodeficiency virus (HIV) from plasma during primary HIV infection. J Med Virol 23:67-73, 1987
3. Albert J, Pehrson PO, Schulman S, et al: HIV isolation and antigen detection in infected individuals and their seronegative sexual partners. AIDS 2:107-111, 1988
4. Allain J-P, Laurian Y, Paul DA, et al: Serological markers in early stages of human immunodeficiency virus infection in haemophiliacs. Lancet 2:1233-1236, 1986
5. Ameisen J-C, Guy B, Chamaret S, et al: Antibodies to the *nef* protein and to *nef* peptides in HIV-1–infected seronegative individuals. AIDS Res Hum Retroviruses 5:279-291, 1989
6. Anonymous: Needlestick transmission of HTLV-III from a patient infected in Africa. Lancet 2:1376-1377, 1984
7. Apperley JF, Rice SJ, Hewitt P, et al: HIV infection due to a platelet transfusion after allogeneic bone marrow transplantation. Eur J Haematol 39:185-189, 1987
8. Balslev E, Thomsen HK, Weismann K: Histopathology of acute human immunodeficiency virus exanthema. J Clin Pathol 43:201-202, 1990
9. Besnier J-M, Barin F, Baillou A, et al: Symptomatic HIV-2 primary infection. Lancet 335:798, 1990
10. Biggar RJ, Johnson BK, Musoke SS, et al: Severe illness associated with appearance of antibody to human immunodeficiency virus in an African. Br Med J 293:1210-1211, 1986
11. Bolognesi DP: Prospects for prevention of and early intervention against HIV. JAMA 261:3007-3013, 1989
12. Bonnetti A, Weber R, Vogt MW, et al: Co-infection with human immunodeficiency virus-type 1 (HIV-1) and cytomegalovirus in two intravenous drug users. Ann Intern Med 111:293-296, 1989
13. Boucher CAB, de Wolf F, Houweling JTM, et al: Antibody response to a synthetic peptide covering a LAV-1/HTLV-IIIB neutralization epitope and disease progression. AIDS 3:71-76, 1989
14. Brehmer-Andersson E, Torssander J: The exanthema of acute (primary) HIV infection. Identification of a characteristic histopathological picture? Acta Derm Venereol (Stockh) 70:85-87, 1990
15. Brew BJ, Perdices M, Darveniza P, et al: The neurological features of early and "latent" human immunodeficiency virus. Aust N Z J Med 19:700-705, 1989
16. Calabresse LH, Proffitt MR, Levin KH, et al: Acute infection with the human immunodeficiency virus (HIV) associated with acute brachial neuritis and exanthematous rash. Ann Intern Med 107:849-851, 1987

17. Carne CA, Tedder RS, Smith A, et al: Acute encephalopathy coincident with seroconversion for anti-HTLV-III. Lancet 2:1206-1208, 1985
18. Casalino E, Bouvet E, Bedos J-P, et al: Acute HIV seroconversion and pneumonitis. AIDS 5:1143-1144, 1991
19. Case records of the Massachusetts General Hospital. Case 33-1989. N Engl J Med 321:454-463, 1989
20. Centers for Disease Control: CDC classification system for human T-lymphotropic virus type III/lymphadenopathy-associated virus infections. MMWR 35:334-339, 1986
21. Centers for Disease Control: Transfusion associated human T-lymphotropic virus type III/lymphadenopathy associated virus infection from a seronegative donor—Colorado. MMWR 35:389-391, 1986
22. Cheingsong-Popov R, Panagiotidi C, Ali M, et al: Antibodies to HIV-1 *nef*(p27): Prevalence, significance and relationship to seroconversion. AIDS Res Hum Retroviruses 6:1099-1105, 1990
23. Cheingsong-Popov R, Panagiotidi C, Bowcock S, et al: Relation between humoral responses to HIV *gag* and *env* proteins at seroconversion and clinical outcome of HIV infection. Br Med J 302:23-26, 1991
24. Clark SJ, Saag MS, Decker WD, et al: High titers of cytopathic virus in plasma of patients with symptomatic primary HIV-1 infection. N Engl J Med 324:954-960, 1991
25. Clerici M, Berzofsky JA, Shearer GM, Tacket CO: Exposure to human immunodeficiency virus type 1—specific T helper cell responses before detection of infection by polymerase chain reaction and serum antibodies. J Infect Dis 164:178-182, 1991
26. Clotet B, Romeu J, Casals A, et al: Spontaneous resolution of *Candida* esophagitis in a seroconverting patient for HIV antibodies. Am J Gastroenterol 83:1433, 1988
27. Cooper DA, Gold J, Maclean P, et al: Acute AIDS retrovirus infection. Definition of a clinical illness associated with seroconversion. Lancet 1:537-540, 1985
28. Cooper DA, Imrie AA, Penny R: Antibody response to human immunodeficiency virus following primary infection. J Infect Dis 155:1113-1118, 1987
29. Cooper DA, Tindall B, Wilson EJ, et al: Characterization of T lymphocyte responses during primary HIV infection. J Infect Dis 157:889-896, 1988
30. Daar ES, Moudgil T, Meyer RD, Ho DD: Transient high levels of viremia in patients with primary human immunodeficiency virus type 1 infection. N Engl J Med 324:961-964, 1991
31. Denning DW, Anderson J, Rudge P, et al: Acute myelopathy associated with primary infection with human immunodeficiency virus. Br Med J 294:143-144, 1987
32. De Ronde A, Reiss P, Dekker J, et al: Seroconversion to HIV-1 negative regulation factor. Lancet 2:574, 1988
33. de Wolf F, Goudsmit J, Paul DA, et al: Risk of AIDS related complex and AIDS in homosexual men with persistent antigenaemia. Br Med J 295:569-572, 1987
34. de Wolf F, Lange JMA, Bakker M, et al: Influenza-like syndrome in homosexual men: A prospective diagnostic study. J R Coll Gen Pract 38:443-446, 1988
35. Ensoli F, Fiorelli V, Mezzaroma I, et al: Plasma viraemia in seronegative HIV-1–infected individuals. AIDS 5:1195-1199, 1991
36. Fox R, Eldred LJ, Fuchs EJ, et al: Clinical manifestations of acute infection with human immunodeficiency virus in a cohort of gay men. AIDS 1:35-38, 1987
37. Gaines H, Albert J, von Sydow M, et al: HIV antigenaemia and virus isolation from plasma during primary HIV infection. Lancet 1:1317-1318, 1987
38. Gaines H, von Sydow M, Parry JV, et al: Detection of immunoglobulin M antibody in primary human immunodeficiency virus infection. AIDS 2:11-15, 1988
39. Gaines H, von Sydow M, Pehrson PO, Lundbergh P: Clinical picture of primary HIV infection presenting as a glandular-fever-like illness. Br Med J 297:1363-1368, 1988
40. Gaines H, von Sydow M, Sonnerborg A, et al: Antibody response in primary human immunodeficiency virus infection. Lancet 1:1249-1253, 1987
41. Gaines H, von Sydow MAE, von Stedingk LV, et al: Immunological changes in primary HIV infection. AIDS 4:995-999, 1990
42. Goudsmit J, de Wolf F, Paul DA, et al: Expression of human immunodeficiency antigen (HIV-Ag) in serum and cerebrospinal fluid during acute and chronic infection. Lancet 2:177-180, 1986
43. Hagberg L, Malmvall B-E, Svennerholm L, et al: Guillan-Barré syndrome as an early manifestation of HIV central nervous system infection. Scand J Infect Dis 18:591-592, 1986

44. Hardy WD, Daar ES, Sokolov RT Jr, Ho DD: Acute neurologic deterioration in a young man. Rev Infect Dis 13:745-750, 1991

45. Ho D, Moudgil T, Alam M: Quantification of human immunodeficiency virus type 1 in the blood of infected persons. N Engl J Med 321:1621-1625, 1989

46. Ho DD, Rota TR, Schooley RT, et al: Isolation of HTLV-III from cerebrospinal fluid and neural tissues of patients with neurologic syndromes related to the acquired immunodeficiency syndrome. N Engl J Med 313:1493-1497, 1985

47. Ho DD, Sarngadharan MG, Resnick L, et al: Primary human T-lymphoptropic virus type III infection. Ann Intern Med 103:880-883, 1985

48. Horsburgh CR Jr, Ou C-Y, Holmberg SD, et al: Human immunodeficiency virus type 1 infection in homosexual men who remain seronegative for prolonged periods. N Engl J Med 321:1679-1680, 1989

49. Hulsebosch HJ, Claessen FAP, van Ginkel CJW, et al: Human immunodeficiency virus exanthem. J Am Acad Dermatol 23:483-486, 1990

50. Imagawa DT, Lee MH, Wolinsky SM, et al: Human immunodeficiency virus type 1 infection in homosexual men who remain seronegative for prolonged periods. N Engl J Med 320:1458-1462, 1989

51. Isaksson B, Albert J, Chiodi F, et al: AIDS two months after primary human immunodeficiency virus infection. J Infect Dis 158:866-868, 1988

52. Jason J, Ou C-Y, Moore JL, et al: Prevalence of human immunodeficiency virus type 1 in hemophiliac men and their sexual partners. J Infect Dis 160:789-794, 1989

53. Jones PD: HIV transmission by stabbing despite zidovudine prophylaxis. Lancet 338:884, 1991

54. Kessler HA, Blaauw B, Spear J, et al: Diagnosis of human immunodeficiency virus infection in seronegative homosexuals presenting with an acute viral syndrome. JAMA 258:1196-1199, 1987

55. Lange JMA, Boucher CAB, Hollak CEM, et al: Failure of zidovudine prophylaxis after accidental exposure to HIV-1. N Engl J Med 322:1375-1377, 1990

56. Lange JMA, Paul DA, de Wolf F, et al: Viral gene expression, antibody production and immune complex formation in human immunodeficiency virus infection. AIDS 1:15-20, 1987

57. Lange JMA, Parry JV, de Wolf F, et al: Diagnostic value of specific IgM antibodies in primary HIV infection. Br Med J 293:1459-1462, 1986

58. Lee T-H, El-Amad Z, Reis M, et al: Absence of HIV-1 DNA in high-risk seronegative individuals using high-input polymerase chain reaction. AIDS 5:1201-1207, 1991

59. Lefrere JJ, Mariotti M, Courouce A-M, et al: Polymerase chain reaction testing of HIV-1 seronegative at-risk individuals. Lancet 335:1400-1401, 1990

60. Lifson AR, Stanley M, Pane J, et al: Detection of human immunodeficiency virus DNA using the polymerase chain reaction in a well characterized group of homosexual and bisexual men. J Infect Dis 161:436-439, 1990

61. Lima J, Ribera A, Garcia-Bragado F, et al: Antiplatelet antibodies in primary infection by human immunodeficiency virus. Ann Intern Med 106:333, 1987

62. Lindhardt BO, Lauritzen E, Ulrich K, et al: Serological markers of primary HIV infection. Scand J Infect Dis 21:491-496, 1989

63. Loche M, Mach B: Identification of HIV-infected seronegative individuals by a direct diagnostic test based on hybridisation to amplified viral DNA. Lancet 2:418-421, 1988

64. Looke DFM, Grove DI: Failed prophylactic zidovudine after needlestick injury. Lancet 335:1280, 1990

65. Ludlam CA, Tucker J, Steel CM, et al: Human T-lymphotropic virus type III (HTLV-III) infection in seronegative haemophiliacs after transfusion of factor VIII. Lancet 2:233-236, 1985

66. Marion SA, Schechter MT, Weaver MS, et al: Evidence that prior immune dysfunction predisposes to human immunodeficiency virus infection in homosexual men. J Acquir Immune Defic Syndr 2:178-186, 1989

67. Mariotti M, Lefrere J-J, Noel B, et al: DNA amplification of HIV-1 in seropositive individuals and in seronegative at-risk individuals. AIDS 4:633-637, 1990

68. Martin DH, Pearson JE, Kumar P, et al: Sequential measurement of beta-2-microglobulin levels, p24 antigen levels, and antibody titers following transplantation of a human immunodeficiency virus-infected kidney allograft. J Acquir Immune Defic Syndr 4:1118-1121, 1991

69. McCune JM, Namikawa R, Shih C-C, et al: Suppression of HIV infection in AZT-treated SCID-hu mice. Science 247:564-566, 1990

70. McMillan A, Bishop PE, Aw D, Peutherer JF: Immunohistology of the skin rash associated with acute HIV infection. AIDS 3:309-312, 1989

71. Mercey DE, Loveday C, Miller RF: Sclerosing cholangitis rapidly following anti-HIV-1 sero-conversion. Genitourin Med 67:239-243, 1991

72. Mittler R, Hoffman M: Synergism between HIV gp120 and gp120 specific antibody in blocking human T cell activation. Science 245:1380-1382, 1989

73. Mosca JD, Bednarik DP, Raj NBK, et al: Herpes simplex virus type-1 can reactivate transcription of latent human immunodeficiency virus. Nature 325:67-70, 1987

74. Paton P, Poly H, Gonnaud P-M, et al: Acute meningoradiculitis concomitant with seroconversion to human immunodeficiency virus type 1. Res Virol 141:427-433, 1990

75. Pedersen C, Dickmeiss E, Gaub J, et al: T-cell subset alterations and lymphocyte responsiveness to mitogens and antigen during severe primary infection with HIV: A case series of seven consecutive HIV seroconverters. AIDS 4:523-526, 1990

76. Pedersen C, Gerstoft J, Lindhardt BO, Sindrup J: *Candida* esophagitis associated with acute human immunodeficiency virus infection. J Infect Dis 156:529-530, 1987

77. Pedersen C, Lindhardt BO, Jensen BL, et al: Clinical course of primary HIV infection: Consequences for subsequent course of infection. Br Med J 299:154-157, 1989

78. Pedersen C, Nielsen CM, Vestergaard BF, et al: Temporal relation of antigenaemia and loss of antibodies to core antigens to development of clinical disease in HIV infection. Br Med J 295:567-569, 1987

79. Pedersen C, Nielsen JO, Dickmeiss E, Jordal R: Early progression to AIDS following primary HIV infection. AIDS 3:45-47, 1989

80. Pezzella M, Mannella E, Mirolo M, et al: HIV genome in peripheral blood mononuclear cells of seronegative regular sexual partners of HIV-infected subjects. J Med Virol 28:209-214, 1989

81. Pezzella M, Rossi P, Lombardi V, et al: HIV viral sequences in seronegative people at risk detected by in situ hybridisation and polymerase chain reaction. Br Med J 298:713-716, 1989

82. Piette AM, Tusseau F, Vignon D, et al: Acute neuropathy coincident with seroconversion for anti-LAV/HTLV-III. Lancet 1:852, 1986

83. Podzamczer D, Casanova A, Santamaria P, et al: Esophageal candidiasis in the diagnosis of HIV-infected patients. JAMA 259:1328-1329, 1988

84. Rabeneck L, Popovic M, Gartner S, et al: Acute HIV infection presenting with painful swallowing and esophageal ulcers. JAMA 263:2318-2322, 1990

85. Raffi F, Boudart D, Billaudel S: Acute co-infection with human immunodeficiency virus (HIV) and cytomegalovirus. Ann Intern Med 112:234-235, 1990

86. Ranki A, Jarvinen K, Valle S-L, et al: Antibodies to recombinant HIV-1 *nef* protein detected in HIV-1 infection as well as in nonrisk individuals. J Acquir Immune Defic Syndr 3:348-355, 1990

87. Ranki A, Valle S-L, Krohn M, et al: Long latency period precedes overt seroconversion in sexually transmitted human immunodeficiency virus infection. Lancet 2:589-593, 1987

88. Reiss P, de Ronde A, Dekker J, et al: Seroconversion to HIV-1 *rev*- and *tat*-gene-encoded proteins. AIDS 3:105-106, 1989

89. Reiss P, de Ronde A, Lange JMA, et al: Antibody response to the viral negative factor *(nef)* in HIV-1 infection: A correlate of levels of HIV-1 expression. AIDS 3:227-233, 1989.

90. Reiss P, Lange JMA, de Ronde A, et al: Antibody response to viral proteins U *(vpu)* and R *(vpr)* in HIV-1 infected individuals. J Acquir Immune Defic Syndr 3:115-122, 1990

91. Ritter J, Chevallier P, Peyramond D, Sepetjan M: Serological markers during an acute HIV-2 infection. Vox Sanq 59:244-245, 1990

92. Roos MTL, Lange JMA, Goede REY, et al: Virus phenotype and immune response in primary human immunodeficiency virus type 1 (HIV-1) infection. J Infect Dis (in press)

93. Ruprecht RM, Chou T-C, Chipty F, et al: Interferon-alpha and 3'-azido-3'-deoxythymidine are highly synergistic in mice and prevent viremia after acute retrovirus exposure. J Acquir Immune Defic Syndr 3:591-600, 1990

94. Ruprecht RM, O'Brien LG, Rossoni LD, et al: Suppression of mouse viraemia and retroviral disease by 3'-azido-3'-deoxythymidine. Nature 323:467-469, 1986

95. Rustin MHA, Ridely CM, Smith MD, et al: The acute exanthem associated with seroconversion to human T-cell lymphotropic virus III in a homosexual man. J Infect 12:161-163, 1986

96. Ruutu P, Suni J, Oksanen K, Ruutu T: Primary infection with HIV in a severely immunosuppressed patient with acute leukemia. Scand J Infect Dis 19:369-372, 1987

97. Saah AJ: Latency preceding seroconversion in sexually transmitted HIV infection. Lancet 2:1402, 1987

98. Sheppard HW, Dondero D, Aron J, Winkelstein W Jr: An evaluation of the polymerase chain reaction in HIV-1 seronegative men. J Acquir Immune Defic Syndr 4:819-823, 1991
99. Sinicco A, Palestro G, Caramello P, et al: Acute HIV-1 infection: Clinical and biological study of 12 patients. J Acquir Immune Defic Syndr 3:260-265, 1990
100. Skolnik PR, Kosloff BR, Hirsch MS: Bidirectional interaction between human immunodeficiency virus type 1 and cytomegalovirus. J Infect Dis 157:508-514, 1988
101. Sonnerborg AB, von Stedingk L-V, Hansson L-O, Strannegard OO: Elevated neopterin and beta$_2$-microglobulin levels in blood and cerebrospinal fluid occur early in HIV-1 infection. AIDS 3:277-283, 1989
102. Steeper TA, Horwitz CA, Hanson M, et al: Heterophil-negative mononucleosis-like illnesses with atypical lymphocytosis in patients undergoing seroconversions to the human immunodeficiency virus. Am J Clin Pathol 89:169-174, 1988
103. Stramer SL, Heller JS, Coombs RW, et al: Markers of HIV infection prior to IgG antibody seropositivity. JAMA 262:64-69, 1989
104. Teeuwsen VJP, Siebelink KHJ, de Wolf F, et al: Impairment of in vitro immune responses occurs within 3 months after HIV-1 seroconversion. AIDS 4:77-81, 1990
105. Terpstra FG, Al BMJ, Roos MTL, et al: Longitudinal study of leukocyte function in homosexual men seroconverted for HIV: Rapid and persistent loss of B cell function after HIV infection. Eur J Immunol 19:667-673, 1989
106. Tersmette M, Gruters RA, de Wolf F, et al: Evidence for a role of virulent HIV variants in the pathogenesis of AIDS obtained from studies on a panel of sequential HIV isolates. J Virol 63:2118-2125, 1989
107. Tersmette M, Lange JMA, de Goede REY, et al: Association between biological properties of human immunodeficiency virus variants and risk for AIDS and AIDS mortality. Lancet 1:983-985, 1989
108. Tindall B, Barker S, Donovan B, et al: Characterization of the acute clinical illness associated with human immunodeficiency virus infection. Arch Intern Med 148:945-949, 1988
109. Tindall B, Cooper DA: Primary HIV infection. Host responses and intervention strategies. AIDS 5:1-14, 1991
110. Tindall B, Gaines H,, Imrie A, et al: Zidovudine in the management of primary HIV infection. AIDS 5:477-484, 1991
111. Tindall B, Hing M, Edwards P, et al: Severe clinical manifestations of primary HIV infection. AIDS 3:747-749, 1989
112. Valle S-L: Febrile pharyngitis as the primary sign of HIV infection in a cluster of cases linked by sexual contact. Scand J Infect Dis 19:13-17, 1987
113. Van Griensven GJP, de Vroome EMM, de Wolf F, et al: Risk factors for progression of human immunodeficiency virus (HIV) infection among seroconverted and seropositive homosexual men. Am J Epidemiol 132:203-210, 1990
114. von Sydow M, Gaines H, Sonnerborg A, et al: Antigen detection in primary HIV infection. Br Med J 296:238-240, 1988
115. von Sydow M, Sonnerborg A, Gaines H, Strannegard O: Interferon-alpha and tumor necrosis factor in serum of patients in varying stages of HIV-1 infection. AIDS Res Hum Retroviruses 7:375-380, 1991
116. Walker CM, Moody DJ, Stites DP, Levy JA: CD8 + lymphocytes can control infection in vitro by suppressing virus replication. Science 234:1563-1566, 1986
117. Ward JW, Bush TJ, Perkins HA, et al: The natural history of transfusion-associated HIV infection: Factors influencing progression to disease. N Engl J Med 321:947-952, 1989
118. Ward JW, Holmberg SD, Allen JR, et al: Transmission of human immunodeficiency virus (HIV) by blood transfusion screened as negative for HIV antibody. N Engl J Med 318:473-478, 1988
119. Winkelstein W Jr, Royce RA: Median incubation time for human immunodeficiency virus (HIV). Ann Intern Med 112:797, 1990
120. Wiselka MJ, Nicholson KG, Ward SC, Flower AJE: Acute infection with human immunodeficiency virus associated with facial nerve palsy and neuralgia. J Infect 15:189-194, 1987
121. Wolinsky SM, Rinaldo CR, Kwok S, et al: Human immunodeficiency virus type 1 (HIV-1) infection a median of 18 months before a diagnostic Western blot. Evidence from a cohort of homosexual men. Ann Intern Med 111:961-972, 1989
122. Yagi MJ, Joesten ME, Wallace J, et al: Human immunodeficiency virus type 1 (HIV-1) genomic sequences and distinct changes in CD8 + lymphocytes precede detectable levels of HIV-1 antibodies in high-risk individuals. J Infect Dis 164:183-188, 1991

6

NATURAL HISTORY AND MANAGEMENT OF THE SEROPOSITIVE PATIENT

MICHAEL CLEMENT, MD
HARRY HOLLANDER, MD

This chapter provides a basic framework from which the clinician can counsel patients about the natural history of HIV infection, stage the disease, and consider antiretroviral therapy and prophylaxis against opportunistic infections. Early intervention therapy with zidovudine before overt immunosuppression or the onset of opportunistic infections is now the standard of care. But crucial issues remain unresolved. The significance of HIV resistance to zidovudine, the role of combination antiretroviral chemotherapy, the timing of prophylaxis against opportunistic infections, and the most cost effective prophylactic agents are unanswered questions. Important clinical research trials are underway to provide some answers, answers we hope will usher in an era in which HIV will be a chronic treatable infection.

NATURAL HISTORY OF HIV INFECTION

The natural history of HIV infection has been studied in homosexual and bisexual men, intravenous drug users, transfusion recipients, and vertically infected children.[1,6,10,17,21,26,30] The cumulative risks of the development of AIDS in these studies differ. In the San Francisco City Clinic cohort 54% of patients progressed to an AIDS diagnosis 11 years after seroconversion.[26] In transfusion recipients 49% develop AIDS after 7 years,[30] and 25% of hemophiliacs develop AIDS 9 years after seroconversion.[10] In one study of 32 vertically infected children six (20%) died within 18 months after birth.[1] The European Collaborative Study[6] of 600 children born to HIV-infected mothers showed that 13% were vertically infected. AIDS developed in 26% of infected children by one year and 17% had died. The differences in progression rates may reflect variations in inoculum size, immunologic state of the individual, or other as yet unidentified cofactors for progression. However, all these studies suggest a progressively increasing risk with time. Whether or not that risk eventually plateaus is still not known. In the San Francisco City Clinic cohort 341 men were infected from 1977 through 1980; 66 (19%) have no signs or symptoms of HIV, and nine (3%) have asymptomatic generalized lymphadenopathy. At present, we cannot conclude that all HIV-infected persons will inevitably progress to end-stage disease (AIDS) and death.

Multiple possible predictors of HIV disease progression have been studied. The most reliable clinical factors are the development of thrush, persistent fever, unexplained diarrhea, and involuntary weight loss.[14,17,19,23] Oral hairy leukoplakia and cutaneous herpes zoster are also important clues to disease progression.[11,23] The presence of generalized lymphadenopathy has not been independently associated with a more rapid disease progression; however, the rapid involution of previously, persistently enlarged lymph nodes is a poor prognostic sign.[17] Age greater than 35 years is also associated with a worse prognosis.[14]

Laboratory markers for disease progression include anemia, neutropenia, CD4+ cell counts, low CD4+ percent, CD4+ :CD8+ ratios, elevated β_2-microglobulin, elevated serum neopterin levels, and p24 antigenemia.[7-9,14,18,20-24,28,31] The CD4+ cell count (expressed as the absolute number, percent of CD4+, or CD4+ :CD8+ ratio) has emerged as the best laboratory predictor of HIV disease progression (see Chapter 3). A number of recent studies have correlated CD4 count with risk of opportunistic infection and death.

Data from the multicenter AIDS cohort study of 1665 seropositive persons without AIDS at the time of enrollment in the study found the highest risk of progressing to *Pneumocystis carinii* pneumonia (PCP) in patients with a CD4+ cell count <200/mm³. Compared to patients with a CD4+ cell count >200/mm³, the relative risk was 4.9. For those with a CD4+ cell count <200/mm³ the presence of thrush, fever, unintentional weight loss, or persistent fatigue increased the risk of developing PCP.[23]

An Australian study stratified the risk of specific opportunistic infections according to CD4+ cell count. Candidiasis and tuberculosis occurred with CD4+ cell counts of 250 to 500; Kaposi's sarcoma, lymphoma, and cryptosporidiosis, with 150 to 200; PCP, *Mycobacterium avium-intracellulare,* herpes simplex virus, toxoplasmosis, cryptococcosis, and esophageal candidiasis with 75 to 125; and cytomegalovirus retinitis with <50.[5] A study from the National Cancer Institute retrospectively looked at the risk of death as a function of CD4+ cell counts in 55 patients. Of 41 deaths, all but one occurred in patients with CD4+ cell counts less than 50 cells/mm³. The median survival time of patients whose CD4+ count had fallen below 50 cells/mm³ was 1 year.[31]

HIV infection alters the natural history of some common infections, most notably syphilis and hepatitis B. Syphilis is discussed in Chapter 24. HIV-induced suppression of cell-mediated immunity resulted in the development of the chronic carrier state of hepatitis B in 23% of HIV-infected persons compared to 4.3% in non–HIV-infected controls in a study from Australia.[2] Patients with depressed CD4 cell counts were more likely to develop chronic HBV infection and less likely to develop clinical icterus than non–HIV-infected persons.

STAGING OF HIV INFECTION

In the staging of HIV infection, a complete baseline physical examination should be done. Repeated routine physical examinations have proved unhelpful in a variety of medical screening settings. Similarly, it is difficult to justify the time and expense

Table 6–1. Essential Portions of the Follow-up Physical Examination

General
Overall well-being
Weight
Skin
Seborrheic dermatitis
Folliculitis
Dermatophytosis
Kaposi's sarcoma
Mouth
Candidiasis (pseudomembranous and erythematous)
Hairy leukoplakia
Aphthous ulcers
Periodontal disease
Lymphatic System
Localized lymphadenopathy*
Splenomegaly
Neurologic or Psychologic Response
Mood or affect
Psychomotor slowing
Eye movement abnormalities
Hyperreflexia (if feasible, simple motor tests such as timed gait and quantifiable neuropsychiatric
    tests such as digit symbol substitution are more sensitive to early neurologic disease than is bedside
    examination)

*Generalized lymphadenopathy does not correlate with increased disease progression.

Table 6–2. Laboratory Markers of HIV Disease Progression

Nonspecific Markers
Decreased hematocrit value
Decreased platelet count
Elevated erythrocyte sedimentation rate
Immunologic Markers
Decreased CD4 lymphocytes
Decreased CD4:CD8 lymphocyte ratio
Elevated serum β_2-microglobulin
Elevated serum neopterin
Elevated serum acid labile interferon
Absent or decreased levels of anti-p24 antibody
HIV-Specific Markers
p24 Antigenemia
Positive serum HIV culture

of repeated full examinations in infected persons. Nevertheless, a focused examination may uncover important new data. The pertinent pieces of the examination with potential findings are listed in Table 6–1. These abridged recommendations pertain only when there has been no change in clinical status. The interval development of significant symptoms dictates a complete re-examination.

Given the explosion of surrogate laboratory markers that (at least retrospectively) correlate with disease progression, a major challenge to clinicians is appropriate laboratory use. Table 6–2 lists some of the tests advocated as markers.

Table 6–3.   Surrogate Markers: How to Decide

Specificity for HIV infection
Correlation with disease progression (sensitivity and predictive value)
Variability of results
   Temporally
   Interlaboratory and intralaboratory
Availability
Cost
Applicability to clinical management

It is tempting to rely heavily on these laboratory tests in the evaluation and staging of patients with HIV disease. However, the clinical presentation of the patient is more predictive of low CD4 + cell counts than a low CD4 + cell count is predictive of clinical symptomatology. The complete history and physical examination remain the most powerful tools in staging patients with HIV infection.

All these tests of surrogate markers suffer from common drawbacks. First, data derived from epidemiologic cohorts have not been validated prospectively for individual patients. Second, normative values often have not been established for these tests in HIV-infected populations or in uninfected risk group members. Finally, laboratory variability and laboratory errors occur; *the reliance on a single mistaken value may have profound implications for an individual.* Thus any laboratory markers must be interpreted carefully in the context of clinical findings and repeated if any question exists about their validity (see Chapter 3).

Three types of test have been used. The hematocrit is an example of the first type: a laboratory value that is abnormal in many disease states. The second type attempts to quantify immunologic deficits or immunologic activation. Enumeration of lymphocyte subsets and measurements of β_2-microglobulin are examples of these surrogate markers. Finally, the third type measures p24 antigenemia and HIV serum culture for direct quantitative evidence of HIV infection.

Which of these tests should be chosen? None of the available surrogate markers is perfect. Table 6–3 presents areas to consider in choosing laboratory markers. Hematocrit determination is inexpensive, universally available, and an essential part of the general evaluation of an HIV-infected individual. Beyond ordering a complete blood count, however, there are a variety of potential strategies. Practically, lymphocyte subsets have been the most widely used of these markers, and the CD4 count should be an essential part of the evaluation of every infected individual. The CD4 count is a requisite before initiating antiretroviral therapy or *P. carinii* prophylaxis. Nevertheless, this measure still has the relative drawbacks of expense, lack of universal availability, diurnal variability, and interlaboratory variability, which make it an imperfect monitoring test. Therefore, insofar as possible, the test should be performed serially in the same laboratory at the same time of the day.

Once the CD4 count is known, other laboratory markers should be used very selectively because currently they seem to have little value in predicting who will or will not respond to antiretroviral therapy. In the large prospective trial of zidovudine in asymptomatic seropositive individuals, p24 antigenemia did not predict a greater response to therapy than for those persons lacking antigen.[29] Surrogate markers may be most helpful in cases in which the CD4 count indicates an intermediate prognosis for disease progression. Such an "intermediate" range might be 200 to 500 CD4 cells. The two best candidates as second-line prognostic markers are β_2-microglobulin and serum neopterin. β_2-Microglobulin determination is a relatively inexpensive test that is widely available; in some studies it has had a higher correlation with disease progression than CD4 counts.[21] β_2-Microglobulin is a low-molecular-weight protein found on the surface of all nucleated cells. It is released into serum with cell activation, and its high concentrations in persons with progression of HIV disease is thought to represent target cell (CD4 +) activation resulting from HIV infection. Its main problem is poor specificity. Serum neopterin is a metabolite of guanosine triphosphate and is increased after activation of macrophages by interferon-γ, which is produced by activated T cells. One epidemiologic study found the combination of CD4 + cell count and neopterin measurements was a powerful predictor of disease progression.[20]

The direct measurement of HIV is still in active development. Three recent studies quantifying plasma viremia have shown direct correlation between plasma virus titer and stage of disease, with the highest viral burden in patients with end-stage disease.[4,12,27] This finding adds strength to the argument for the early initiation of antiretroviral therapy in the hope of decreasing or limiting the growth of plasma viremia. Although use of HIV p24 antigen is advocated by some as a sensitive marker of disease progression, poor correlation between HIV plasma viremia and elevation of p24 antigen was found in one study.[4] Because of its expense and relatively low sensitivity, routine p24 antigen testing is not recommended. Furthermore, fewer than 70% of patients with full-blown AIDS will have p24 antigenemia, so this is not a highly sensitive marker of active disease. A final caveat is that approximately half of individuals without measurable antigenemia appear to have serum antigen bound in circulating immune complexes.[18] The prognostic significance of this finding is unknown.

Table 6–4.   Staging and Treatment of HIV Infection

Early Stage Disease (CD4 + count >500 cells/mm³)
No treatment currently is indicated; monitor CD4 every 3-6 months.
Update immunizations.
Middle Stage Disease (CD4 + count of 200-500 cells/mm³)
Prescribe zidovudine, 500 mg/day (divided in three doses).
Monitor complete blood count results every 2 weeks for 1 month, then once a month for 2 months, then every 2 months if patient is stable.
Monitor CD4 counts every 3 months.
Do not start zidovudine therapy in an asymptomatic individual without documentation of antibody positivity.
Do not start zidovudine therapy at first patient visit.
Later Stage Disease (CD4 + count <200 cells/mm³)
Prescribe zidovudine, 500 mg/day, although higher dose may be used if clinical situation warrants (e.g., in patients with AIDS dementia complex).
Monitor the same as with middle stage disease; obtain other laboratory values as indicated by patient's clinical condition.
Initiate *Pneumocystis carinii* pneumonia prophylaxis.
   Trimethoprim/sulfamethoxazole (one double-strength tablet daily)
or
   Inhaled pentamidine (300 mg monthly)
or
   Dapsone (50-100 mg daily)

Thus there are still many questions remaining in the area of disease monitoring. Both clinical and laboratory assessment are important components, but the optimum visit interval and laboratory use have not yet been determined. One approach is to stratify asymptomatic individuals on a basis of complete blood count and CD4 studies. For those with normal results, an initial follow-up frequency of 3 to 6 months may be adequate. In contrast, individuals with low, intermediate, or rapidly declining CD4 values might be seen every 2 to 3 months, with a shorter follow-up period if additional surrogate markers such as β_2-microglobulin are abnormal. Once the decision is made to embark on medical therapy, follow-up recommendations intensify accordingly.

Our current approach to the staging of HIV infection is illustrated in Table 6-4.

INSTITUTION OF ANTIRETROVIRAL THERAPY

Although this topic is discussed in more detail in Chapter 7 and data are rapidly evolving, this section briefly reviews the arguments for and against early institution of antiviral therapy in asymptomatic seropositive patients.

The strongest rationale for the early initiation of antiretroviral therapy is epidemiologic data that show that the majority of infected people will ultimately become ill as a result of HIV's effects. There is also strong evidence that zidovudine, which has significant toxicity in advanced disease, is better tolerated by individuals who are healthier at the start of therapy. In asymptomatic seropositive individuals with a CD4 + cell count <500 cells/mm^3, progression rates to symptomatic disease or death were cut in half by administering zidovudine (500 mg/day).[29]

The drawbacks of early antiretroviral therapy involve three very different considerations. The first is the cost of such long-term therapy to individuals, their insurers, and society. Second, many clinical trials do not provide data about long-term toxicity of these agents. For example, the myopathy associated with zidovudine was not appreciated until several years after the initial placebo-controlled trial was finished. It should be anticipated that zidovudine and other antiretroviral agents will be associated with other idiosyncratic, unexpected side effects over time, especially when these agents are used in combination. Finally, there is the issue of development of drug resistance by HIV. To date, the only examples of resistance have occurred in people with advanced disease after prolonged low-dose exposure to zidovudine.[16] In theory, chronic low-dose therapy could provide a favorable milieu for resistant HIV to occur. However, treating HIV earlier in the course of the infection when the overall viral burden is lower has resulted in a decreased incidence of resistance,[25] and the current standard of care for the initiation of zidovudine at 500 mg per day when the CD4 + is <500 remains reasonable. However, the decision to initiate antiretroviral therapy in an asymptomatic seropositive person must be individualized and discussed fully with each patient.

PROPHYLAXIS OF OPPORTUNISTIC INFECTIONS

Experience with *P. carinii* has reinforced the principle that, when possible, prophylaxis of opportunistic infection should be attempted in patients with HIV

**Table 6–5.   Critical Issues in
Opportunistic Infection Prophylaxis**

Likelihood of reactivation of the infection
Availability of effective, bioavailable antimicrobials
Acceptable long-term toxicity profile
Compatibility with other therapies, particularly antiretrovirals
Development of drug resistance
Cost of therapy

infection (see Chapter 17). Table 6–5 lists issues to consider when planning pro-phylactic therapy. Several uncertainties are identified in the table. First, data to allow prediction of a given infection in HIV-infected individuals are limited.[5,23] Thus improved diagnosis and staging are fundamental in the planning of rational prophylaxis. Second, efficacy or lack thereof in other treatment settings does not necessarily predict the outcome of prophylaxis; an example is the trend toward decreased cytomegalovirus (CMV) infection in HIV-infected persons receiving high doses of acyclovir. Third, prophylaxis may lead to undesirable therapeutic trade-offs. For example, use of a highly effective antimicrobial that has synergistic toxicity with an antiretroviral could, on balance, be detrimental. Fourth, the past several years have demonstrated the clinical significance of antimicrobial resistance in this population. Whether the use of prophylactic therapy merits risking the development of resistance that could render later therapy useless must be considered. This is particularly germane for infections treatable with only one or few efficacious agents. Finally, cost of therapy is a major consideration. Given these competing issues, it should be anticipated that, at present, there are no ideal prophylactic agents.

VACCINATION

Several bacterial and viral infections may be preventable by vaccination. Clinical efficacy data are not available, but the majority of people with early HIV disease (CD4 + cell count >500 cells/mm^3) will mount an appropriate antibody response to some serotypes represented in pneumococcal vaccine.[13] Since the incidence of adverse effects is no higher in this population, polyvalent pneumococcal vaccine should be administered to each HIV-infected person at the time of first contact. The need for a booster is unknown. Since data on the antibody response to *Hae-mophilus influenzae* type B vaccine do not exist and the serotype distribution to *H. influenzae* in HIV-seropositive individuals is unknown, widespread use of this vaccine cannot be generally recommended (see Chapter 22).

Seasonal influenza vaccination is recommended, although one study demonstrated poor antibody responses to immunization, even in asymptomatic HIV-infected in-dividuals.[22] However, there is no evidence that influenza is more severe in the presence of concomitant HIV infection or that vaccination prevents disease. Finally, recombinant hepatitis B vaccine should be administered to those who have no prior exposure and who might continue behaviors that place them at risk for hepatitis B infection. Antibody to hepatitis B surface antigen declines more rapidly in an HIV-infected cohort, but the need for rechecking serology and booster doses has not been evaluated.[3]

Table 6–6.   Basic Care of Patients With Early HIV Disease

Relevant Historical Questions
Estimate time of initial infection.
Establish risks for acquisition with open, nonjudgmental questions.
Review current sexual practices (with emphasis on "safer sex") and current or past drug use.
Obtain past medical history, especially about sexually transmitted diseases, Papanicolaou smears, immunizations, and purified protein derivative (tuberculin) status.
Obtain social history—travel, current social supports, questions about pets, insurance status, durable power of attorney, will, and employment.
Monitoring
Obtain complete baseline history and physical examination; perform directed interval interview and examination approximately every 6 months.
Perform baseline complete blood count and absolute CD4 cell count, with repetition approximately every 6 months.
Diagnosis and Treatment of Occult Infection
Measure baseline purified protein derivative (PPD).*
Perform baseline rapid plasma reagin test and fluorescent treponemal antibody absorption (FTA-ABS) test or microhemiagglutination assay–*Treponema pallidum* (MHA-TP) test if negative.
Health Care Maintenance
Assess for ongoing counseling needs, and refer for significant psychiatric or social problems.
Administer pneumococcal vaccine.
Administer hepatitis B vaccine if no prior exposure.
Administer yearly influenza vaccine.

*See Chapter 18 for discussion of the limitations of tuberculin skin testing.

SUMMARY

Although more attention is being paid to the delivery of adequate care early in the course of HIV disease, many questions still remain. It is hoped that patients with HIV infection will have their care optimized and disease progression slowed by a combination of monitoring, preventive therapy, and well-timed intervention with antiretroviral agents. It is increasingly clear that decisions made in the course of treating individuals cannot be made in a vacuum without consideration of the changing ecology of HIV infection and the potential costs of therapy to society. Practitioners must have the flexibility to manage individuals according to their unique needs. Table 6–6 summarizes the main points previously discussed and proposes a basic level of care for those with early HIV disease, but these guidelines probably will soon change as more clinical questions are resolved and rapid drug development continues.

REFERENCES

1.   Blanche S, Rouzioux C, Moscato M-L, et al: A prospective study of infants born to women seropositive for human immunodeficiency virus type 1. N Engl J Med 320:1643-1648, 1989
2.   Bosworth NJ, Cooper DA, Donovan B: The influence of human immunodeficiency virus type I infection on the development of the hepatitis B virus carrier state. J Infect Dis 163:1138-1140, 1991
3.   Collier AC, Corey L, Murphy VL, Handsfield HH: Antibody to human immunodeficiency virus and suboptimal response to hepatitis B vaccination. Ann Intern Med 109:101-105, 1988

4. Coombs RW, Collier AC, Allain J-P, et al: Plasma viremia in human immunodeficiency virus infection. N Engl J Med 321:1626-1631, 1989
5. Crowe SM, Carlin JB, Stewart KI, et al: Predictive value of CD4 lymphocyte numbers for the development of opportunistic infections and malignancies in HIV-infected persons. J AIDS 4:770-776, 1991
6. European Collaborative Study: Children born to women with HIV-1 infection: Natural history and risk of transmission. Lancet 337:253-260, 1991
7. Eyster ME, Ballard JO, Gail MH, et al: Predictive markers for the acquired immunodeficiency syndrome (AIDS) in hemophiliacs: Persistence of p24 antigen and low T4 cell count. Ann Intern Med 110:963-969, 1989
8. Fahey JL, Taylor JMG, Detels R, et al: The prognostic value of cellular and serologic markers in infection with human immunodeficiency virus type 1. N Engl J Med 332:166-172, 1990
9. Goedert JJ, Biggar RJ, Melbye M, et al: Effect of T4 count and cofactors on the incidence of AIDS in homosexual men infected with the human immunodeficiency virus. JAMA 257:331-334, 1987
10. Goedert JJ, Kessler CM, Aledort LM, et al: A prospective study of human immunodeficiency virus type 1 infection and the development of AIDS in subjects with hemophilia. N Engl J Med 321:1141-1148, 1989
11. Greenspan D, Greenspan JS, Hegarst NG, et al: Relation of oral hairy leukoplakia to infection with the human immunodeficiency virus and risk of developing AIDS. J Infect Dis 155:475-481, 1987
12. Ho DD, Moudgil T, Alam M: Quantitation of human immunodeficiency virus type 1 in the blood of infected persons. N Engl J Med 321:1621-1625, 1989
13. Juan K-L, Ruben FL, Rinaldo CR, et al: Antibody responses after influenza and pneumococcal immunization in HIV-infected men. JAMA 257:2047-2050, 1987
14. Kaslow RA, Phair JP, Friedman HB: Infection with the human immunodeficiency virus: Clinical manifestations and their relationship to immune deficiency—a report from the multicenter AIDS cohort study. Ann Intern Med 107:474-480, 1987
15. Lange JM, Paul DA, Huisman HG, et al: Persistent HIV antigenemia and decline of HIV core antibodies associated with transition to AIDS. Br Med J 293:1459-1462, 1986
16. Larder BA, Darby G, Richman DD: HIV with reduced sensitivity to zidovudine (AZT) isolated during prolonged therapy. Science 243:1731-1734, 1989
17. Lifson AR, Rutherford GW, Jaffe HW: The natural history of human immunodeficiency virus infection. J Infect Dis 158:1360-1367, 1988
18. McHugh TM, Sites DP, Busch MP, et al: Relationship of circulating levels of HIV antigen, anti-p24 antibody and HIV containing immune complexes in patients infected with HIV. J Infect Dis 158:1088-1091, 1988
19. Melbye R, Biggar R, Ebbesen P, et al: Long-term seropositivity for human T-lymphotrophic virus type III in homosexual men without the acquired immunodeficiency syndrome: Development of immunologic and clinical abnormalities. Ann Intern Med 104:496-500, 1986
20. Melmed RN, Taylor JMG, Detels R, et al: Serum neopterin changes in HIV infected subjects: Indicator of significant pathology, CD4 T cell changes and development of AIDS. J AIDS 2:70-76, 1989
21. Moss AR, Bacchetti P, Osmond D, et al: Seropositivity for HIV and the development of AIDS or AIDS related condition: Three year follow up of the San Francisco General Hospital cohort. Br Med J 296:745-750, 1988
22. Nelson KE, Clements ML, Miotti P, et al: The influence of human immunodeficiency virus (HIV) infection on antibody responses to influenza vaccines. Ann Intern Med 109:383-388, 1988.
23. Phair J, Munoz A, Detels R, et al: The risk of *Pneumocystis carinii* pneumonia among men infected with human immunodeficiency virus type 1. N Engl J Med 322:161-165, 1990
24. Polk BF, Fox R, Brookmeyer R, et al: Predictors of the acquired immunodeficiency syndrome developing in a cohort of seropositive homosexual men. N Engl J Med 316:61-66, 1987
25. Richman DD, Grimes JM, Lagakos SW: Effect of stage of disease and drug dose on zidovudine susceptibilities of isolates of human immunodeficiency virus. J AIDS 3:743-746, 1990
26. Rutherford GW, Lifson AR, Hessol NA, et al: Course of HIV-1 infection in a cohort of homosexual and bisexual men: An 11 year follow-up study. Br Med J 301:1183-1188, 1990
27. Saag MS, Crain MJ, Decker D, et al: High-level viremia in adults and children infected with human immunodeficiency virus: Relation to disease stage and CD4 + lymphocyte levels. J Infect Dis 164:72-80, 1991

28. Taylor JMG, Fahey JL, Detels R, Giorgi JV: CD4 percentage, CD4 number, and CD4:CD8 ratio in HIV infection: Which to choose and how to use. J AIDS 2:114-124, 1989
29. Volberding PA, Lagakos SW, Koch MA, et al: Zidovudine in asymptomatic human immunodeficiency virus infection. A controlled trial in persons with fewer than 500 CD4-positive cells per cubic millimeter. N Engl J Med 322:941-949, 1990
30. Ward JW, Bush TJ, Perkins HA, et al: The natural history of transfusion-associated infection with human immunodeficiency virus. Factors influencing the rate of progression to disease. N Engl J Med 321:947-957, 1989
31. Yarchoan R, Venzon DJ, Pluda JM, et al: CD4 count and the risk for death in patients infected with HIV receiving antiretroviral therapy. Ann Intern Med 115:184-189, 1991

7

TREATMENT OF HIV INFECTION

MARGARET A. FISCHL, MD

Drug development for anti-HIV therapies hinges on knowledge of the replication cycle of the human immunodeficiency virus type 1 (HIV-1). Infection with HIV begins with the binding of the envelope protein gp120 to the cellular receptor CD4. The viral core can then enter cells. Once in cells, the RNA genome of the virus is converted to a DNA copy via reverse transcriptase. A complementary-strand DNA copy of viral genomic RNA is made, and then a second, double-stranded DNA copy is made. This linear, double-stranded provirus is integrated into host chromosomes and transcribed into mRNA. mRNA is then translated to make precursor proteins, which are specifically cleaved to form mature viral particles that reassemble with viral genome RNA to form new infectious viral particles. Thus replication of HIV begins with binding to cells and integration into host-cell DNA. Transcription of HIV mRNA occurs with production of infectious virions. Agents that block the initial phases of viral replication should prevent infection of new cells but will not affect chronically infected cells. Agents that block the later phases of viral replication should block the chronic infection of cells but will not prevent uninfected cells from becoming infected.

A number of compounds under evaluation or development interfere with HIV replication. The best known of these agents are the dideoxynucleosides, which are potent inhibitors of HIV in vitro. As 5′-triphosphates, these agents exert anti-HIV activity at the reverse transcriptase level. Two mechanisms may contribute to dideoxynucleoside effects on reverse transcriptase. As triphosphates, they compete with cellular dideoxynucleoside-5′-triphosphates, which are essential substrates for the formation of proviral DNA by reverse transcriptase. They also act as chain terminators in the synthesis of proviral DNA. Mammalian DNA polymerase-α is relatively resistant to the effects of this class of drugs, which accounts for the select anti-HIV activity of these compounds. However, mammalian DNA polymerase-γ, found in mitochondria, and DNA polymerase-β are sensitive to these compounds, which may account for their toxicities. HIV infection is a chronic viral infection in which titers of circulating virus are higher when the disease is more advanced.[2,12] In addition, increasing viral burden, especially in CD4 cells, is directly associated with a progressive decline in CD4 cell counts and deteriorating clinical course in infected patients.[25] Since nucleosides prevent infection of new cells, their use early

97

in the course of HIV infection, when the viral burden is low, is likely to result in better clinical benefits. Compounds approved or under evaluation include zidovudine (Retrovir, AZT), zalcitabine (dideoxycytidine, ddC), didanosine (dideoxyinosine, ddI), didehydrodideoxythymidine (D4T), and phosphonoformate (foscarnet).

The target cells of HIV express the CD4 receptor. The region of CD4 that binds directly with the gp120 envelope protein of the virus has been mapped. Fragments of the CD4 molecule that exist in a soluble form can be used as viral inhibitors. Soluble CD4 can prevent HIV from binding to the cellular receptor. Anti-idiotypic antibodies to CD4, which mimic the CD4 molecule, should have similar effects. Soluble recombinant CD4, however, is not very stable in the blood and necessitates continuous infusion of the compound. The binding region of the CD4 molecule has been combined in a chimeric molecule containing an antibody chain (IgG), which has resulted in a more stable compound. Unfortunately, preliminary data involving soluble CD4 and the chimeric molecule have not demonstrated efficacy of these compounds in vivo.

HIV has several genes to moderate or down-regulate viral expression to prevent killing of infected host cells and persistent viral infection. At least three genes, *tat*, *nef*, and *rev*, have been identified as having a direct role in regulation. The *tat* gene turns on all proteins forming the structure of viral particles and regulates growth; *nef* down-regulates both sets of proteins; *rev* is a differential regulator, and a threshold of *rev* is required for expression of viral structural proteins. When *rev* is overexpressed, it will shut down the other two proteins. The regulator genes of HIV are potential targets for inhibiting viral replication. Developing chronically infected cells cultured with an antisense oligonucleotide construct derived from the coding sequence of the *tat* and *rev* genes should result in a reduction of viral expression. Such compounds may also inhibit the replication of HIV in a manner that is not sequence specific. Several phase I studies of one *tat* gene inhibitor drug are underway.

ZIDOVUDINE

Zidovudine is a thymidine analog that inhibits the replication of HIV in vitro. Zidovudine is phosphorylated by cellular enzymes to the 5'-triphosphate, which interferes with HIV RNA-dependent DNA polymerase (reverse transcriptase) and elongation of the viral DNA chain.

On the basis of the pharmacologic properties of zidovudine, the initial dose tested in clinical trials for the treatment of patients with advanced HIV disease was 250 mg given orally every 4 hours (1500 mg, total daily dose).[8] The current recommended dose is 100 mg every 4 hours (600 mg, total daily dose) for symptomatic patients with HIV infection and 100 mg every 4 hours while awake (500 mg, total daily dose) for patients with asymptomatic infection.

A study sponsored by the National Institutes of Health (NIH) AIDS Clinical Trials Group (ACTG) demonstrated that a reduced dose of zidovudine (100 mg every 4 hours) was as effective and less toxic than the originally tested dose (250 mg every 4 hours).[6] A statistically significant better 18-month survival rate ($p = 0.012$) and no differences in the time to development of an opportunistic infection, change in CD4 cells, or decrease in serum HIV antigen levels were noted. In addition, a significantly lower incidence of hematologic toxicity, including both anemia and neutropenia, was noted among patients receiving the lower dose of zidovudine. The absence of differences between the two treatment groups and a better 18-month survival rate demonstrate that the reduced dose of zidovudine is effective. Similarly, another ACTG study revealed no difference in progression rates to AIDS or advanced AIDS-related complex (ARC) and significantly less toxicity in asymptomatic subjects with HIV infection who received 100 mg of zidovudine every 4 hours while awake (500 mg, total daily dose) as compared with 300 mg every 4 hours while awake (1500 mg, total daily dose).[31]

Based on these data, a lower daily dose of zidovudine (500 to 600 mg) should be used when treating patients with HIV infection. Since HIV infection is a chronic viral infection and zidovudine cannot completely eradicate infection, use of a higher induction dose when treating patients with advanced HIV disease does not appear warranted at this time. Although the serum half-life of zidovudine is 1 hour, the intracellular half-life of the 5'-triphosphate approaches 3 hours. Thus it may also be possible to increase the dosing interval to every 8 hours. The optimum dose of zidovudine for the treatment of patients with AIDS dementia complex is not known. Although lower doses have been associated with measurable improvement in cognitive function tests, systematic evaluation of lower doses in the treatment of AIDS dementia complex has not been completed.

Zidovudine is beneficial in the treatment of patients with advanced HIV disease[3,6-8,21,28,29] (Table 7–1), and beneficial effects have been seen among patients with a variety of AIDS-defining opportunistic infections. However, certain opportunistic infections remain difficult to treat, and patients who are terminally ill with these types of infections may not respond as well. Median survival time for patients with AIDS who are receiving zidovudine is approximately 124 weeks,[3,7,29] an almost twofold to threefold better outcome than survival estimates from historical controls, suggesting that short-term therapy provides continuing benefits to these patients. However, an increasing frequency of opportunistic infections, mortality, and wasting has been noted during long-term follow-up. Since zidovudine cannot eradicate HIV infection or result in sustained immunologic improvements, progressive HIV disease is likely to occur sometime during the treatment of patients with advanced HIV disease. Therefore patients who have advanced HIV disease and develop progressive HIV infection as manifested by recurrent opportunistic infections, wasting, or deterioration in immune function should be considered for alternative therapy. Currently, didanosine (ddI) has been approved by the Food and Drug Administration (FDA) for these indications. Zalcitabine (ddC) is also available through an expanded access program.

Table 7–1. Beneficial Effects Associated with Zidovudine Therapy

Prolonged survival	Increased CD4 cell numbers
Decreased frequency and severity of opportunistic infections	Increased CD8 cell numbers
	Increased skin-test reactivity
Delayed progression to AIDS	Decreased serum and cerebrospinal fluid p24 antigen levels
Delayed progression to AIDS-related complex	
Weight gain	Delayed development of serum p24 antigen
Improved performance status	Increased platelet counts
Improved cognitive or neurologic function	

Zidovudine benefits patients with asymptomatic HIV infection[31] who have a CD4 cell count <500 cells/mm³ and patients with mildly symptomatic HIV infection[9] who have a CD4 cell count <500 cells/mm³. In a randomized, placebo-controlled trial 1338 patients with asymptomatic HIV infection and ≤500 CD4 cells/mm³ received either placebo (n = 428), zidovudine at a daily dose of 500 mg (n = 453), or zidovudine at a daily dose of 1500 mg (n = 457).[31] The median follow-up period was 55 weeks. The rates of disease progression per 100 person years were 7.6 in the placebo group, 3.6 in the 500 mg/day zidovudine group ($p = 0.01$), and 4.3 in the 1500 mg/day zidovudine group ($p = 0.10$).

In another ACTG study 711 patients with mildly symptomatic HIV and ≥200 CD4 cells/mm³ received placebo (n = 351) or zidovudine (n = 360) at a daily dose of 1200 mg.[9] The median follow-up period was 11 months. The rates of disease progression were 14.7 for placebo recipients and 5.0 for zidovudine recipients. On the basis of these data, patients with asymptomatic and symptomatic HIV infection who have a CD4 cell count <500 cells/mm³ should be considered candidates for zidovudine therapy. Since CD4 cell counts are subject to considerable intrapatient variability, patients with either asymptomatic or symptomatic HIV infection should have two documented CD4 cell counts below 500 cells/mm³, especially patients with CD4 cell counts close to 500 cells/mm³. General guidelines for the initiation of zidovudine therapy in patients with asymptomatic or mildly asymptomatic HIV infection, adopted from a State-of-the-Art Conference,[27] are outlined in Figure 7-1.

Zidovudine has been administered to patients with HIV-related neurologic disease, including dementia, peripheral neuropathy, and myelopathy.[35] Patients with dementia improve in neurologic dysfunction as assessed by clinical evaluations, neuropsychologic testing, or positron-emission tomographic scans. Improvements have been noted soon after the initiation of zidovudine, and in approximately 50% of patients sustained improvements for up to 18 months have been described. In a subgroup of patients neurologic dysfunction reappears within several months of initiation of therapy. Less promising benefits have been described among patients with HIV-related peripheral neuropathy and myelopathy.

Autoimmune thrombocytopenia has been described among patients with HIV infection. Administration of zidovudine increases the mean platelet count within 1 to 2 weeks after the initiation of therapy.[11,20] This rapid increase in platelet count suggests that zidovudine therapy may lead to diminished clearance of immuno-globulin-coated platelets or, alternatively, may stimulate platelet production by interfering with HIV infection in the bone marrow. Among patients with HIV-related autoimmune thrombocytopenia, a substantial improvement in the platelet count has been noted in at least 50% of patients receiving zidovudine, suggesting a beneficial effect of zidovudine in the treatment of HIV-associated autoimmune thrombocytopenia.

The most common opportunistic infection noted among patients receiving zidovudine is *Pneumocystis carinii* pneumonia. The greatest risk for recurrent *P. carinii* infection is within the first 9 months after diagnosis. Hemoglobin concentration, number of CD4 cells, and time interval since the diagnosis of *P. carinii* pneumonia correlate with the early development of recurrent *P. carinii* pneumonia after initiation of zidovudine therapy. Concomitant therapy with zidovudine and an antimicrobial agent effective in the prevention of *P. carinii* pneumonia is likely to improve survival benefits further. Patients receiving zidovudine who are at an

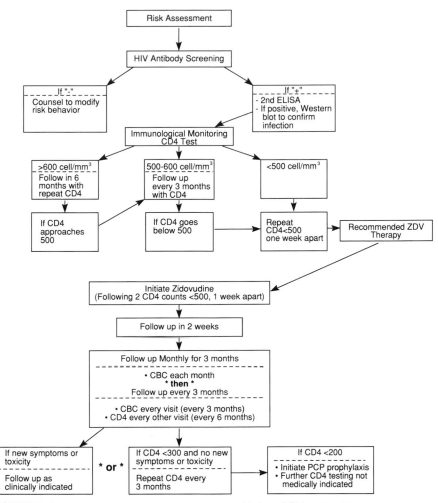

FIGURE 7–1. NIAID 1990 General Guidelines for Initiation of Zidovudine Therapy in Early HIV Disease.

increased risk for *P. carinii* pneumonia should receive chemoprophylactic therapy for the prevention of *P. carinii* infection. Any of the currently effective antimicrobial agents can be used as long as patients are monitored carefully (see Chapter 17). If additive toxicities occur and if lower doses of zidovudine are not tolerated, another antimicrobial agent for the prevention of *P. carinii* pneumonia should be chosen.

Adverse reactions reported during the first several weeks of zidovudine therapy include headache, insomnia, nausea, vomiting, abdominal discomfort, diarrhea, malaise, myalgias, rash, and fever[22] (Table 7–2). Headache, nausea, and malaise are the most common early adverse experiences, especially in patients with early HIV infection. Symptoms generally subside with ongoing therapy. Occasionally symptoms will persist or be severe enough to require temporary interruption of

Table 7–2.   Adverse Experiences Associated with Zidovudine Therapy

SYMPTOM	INTERVAL (WK)	SYMPTOM	INTERVAL (WK)
Malaise or fatigue	1-4	Macrocytosis	4-12
Nausea or vomiting	1-4	Anemia	4-12
Abdominal discomfort	1-4	Neutropenia	4-24
Headaches	1-4	Hepatoxicity (uncommon)	>24
Confusion	1-2	Myopathy	>24
Fever or rash (rare)	1-2	Nail pigmentation	>24

therapy. Rarely must zidovudine therapy be discontinued. Rare reports of rash and fever have been described that necessitate discontinuing zidovudine therapy. Anaphylaxis has not been noted.

An association has been described between long-term zidovudine therapy and the development of a myopathy characterized by myalgias, proximal muscle weakness, wasting, and elevation in serum creatine kinase values.[4] Development of myopathy is associated with prolonged therapy and has not been described during the first 6 months of treatment. The lower extremities are disproportionately affected. Temporary interruption of therapy and use of nonsteroidal anti-inflammatory agents may be helpful.

The major toxicity or adverse reaction associated with zidovudine administration is bone marrow toxicity.[22] Anemia, neutropenia and, less commonly, thrombocytopenia (see Chapter 9) have been described. Macrocytosis with moderate elevations in the mean corpuscular volume (MCV) of 25 to 40 units has been seen in approximately 75% of patients receiving zidovudine. Increases in the MCV can be appreciated as early as 6 to 8 weeks after initiation of therapy and are most prominent after 16 to 24 weeks of therapy. In the majority of patients this macrocytosis is not associated with anemia; if anemia occurs, it is frequently mild, and reductions in the dose of zidovudine may not necessarily be required.

In a subgroup of patients a more severe anemia secondary to suppression of erythropoiesis has been noted.[32] Occasionally, a mild-to-moderate elevation in the MCV also occurs. Serum folate levels are generally normal or elevated, and vitamin B$_{12}$ levels are normal to low normal. The reticulocyte count is frequently depressed (to <0.5%) and may be the first sign of bone marrow toxicity and developing anemia. A decrease or absence of red cell precursors is frequently seen on bone marrow evaluation. Erythropoietin levels commonly are elevated, suggesting that the erythroid hypoplasia or aplasia seen is not due to an interference with erythropoietin production. These findings suggest that zidovudine may inhibit commitment of cells into the erythroid line or may have a direct toxic effect on committed erythroid stem cells. Interruption of therapy results in increases in the level of hemoglobin and resolution of erythroid hypoplastic or aplastic findings in the bone marrow. However, in one third of patients with advanced HIV disease, blood transfusions may be needed, and in 10% of patients repeated blood transfusions may be necessary to maintain patients on long-term zidovudine therapy. Several studies have demonstrated that use of epoetin alfa (recombinant human erythropoietin [r-HuEPO]) is safe and decreases blood transfusion needs in patients receiving zidovudine whose endogenous erythropoietin levels are not elevated.[5] Lower doses of zidovudine are also helpful in decreasing the incidence and severity of anemia. Patients with anemia should receive no more than 500 to 600 mg of zidovudine per day. The blood counts of patients with advanced HIV disease receiving zidovudine should be monitored every 2 to 3 weeks for the first 1 to 3 months of zidovudine therapy and monthly thereafter if no toxicities are noted. In contrast, patients with mildly symptomatic or asymptomatic HIV infection experience considerably less hematologic toxicity. Serious anemia, for example, was noted in only 5% of patients with mildly symptomatic HIV infection[9] and in 1% of patients with asymptomatic HIV infection.[31] Blood counts in this population of patients should be monitored approximately every 3 months if no toxicities are noted (see Figure 7–1).

Neutropenia has also been described with zidovudine therapy and is usually the dose-limiting factor for long-term treatment. Neutropenia can be seen as early as 4 weeks but is most common after 12 weeks of therapy. Mild-to-moderate neutropenia (neutrophil count, 750 to 1000/mm^3) occurs in the majority of patients with advanced HIV disease during initial therapy with 1000 to 1500 mg/day and is typically well tolerated. Moderate to more severe neutropenia (cell count, 500 to 750/mm^3) occurs in 50% of patients and is more common among patients with advanced HIV disease receiving zidovudine for more than 16 to 24 weeks, especially among those patients also receiving other medications known to cause neutropenia (see Chapter 9). Initiating therapy at lower doses (500 to 600 mg/day) is essential in limiting neutropenia. Among patients with earlier manifestations of HIV infection who receive zidovudine, the incidence of serious neutropenia is substantially lower. Among patients with mildly symptomatic HIV infection who had 200 to 500 CD4 cells/mm^3, only 4% developed serious neutropenia while receiving 1200 mg per day of zidovudine. Among patients with asymptomatic HIV infection and <500 CD4 cells/mm^3, serious neutropenia occurred in only 1.8% of patients receiving 500 mg per day of zidovudine.

Zidovudine inhibits replication of HIV in vitro at concentrations of <0.1 μmol/L (<0.37 μg/ml). The development of reduced viral susceptibility after 6 months or more of zidovudine therapy has been demonstrated in HIV isolates from patients with AIDS and ARC, using a plaque assay with CD4+ HeLa cells.[16] Sequential isolates typically showed a stepwise decrease in susceptibilities over time. Isolates obtained from patients late in therapy demonstrated a 100-fold increase in median infective dose (ID$_{50}$) values. Cross-resistance to other nucleosides without a 3'azido moiety (ddC, ddI, d4T) or nonnucleoside anti-HIV drugs has not been seen. No apparent correlation between reduced susceptibility in vitro and clinical outcome has been documented to date. However, further careful, prospective studies are still needed. The molecular mechanisms of zidovudine resistance are unclear, although specific mutations in the reverse transcriptase gene have been described in resistant isolates.[17] In contrast to isolates from patients with AIDS and ARC, isolates from patients with mildly symptomatic or asymptomatic HIV infection and <500 CD4 cells/mm^3 showed both slower rates and lower levels of resistance to zidovudine during long-term follow-up.[23] In addition, patients receiving lower daily doses of zidovudine at both early and later stages of HIV disease did not develop resistance more readily than patients receiving higher doses of zidovudine.[23]

DIDANOSINE

Didanosine (dideoxyinosine, ddI) is a nucleoside analog that inhibits the replication of HIV in vitro. After single oral doses of 0.8 to 22.8 mg/kg, its mean half-life is 1.6 hours. The mean steady-state plasma peak concentration after oral administration of didanosine is 244 to 4163 ng/ml. The mean bioavailability is 40% in dose ranges of 0.8 to 10.2 mg/kg. Administration with a meal can decrease absorption. Didanosine is rapidly degraded at an acidic pH. All oral formulations contain buffering agents designed to increase the pH of the stomach. The drug should be taken on an empty stomach. The absorption of certain medications (e.g., dapsone, ketoconazole) can be affected by the co-administration of didanosine (see Chapter 9).

Approximately 90 patients have been treated with didanosine in phase I studies at dosages ranging from 0.8 to 66.0 mg/kg per day. Decreasing serum p24 antigen levels were noted in approximately 50% of patients who could be evaluated, and increases in the number of CD4 cells were noted in approximately one third.[24] Overall, 22% of patients receiving didanosine had an increase of 50 cells/mm^3 in the CD4 cell count during therapy compared with 2% to 12% of historical controls. In one phase I study 17 patients with AIDS and 20 with ARC were treated twice daily with drug doses ranging from 0.4 to 66 mg/kg per day.[15] Duration of treatment ranged from 2 to 44 weeks. The maximum tolerated dose (MTD) of oral didanosine was estimated as 12 mg/kg/day. The administration of didanosine was associated with statistically significant decreases in serum HIV antigen levels and increases in CD4 cells at 2 to 20 weeks of therapy. In another study 17 patients with AIDS and 17 with ARC were treated with a single daily dose of didanosine ranging from 1.6 to 30.4 mg/kg/day.[1] The MTD was estimated as 20.4 mg/kg/day. Treatment with didanosine was associated with a mean increase in CD4 cells from 125 cells/mm^3 before treatment to 182 cells/mm^3 at 10 weeks ($p = 0.005$). Serum HIV antigen levels decreased by 50% in 14 of 19 patients. Interim analyses of an ongoing ACTG randomized trial comparing didanosine to zidovudine in patients previously treated with zidovudine demonstrated a mean 11% increase in CD4 cell counts among didanosine recipients after 12 weeks, compared with a 3.2% decrease among zidovudine recipients.

Based on these preliminary findings, didanosine was approved by the FDA for the treatment of patients with advanced HIV infection who are intolerant of zidovudine therapy or who have demonstrated serious clinical or immunologic deterioration during zidovudine therapy. Thus patients who have advanced HIV disease and develop progressive HIV infection as manifested by recurrent opportunistic infections, wasting, or deterioration in immune function should be considered for didanosine therapy.

Didanosine is available as a chewable, dispersible buffered tablet or a buffered powder for oral solution. Didanosine should be taken on an empty stomach every 12 hours. The chewable, dispersible buffered tablet has a slightly better oral bioavailability and should be administered at lower doses than the buffered powder[30] (Table 7–3). To decrease problems with dryness of the mouth, chewable tablets can be dispersed in at least 1 ounce of water and drunk immediately, followed by 4 ounces of water.

The major toxicities associated with didanosine therapy include peripheral neuropathy, pancreatitis, hyperamylasemia, increases in serum urate levels, and diar-

Table 7–3.   **Adult Dosing for Didanosine**

PATIENT WEIGHT (kg)	CHEWABLE TABLETS (mg twice daily)	BUFFERED POWDER (mg twice daily)
≥75	300	375
50-74	200	250
35-49	125	167

Data from VIDEX (Didanosine). Package insert. Bristol Laboratories, 1991.[30]

rhea.[1,15,34] Hepatic toxicity causally related to didanosine administration has been reported less frequently. In addition, rare cases of electrolyte imbalances, especially low potassium levels, and cardiac arrhythmias have been noted. The most common toxicity associated with didanosine therapy is diarrhea apparently related to the citrate-phosphate buffer that is being used with the current formulations. Adequately dispersing the chewable tablet and mixing the powder solution in larger volumes of water may decrease problems associated with the buffer.

The major dose-limiting toxicity is painful sensorimotor peripheral neuropathy. The occurrence of peripheral neuropathy was more common and occurred early in the course of treatment among patients receiving higher daily doses of didanosine, typically exceeding 12 mg/kg/day. Among 79 patients receiving more than 12.5 mg/kg/day of didanosine, 27 patients (34%) developed serious peripheral neuropathy requiring dose modification. Among 91 patients who received 12.5 mg/kg/day or less, 11 patients (12%) developed serious peripheral neuropathy requiring dose modifications. Peripheral neuropathy is more common among patients with a history of peripheral neuropathy and among those receiving neurotoxic medications. The peripheral neuropathy typically consisted of tingling, burning, or aching in the lower extremities, particularly the feet. Initially, discomfort was noted while walking, but in more advanced cases, it interfered with sleep and routine daily activities. After prompt interruption of therapy, symptoms gradually resolved over a period of several weeks. Patients should be counseled about the symptoms of peripheral neuropathy, and therapy should be interrupted if signs and symptoms of peripheral neuropathy develop. In mild-to-moderate cases didanosine may be tried at lower doses after symptoms resolve. Drugs known to cause peripheral neuropathy should be used cautiously.

Pancreatitis has also been associated with didanosine therapy. In phase I studies 21 patients (27%) receiving more than 12.5 mg/kg/day of didanosine and eight patients (9%) receiving ≤12.5 mg/kg/day of didanosine developed pancreatitis. In an expanded access program a lower incidence of pancreatitis (5%) has been reported.[30] Onset of abdominal pain with or without nausea or vomiting should alert the physician to the possible presence of pancreatitis. Didanosine treatment should be stopped in patients who experience any signs or symptoms of pancreatitis until a diagnosis of pancreatitis can be excluded. In some patients symptoms can be rather sudden in onset, and in less than 0.4% of the cases described, a fulminate course with death has occurred. Monitoring serum amylase or lipase may be helpful. However, elevation in serum amylase may not necessarily occur before an episode of pancreatitis. In addition, asymptomatic elevation in serum amylase has been described. Patients who continue to have progressive increases in serum amylase levels should stop receiving the drug and should be carefully followed. In a subset of patients, fractionation of serum amylase has noted predominately an elevation in the salivary component. A number of cases of parotid gland enlargement and pain have been described. Pancreatitis was correlated with a prior history of pancreatitis and advanced HIV disease. Patients receiving didanosine should be advised to limit alcohol consumption and avoid drugs associated with pancreatitis. Didanosine use should be interrupted in patients receiving treatment for *P. carinii* pneumonia with intravenous pentamidine.

ZALCITABINE

Zalcitabine (dideoxycytidine, ddC) inhibits replication of HIV at concentrations of 0.01 to 0.5 μmol/L in vitro. Zalcitabine, with a mean half-life of approximately 1 hour, is absorbed rapidly from the gastrointestinal tract. Mean steady-state plasma peak concentrations of zalcitabine after oral administration of 0.03 mg/kg of body weight is 0.1 to 0.2 μmol/L. Zalcitabine has been detected in cerebrospinal fluid (CSF), although penetration into the CSF is not optimum. Current doses under investigation include 0.01 mg/kg every 8 hours and 0.005 mg/kg every 8 hours.

In phase I studies zalcitabine doses of 0.03 to 0.06 mg/kg given every 4 hours resulted in decreases in serum p24 antigen levels and increases in the number of CD4 cells in the majority of patients.[19,33] At lower doses of zalcitabine tested (0.01 to 0.005 mg/kg every 4 hours), decreases in serum p24 antigen levels and increases in CD4 cells still occurred but were less prominent.

Recent data from a large multicenter study comparing the effectiveness and toxicity of zalcitabine to zidovudine in patients with advanced HIV disease who received little or no zidovudine were released by Hoffman-La Roche.[13] A total of 635 patients (320 zalcitabine recipients and 315 zidovudine recipients) were followed for a median treatment time of 10.2 and 12.4 months, respectively. There was a significantly greater mortality rate among zalcitabine recipients compared to that of zidovudine recipients ($p = 0.007$). The projected 1-year probability of survival was 85% for zalcitabine recipients and 92% for zidovudine recipients. No differences in time to an AIDS-defining opportunistic infection or malignancy were noted between the two groups. This inferiority of zalcitabine monotherapy to zidovudine has been seen only in this trial. No such inferiority has been noted with zalcitabine therapy among patients who have received more than 3 months of previous zidovudine therapy or among combination therapy trials.

The major toxicities of zalcitabine are outlined in Table 7-4. The initial toxicities associated with zalcitabine include maculovesicular cutaneous eruptions, aphthous oral ulcerations, and fevers during the first 1 to 4 weeks of therapy. The occurrence of this constellation of symptoms was both less frequent and less severe at lower daily doses of zalcitabine ($\leq$0.01 mg/kg/day). Resolution of these symptoms is also common without interruption of therapy. Administration of antihistamines, acetaminophen, or nonsteroidal anti-inflammatory drugs may be helpful. For associated mucositis or stomatitis, patients can gargle with a solution containing dexamethasone sodium phosphate.

The major dose-limiting toxicity of zalcitabine is a painful sensorimotor peripheral neuropathy involving predominantly the lower extremities. Phase I studies have shown that the incidence of peripheral neuropathy is correlated with the daily and

Table 7–4.   Observed Toxicity With Zalcitabine Administration

TYPE OF TOXICITY	INCIDENCE OF TOXICITY AT DIFFERENT DOSES			
	0.06 mg/kg	0.03 mg/kg	0.01 mg/kg n(weeks ± S.D.)	0.005 mg/kg
Hematologic				
Neutropenia	3(5.7 ± 7.1)	1(5.0)	1(5.0)	1(18.5)
Thrombocytopenia	1	0	1(3.0)	0
Anemia	1(5.0)	0	0	0
Dermatologic				
Stomatitis				
Severe	4(1.0 ± 0.0)	2(2.5 ± 2.1)	2(4.0)	1(2.0)
Mild	12(2.6 ± 1.7)	9(1.7 ± 1.4)	7(2.7 ± 1.7)	6(8.2 ± 4.3)
Rashes				
Severe	4(3.0 ± 1.4)	2(6.0 ± 2.8)	2(7.0 ± 7.1)	1(8.0)
Mild	11(4.5 ± 3.0)	7(3.3 ± 2.3)	6(5.5 ± 2.8)	6(2.8 ± 2.6)
Arthritis/Arthralgia	13(4.1 ± 3.1)	11(3.6 ± 4.2)	3(4.0 ± 1.5)	8(4.6 ± 4.9)
Neurologic				
Peripheral neuropathy	14(7.4 ± 1.8)	15(8.2 ± 2.7)	8(11.8 ± 2.9)	2(17.5 ± 8.5)
Other				
Fever (>38° C)	15(3.0 ± 2.3)	15(1.7 ± 1.0)	9(3.7 ± 2.6)	10(2.8 ± 2.7)

Reproduced with permission from Merigan TC, Skowron G, Bozzette SA, et al: Circulating p24 antigen levels and responses to dideoxycytidine in human immunodeficiency virus (HIV) infections. A phase I and II study. Ann Intern Med 110:189-194, 1989.

cumulative dosages of zalcitabine.[19,33] Overall, approximately 10% of patients receiving the current test doses of zalcitabine experience moderate-to-severe peripheral neuropathy. The first symptoms of drug-related peripheral neuropathy are pain or discomfort in the feet, followed by a burning sensation or numbness. Loss of a deep tendon reflex may be an important sign of early peripheral neuropathy. Motor abnormalities are uncommon but may occur if therapy is continued. Patients should be instructed to call their physicians if they experience any pain, burning, or other types of foot or hand discomfort. If zalcitabine treatment is stopped at the first sign of peripheral neuropathy, the condition typically resolves over several weeks. The patient should be warned that symptoms may worsen before they improve. If the neuropathy is mild and resolves completely after discontinuing zalcitabine, it may be possible to reinstitute therapy at lower doses. Switching to didanosine is not recommended because of overlapping neurotoxicity.

On rare occasions zalcitabine use has been associated with pancreatitis. Patients who have had previous episodes of pancreatitis apparently are at an increased risk for its development while receiving zalcitabine. Zalcitabine therapy should be interrupted temporarily at the first sign or symptom of pancreatitis until a definitive diagnosis can be excluded. In a few patients zalcitabine therapy has been associated with marked elevations in plasma glucose levels. The association of these elevations with zalcitabine therapy is unknown. Patients who have diabetes and HIV infection have experienced no unusual problems with glucose control while receiving zalcitabine.

The combination of zalcitabine and zidovudine in vitro has a synergistic inhibitory activity against HIV. Two phase I studies evaluating the combination[18] and alternation[26] of both drugs have been completed.

COMBINATION THERAPIES

Combination microbial therapy and cancer chemotherapy have been used successfully to treat bacterial infections, fungal infections, viral infections, and a variety of malignancies. Although zidovudine is effective in the treatment of HIV infection, limitations in its use have occurred because of disease progression, toxicity, and potential adverse consequences of the emergence of resistant mutants. The use of combination therapies in patients with HIV infection therefore appears logical and may allow for delays in the development of reduced sensitivity and enhanced effectiveness of anti-HIV activity. Several drug combinations in vitro have synergistic inhibitory activity against HIV, including zidovudine and interferon alfa, *rs*CD4 and zidovudine, castanospermine or deoxynojirmycin (n-butyl DNJ) (glycosylation inhibitors) and zidovudine, and zalcitabine and zidovudine. Possible synergistic or additive inhibitory activity in vitro has also been shown for combination therapies with acyclovir and zidovudine and didanosine and zidovudine. In contrast, antagonistic inhibitory activity against HIV has been seen with ribavirin and zidovudine.

Several studies have found that combined daily doses of 1200 mg of zidovudine and up to 5 g of acyclovir do not result in a substantial alteration of the pharmacokinetics of zidovudine. Short courses of combined therapy apparently are tolerated without additive toxicities. However, no definitive data are available that demonstrate an advantage for use of combination therapy over high doses of monotherapy with zidovudine. With the demonstration that lower daily doses of zidovudine may be more effective than higher doses, combination studies of acyclovir and lower daily doses of zidovudine are needed.

The combination of 4 to 18 million units of interferon alfa and 600 mg/day of zidovudine in patients with HIV-associated Kaposi's sarcoma is relatively well tolerated. The major adverse reactions seen to date include anemia, neutropenia, and hepatotoxicity. Increases in the number of CD4 cells, suppression of serum p24 antigen, and antitumor responses have been noted.[10,14] Antitumor responses apparently are greater with the combination than with high dose interferon alfa monotherapy. Low daily doses of interferon alfa (1 to 9 million units) and zidovudine in combination are being evaluated in the treatment of patients with early manifestations of HIV infection.

Studies evaluating the combination of other nucleoside anti-HIV drugs, including zalcitabine, didanosine, and zidovudine, are also in progress. Preliminary data from several of these trials would indicate enhanced antiviral activity of combination therapies with zalcitabine, didanosine, and zidovudine. Recent data from a phase I to II trial of escalating dose combinations of zidovudine and zalcitabine among patients with advanced HIV disease demonstrated enhanced antiviral effects as manifested by increases in CD4 cells and suppression of serum p24 antigen.[18] Patients were assigned randomly to five dosage regimens of zidovudine (150 mg, 300 mg, 600 mg) and zalcitabine (0.03 mg, 0.01 mg) and one monotherapy regimen of zidovudine (150 mg). Fifty–six patients were followed for a median of 40.6 weeks. Episodes of serious hematologic toxicity were infrequent (17.9%). Severe peripheral neuropathy occurred in two patients. The mean maximum increase in CD4 cells exceeded 109 cells/mm^3, and 69% of patients receiving combinations containing 300 or 600 mg of zidovudine had an increase of 50 cells/mm^3 or more in CD4 cell counts during treatment. Regimens containing 600 mg of zidovudine were also more likely to result in persistent increases in CD4 cells beyond 1 year. Based on these data, combination therapy with zidovudine and zalcitabine at the doses tested was tolerated well, and combination therapy appeared to produce more substantial and sustained effects compared with other study regimens and with results of previous trials of zidovudine monotherapy. Although these results are very promising, confirmation of them in larger clinical trials is needed. Currently, zidovudine (600 mg) and zalcitabine (0.01 mg) are being tested in patients with advanced HIV disease and in those with asymptomatic or symptomatic HIV infection and a CD4 cell count >200 cells/mm^3.

In another study alternating and intermittent regimens of zidovudine and zalcitabine were elevated in patients with AIDS and ARC. Patients were randomly assigned to one of seven treatment regimens of alternating or intermittent zidovudine (200 mg every 4 hours) or zalcitabine (0.01 or 0.03 mg/kg every 4 hours). Hematologic toxicities were lower among patients receiving weekly or monthly regimens containing zidovudine compared with a regimen of continuous zidovudine. Monthly regimens and regimens with lower doses of zalcitabine resulted in a lower incidence of peripheral neuropathy. Sustained increases in CD4 cells were seen with the alternating regimens as compared with the continuous regimen of zidovudine. Alternating therapy with zidovudine and zalcitabine appeared to result in less toxicity and enhanced antiviral activity and may play a role in the treatment of patients with advanced HIV disease. Further studies evaluating this approach are needed.

REFERENCES

1. Cooley TP, Kunches LM, Saunders CA, et al: Once-daily administration of 2',3'-dideoxyinosine (ddI) in patients with the acquired immunodeficiency syndrome and AIDS-related complex: Results of a phase I trial. N Engl J Med 322:1340-1345, 1990
2. Coombs RW, Collier AC, Allain JP, et al: Plasma viremia in human immunodeficiency virus infection. N Engl J Med 321:1626-1631, 1989
3. Creagh-Kirk T, Doli P, Andrews E, et al: Survival experience among patients with AIDS receiving zidovudine: Follow-up of patients in a compassionate plea program. JAMA 260:3009-3015, 1988
4. Dalakas MC, Illa I, Pezeshkpour GH, et al: Mitochondrial myopathy caused by long-term zidovudine therapy. N Engl J Med 322:1098-1115, 1990
5. Fischl MA, Galpin JE, Levine JC, et al: Recombinant human erythropoietin for patients with AIDS treated with zidovudine. N Engl J Med 322:1498-1493, 1990
6. Fischl MA, Parker CR, Pettinelli C, et al: A randomized controlled trial of a reduced daily dose of zidovudine in patients with the acquired immunodeficiency syndrome. N Engl J Med 323:1009-1014, 1990
7. Fischl MA, Richman DD, Causey DM, et al: Prolonged zidovudine therapy in patients with AIDS and advanced AIDS-related complex. JAMA 262:2405-2410, 1989
8. Fischl MA, Richman DD, Grieco MH, et al: The efficacy of azidothymidine (AZT) in the treatment of patients with AIDS and AIDS-related complex: A double-blind, placebo-controlled trial. N Engl J Med 317:185-191, 1987
9. Fischl MA, Richman DD, Hansen N, et al: The safety and efficacy of zidovudine (AZT) in the treatment of subjects with mildly symptomatic human immunodeficiency virus type 1 (HIV) infection: A double-blind, placebo-controlled trial. Ann Intern Med 112:727-737, 1990
10. Fischl MA, Uttamchandani RB, Resnick L, et al: A phase I study of recombinant human interferon-alfa$_{2a}$ or human lymphoblastoid interferon-alfa$_{n1}$ and concomitant zidovudine in patients with AIDS-related Kaposi's sarcoma. J Acquir Immune Defic Syndr 4:1-10, 1991
11. Hirschel B, Glauser MP, Chave DR, Tauber M: Zidovudine for the treatment of thrombocytopenia associated with human immunodeficiency virus (HIV). Ann Intern Med 109:718-721, 1988

12. Ho DD, Moudgil T, Alam M: Quantitation of human immunodeficiency virus infection. N Engl J Med 321:1621-1625, 1989

13. Hoffman-La Roche: Letter to investigators. 1991

14. Krown SE, Gold JWM, Niedzwiecki D, et al: Interferon-alfa with zidovudine: Safety, tolerance and clinical and virologic effects in patients with Kaposi sarcoma associated with the acquired immunodeficiency syndrome (AIDS). Ann Intern Med 112:812-821, 1990

15. Lambert JS, Seidlin M, Reichman RC, et al: 2',3'-dideoxyinosine (ddI) in patients with the acquired immunodeficiency syndrome or AIDS-related complex: A phase I trial. N Engl J Med 322:1333-1340, 1990

16. Larder BA, Darby G, Richman DD: HIV with reduced sensitivity to zidovudine (AZT) isolated during prolonged therapy. Science 243:1731-1734, 1989

17. Larder BA, Kemp DS: Multiple mutations in the HIV reverse transcriptase confer high level resistance to zidovudine (AZT). Science 246:1115-1118, 1989

18. Meng TC, Fischl MA, Boota AM, et al: Combination therapy with zidovudine and dideoxycytidine in patients with advanced HIV infection: A phase I/II study. Ann Intern Med 116:13-20, 1991

19. Merigan TC, Skowron G, Bozzette SA, et al: Circulating p24 antigen levels and responses to dideoxycytidine in human immunodeficiency virus (HIV) infections. A phase I and II study. Ann Intern Med 110:189-194, 1989

20. Oksenhendler E, Bierling P, Ferchal F, et al: Zidovudine from thrombocytopenic purpura related to human immunodeficiency virus (HIV) infection. Ann Intern Med 110:365-368, 1989

21. Pinching AJ. Helbert M, Peddle B, et al: Clinical experience with zidovudine for patients with acquired immunodeficiency syndrome and acquired immunodeficiency syndrome-complex. J Infect Dis 18:33-40, 1989

22. Richman DD, Fischl MA, Grieco MH, et al: The toxicity of azidothymidine (AZT) in the treatment of patients with AIDS and AIDS-related complex: A double-blind, placebo-controlled trial. N Engl J Med 317:192-197, 1987

23. Richman DD, Grimes JN, Lagakos SW: Effect of stage of disease and drug dose on zidovudine susceptibilities of isolates of human immunodeficiency virus. J Acquir Immune Defic Syndr 3:743-746, 1990

24. Rozencweig M, McLaren C, Beltangady M, et al: Overview of phase I trials of 2',3'-dideoxyinosine (ddI) conducted on adult patients. Rev Infect Dis 129(suppl 5):S570-S575, 1990

25. Schnittman SM, Greenhouse JJ, Psallidopoulos MC, et al: Increasing viral burden in CD4+ cells from patients with human immunodeficiency virus (HIV) infection reflects rapidly progressive immunosuppression and clinical disease. Ann Intern Med 113:438-443, 1990

26. Skowron G, Merigan TC, 047 Study Group of the AIDS Clinical Trials Group: Phase II trial of alternating and intermittent regimens of zidovudine (ZDV) and 2',3'-dideoxycytidine (ddCO) in ARC and AIDS. In Program and Abstracts of the Sixth International Conference on AIDS. San Francisco, 1990

27. Sponsored by the National Institute of Allergy and Infectious Diseases: State-of-the-art conference on azidothymidine therapy for early HIV infection. Am J Med 89:335-344, 1990

28. Stambuck D, Hawkins D, Gazzard BG: Zidovudine treatment of patients with acquired immunodeficiency syndrome and acquired immunodeficiency syndrome-complex. St. Stephen's Hospital experience. J Infect Dis 18:41-51, 1989

29. Swanson CE, Cooper DA, Australian Zidovudine Study Group: Factors influencing outcome of treatment with zidovudine of patients with AIDS in Australia. AIDS 4:749-757, 1990

30. VIDEX (Didanosine). Package insert. Bristol Laboratories, 1991

31. Volberding PA, Lagakos SW, Koch MA, et al: Zidovudine in asymptomatic human immunodeficiency virus infection: A controlled trial in person with fewer than 500 CD4-positive cells per cubic millimeter. N Engl J Med 322:941-949, 1990

32. Walker RE, Parker RL, Kovacs JA, et al: Anemia and erythropoiesis in patients with the acquired immunodeficiency syndrome (AIDS) and Kaposi's sarcoma treated with zidovudine. Ann Intern Med 108:372-376, 1988

33. Yarchoan R, Perno CF, Thomas RV, et al: Phase I studies of 2',3'-dideoxycytidine in severe human immunodeficiency virus (HIV) infection as a single agent and alternating with zidovudine (AZT). Lancet 1:76-81, 1988

34. Yarchoan R, Pluda JM, Thomas RV, et al: Long-term toxicity/activity profile of 2',3'-dideoxyinosine in AIDS and AIDS-related complex. Lancet 2:526-529, 1990

35. Yarchoan R, Thomas R, Grafman J, et al: Long-term administration of 3'-azido-2',3'-dideoxythymidine to patients with AIDS-related neurologic disease. Ann Neurol 23(suppl):S82-S87, 1988

8

DEALING WITH ALTERNATIVE THERAPIES FOR HIV

DONALD I. ABRAMS, MD

Despite a decade of progress in understanding the molecular virology and pathophysiology of the human immunodeficiency virus (HIV), the disease caused by infection with this novel retrovirus remains incurable. As increasing numbers of individuals have taken heed and have determined that they are, in fact, infected with the retrovirus although currently clinically asymptomatic, a large population of people who view themselves as "ticking time bombs" has developed. In the United States the male homosexual community continues to have the highest incidence of HIV infection. This group had been organized politically into an effective interest group during the previous decades when the goal was to obtain civil rights. With the advent of the HIV epidemic, many in the community shifted their attention toward treatment activism.[3] Baffled by the continued lack of effective therapies, they started an alternative treatment movement that has grown to the point at which most practicing providers caring for patients with HIV infection are likely to have interacted with patients who have chosen alternative therapies.

The alternative therapy movement is not unique to patients with HIV disease. A recent *Time*/CNN poll by Yankelovich Clancy Schulman found that 30% of 500 people questioned in a telephone survey have tried some form of unconventional therapy, half of them within the year before the survey.[50] Among those who responded that they had never sought help from a practitioner of alternative medicine, 62% stated that they would consider seeking medical help from an alternative doctor if conventional medicine failed to help them. Of those who had sought help from a practitioner of alternative medicine, 84% responded that they would go back to an alternative doctor. It is believed alternative medicine is already a $27 billion per year industry that "reflects a gnawing dissatisfaction with conventional or allopathic medicine."

Use of alternative therapies has been studied extensively in patients with malignant diseases. Research has documented that increased use of unorthodox treatments is related to disillusionment with standard medical practice.[12] Higher use of alternative therapies is noted among patients with diseases for which treatment is limited. Another factor apparently affecting the use of other than conventional therapies is the patient's having the necessary skills to obtain the information about the treatment and to follow complex regimens. Those using these treatments are often well-educated individuals with high socioeconomic status. The *Time* cover story on alternative medicine points out that the "baby boom generation, which is just beginning to show the wear and tear of middle age" is a group that would be particularly prone toward dabbling in alternative treatment because this group has frequently been known to challenge authority and has desired an active role in decision making throughout its maturation. The bulk of individuals infected with HIV belongs to this generation.

Whether or not people with HIV infection are more frequent users of alternative therapy is difficult to assess. A survey of hospitalized patients in Chicago reported in 1984 that among patients with general medical problems, 5% had used alternative therapies.[23] In a similar subset of hospitalized cancer patients 7% reported using alternative approaches in addition to their conventional medical treatment. Among the 50 AIDS patients interviewed as part of this study, 18% stated that they were using alternative therapies.

Patients with AIDS and HIV infection have been quite vocal in their demands to have wider access to experimental treatments. Protocol design, sample size limitations, and geographic restrictions often make it difficult for each person with HIV infection to participate in orthodox clinical trials of investigational agents. "Alternative" in the term *alternative therapies* thus has taken on two different meanings in the era of HIV disease. Some therapies have been considered as alternative to orthodox therapies. In addition, alternative acquisition of orthodox therapies has also occurred. With the availability of a licensed antiretroviral agent in 1986, some in the alternative therapy movement believed that a better term for self-administered treatment was *complementary therapy,* chosen as a supplement and not as an alternative to licensed antiretroviral agents. Others have chosen as the term for these treatment regimens, *unorthodox* or *unproved.* Often these treatments are obtained through elaborate and clandestine, frequently international networks, leading to the term *underground* as yet another synonym for this ever-increasing group of therapies.

The history of the alternative therapy movement commences shortly after the recognition of HIV as the causative agent of AIDS. Once the enemy was known, expectations ran high that a cure would be available within 1 or 2 years at the most; in view of the conquest of modern medicine over Legionnaires' disease and toxic shock syndrome, expectations ran high, for a society that had put men on the moon should certainly be able to devise technology to combat a minute retrovirus in a short period of time. By 1985, however, disappointment began to emerge. Although substantial progress had been made in understanding the structure and function of the virus itself, no progress was seen in the search for effective antiviral therapies. Numerous agents had demonstrated some in vitro activity against the retrovirus, but the question was asked, "Why were they taking so long to enter clinical trials?" For those compounds that were being investigated in clinical trials, it was unclear why the number of potential participants was so limited and why the inclusion and exclusion criteria seemed so stringent. It was out of this climate of frustration and despair that community activists began to pursue some of the first alternative regimens for HIV disease.

Vitamin C was one of the first interventions proposed as a potential alternative therapy.[4] Rationale was based on anecdotal observations of broad antiviral activity and in vitro activity against a human retrovirus.[9] High doses (up to 50 g/day) were administered by either oral routes or intravenous infusion. Patients were advised to escalate their vitamin C intake to "bowel tolerance"—to ingest as much ascorbate as possible without developing completely intolerable diarrhea. As many of the advocates of ascorbate therapy died secondary to progression of their AIDS-related illness, enthusiasm for further pursuit of this agent waned in the community.

Another of the early AIDS alternative treatments that achieved prominence was the chemical dinitrocholorobenzene (DNCB). DNCB is used as a topical sensitizer and an agent for testing for anergy. It also is effective in the treatment of common warts and alopecia areata.[16,24] A community dermatologist in San Francisco reported observing an increase in the CD4 lymphocyte number in patients repeatedly painted with sensitizing quantities of DNCB in a 1% concentration dissolved in acetone while experimenting with the compound as a potential therapy for patients with AIDS-related Kaposi's sarcoma.[40] Word spread throughout the community that the dermatologist was seeing improvement in immune function. Because DNCB was a widely available chemical, a group purchased the compound in kilogram quantities from photographic supply houses and produced the treatment solution in bulk. It was subsequently distributed to individuals interested in DNCB's potential immunomodulating effect and its activity against Kaposi's sarcoma. A network of similar buyers' groups took shape, thereby creating an infrastructure for drug distribution of alternative treatments on a national level. These "guerilla clinics" became the forerunners of the current "buyers' clubs" that continue in the current for-profit distribution of potentially therapeutic agents for patients with HIV infection.

Coincident with the increasing use of vitamin C and DNCB in the community, clinical investigators in AIDS trial centers were studying immunomodulators and potential antiretrovirals in clinical trials. In 1985 studies of isoprinosine and ribavirin were launched in a number of medical centers in high-impact HIV endemic areas.[36,48] Soon it became known that these same agents were widely available through over-the-counter sales in Mexican pharmacies. Individuals began to cross the border to obtain their own supply of drugs from the nearby pharmacies. The pharmaceutical industry realized the profit potential, and responding to the increased demand, prices in Tijuana pharmacies for isoprinosine and ribavirin tripled within a year. Occasional skirmishes were reported between border agents and infected importers with their contraband of hope, stories reminiscent of the Laetrile saga of decades past.

With the advent of clinical trials investigating dextran sulfate in 1987, similar widespread importation of this over-the-counter agent available from Japanese pharmacies began to occur. The agent was widely available as a drug to lower cholesterol. Increasing use of "street" dextran sulfate threatened to hamper the interpretation of data from patients participating in the phase I studies.[2] Patients receiving the lowest dose in the official trial reportedly supplemented it with street-obtained dextran sulfate to achieve a dose they believed might have more potential for antiviral efficacy. As the Japanese government became aware of the increased demand for dextran sulfate from its pharmacies, it threatened to impose a shutdown on exports. Accusations and allegations flew back and forth and AIDS activists threatened to stage embassy demonstrations. At this point the Food and Drug Administration (FDA), also reacting to the controversy that had surrounded isoprinosine and ribavirin importation, announced a new policy allowing the importation of drugs from foreign countries for personal use. The FDA decision allowed individuals to obtain up to a 3 months' supply of a particular agent for use under the direction of a monitoring physician. The alternative therapies movement had affected the FDA regulatory system for the first, but certainly not the last, time.

Zidovudine was approved in late 1986 for use in patients with symptomatic HIV disease and <200/mm³ CD4 cells[18] (see Chapter 7). This made an orthodox treatment available by prescription to patients for the first time. There was a brief slowdown in interest in alternatives. However, when it became clear that newer and possibly better antiviral agents would not soon be released, the alternative movement surged again from 1987 through 1989. In 1989 results of large clinical trials demonstrated that zidovudine prevented progression to advanced HIV disease in patients treated earlier in their course of infection.[19,49] This led to the approval of the drug for patients with <500/mm³ CD4 cells, allowing increased numbers of individuals to obtain a licensed agent by prescription from their provider. At the same time the expanded access program for dideoxyinosine (ddI) was initiated, allowing access to patients who had failed or progressed on zidovudine to another potentially beneficial therapeutic agent. The realization of the strength of the alternative therapies movement and the fact that the treatment activists would likely gain access to ddI in an unmonitored fashion even in the absence of the "parallel track" was probably one of the factors that encouraged the initiation of such expanded access programs for speedier delivery of drugs to interested individuals while they were still in early stages of conventional clinical trials.

In 1991, just 3 years after it entered phase I clinical trials in humans, dideoxyinosine was approved by the FDA as the second antiretroviral agent for patients with HIV disease.[13,33,52] Even with antiretroviral therapies available by prescription, individuals with HIV infection continue to use alternative treatments. The extent of use remains unknown and is probably geographically variable and related to numerous factors. Greenblatt et al.,[21] reporting on polypharmacy among patients attending an AIDS clinic, gave one of the most extensive accounts of use of unorthodox treatments in this patient population. One hundred ninety-seven randomly selected individuals receiving care at the University of California San Francisco AIDS Clinic were identified in the period between October 1988 and January 1989. Participating individuals were interviewed by telephone every 4 months and were asked questions about the use of five classes of drugs: prescribed, over-the-counter, investigational, recreational, and unorthodox. The patient population surveyed was in itself probably somewhat biased because these individuals were seeking care at a university-based clinic known to participate in orthodox clinical trials of investigational agents for patients with HIV disease. The demographics of the participant group reflect the demographics of HIV infection in San Francisco at that time. Ninety-seven percent of the respondents were males, with the majority white and infected through homosexual sexual contact. Of the participants, 55% were diagnosed with AIDS, 28% were diagnosed with AIDS-related complex, and 17% were asymptomatic. Fifty percent of the respondents were college graduates, with an additional 20% having graduate degrees. Greenblatt et al. found that, in addition to obtaining medication, treatment, and drugs from their primary providers, 40% of participants received a prescription medication from a practitioner other than their primary health care provider. Eleven percent of the cohort reported receiving medication from an unorthodox provider. Use of prescription drugs was reported by 96% of the respondents, who used a mean of 4.8 drugs. Thirty-one percent of the participants had participated in an investigational trial. Twenty-nine percent reported use of alternative treatments. The unorthodox treatments most widely used were megadose vitamin C, AL-721, ribavirin, and dextran sulfate.

Use of prescription medication and unorthodox treatment were both associated with stage of illness, with AIDS patients more likely to use these modalities when compared to those who were still asymptomatic. In an analysis investigating the association between clinical and individual characteristics and use of different kinds of treatments, Greenblatt et al.[21] reported that the number of HIV-related symptoms directly correlated with the number of prescribed drugs used. The number of unorthodox treatments was correlated significantly with greater educational attainment but not with the number or duration of symptoms. They point out that users of unorthodox treatments were half as likely as nonusers to state that their primary provider was aware of all the medication and treatments that they were using. This underlines the importance of the provider's maintaining a direct line of communication with the patient, fully understanding a patient's symptomatology, and appreciating the potential drug interactions. Primary providers caring for patients with HIV infection must become cognizant and conversant with the use of potential alternative therapies.

CURRENTLY USED ALTERNATIVE THERAPIES

The popularity of a number of the alternative treatments has waxed and waned over the last decade. However, a few are still used to an appreciable extent within the community (Table 8–1). Others are becoming more widely touted as complementary treatments (Table 8–2). Providers should be aware of these agents, their rationale for use, and their potential toxicities. With increasing frequency, agents initially chosen as alternatives have begun to enter orthodox clinical trials through university centers or the government-sponsored AIDS Clinical Trial Group (ACTG) program of the National Institutes of Allergy and Infectious Diseases (NIAID).

Table 8–1.   Alternative Therapies Still in Current Use

AGENT	NATURE OF AGENT	SUGGESTED ACTIVITY	POTENTIAL SIDE EFFECTS
AL-721	Lipid mixture	Antiviral via membrane interaction	Nausea, abdominal pain, increased cholesterol
Naltrexone	Narcotic antagonist	Immune modulator via endorphins	None reported
Disulfiram (Antabuse)/ diethyl-dithiocarbamate (DTC)	Alcohol deterrent	Immune modulator	ETOH reaction, bad taste, drug metabolism alteration
Compound Q (GLQ223)	Chinese cucumber extract	Antiretroviral	Influenza symptoms, myalgias, throat pain, central nervous system effects

Table 8–2.   Alternative Therapies with Increased Current Use

AGENT	NATURE OF AGENT	SUGGESTED ACTIVITY	POTENTIAL SIDE EFFECTS
Hypericin	Herbal tea	Antiretroviral	Photosensitivity, elevated LFTs
Oral alpha interferon	Human cytokine on a wafer	Immunomodulator, antiretroviral	Rare influenza symptoms
NAC	Cysteine precursor, mucolytic, acetaminophen antidote	Antiretroviral via tumor necrosis factor (TNF)	None reported
Pentoxifylline	Approved vasodilator	Antiretroviral via TNF inhibition	Nausea, agitation

AL-721

AL-721 is a mixture containing 70% neutral lipids, 20% phosphatidylcholine, and 10% phosphatidyldiethanolamine.[35] These components are extracted by acetone from egg yolks and were reported to have in vitro activity against HIV.[45] A postulated mechanism of antiviral activity was through alteration of the cholesterol of the lymphocyte membrane and the viral envelope; the critical receptor binding could not occur, thus aborting the infection of target lymphocytes.

An early trial of AL-721 evaluated the use of 10 g twice daily in eight patients with lymphadenopathy or AIDS-related complex.[22] Preliminary reports suggested possible antiretroviral activity. However, long-term follow-up showed no prevention of disease advancement. Subsequently, an open-label, dose-ranging trial of AL-721 in a similar patient population was initiated through the ACTG process.[39] Forty-two patients were enrolled in this dose-escalating clinical trial. Toxicities were confined predominately to the gastrointestinal tract, with 70% of the patients experiencing mild or moderate diarrhea and an additional 40% to 50% experiencing nausea or abdominal pain. A substantial increase in serum cholesterol levels was observed. Patients participating also had a modest weight gain. No antiviral or immunorestorative effects were noted in ACTG protocol 022. Enthusiasm for egg lipid substances in the alternative treatment community has waned over the past few years.

Naltrexone

Naltrexone is a narcotic antagonist that increases serum endorphin levels. Endorphins are probably a link between the brain and the immune system, with lymphocytes reportedly having opiate receptors that respond to these agents.[51] Low-dose naltrexone may increase the number and sensitivity of the opiate receptors of the lymphocytes. In a placebo-controlled trial initiated in 1985, an AIDS clinical investigator noted that patients on extremely low doses of naltrexone at bedtime appeared protected from the development of opportunistic infections.[7] Patients who responded also had a significant drop in their endogenous level of serum alpha interferon. During the course of the trial five of 16 patients in the placebo group developed major opportunistic infections, compared with none of the 22 on naltrexone. In addition, patients receiving the treatment showed no deterioration in their helper T-cell function, whereas those receiving a placebo reportedly did. No untoward side effects or toxicities have been reported.

Naltrexone is available in 50 mg tablets. A collaborating pharmacist generally concocts a dilute solution so that patients can take the extremely low dose, 1.75 mg, at bedtime. Advocates claim that it should be taken "no earlier than 9 PM, as it works in large part by boosting beta endorphin production, which peaks in the early morning hours."[6] Results of the naltrexone trials to date have been reported only as abstracts without publication in a peer-reviewed journal.

Disulfiram

Diethyl-dithiocarbamate (DTC) entered clinical trials in France in 1985 as a potential immunomodulator. This chelating agent had shown some efficacy in patients with malignant disease.[43] Early reports of the European DTC trials suggested a potential immune augmenting effect in patients with HIV infection.[34] As clinical trials were initiated in the United States, the alternative treatment movement discovered that raw DTC could be purchased or produced for self-administration. Individuals began to take rectally administered DTC in enema form or in suppositories. Others developed techniques to produce enteric-coated capsules so that the homemade DTC could be taken orally without destruction by gastric acidity. One of the drawbacks of the do-it-yourself compound was that it was more likely to produce an offensive garbagelike smell in the individuals receiving the treatment. It soon was realized that disulfiram (Antabuse) is metabolized in part to diethyl-dithiocarbamate. The exact percentage of disulfiram that is converted to DTC in the bloodstream is uncertain. This information, in conjunction with anecdotal reports that alcoholics with HIV infection who took disulfiram retained normal numbers of CD4-positive lymphocytes, led to the initiation of underground acceptance of disulfiram as an alternative treatment regimen.[8] Activists recommend that individuals take 500 mg of disulfiram orally two times a week. The main toxicity is the disulfiram-alcohol reaction. A metallic or garliclike taste has also been reported frequently. Physicians should be aware that disulfiram decreases the rate of metabolism of certain drugs and therefore may increase blood levels and possible clinical toxicity of some substances (see Chapter 9).

Although extensive use of disulfiram has occurred, the clinical trials evaluating DTC in carefully monitored studies have produced equivocal results.[25] Most recently the pharmaceutical manufacturer has withdrawn DTC from further clinical trials because a large placebo-controlled study of asymptomatic patients demonstrated no protection from disease progression and suggested, in fact, that perhaps patients on drugs were more likely to develop advanced HIV disease than those receiving placebo.[1]

Compound Q (GLQ223)

A purified extract from the root tuber of a Chinese cucumber *(Trichosanthes kirilowii),* compound Q (GLQ223) has been demonstrated in in vitro studies to kill HIV-infected macrophages and block replication of virus in T-helper lymphocytes.[37] In China the root itself has been used for centuries as an abortifacient and more recently in the treatment of choriocarcinomas. As phase I trials of compound Q were commencing in the United States, treatment activists were obtaining a similar product from a manufacturer in Shanghai. Sufficient quantities of compound Q were exported to establish a treatment network in four U.S. cities, and patients were given vials of the substance to bring to their collaborating physicians. The provider was asked to inject them with the substance, thereby forgoing the need for the physician to obtain regulatory approval to participate in this "treatment experience." Extensive information was collected by the collaborating physicians to accumulate a database on the toxicity and efficacy of the agent.[11] The community network had treated 35 patients with a fixed dose, whereas the phase I protocol had just begun evaluation of its first four patients who were receiving one twentieth of the community-regimen dose.[28]

News of the underground network's delivering compound Q to interested parties was revealed in the national media when one of the study participants died. Reports of additional individuals sustaining significant adverse effects accompanied the reported fatality. The FDA intervened, asking that the unsanctioned AIDS drug trial come to an end. Citing the lack of speed in the testing of new and experimental agents for HIV infection, the treatment activists maintained that they had successfully challenged academic medicine, the government's clinical trials program, and the FDA with this treatment experience. After further negotiations, the FDA granted a treatment IND (investigational new drug) to the community network group. Continued parallel trials of compound Q currently occur in orthodox trial centers and in the community-based network.

Compound Q, unlike some of the previously mentioned alternative therapies, is not without potential for serious toxicity. Many patients experience influenza-like symptoms, which occur for days after their intravenous injections. Elevated creatine phosphokinase levels may accompany the myalgias. Throat pain is common. Central nervous system (CNS) toxicities, including stupor and coma, have been reported in some patients. Those patients with evidence of pre-existent HIV-related CNS disease are more likely to experience the untoward CNS effects. These symptoms generally respond to acetaminophen therapy.

Hypericin

Hypericin and pseudohypericin are aromatic polycyclic diones extracted from the herb *Hypericum triquetrifolium* Turra (St. John's wort). St John's wort has been used frequently by herbalists, especially in Germany and the Soviet Union, as an antidepressant for several years. Early studies demonstrated that a single dose of hypericin before exposure to Friend leukemia virus protected mice from the disease.[38] Subsequently hypericin has been shown to inhibit the assembly and budding of HIV virions from infected cells in vitro. Early preliminary findings led to increased use of the herbal tea as a potential antiretroviral agent.

Twenty-six patients self-medicating with over-the-counter hypericin containing herbal extracts were monitored by a community-based group over a 4-month period of observation.[14] Routine blood chemistries demonstrated reversible elevation in liver function test results. Photosensitivity may also be an adverse reaction. A 13% increase in CD4-positive lymphocytes in patients who had not previously taken zidovudine was observed, suggesting to the investigators that further studies of hypericin were warranted. A synthetic version of hypericin has now been produced, which is being evaluated in a phase I dose-escalating trial conducted at New York University, and subsequent trials will be coordinated through the ACTG.

Oral Alpha Interferon

Alpha interferon generally has been used as a parenteral agent because it was believed that oral administration leads to destruction of the active moieties. The AIDS treatment world was therefore surprised by a report of possible efficacy of low-dose oral natural human alpha interferon (KEMRON) in a study conducted in HIV-infected patients in Kenya.[31] Investigators used an extremely low-dose preparation (2 units/kg/day) that was held in the mouth for sustained mucosal absorption. Evaluating 40 patients over 6 weeks of treatment, the researchers reported that all symptomatic patients reported dramatic relief of constitutional symptoms, with weight gain and CD4 cell count increases accompanying therapy. In an attempt to reproduce these findings, the World Health Organization (WHO) assisted in developing a multicenter 28-day trial using the same interferon preparation used in the Kenyan study. Multiple logistic problems, however, led to a paucity of data that could be evaluated from this 108-patient trial. Subsequently a number of trials in the United States have been initiated to confirm the initial KEMRON findings. Unfortunately, access to the specific preparation used in the first study has been difficult, and other interferon preparations are being used. To date, none of the studies has demonstrated significant increases in CD4-positive lymphocyte numbers, although stabilization of counts compared to those of placebo-treated patients has been suggested.[29] Anecdotal reports of increased energy and weight gain have been generated. No significant adverse reactions are said to result from oral administration of low dose alpha interferon although a few instances of influenza-like symptoms have occurred.

Cysteine Precursors

Cysteine, an essential amino acid, is utilized in the biosynthesis of the peptide glutathione. Patients with HIV infection have decreased intracellular glutathione.[10] N-acetylcysteine (NAC) is the N-acetyl derivative of cysteine. It is available in aerosolized form as a mucolytic treatment for bronchitis in Europe. It is administered systemically in the United States for management of acetaminophen overdosage. OTC (2-oxothiazolidine-4-carboxylate, procysteine) is a precursor of cysteine as well.

It is believed that these cysteine precursors may indirectly inhibit HIV replication by raising intracellular glutathione levels.[44] In vitro cysteine and NAC raise intracellular glutathione and inhibit HIV-1 replication in persistently infected cell lines.[30]

This may occur by blocking the effects of tumor necrosis factor (TNF) in HIV-infected cells. TNF levels are elevated in people with HIV infection and may be associated with accelerated HIV replication.[20,32]

Early clinical trials are currently underway evaluating NAC in phase I dose-ranging and pharmacokinetic studies and in placebo-controlled efficacy trials. With the agent widely available in Europe, importation has occurred, and extensive use is being reported in the buyers' club market. The agent is essentially nontoxic. Stomatitis, nausea, vomiting, and fever have been reported infrequently.

Pentoxifylline

Pentoxifylline (Trental) is a trisubstituted derivative of xanthine that is approved for the treatment of patients with intermittent claudication and peripheral vascular disease. A reduction of HIV replication in vitro in acutely infected peripheral blood mononuclear and T cells has been reported with the addition of pentoxifylline to the systems.[17] It is believed that the agent indirectly inhibits HIV, possibly through suppression of TNF.[46] Pentoxifylline may upregulate cyclic AMP, which downregulates TNF. TNF increases HIV infection in chronically infected T cells; therefore repression of TNF may lead to reduced viral replication. With preliminary reports of possible antiretroviral activity, use of this currently licensed and available agent has increased in the alternative therapies community. Controlled clinical trials, including one sponsored through the ACTG mechanism, are commencing. The major reported side effects are nausea and agitation, which are known toxicities of pentoxifylline when used for peripheral vascular disease.

Chinese Herbs and Acupuncture

A significant number of individuals with HIV infection seek alternative therapies from other than Western health care providers. Specifically in the San Francisco Bay Area where much traditional Chinese medicine is practiced by the large local Asian community, patients with HIV infection in various stages have taken advantage of the abundance of providers as an alternative to Western medicine. These therapies are generally sought, not specifically as antiretroviral or immunomodulatory interactions, but as treatment for certain clinical or systemic manifestations of HIV disease, including wasting, nausea, sleep disturbances, and pain syndromes. Anecdotal reports of effectiveness of these interventions in patients who have failed previous attempts at Western treatments are abundant. Recognition of the widespread use of these interventions is evidenced by the inclusion of the following statement regarding concomitant medications in an ACTG protocol comparing combinations of nucleoside analogue antiretroviral agents[5]: "Alternative therapies such as vitamins, acupuncture, herbal therapies, and visualization techniques will be permitted. Participants should, however, report the use of these therapies; alternative therapies will be recorded but not keyed."

ACQUISITION OF ALTERNATIVE THERAPIES

Although many individuals procure their alternative therapies on their own, an increasing number are using the services of the buyers' club. A cottage industry appears to be developing based on importation and resale of desirable alternative treatments. Initially established as centers for sale of vitamins and herbal remedies to patients interested in restoring immune function, the buyers' clubs have now moved on to the business of providing patients with a veritable menu of desired alternative regimens and orthodox agents acquired through alternative means. The PWA Health Group in New York City, for example, list lipids, hypericin, oral alpha interferon, isoprinosine, itraconazole, NAC, ribavirin, and ddC in its December 1991 offerings.[26] In addition, the PWA Health Group also provides azithromycin, clarithromycin, DTC (Imuthiol), pentamidine, and primaquine; however, these items require a prescription from a health care provider.

Numerous health care providers have taken advantage of the ease of acquisition of agents through the buyers' club mechanism instead of doing the copious amounts of paperwork and monitoring required to obtain similar agents through expanded access programs. Despite the fact that the drugs available through expanded access programs are free of charge to the patient, many prefer the ease of obtaining agents through the buyers' club. For some agents such as pentamidine, the buyers' club may offer a rate that is less than half what it would cost to obtain the drug by prescription through an orthodox pharmacy. These practices, however, have recently brought the club movement to the attention of the FDA. There are concerns these organizations may possibly be profiteering from their sales of AIDS drugs. As yet, there has been no formal investigation or comment from the FDA on the activities of the buyers' clubs.

Individuals with HIV infection and their providers obtain information about which alternative treatments are currently being used through a number of regular publications. As an infrastructure for distribution of alternatives was established and with an increasing number of complementary treatments from which to choose, a need for information dissemination arose. Organizations and publications devoted entirely to the spread of up-to-date information on available underground treatments began to appear in 1987. Project Inform, a community-based group of AIDS activists, was one of the first organizations established to provide such information. Using a 24-hour hotline and monthly newsletter, Project Inform quickly became one of the major clearinghouses for the alternative treatment movement.[41]*

AIDS Treatment News, a biweekly update of AIDS treatment information, was first published in 1987.[27] With a current circulation of 5000, the newsletter informs readers of both alternative and experimental treatments. *Treatment Issues, the Gay Men's Health Crisis Newsletter of Experimental AIDS Therapies,* also appeared in 1987.[47] It cautions subscribers that "describing an experimental therapy should not be misconstrued as recommending it. All new treatments should be conducted under a physician's care." Ironically, however, with increased availability of these sophisticated publications geared at the consumer population, the providing physicians were frequently ignorant of the particular new agent about which their patient was inquiring as a potential therapeutic intervention. Focused at the health care provider in addition to the consumer is the *AIDS/HIV Treatment Directory.*[1] This quarterly directory reviews both orthodox and unorthodox agents that are currently in both early and later stages of clinical development.

As the second decade of dealing with the HIV virus and its disease manifestations

---

*Project Inform national hotline, 1-800-822-7422; California hotline, 1-800-334-7422.

**Table 8–3.   Providers' Attitudes Toward
Alternative Therapies in Their
HIV Patient Population**

Remain unaware
Ignore
Condemn
Acknowledge
Monitor
Encourage
Refer

is entered, the introduction of increasing numbers of alternative treatments into the patient community can be expected. The practitioners caring for patients with this life-threatening disease have a number of options with regard to their ultimate approach to the use of alternative treatments in their patient populations (Table 8–3). Some providers may remain unaware of the use of alternatives, and some may choose to ignore that their patients are using unprescribed agents. Often patients fear that they cannot be forthcoming with their provider, being concerned about possible condemnation for not being fully content or confident with medications prescribed by their primary care physician. Condemning a patient's use of alternative treatment regimens without trying to understand what motivates the individual to seek these options is counterproductive in establishing and maintaining trust in the patient-doctor relationship.

Physicians should acknowledge the possibility that their patients are using alternative therapies. In taking a history they should stress in a nonjudgmental manner the need to understand all medications and substances their patients are ingesting so they can best be able to evaluate the patient's clinical condition and determine what, in fact, may be the adverse effects of potential treatments. In some situations providers enter into a partnership with the patient and choose to assist in monitoring their use of alternative treatments. The Community Consortium, a group of San Francisco Bay Area HIV care providers engaged in conducting community-based clinical trials, established an Alternative Treatment Database in 1988. The goal of this observational study was to collect information on various alternative regimens being used by patients in the community. The hope was that, by using a set of standardized case report forms to monitor physical examinations, laboratory data, and adverse experiences, more could be learned about various alternatives being used by the population. After the inception of the HIV Alternative Treatment Database, zidovudine became available for patients with <500 CD4 cells, and ddI became available on an expanded access program. Their availability diminished the need, in part, for patients to seek alternative treatment. Many patients in the community who were using unorthodox regimens may not have been cared for by providers enrolling patients onto the Consortium clinical trials. Therefore the study was terminated after enrolling only 40 patients onto this observational database.

Some providers have taken an even more active stance in their approach to the use of alternative treatments by their patients. Often discouraged by the slow pace of drug development for HIV disease and enthusiastic about early in vitro reports of activity, some providers have encouraged the use of unorthodox, unproved treatments by their patients, especially for patients with advanced disease whose life span may not permit them to survive until actual clinical trials of an agent commence or to benefit from the result of such studies. In such situations providers may encourage patients to seek alternative therapies and in fact refer them to a buyers' club to obtain the agents. Referrals by providers to alternative sources to obtain drugs otherwise available through expanded access programs have been made to minimize necessary paperwork for the physician. In addition, the discounts available on some agents through the buyers' club have led physicians to refer patients to the alternative sources of obtaining a licensed medication.

POTENTIAL RISK OF ALTERNATIVE THERAPIES

HIV prefers to target cells of the immune system that are stimulated in some fashion. The effect of many alternative treatments on the status of the immune system remains unknown at this time (Table 8-4). Therefore care must be taken that agents not activate lymphocytes, thus making them more susceptible to HIV infection. On the other hand, some substances may also suppress cellular or other aspects of the immune system and may ultimately prove detrimental to patients with HIV infection. For this reason it is desirable that individuals be cautioned against taking underground complementary therapies in the absence of monitoring by their physician.

Greenblatt et al.[21] clearly demonstrates the potential risk of alternative therapies with regard to possible interaction of these agents with prescribed medications or over-the-counter therapeutics that patients are using. If a patient is participating in a clinical trial to investigate another experimental agent and is not fully reporting alternative treatments being ingested, data could be invalidated.

A potential risk of use of alternative therapies has recently come to light. Clarithromycin is a new macrolide antibiotic with promising activity against *Mycobacterium avium-intracellulare* infection (see Chapter 18).[15] It was approved in a number of European nations before entering clinical trials in the United States. Widespread importation and distribution of clarithromycin by underground routes was ongoing before the release of the drug through the expanded access program established by the pharmaceutical sponsor. The expanded access protocol, however, stipulated that patients participating must have no prior exposure to clarithromycin. Thus those who had obtained the drug under their own devices were not eligible

**Table 8–4. Potential Risks of
Alternative Therapies**

Immune stimulation or suppression
Interaction with prescribed medications
Invalidation of data if enrolled in clinical trial
Prohibition from participation in orthodox clinical trial
Potential strain on patient-provider relationship
Financial considerations
Potential for fraud and quackery

for the compassionate-use protocol. The pharmaceutical manufacturer responded to the concerned community and established a supplemental protocol for patients with prior clarithromycin experience, thus recognizing the existence of the underground distribution network and not penalizing those who had the advance opportunity to use the drug.

Patients in their desire to obtain a potentially useful intervention, often coupled with desperation resulting from their declining clinical status, may be willing to pay a significant cost for alternative treatment. The financial risk is coupled with the possibility that the agent may have very little chance of producing a positive effect. The dilemma was summarized in describing why a task force to investigate AIDS consumer fraud and quackery was established by the California State Attorney General's Office: "With so much unknown about AIDS, and with existing treatments so unsatisfactory, it will be hard to find consensus on how to distinguish legitimate, unproven and unconventional treatment attempts from unconscionable schemes to exploit people's desperation."[27]

POTENTIAL BENEFITS OF ALTERNATIVE THERAPIES

Despite significant progress made in the past decade, there still is no cure for HIV infection. Individuals infected with the virus undergo decimation of their cellular immune system and ultimately develop life-threatening opportunistic infections or malignancies. Numerous potential antiretroviral, immunomodulatory, and antibiotic regimens are under study through NIAID's ACTG and Community Programs for Clinical Research on AIDS (CPCRA) mechanisms. Other agents are being tested as pilot studies in academic medical centers and AIDS treatment clinics nationwide and throughout the world. However, AIDS currently is the second leading cause of death in the United States in men age 25 to 44 and has become the leading cause of death in women in this age group in New York City. Knowing this grave prognosis, individuals in earlier stages of HIV infection and their advocates are anxious to expedite evaluation and approval of potentially efficacious agents.

The alternative therapies movement offers the possibility for evaluation of increased numbers of potentially useful drugs. Even in the absence of careful monitoring and protocol analysis, should one of the alternatives turn out to be the "magic bullet," it is likely that this would not go unrecognized. As the alternative treatment movement has matured, however, increased interest in scientific method and clinical trials design has been demonstrated by its advocates. Often these spokespersons for the alternative treatment movement are very helpful in educating their peers and their community about the necessity of following clinical protocols for drug evaluation. Increasing collaboration is being observed between the AIDS treatment activists and the medical establishment. Much of this has been due to the energy of the AIDS Coalition to Unleash Power (ACT UP), a group instrumental in increasing awareness about the sense of urgency to develop and promote expedited drug development for patients with HIV disease.

The impact of the alternative therapy movement can already be appreciated (Table 8–5). Drug approval is accelerating. The recent approval of ddI came slightly more than 3 years after the drug entered phase I clinical trials. This recommendation for

**Table 8−5.   Impact of the Alternative
Therapy Movement**

Importation for personal use allowed
Buyers' club industry established
Parallel track and expanded access mechanisms created
Protocols for patients with prior drug exposure designed
Drug approval by FDA accelerated

approval was historic in many aspects. The data presented to the FDA were predominately information from phase I studies. The phase I trials were given a phase II aspect by comparison to historical control groups. For the first time in the approval of HIV therapeutics, a surrogate marker, the CD4 cell count, was used instead of clinical events or survival as the basis for determining that the drug had biologic activity. An ongoing ACTG clinical trial was partially unblinded while it was still in progress to provide supporting information to the FDA during the IND application review process. Dideoxyinosine was approved simultaneously for both adult and pediatric populations—another first in AIDS drug approval.

The FDA has already responded to the alternative treatment movement in a number of ways over the past decade. Allowing personal use importation, sanctioning the parallel track–expanded access program, coexisting with the buyers' club industry, and conducting timely reviews for accelerated approval are all demonstrations that the regulatory agency is not responding in a vacuum. Despite these steps in a positive direction, the Council on Competitiveness has recently suggested that the FDA move even faster. A statement from the Office of the Vice President of the United States described the new accelerated approval process[42]: "The administration's major reforms in the FDA's drug approval process will cut years off the review process. They will also save millions of lives and billions of dollars. Under these reforms, patients with serious and life-threatening diseases will benefit from earlier access to important new drugs. Unnecessary regulatory burdens will be eased. And American competitiveness will be strengthened."

Whether arising from competitiveness or cooperation, hopefully more effective therapies for HIV infections and their manifestations will emerge in the upcoming decade. The alternative therapies movement has encouraged strides in modernizing and accelerating the drug approval process that will benefit patients with AIDS and HIV infection as well as those with other serious and life-threatening diseases. Providers caring for patients with HIV infection should make every attempt to inform themselves about complementary therapies that may be in use in their community. Establishing trusting and open communication will allow the health professionals to enter a caring partnership with their patients, including those who may be empowering themselves in the presence of this relentless scourge by using alternative treatments.

ACKNOWLEDGMENT

Thanks to Rosemary Bell for preparation of this manuscript.

REFERENCES

1. Abrams D, Grieco M: AIDS/HIV treatment directory. Am Found AIDS Res (AmFAR) 5(2):19, 1991
2. Abrams D, Kuno S, Wong R, et al: Oral dextran sulfate (UA001) in the treatment of the acquired immunodeficiency syndrome (AIDS) and AIDS-related complex. Ann Intern Med 110:183-188, 1989
3. Abrams DI: Alternative therapies. In Repoza NP (ed): HIV infection and disease; monographs for physicians and other health care workers. 1989, Chicago, AMA Press, 1989, pp 163-175
4. Abrams DI: Alternative therapies in HIV infection. AIDS 4:1179-1187, 1990
5. ACTG 175: A randomized, double-blind phase II/III trial of monotherapy vs. combination therapy with nucleoside analogues in HIV-infected persons with CD4 cells $\geq$200 and $\leq$500/mm^3. 1991, 20
6. Bihari B: Management of HIV disease: one physician's approach. Bull Exp Treatments AIDS 10-27, November 1991
7. Bihari B, Drury F, Ragone V, et al: Low-dose naltrexone in the treatment of AIDS: Long term follow-up results. Fifth International Conference on AIDS. (Abstract M.C.P. 62.) Montreal, June 1989
8. Bihari B, Seaman J: Disulfiram in the treatment of AIDS related illness. Fourth International Conference on AIDS. (Poster 3042.) Stockholm, June 1988
9. Blakeslee JR, Yamamoto N, Hinuma Y: Human T-cell leukemia virus I induction by 5-iodo-2'-deoxyuridine and N-methyl-N-nitro-N-nitrosoguanidine: Inhibition by retinoids, L-ascorbic acid, and DL-a tocopherol. Cancer Res 45:3471-3476, 1985
10. Buhl R, Ari Jaffe H, Holroyd KS, et al: Systemic glutathione deficiency in symptom-free HIV-seropositive individuals. Lancet 2:1294-1298, 1989
11. Byers VS, Levin AS, Waites LA, et al: A phase I/II study of trichosanthin treatment of HIV disease. AIDS 4:1189-1196, 1990
12. Cassileth BR, Lusk EJ, Strouse TB, Bodenheimer BJ: Contemporary unorthodox treatments in cancer medicine: A study of patients, treatments and practitioners. Ann Intern Med 101:105-112, 1984
13. Cooley TP, Kunches LM, Saunders CA, et al: Once-daily administration of 2,3-dideoxyinosine (ddI) in patients with the acquired immunodeficiency syndrome or AIDS-related complex: Results of a phase I trial. N Engl J Med 322:1340-1345, 1990
14. Cooper WC, James J: An observational study of the safety and efficacy of hypericin in HIV + subjects. Sixth International Conference of AIDS. San Francisco, June 1990
15. Dautzenberg B, Truffot C, Legris S, et al: Activity of clarithromycin against *Mycobacterium avium* infection in patients with AIDS. Ann Rev Respir Dis 44:564-569, 1991
16. Eriksen K: Treatment of the common wart by induced allergic inflammation. Dermatoligica 160:161-166, 1980
17. Fazely F, Dezube BJ, Allen-Ryan J, et al: Pentoxifylline (Trental) decreases the replication of the human immunodeficiency virus type 1 in human peripheral blood mononuclear cells and in cultured T cells. Blood 77:1653-1656, 1991
18. Fischl MA, Richman DD, Grieco MH, et al: Azidothymidine (AZT) in the treatment of patients with AIDS and AIDS-related complex. A double-blind, placebo-controlled trial. N Engl J Med 317:185-191, 1987
19. Fischl MA, Richman DD, Hansen N, et al: The safety and efficacy of zidovudine (AZT) in the treatment of subjects with mildly symptomatic human immunodeficiency virus type 1 (HIV) infection. A double-blind, placebo-controlled trial. Ann Intern Med 112:727-737, 1990
20. Folks TM, Clouse KA, Justement J, et al: Tumor necrosis factor alpha induces expression of human immunodeficiency virus in a chronically infected T cell clone. PNAS 86:2365-2368, 1989
21. Greenblatt RM, Hollander H, McMaster JR, Henke CJ: Polypharmacy among patients attending an AIDS clinic: Utilization of prescribed unorthodox, and investigational treatments. J Acquir Immune Defic Syndr 4:136-143, 1991
22. Grieco MH, Lange M, Klein EB, et al: Open study of Al 721 in HIV infected subjects with generalized lymphadenopathy syndrome (LAS). Third International Conference on AIDS. (Abstract T.P. 223.) Washington DC, June 1987
23. Hand R: Alternative therapies used by patients with AIDS. N Engl J Med 320:672-673, 1989

24. Happle R: Antigenic competition as a therapeutic concept for alopecia areata. Arch Dermatol Res 267:109-114, 1980
25. Hersh E, Brewton G, Abrams D, et al: Ditiocarb sodium (di-ethyl dithiocarbamate) therapy in patients with asymptomatic HIV infection and AIDS. JAMA 265:1538-1544, 1991
26. Hodel D, Franke-Ruta G: Crackdown crackup! Notes from the underground. PWA Health Group Newsletter 12:1-6, 1991
27. James JS: AIDS Treatment News No 31, June 5, 1987
28. Kahn JO, Kaplan LD, Gambertoglio JG, et al: The safety and pharmacokinetics of GLQ223 in subjects with AIDS and AIDS-related complex: A phase I study. AIDS 4:1197-1204, 1990
29. Kaiser G, Jaeger M, Birkmann J, et al: Oral natural low-dose human alpha interferon (HuIFN) in 30 patients with human immunodeficiency virus (HIV-1) infection. A double blind placebo-controlled trial. Seventh International Conference on AIDS. (W.B. 2140.) Florence, 1991
30. Kalebic T, Kinter A, Poli G, et al: Suppression of human immunodeficiency virus expression in chronically infected monocytic cells by glutathione, glutathione ester and N-acetylcysteine. PNAS 88:986-990, 1991
31. Koech DK, Obel AO, Minowada J, et al: Low dose oral alpha-interferon for patients seropositive for human immunodeficiency virus type-1. Mol Biother 2:91-95, 1990
32. Lahdevirta J, Maury CP, Teppo AM, Repo H: Elevated levels of circulating cachectin/tumor necrosis factor in patients with acquired immunodeficiency syndrome. Am J Med 85:289-291, 1988
33. Lambert JS, Seidlin N, Reichman RC, et al: 2′,3′-dideoxyinosine (ddI) in patients with the acquired immunodeficiency syndrome or AIDS-related complex: A phase I trial. N Engl J Med 322:1333-1340, 1990
34. Lang J-M, Touraine J-L, Trepo C, et al: Randomised, double-blind, placebo-controlled trial of dithicarb sodium (Imuthiol) in human immunodeficiency virus infection. Lancet 2:702-706, 1988
35. Lyte M, Shinitsky M: A special lipid mixture for membrane fluidization. Biochim Biophys Acta 812:133-138, 1985
36. McCormick JB, Getchell JP, Mitchell SW, et al: Ribavirin suppresses replication of lymphade-nopathy-associated virus in cultures of human adult T-lymphocytes. Lancet 2:1367-1369, 1984
37. McGrath MS, Hwang KM, Caldwell SE: GLQ 223: An inhibitor of human immunodeficiency virus replication in acutely and chronically infected cells of lymphocyte and mononuclear phagocyte lineage. Proc Natl Acad Sci U S A 86:2844-2848, 1989
38. Meruelo D, Lavie G, Lavie D: Therapeutic agents with dramatic anti-retroviral activity and little toxicity at effective doses: Aromatic polycyclic diones hypericin and pseudo-hypericin. Proc Natl Acad Sci U S A 85:5232-5234, 1988
39. Mildvan D, Armstrong D, Antoniskis D, et al: An open label dose-ranging trial of Al 721 in PGL and ARC. Fifth International Conference on AIDS. (Abstract W.P.B. 312.) Montreal, June 1989
40. Mills BL: Stimulation of T-cellular immunity by cutaneous application of dinitrochlorobenzene. J Am Acad Dermatol 6:1089:1090, 1986
41. P.I. Perspective. (Quarterly) Project Inform.
42. Quayle D: Council on competitiveness fact sheet. Improving the nation's drug approval process. November 1991.
43. Renoux G, Renoux M, LeMarie E, et al: Sodium diethyldithiocarbamate (Imuthiol) and cancer. Adv Exp Med Biol 166:223-239, 1983
44. Roderer M, Stahl FJI, Raju PA, et al: Cytokine-stimulated human immunodeficiency virus replication is inhibited by N-acetyl-L-cysteine. PNAS 87:4884-4888, 1990
45. Sarin PS, Gallo RC, Scheer DI, et al: Effects of a novel compound (AL721) on HTLV-III infectivity in vitro. N Engl J Med 313:1289-1290, 1985
46. Strieter RM, Remick DG, Ward PA, et al: Cellular and molecular regulation of tumor necrosis facter-alpha production by pentoxifylline. Biochem Biophys Res Commun 155:1230-1236, 1988
47. Treatment Issues: The GMHC newsletter of experimental AIDS therapies. New York, GMHC.
48. Tsang PH, Tangnavarad S, Solomon S, Bekesi JG: Modulation of T- and B-lymphocyte functions by isoprinosine in homosexual subjects with prodomata and patients with acquired immune deficiency syndrome (AIDS). J Clin Immunol 4:469, 1984
49. Volberding PA, Lagakos SW, Koch MA, et al: Zidovudine in asymptomatic human immunode-ficiency virus infection. A controlled trial in persons with fewer than 500 CD4-positive cells per cubic millimeter. N Engl J Med 322:941-949, 1990

50. Wallis C: Why new age medicine is catching on. Time 38(18):68-76, 1991
51. Wybran J, Appelboom T, Famaey JP, Govaerts A: Suggestive evidence for receptors for morphins and methionine-enkephalin on normal human blood T lymphocytes. J Immunol 123:1068-1070, 1979
52. Yarchoan R, Mitsuya M, Thomas RV, et al: In vivo activity against HIV and favorable toxicity profile of 2′,3′-dideoxyinosine. Science 245:412-415, 1989

9

DRUG INTERACTIONS AND TOXICITIES IN PATIENTS WITH AIDS

BELLE L. LEE, Pharm D
SHARON SAFRIN, MD

The potential for drug interactions leading to adverse reactions is great in patients with AIDS, since multiple drugs are commonly prescribed to these patients. In addition, patients with AIDS have a higher incidence of adverse reactions to drugs that are commonly used in the treatment of opportunistic infections than non-AIDS patients have. As a result of the high rate of adverse reactions, use of currently available drugs often is limited. An appreciation of the potential drug interactions and knowledge of the most frequently occurring adverse reactions can increase the chance of a successful therapeutic response.

DRUGS USED TO TREAT *PNEUMOCYSTIS CARINII* PNEUMONIA (see Chapter 17)

Trimethoprim-Sulfamethoxazole, Trimethoprim-Dapsone

Trimethoprim-sulfamethoxazole therapy has been associated with adverse effects in up to 100% of patients with AIDS.[24,36,70] Medina et al.[49] reported that 57% of patients with AIDS receiving trimethoprim-sulfamethoxazole developed major toxicity requiring a change of therapy to pentamidine as compared to 30% of those receiving trimethoprim-dapsone (Table 9–1). The incidence of minor toxicities was equal in both groups, with 2.7 reactions occurring per patient, but mild elevation of alanine aminotransferase or aspartate aminotransferase levels (to five times normal) or neutropenia (<50% baseline value) was more common in the group assigned to trimethoprim-sulfamethoxazole. Hyperkalemia (5 to 6.1 mmol/L) occurred sig-

Portions of this chapter appeared previously in *Clinical Infectious Diseases,* March 1992, published by The University of Chicago Press, and *Current Opinion in Infectious Diseases,* April 1992, published by Current Science.

Table 9–1. Outcome of Treatment and Major Adverse Drug Reactions Requiring Discontinuation of Study Drugs*

VARIABLE	TRIMETHOPRIM-DAPSONE (N = 30) No. (%)	TRIMETHOPRIM-SULFAMETHOXAZOLE (N = 30) No. (%)
Treatment failure	2 (7)	3 (10)
Adverse reaction	9 (30)	17 (57)[†]
ALT or AST greater than five times normal	1 (3)	6 (20)[‡]
Neutropenia (<750 neutrophils/μl)	1 (3)	5 (17)[§]
Thrombocytopenia (<40.000 platelets/μl)	1 (3)	1 (3)
Intolerable rash	3 (10)	3 (10)
Nausea and vomiting	2 (7)	2 (7)
Decline in hematocrit concentration by ≥25%	0 (0)	0 (0)
Methemoglobinemia >20%	1 (3)	0 (0)
Days to onset of reaction—mean (range)	10.3 (9-13)	12.5 (8-17)

Reprinted with permission from Medina I, Mills J, Leoung G, et al: N Engl J Med 323:778, 1990.
*P, ≥0.1 for all comparisons between groups except as noted; ALT denotes alanine aminotransferase and AST, aspartate aminotransferase.
[†]*P*, 0.025.
[‡]*P*, 0.05.
[§]*P*, 0.08.

nificantly more frequently in the trimethoprim-dapsone group, occurring in 16 (53%) of these patients as compared to six (20%) of the trimethoprim-sulfamethoxazole patients (*p* <0.001).

Concurrent use of dapsone and trimethoprim increases the plasma concentrations of both drugs, possibly as a result of an inhibition or competition of renal secretion of these drugs.[45] Rifampin can decrease the half-life of dapsone as a result of enzyme induction, and probenecid can cause a significant reduction in the urinary excretion of dapsone.[74] Drug interactions reported with use of trimethoprim-sulfamethoxazole include warfarin (increased prothrombin time),[55] procainamide (decreased clearance of procainamide),[35] and phenytoin (increased half-life of phenytoin).[71] The prothrombin time or the concentrations of these drugs should be monitored closely when they are given concurrently with trimethoprim-sulfamethoxazole.

Pentamidine

The use of intravenous pentamidine is limited by the high frequency of adverse reactions. Nephrotoxicity can range from mild azotemia to severe tubular necrosis.[38] Both hypoglycemia and hyperglycemia have been associated with pentamidine therapy; the latter often is not reversible. This toxicity probably is caused by a direct cytolytic effect of pentamidine on the beta islet cells of the pancreas. One report found the risk of hypoglycemia is increased with higher doses of pentamidine, prolonged therapy, or retreatment within 3 months.[69] Other complications include elevation in liver enzymes, hyperkalemia, leukopenia, thrombocytopenia, acute pancreatitis, and ventricular arrhythmias.[58,70] Rapid infusion of pentamidine can result in a precipitous drop in blood pressure.

Aerosolized pentamidine is generally free of all but local (bronchospastic) complications; however, acute pancreatitis[26] and mild hypoglycemia have been reported in association with this therapy. In addition, an increased risk of spontaneous pneumothorax has occurred.[52]

Clindamycin

Gastrointestinal side effects, particularly diarrhea and nausea, are the most frequent adverse reactions associated with use of clindamycin. In retrospective and prospective studies the frequency of clindamycin-associated diarrhea has varied from 0.3% to 21% and of pseudomembranous colitis, from 1.9% to 10%.[37] Diarrheal side effect is more common with oral than with parenteral therapy. Rash may also occur in association with clindamycin therapy; in clinical trials of the combination of clindamycin with primaquine for the treatment of acute *Pneumocystis carinii* pneumonia, rash was the most common side effect (61%), followed by diarrhea (17%), elevation in serum transaminases, and mild methemoglobinemia.[5,57] In only 2% were these side effects dose limiting. A recent trial of clindamycin for prophylaxis against *Toxoplasma gondii* infection in 52 HIV-infected patients with a CD4 cell count <200 mm^3 was halted prematurely because of diarrhea (30.8%) and rash (21.2%).[31] Although isolated cases of reversible neutropenia have been reported with use of clindamycin, this drug is generally not myelosuppressive and apparently does not enhance zidovudine hematologic toxicity. Mean half-life, peak concentration, and area under the curve of zidovudine are unchanged by clindamycin.[32]

Use of neuromuscular blocking agents in combination with clindamycin may result in skeletal muscle weakness and/or respiratory depression caused by enhancement of neuromuscular blockade.[67] Use of kaolin- or attapulgite-containing antidiarrheals can decrease oral absorption of clindamycin; any antiperistaltic agent can prolong or worsen pseudomembranous colitis by delaying the elimination of toxin. Erythromycin can displace clindamycin from its ribosomal binding site; therefore concurrent use is not recommended.

Primaquine

Hemolysis can occur with administration of primaquine and is particularly severe in patients with substantial deficiency of the glucose-6-phosphate dehydrogenase enzyme. Methemoglobinemia may also result, particularly with the use of high doses of primaquine or in patients with NADH methemoglobin reductase deficiency. More rarely, granulocytopenia or gastrointestinal disturbances occur.[48]

DRUGS USED TO TREAT FUNGAL INFECTIONS
(see Chapter 19)

Fluconazole

Fluconazole given either orally or intravenously is generally well tolerated. In approximately 4000 patients treated with fluconazole, the overall incidence of side effects was 16%.[25] Hepatotoxicity and exfoliative skin disorders are rare occurrences with fluconazole treatment.

There are several potential drug interactions with fluconazole.[44] Coadministration of fluconazole and cyclosporin A may lead to the accumulation of cyclosporin A, and monitoring of cyclosporine A level is recommended.[44] Rifampin decreases the half-life of fluconazole; thus increasing the dosage of fluconazole may be necessary when coadministered with rifampin.[11,44] Concomitant administration of fluconazole and phenytoin results in a clinically significant increase in the phenytoin concentrations.[7,44] Serum concentrations of phenytoin therefore should be closely monitored, and the necessity of modifying the dosage of phenytoin for patients being treated with fluconazole should be anticipated. Concurrent use of fluconazole with tolbutamide, chlorpropamide, glyburide, and glipizide[25,44] has increased the plasma concentrations of these sulfonylureas, and hypoglycemia has been noted; blood glucose concentrations should be monitored, and reduction in the dose of the oral hypoglycemic may be necessary. Concurrent use of warfarin with fluconazole may decrease the metabolism of warfarin, resulting in an increase in prothrombin time.[44] Prothrombin time must be carefully monitored in patients receiving warfarin or a coumarin-type anticoagulant.

Ketoconazole

Nausea and vomiting commonly occur with ketoconazole administration. The drug may be given with food, but absorption is reduced. Reversible hepatitis has been observed and apparently is not dose related. Adrenal suppression and gynecomastia have been reported and probably are due to inhibition of steroid synthesis.[4]

Plasma levels of ketoconazole are markedly reduced when the drug is administered with either cimetidine or antacids.[6,44] Since bioavailability of oral ketoconazole is reduced in patients with AIDS, largely as a result of gastric hypochlorhydria,[41] drug administration should occur at least 2 hours before antacid administration or in an acidic fluid such as fruit juice. Coadministration of cyclosporin A and ketoconazole significantly increases the serum levels and prolongation of the half-life of cyclosporin A.[44] Coadministration of ketoconazole and phenytoin may alter the disposition of both drugs.[44] Concomitant administration of rifampin and ketoconazole results in a marked decrease (80%) in ketoconazole levels,[44] so coadministration of the two should be avoided.

Amphotericin B (Liposomal and Lipid Complex)

Liposomal and lipid-complex drug delivery systems are being developed to enhance the therapeutic activity and to decrease the toxicity of amphotericin B. Toxic reactions associated with both amphotericin B and liposomal amphotericin B therapy in humans include fever, chills, nausea, electrolyte imbalance, and renal toxicity (Table 9–2). Liposomal amphotericin B infusion may also lead to cardiopulmonary toxic effects.[47]

Caution must be taken to monitor the serum potassium concentration when digitalis and amphotericin are coadministered. Carbenicillin or ticarcillin given concomitantly with amphotericin B may also exacerbate hypokalemia. Amphotericin

Table 9–2.   Antifungal Medications

DRUG	SIDE EFFECTS	INTERACTIONS
Fluconazole	Nausea Headache Skin rash Abdominal pain Vomiting/diarrhea	Serum levels of cyclosporin A, phenytoin, and oral hypoglycemics increase Rifampin decreases half-life of fluconazole Metabolism of warfarin decreases and prothrombin time increases
Ketoconazole	Nausea Vomiting Hepatitis Adrenal suppression Gynecomastia	Cimetidine and antacids decrease plasma levels of ketoconazole Cyclosporin A levels increase
Amphotericin B	Fever Chills Nausea Electrolyte disturbances Renal toxicity	Hypokalemia may develop when administered in combination with digitalis, carbenicillin, and ticarcillin Additive renal toxicity with aminoglycosides
Flucytosine	Nausea Vomiting Agranulocytosis Aplastic anemia	Additive hematologic toxicity when administered in combination with other bone marrow toxic drugs.

B administered with either miconazole or ketoconazole may be less effective than amphotericin alone.[66] Nephrotoxicity attributed to the concurrent use of gentamicin and amphotericin B has been described in four patients.[65] Both antibiotics are nephrotoxic and may have additive toxic effects when given in combination.

Flucytosine

Nausea and vomiting occur frequently with flucytosine administration; spacing ingestion in 5- to 10-minute intervals may help alleviate this problem. The hematologic toxicity is believed to be dose related, and excessive serum levels are associated with signs of bone marrow toxicity. Agranulocytosis and aplastic anemia have been reported. Hepatic necrosis has been reported but is rare and is apparently dose related also.[4]

DRUGS USED TO TREAT TOXOPLASMOSIS (see Chapter 21)

Pyrimethamine, Sulfadiazine

Treatment with pyrimethamine and sulfadiazine for *Toxoplasma* encephalitis is effective in 80% to 90% of patients.[14,46] Unfortunately, toxicity develops in 60% to 70% of patients and has resulted in the discontinuation of therapy in 30% to 45% of patients.[27,46] Adverse reactions include severe rash, leukopenia, thrombocytopenia, and elevated liver enzyme levels.[27,46] Because therapy for toxoplasmosis in patients with AIDS is lifelong, bone marrow toxicity may also preclude therapy with antiviral agents such as zidovudine. In addition, there is some evidence that zidovudine antagonizes the antitoxoplasma activity of pyrimethamine.[30] Sulfadiazine-induced crystalluria has been described in patients with AIDS.[51]

Serious pancytopenia and megaloblastic anemia have been reported in patients under treatment with pyrimethamine and either trimethoprim-sulfamethoxazole or other sulfonamides.[65] The additive adverse reactions seem to reflect a depression of the normal folate metabolism caused by the combined actions of both drugs. Hematologic parameters should be monitored closely if both drugs are given simultaneously.

Clindamycin

See under "Drugs Used to Treat *Pneumocystis carinii* Pneumonia."

DRUGS USED TO TREAT *MYCOBACTERIUM TUBERCULOSIS* INFECTION (see Chapter 18)

Isoniazid

Isoniazid frequently causes a rise in serum transaminases, although clinical hepatitis is rare. The frequency of hepatotoxicity rises proportionally with the age of the individual ($\leq 0.3\%$ in persons <35 years of age, $\leq 2.3\%$ in persons >50 years of age); in addition, risk is increased in persons who are rapid acetylators of the drug, in those who ingest alcohol daily, (Table 9–3),[33] and in those with pre-existing liver disease who are taking rifampin concomitantly.

A pyridoxine-responsive peripheral neuropathy may occur; frequently it is greater in persons who acetylate the drug slowly[62] or who are malnourished. Rash and nausea may occur occasionally. Use of aluminum-containing antacids may decrease the absorption of isoniazid. Inhibition of hepatic microsomal enzymes by isoniazid can result in elevation of phenytoin, carbamazepine, coumarin-like anticoagulants, benzodiazepines, and theophylline serum levels.[37,67] Flushing may occur in some patients who ingest certain fish or cheese while receiving isoniazid because of inhibition of histamine metabolism by isoniazid.[37] Isoniazid may cause niacin deficiency by inhibiting niacin incorporation into nicotinamide adenine dinucleotide (NAD).[67] Increased metabolism of isoniazid, with resultant decreased effectiveness, may occur with alcohol ingestion or with concurrent use of prednisolone.

Rifampin

Hepatotoxicity caused by rifampin administration is relatively uncommon, occurring in $\leq 1\%$ of patients.[23] In the early weeks of therapy interference with excretion by rifampin may cause a transient elevation in serum bilirubin. A hypersensitivity syndrome comprised of flushing, fever, redness of the eyes, and thrombocytopenia may occur, generally within 3 hours of the ingestion of the drug,

Table 9–3.   Antimycobacterial Medications

DRUG	SIDE EFFECTS	INTERACTIONS
Isoniazid	Elevated liver function test results, especially with increasing age or daily alcohol intake	Absorption decreases with aluminum-containing antacids
	Peripheral neuropathy Nausea Rash	Serum levels of carbamazepine, coumarin, benzo-diazepines, theophylline, phenytoin elevate
Rifampin	Elevated liver function test results	Serum levels of ketoconazole and fluconazole decrease
	Discoloration of body secretions	Half-life of tolbutamide and of trimethoprim decreases
	Hypersensitivity syndrome	Serum levels of oral contraceptives, corticosteroids, cyclosporine, coumarin, methadone, theophylline, digoxin, levothyroxine, quinidine, propranolol, dapsone decrease
		Absorption with aminosalicylates decreases
Ethambutol	Retrobulbar neuritis Hyperuricemia	
Pyrazinamide	Elevated liver function test results	Half-life of probenecid increases
	Hyperuricemia Arthralgia Nausea	
Ciprofloxacin	Nausea	Serum levels of theophylline increase
	Diarrhea	Absorption with magnesium- or aluminum-containing antacids or with sucralfate decreases
Clofazimine	Skin discoloration Nausea Retinal degeneration	

particularly in patients receiving intermittent therapy.[23] Rifampin causes a reddish discoloration of body fluids such as urine, tears, and sweat.

Although early reports suggested that antituberculous medications were tolerated as well in HIV-infected patients as in others, more recent investigators have reported an increased frequency of adverse effects, particularly in association with rifampin administration. In one study adverse drug reactions to antituberculous medications occurred more frequently in patients with AIDS than in non-AIDS patients (26% versus 3%).[9] Another study found a frequency of side effects of 39% in HIV-infected patients compared with 22% of seronegative controls; the most frequent side effects were elevation in serum transaminase levels and fever.[63] In a third study 18% of patients required an alteration in antituberculous therapy because of adverse effects, substantially higher than the 3.7% rate reported from the same clinic in non–HIV-infected patients.[60] Twelve percent of adverse reactions were believed associated with rifampin therapy and consisted primarily of rash and hepatitis. In one patient life-threatening anaphylaxis was reported in association with ingestion of rifampin.[72] Nearly all major side effects occurred during the first 2 months of therapy.[60]

The area under the curve (AUC) of ketoconazole decreases by >80% when administered concurrently with rifampin, and serum levels of ketoconazole decrease,[18] causing the Food and Drug Administration to recommend that the two drugs not be administered together.[44] Concurrent administration of fluconazole with rifampin also results in a decrease in the AUC and half-life of fluconazole[11]; however, the magnitude of change is considerably smaller (~23%). Thus administering fluconazole together with rifampin is acceptable, although an increase in the dosage of fluconazole may be necessary.[44]

The half-life of oral hypoglycemic agents such as tolbutamide is shortened with concurrent administration of rifampin.[37] Induction of liver enzymes by rifampin may cause increased metabolism of oral contraceptive agents, corticosteroids, cyclosporine, coumarin-like anticoagulants, methadone, theophylline, levothyroxine, digoxin, quinidine, and propranolol, so that close observation, monitoring of serum levels if possible, and adjustment of dosage of these agents or identification of alternative agents for a given indication may be necessary in the patient receiving rifampin.[37] A similar mechanism of interaction may cause a sevenfold to tenfold decrease in serum levels of dapsone when administered concurrently with rifampin; however, this decrease was not believed to be clinically important when its use was evaluated in patients with leprosy.[56]

Aminosalicylates may impair the absorption of rifampin, resulting in decreased serum concentrations; for this reason ingestion of the two should be separated by at least 6 hours. Concurrent use of rifampin and trimethoprim may significantly increase the rate of clearance and shorten the elimination half-life of trimethoprim.[65]

Ethambutol

Retrobulbar neuritis is the main complication of ethambutol therapy; symptoms include central scotomata, red-green color blindness, and blurred vision. This complication is dose related, occurring in ~5% of patients receiving 25 mg/kg/day and rarely if at all in patients receiving 15 mg/kg/day.[61] It apparently is not related to the cumulative dose of drug administered. Hyperuricemia occasionally occurs.

Pyrazinamide

The most important side effect associated with pyrazinamide therapy is hepatotoxicity; however, the risk for it is small and is related to administration of large doses of the drug (40 to 50 mg/kg/day) for prolonged periods of time. There is no apparent additive risk for hepatotoxicity when pyrazinamide is administered in combination with isoniazid and rifampin. The other main side effect is arthralgia, associated with the increased serum levels of uric acid due to suppression of urinary secretion and excretion. Acute gouty arthritis, however, is rare. Nausea and/or vomiting may occur, although rarely.[1]

Pyrazinamide causes a prolonged half-life of probenecid, so its suppression of urate excretion may be neutralized. Rifampin may enhance the renal excretion of uric acid, both in the presence and absence of pyrazinamide.[65]

DRUGS USED TO TREAT *MYCOBACTERIUM AVIUM* COMPLEX INFECTION (see Chapter 18)

Rifampin

See under "Drugs Used to Treat *Mycobacterium Avium Tuberculosis* infection."

Ethambutol

See under "Drugs Used to Treat *Mycobacterium tuberculosis* infection."

Ciprofloxacin

Nausea, vomiting, diarrhea, and abdominal pain are the most common adverse reactions associated with ciprofloxacin treatment (up to 10%).[8] Stimulatory effects on the central nervous system such as anxiety, nervousness, insomnia, euphoria, and tremor occur in 1% to 4% of patients. Seizures have been reported with ciprofloxacin, and it should be used with caution in epileptic patients. Hallucinations are reported rarely in patients administered ciprofloxacin. Theophylline serum levels can markedly increase in some patients with concurrent use of ciprofloxacin[8]; therefore theophylline levels should be monitored in patients who receive theophylline and ciprofloxacin concurrently. Simultaneous administration of antacids containing magnesium and/or aluminum hydroxide with ciprofloxacin leads to a reduction in the bioavailability of the latter.[53] It is believed that ciprofloxacin forms insoluble chelates with aluminum and magnesium ions in the gut, reducing absorption. This interaction is of potential concern not only in patients using antacids for gastrointestinal symptoms, but also in patients with compromised renal function and on hemodialysis or continuous ambulatory peritoneal dialysis who utilize antacids as phosphate binders. Sucralfate can significantly reduce ciprofloxacin concentrations, and the two drugs should not be administered concurrently.[22]

Clofazimine

Clofazimine therapy is generally tolerated well in the doses administered to treat *M. avium* complex infection (50 to 100 mg daily). Adverse reactions include a reversible discoloration of the skin and body fluids, gastrointestinal intolerance, and visceral deposition of crystal.[29] Generalized retinal degeneration believed due to clofazimine has been described recently, so visual acuity should be closely monitored in patients receiving long-term therapy.[13] In six male patients with leprosy who received rifampin in conjunction with clofazimine, a statistically significant reduction in the rate of rifampin absorption and time to reach maximum serum concentration was noted[21]; however, since bioavailability was unaffected, the interaction probably is not clinically significant.

DRUGS USED FOR CYTOMEGALOVIRUS INFECTION (see Chapter 23)

Ganciclovir

The most frequent toxicities occurring with ganciclovir therapy are those involving the hematopoietic system; in particular, neutropenia and/or thrombocytopenia may occur and are generally reversible with discontinuation of ganciclovir therapy. Although the incidence of lowering of the granulocyte count is approximately 40%, this is a dose-limiting problem in <20% of individuals.[67] Thrombocytopenia may also occur, although less frequently (incidence, ~20%; dose-limiting frequency, 5% to 10%).

In several reports coadministration of ganciclovir with zidovudine has resulted in additive hematologic toxicity[28,50]; many patients are unable to tolerate these two drugs in combination. Less frequent drug interactions include the occurrence of generalized seizures in six patients receiving imipenem-cilastatin concurrently with ganciclovir and a reduction in renal clearance because of inhibition of renal tubular secretion by probenecid.

Table 9-4.   Antiviral Medications

DRUG	SIDE EFFECTS	INTERACTIONS
Zidovudine	Neutropenia Anemia	Additive hematologic toxicity when administered in combination with ganciclovir Probenecid increases zidovudine serum levels
Dideoxyinosine (ddI)	Pancreatitis Peripheral neuropathy Diarrhea Transaminase elevation	May cause decreased absorption of drugs that require gastric acidity (e.g., dapsone, ketoconazole) May cause decreased absorption of tetracycline or quinolone antibiotics
Acyclovir	Nausea Nephrotoxicity Neurologic toxicity	
Ganciclovir	Neutropenia Thrombocytopenia	Additive hematologic toxicity when administered in combination with azido-chymidine (AZT) Increases risk of seizures when administered in combination with imipenem-cilastatin
Foscarnet	Nephrotoxicity Hypocalcemia/hypercalcemia Hyperphosphatemia Anemia Nausea/vomiting Transaminase elevation Neurologic toxicity Penile ulcerations	Possible additive nephrotoxicity when administered in combination with other nephrotoxic agents Increases risk of hypocalcemia when administered with pentamidine

Foscarnet

The spectrum of potential toxicities associated with foscarnet therapy is broad (Table 9–4). Impairment in renal function is the most common dose-limiting toxicity, is generally reversible, and is often associated with proteinuria. Postmortem studies of patients with acute renal failure occurring in association with foscarnet therapy have demonstrated acute tubular necrosis or tubular interstitial nephritis.[54] In several patients crystals have been demonstrated in the glomerular capillaries.[3] Polydipsia and polyuria due to nephrogenic diabetes insipidus have also been described.[19] Recent investigations have suggested that careful adjustment of dosage according to serial serum creatinine and weight determinations and hydration with normal saline solution as an adjunct to foscarnet infusion may prevent renal toxicity in most patients.[16] In addition, the avoidance of concomitant administration of other drugs with nephrotoxic potential such as pentamidine, aminoglycosides, and amphotericin B has been recommended.

Serum calcium levels may either rise or decrease during foscarnet administration; chelation of ionized calcium is believed to occur, especially after larger doses. Concomitant treatment with pentamidine administration in one case series of four patients resulted in severe symptomatic hypocalcemia.[73] Also, hyperphosphatemia is a relatively common occurrence in patients receiving foscarnet (although generally not a cause of adverse symptoms); possible explanations include the replacement of phosphorous in bone by foscarnet and the inhibition of sodium and phosphate transport across renal tubular membranes.[10]

DRUGS FOR HERPES SIMPLEX AND VARICELLA ZOSTER VIRUS INFECTION (see Chapter 23)

Acyclovir

Acyclovir is, in general, a remarkably well-tolerated agent. When administered orally (2 to 4 g/day), the most frequent adverse effects are nausea (2% to 8%) and headache (0.6% to 6%); rarely are side effects dose limiting. High-dose intravenous infusion has been associated with transient rises in serum creatinine concentration. Dehydration, pre-existing renal insufficiency, and high-dose bolus infusion may predispose the patient to precipitation of the drug in the renal tubules, causing a reversible crystalline nephropathy.[17] Gastrointestinal symptoms may be associated with intravenous infusion as well, particularly when peak serum levels of acyclovir exceed 25 μg/ml.[2] Also, encephalopathic and/or neuropsychiatric changes have been sporadically noted in patients receiving intravenous acyclovir (~1%).[68]

Foscarnet

See under "Drugs Used to Treat Cytomegalovirus Infection."

ANTIRETROVIRAL AGENTS

Zidovudine

The major toxicities associated with zidovudine are neutropenia and anemia.[20] They are inversely related to the CD4 lymphocyte count, hemoglobin concentration, and granulocyte count and directly related to dosage and duration of therapy.[12] Significant anemia most commonly occurs after 4 to 6 weeks of therapy; other toxic symptoms include malaise or fatigue, dyspepsia, nausea, vomiting, and bloating.[20] Macular edema was described in one patient who was treated with zidovudine.[42]

The combination of zidovudine and ganciclovir is poorly tolerated in patients with AIDS and serious cytomegalovirus disease, with 82% developing severe to life-threatening hematologic toxicity.[28] It is thought that the toxicity is not a result of pharmacologic interaction but of a combined myelosuppressive toxicity of the two drugs; therefore close monitoring of hematologic parameters should accompany concurrent administration.

Probenecid inhibits hepatic glucuronidation and secretion of zidovudine through the renal tubules, resulting in increased serum concentrations and a prolonged elimination half-life.[15] These results may increase the risk of toxicity or permit a reduction in daily zidovudine dosage; however, one small trial observed a very high incidence of rash in patients receiving probenecid concurrently with zidovudine.[34]

2′,3′-Dideoxyinosine (ddI)

The major clinical toxicities associated with ddI therapy include pancreatitis and peripheral neuropathy. In a phase I study[43] reversible neuropathy was related to both daily dosage and to total dose of drug administered. The incidence of neuropathy was 34% of all phase I patients treated with doses at or below the currently recommended dose but 14.2% in controlled trials. In one study acute pancreatitis occurred in 5 of 37 (13.5%) patients[43] and was not clearly related to the dose of ddI. In the U.S. Expanded Access Program, 13.8% of 166 persons developed pancreatitis, of whom two died.[64] However, in randomized controlled trials, frequency of pancreatitis has been lower, approximately 2.3%. Predisposing factors to the development of pancreatitis with administration of ddI include a prior history of pancreatitis, advanced HIV disease, and low CD4 count ($<50/mm^3$). Preliminary reports suggest that concurrent administration of ganciclovir with ddI may increase the frequency of acute pancreatitis; however, this has not been well documented. Optic neuritis[39] and fulminant hepatitis[40] have been associated with ddI therapy. Other dose-limiting toxicities include elevation in liver function test results and abdominal pain. Diarrhea may occur but does so less frequently with the new buffered tablets than with the powdered preparation.

The manufacturers of ddI recommend that drugs that require an acidic environment for absorption (e.g., ketoconazole, dapsone) be ingested at least 2 hours before ddI because the buffered vehicle for ddI (i.e., a magnesium-aluminum antacid) produces an acutely alkaline gastric environment that may decrease the absorption of other drugs. Also, it is recommended that ddI not be ingested concurrently with tetracycline or the quinolone antibiotics because of concerns about their decreased absorption.

Because food reduces the bioavailability of ddI twofold, it is recommended that ddI be given under fasting conditions.[59]

REFERENCES

1. Alford RH: Antimycobacterial agents. In Mandell GL, Douglas RG, Bennett JE, eds. Anti-Infective Therapy. New York, John Wiley & Sons, 1985, p 290
2. Bean B, Aeppli D: Adverse effects of high-dose intravenous acyclovir in ambulatory patients with acute herpes zoster. J Infect Dis 151:362, 1985
3. Beaufils H, Deray G, Katlana C, et al: Foscarnet and crystals in glomerular capillary lumens (letter). Lancet 336:755, 1990
4. Bennett JE: Antifungal agents. In Mandell GL, Douglas RG, Bennett JE, eds. Anti-Infective Therapy. New York, John Wiley & Sons, 1985, pp 307-324
5. Black JR, Feinberg J, Murphy RL, et al: Clindamycin and primaquine as primary treatment for mild and moderately severe *Pneumocystis carinii* pneumonia in patients with AIDS Eur J Clin Microbol Infect Dis 10:204-207, 1991
6. Blum RA, D'Andrea DT, Florentino BM, et al: Increased gastric pH and the bioavailability of fluconazole and ketoconazole. Ann Intern Med 114:755-757, 1991
7. Blum RA, Wilton JH, Hilligoss DM et al: Effect of fluconazole on the disposition of phenytoin. Clin Pharmacol Ther 49:420-425, 1991
8. Campoli-Richards DM, Monk JP, Price A, et al: Ciprofloxacin. A review of its antibacterial activity, pharmacokinetic properties and therapeutic use. Drugs 35:373-447, 1988
9. Chaisson RE, Schecter GF, Theuer CP, et al: Tuberculosis in patients with the acquired immunodeficiency syndrome: Clinical features, response to therapy and survival. Am Rev Respir Dis 136:570-574, 1987
10. Chrisp P, Clissold SP: Foscarnet: A review of its antiviral activity, pharmacokinetic properties and therapeutic use in immunocompromised patients with cytomegalovirus retinitis. Drugs 41:104-129, 1991
11. Coker RJ, Tomlinson DR, Parkin J, et al: Interaction between fluconazole and rifampicin. Br Med J 301:818, 1990
12. Collier AC, Bozzette S, Coombs RW, et al: To examine the vivo effect of acyclovir and a range of doses of zidovudine. N Engl J Med 323:1015-1021, 1990
13. Cunningham CA, Friedberg DN, Carr RE: Clofazamine-induced generalized retinal degeneration. Retina 10(2):131-134, 1990
14. Dannenman B, McCutchan JA, Israelski DM, et al: Treatment of toxoplasmic encephalitis in patients with AIDS. Ann Intern Med 116:33-43, 1992
15. De Miranda P, Good SS, Yarchoan R, et al: Alteration of zidovudine pharmacokinetics by probenecid in patients with AIDS or AIDS-related complex. Clin Pharmacol Ther 46:494-499, 1989
16. Deray G, Katlama C, Dohin E: Prevention of foscarnet nephrotoxicity (letter). Ann Intern Med 113:332, 1990
17. Dorsky DI, Crumpacker CS: Drugs five years later: Acyclovir. Ann Intern Med 107:859-874, 1987
18. Engelhard D, Stutman HR, Marks MI: Interaction of ketoconazole with rifampin and isoniazid. N Engl J Med 311:1681-1683, 1984
19. Farese RV Jr, Schambelan M, Hollander H, et al: Nephrogenic diabetes insipidus associated with foscarnet treatment of cytomegalovirus retinitis. Ann Intern Med 112:955-956, 1990
20. Fischl MA, Parker CB, Pettinelli C, et al: A randomized controlled trial of a reduced daily dose of zidovudine in patients with the acquired immunodeficiency syndrome. N Engl J Med 323:1009-1014, 1990

21. Garrelts JC: Clofazamine: A review of its use in leprosy and *Mycobacterium avium* complex infection. DICP 25:525-531, 1991

22. Garrelts JC, Godley PJ, Peterie JD, et al: Sucralfate significantly reduces ciprofloxacin concentrations in serum. Antimicrob Agents Chemother 34:931-933, 1990

23. Girling DJ: Adverse reactions to rifampicin in antituberculosis regimens. J Antimicrob Chemother 3:115, 1977

24. Gordin FM, Simon GL, Wofsy CB, Mills J: Adverse reactions to trimethoprim-sulfamethoxazole in patients with acquired immunodeficiency syndrome. Ann Intern Med 100:495-499, 1984

25. Grant SM, Clissold SP: Fluconazole. A review of its pharmacodynamics and pharmacokinetic properties, and therapeutic potential in superficial and systemic mycoses. Drugs 39(6):877-916, 1990

26. Hart CC: Aerosolized pentamidine and pancreatitis. Ann Intern Med 111:691, 1989

27. Haverkos HO: Assessment of therapy for toxoplasma encephalitis. The TE Study Group. Am J Med 82:907, 1987

28. Hochster H, Dieterich D, Bozzette S, et al: Toxicity of combined ganciclovir and zidovudine for cytomegalovirus disease associated with AIDS. Ann Intern Med 113:111-117, 1990

29. Hudson V, Cox F, Taylor L, et al: Pulmonary clofazamine crystals in a child with acquired immunodeficiency syndrome and disseminated *Mycobacterium avium-intracellulare* infection. Pediatr Infect Dis J 7(12):880-882, 1988

30. Israelski DM, Tom C, Remington JS: Zidovudine antagonizes the action of pyrimethamine in experimental infection with *Toxoplasma gondii*. Antimicrob Agents Chemother 33:30-34, 1988

31. Jacobson MA, Besch CL, Child C, et al: Randomized study of clindamycin or pyrimethamine prophylaxis for toxoplasmic encephalitis in patients with advanced HIV disease. Thirty-first Interscience Conference on Antimicrobial Agents and Chemotherapy. Abstract 298. Chicago, 1991

32. Jones DR, Black JR: Evaluation of pharmacokinetic interactions between the combination of primaquine plus clindamycin and zidovudine. Sixth International Conference on AIDS. (Abstract Th.B. 400.) San Francisco, 1990

33. Kopanoff DE, Snider DE Jr, Caras GJ: Isoniazid-related hepatitis: A U.S. Public Health Service cooperative surveillance study. Am Rev Respir Dis 117:991-1001, 1978

34. Kornhauser DM, Petty BG, Hendrix CW, et al: Probenecid and zidovudine metabolism. Br Med J 2:473-475, 1989

35. Kosoglou T, Rocci ML Jr, Vlasses PH: Trimethoprim alters the disposition of procainamide and N-acetylprocainamide. Clin Pharmacol Ther 44:467-477, 1988

36. Kovacs JA, Hiemenz JW, Macher AM, et al: *Pneumocystis carinii* pneumonia: A comparison between patients with the acquired immunodeficiency syndrome and patients with other immunodeficiencies. Ann Intern Med 100:663-671, 1984

37. Kucers A, Bennett N: The Use of Antibiotics. A Comprehensive Review With Clinical Emphasis, ed 4. Philadelphia, JB Lippincott Co, 1987

38. Lachaal M, Venuto RC: Nephrotoxicity and hyperkalemia in patients with acquired immunodeficiency syndrome treated with pentamidine. Am J Med 87:260-263, 1989

39. Lafeuillade A, Aubert L, Chaffanjon P, Quilichini R: Optic neuritis associated with dideoxyinosine. Lancet 337:615-616, 1991

40. Lai KK, Gang DL, Zawacki JK, Cooley TP: Fulminant hepatic failure associated with 2',3'-dideoxyinosine (ddI). Ann Intern Med 115:283-284, 1991

41. Lake-Bakaar G, Tom W, Lake-Bakaar D, et al: Gastropathy and ketoconazole malabsorption in the acquired immunodeficiency syndrome (AIDS). Ann Intern Med 109:471-473, 1988

42. Lalonde RG, Deschenes JG, Seamone C. Zidovudine-Induced macular edema. Ann Intern Med 114:297-298, 1991

43. Lambert JS, Seidlin M, Reichman RC, et al: 2',3'-Dideoxyinosine (ddI) in patients with the acquired immunodeficiency syndrome or AIDS-related complex. N Engl J Med 322:1333-1340, 1990

44. Lazar JD, Wilner KD: Drug interactions with fluconazole. Rev Infect Dis 12:327-333, 1990

45. Lee BL, Medina I, Benowitz NL, et al: Dapsone, trimethoprim and sulfamethoxazole plasma levels during treatment of *Pneumocystis* pneumonia in patients with acquired immunodeficiency syndrome: Evidence of drug interactions. Ann Intern Med 110:606-611, 1989

46. Leport C, Raffi F, Matheron S, et al: Treatment of central nervous system toxoplasmosis with pyrimethamine/sulfadiazine combination in 35 patients with the acquired immunodeficiency syndrome. Am J Med 84:94, 1988

47. Levine S, Walsh T, Martinez A, et al: Cardiopulmonary toxicity after liposomal amphotericin B infusion. Ann Intern Med 114:664-666, 1991

48. Marr JJ: Antiparasitic agents. In Mandell GL, Douglas RG, Bennett JE (eds). Anti-Infective Therapy. New York, John Wiley & Sons, 1985, pp 383-384

49. Medina I, Mills J, Leoung G, et al: Oral therapy for *Pneumocystis carinii* pneumonia in the acquired immunodeficiency syndrome. A controlled trial of trimethoprim-sulfamethoxazole versus dapsone-trimethoprim. N Engl J Med 323:776-782, 1990

50. Millar AB, Miller RF, Patou G, et al: Treatment of cytomegalovirus retinitis with zidovudine and ganciclovir in patients with AIDS: Outcome and toxicity. Genitourin Med 66:156-158, 1990

51. Molina J, Belenfant X, Doco-Lecompte T, et al: Sulfadiazine-induced crystalluria in AIDS patients with toxoplasma encephalitis. AIDS 5:587-589, 1991

52. Newsome GS, Ward DJ, Pierce PF: Spontaneous pneumothorax in patients with acquired immunodeficiency syndrome treated with prophylactic aerosolized pentamidine. Arch Intern Med 150:2167-2168, 1990

53. Nix DE, Watson WA, Lener ME, et al: Effects of aluminum and magnesium antacids and ranitidine on the absorption of ciprofloxacin. Clin Pharmacol Ther 46:700-705, 1989

54. Nyberg G, Blohme I, Persson H, Svalander C: Foscarnet-induced tubulointerstitial nephritis in renal transplant patients. Transplant Proc 22:241, 1990

55. O'Reilly RA, Motley CH: Racemic warfarin and trimethoprim-sulfamethoxazole interaction in humans. Ann Intern Med 91:34-36, 1979

56. Pieters FA, Woonick F, Zuidema J: Influence of once-monthly rifampicin and daily clofazamine on the pharmacokinetics of dapsone. Eur J Clin Pharmacol 34:73-76, 1988

57. Ruf B, Rohde I, Pohle HD: Efficacy of clindamycin/primaquine versus trimethoprim/sulfamethoxazole in primary treatment of *Pneumocystis carinii* pneumonia. Eur J Clin Microbiol Infect Dis 10:207-210, 1991

58. Sands M, Kron MA, Brown RB: Pentamidine: A review. Rev Infect Dis 7:625-634, 1985

59. Shyu WC, Knupp CA, Pittman KA, et al: Food-induced reduction in bioavailability of didanosine. Clin Pharmacol Ther 50:503-507, 1991

60. Small PM, Schecter GF, Goodman PC, et al: Treatment of tuberculosis in patients with advanced human immunodeficiency virus infection. N Engl J Med 324:289-294, 1991

61. Snider DE Jr: Pyridoxine supplementation during isoniazid therapy. Tubercle 61:191, 1980

62. Snider DE Jr, Long MW, Cross FS, Farer LS: Six-months isoniazid-rifampicin therapy for pulmonary tuberculosis. Report of a United States public health service cooperative trial. Am Rev Respir Dis 129:573, 1984

63. Soriano E, Mallolas J, Gatell JM, et al: Characteristics of tuberculosis in HIV-infected patients: A case control study. AIDS 2:429-432, 1988

64. Steinberg JP, Gunthel CJ, White RL, et al: Outcomes and toxicities on 2',3'-dideoxyinosine (ddI) in the expanded access program. Thirty-first Interscience Conference on Antimicrobial Agents and Chemotherapy. Abstract 707. Chicago, 1991

65. Stockley IH: Drug Interactions. A Source Book of Drug Interactions, Their Mechanisms, Clinical Importance and Management, ed 2. Oxford, Blackwell Scientific Publications, 1991

66. Sud IJ, Feingold DS: Effect of ketoconazole on the fungicidal action of amphotericin B in *Candida albicans*. Antimicrob Agents Chemotherapy 23:185-187, 1983

67. USP DI: Drug Information for the Health Care Professional, ed 11, vols IA and IB. The United States Pharmacopeial Convention, 1991

68. Wade JC, Meyers JD: Neurologic symptoms associated with parenteral acyclovir treatment after marrow transplantation. Ann Intern Med 98:921, 1983

69. Waskin H, Stehr-Green JK, Helmick CG, Sattler FR: Risk factors for hypoglycemia associated with pentamidine therapy for *Pneumocystis* pneumonia. JAMA 260:345-347, 1988

70. Wharton JM, Coleman DL, Wofsy CT, et al: Trimethoprim-sulfamethoxazole or pentamidine for *Pneumocystis carinii* pneumonia in the acquired immunodeficiency syndrome. Ann Intern Med 105:37-44, 1986

71. Wilcox JB: Phenytoin intoxication and co-trimoxazole (letter). NZ Med J 94:235-236, 1981

72. Wurtz RM, Abrams D, Becker S, et al: Anaphylactoid drug reactions to ciprofloxacin and rifampicin in HIV-infected patients (letter). Lancet 1:955-956, 1989.
73. Youle MS, Clarbour J, Gazzard B, Chanas A: Severe hypocalcemia in AIDS patients treated with foscarnet and pentamidine (letter). Lancet 1:1455-1456, 1988
74. Zuidema J, Hilbers-Modderman ESM, Merkus FWHM: Clinical pharmacokinetics of dapsone. Clin Pharmacokinet 11:299-315, 1936

10

DERMATOLOGIC CARE IN THE AIDS PATIENT

TIMOTHY G. BERGER, MD

Skin disease is an extremely common complication of HIV infection, affecting up to 90% of persons.[4] Some of the skin conditions also are commonly seen in uninfected persons (e.g., seborrheic dermatitis) but are of increased severity in the HIV-infected person. Other skin diseases are relatively unique to HIV infection (e.g., Kaposi's sarcoma [KS]). The average HIV-infected patient has at least two and often more different skin conditions simultaneously. It is useful to classify the cutaneous disorders seen with HIV disease as either infectious disorders, hypersensitivity disorders and drug reactions, or neoplasms. The treatment of these conditions is summarized in Table 10–1.

INFECTIOUS CUTANEOUS DISORDERS

Bacterial Infections

Staphylococcus aureus is the most common cutaneous bacterial pathogen.[6] The following patterns of staphylococcal infection may be seen: folliculitis, bullous impetigo, ecthyma, abscesses, hidradenitis suppurativa-like plaques, and cellulitis. Folliculitis is the most common form of staphylococcal infection seen in HIV-infected persons (Figure 10–1). The central trunk, groin, and face are the most common sites of infection. The primary lesion is a follicular pustule, but lesions may be almost urticarial. Many HIV-infected patients with staphylococcal folliculitis of the trunk have severe pruritus, which represents one of the more treatable pruritic eruptions seen in HIV disease.[6] Often many of the lesions are excoriated, and the patient must be carefully examined for a primary lesion adequate for culture. Bullous impetigo is quite common in the groin and axillae, presenting as flaccid blisters that quickly rupture, leaving small superficial erosions with a peripheral scale. The lesions are usually asymptomatic and occur more common during hot, humid weather. Ecthyma is a punched out ulcer with a sharp border. The base may be purulent or may be covered with a thick, adherent crust (Figure 10–2). Lesions are most common on the lower legs, commonly overlying a pre-existing dermatitis. Violaceous, tender cystic plaques and nodules in the axillae and groin may be due

145

Table 10–1.   Diagnosis and Treatment of Skin Conditions Commonly Seen with HIV Infection

CONDITION	MORPHOLOGY	LOCATION
Staphylococcal folliculitis	Erythematous follicular pustules or papules; may be pruritic	Face, trunk, groin
Bacillary angiomatosis	Friable, vascular papules, cellulitic plaques, subcutaneous nodules	Skin, bone, liver, spleen, lymph node
Herpes zoster (shingles)	Grouped vesicles on erythematous bases	Dermatomal distribution; may spill onto adjacent dermatomes
Herpes simplex	Grouped vesicles on erythematous bases, rapidly evolving into superficial mucocutaneous ulcerations or fissures; necrotizing ulcers may be seen when chronic	Face, hand, or anogenital area
Molluscum contagiosum	2-5 mm pearly flesh-colored papules, often with central umbilication	Face, anogenital area
Insect bite reactions	Erythematous, urticarial papules	Scabies: axillae, groin, finger webs Fleas: lower legs Mosquitoes: upper and lower extremities
Photosensitivity	Eczematous eruption	Face (tip of nose), extensor forearms, neck
Eosinophilic folliculitis	Urticarial follicular papules	Trunk, face
Seborrheic dermatitis	Fine, white scaling without erythema (dandruff) to patches and plaques of erythema with indistinct margins and yellowish, greasy scale	Scalp, central face, eyebrows, nasolabial and retroauricular folds, chest, upper back, axillae, groin
Psoriasis and Reiter's syndrome	Sharply marginated plaques with a silvery scale	Elbows, knees, lumbosacral area

TREATMENT	DURATION
Dicloxacillin, 500 mg PO q.i.d., *or* other penicillinase-resistant antistaphylococcal antibiotic	7-21 days
Refractory: add rifampin, 600 mg q.d. to above	First 5 days of antibiotic therapy with above
Erythromycin, 500 mg q.i.d.	Skin: 8 wk
or	
Doxycycline, 100 mg b.i.d.	Visceral: unknown, but consider 8-16 wk
Acute: acyclovir, 800 mg PO 5 times per day	7-10 days
Dissemination, severe immunosuppression, or involvement of ophthalmic branch of trigeminal nerve: acyclovir, 10 mg/kg IV q8h (corrected for creatinine clearance)	Give IV until no new blisters for 72 hr, then finish orally as above
Acute: acyclovir, 200-400 mg PO 5 times per day	7-10 days or until ulcers healed
Oral acyclovir failure or dissemination: acyclovir, 5 mg/kg IV q8hr (corrected for creatinine clearance)	
Maintenance: acyclovir, 200 mg PO t.i.d. or 400 mg, PO b.i.d.	Indefinitely
Acyclovir resistance: foscarnet	
Cryotherapy	For all treatments: repeat at 2- to 3-wk intervals until resolved
or	
Topical cantharidin sparingly, applied for 4-6 h to nonanogenital lesions and then washed off	
or	
Electrosurgery	
or	
Curettage	
Scabies: lindane 1% lotion for 12 hr; permethrine (Elimite) 5% lotion for 12 hr	Twice, 1 wk apart
Fleas, mosquitoes:	Constant, regular use
1. Insect repellants	
2. Antihistamines	
3. Insecticide spray of environment (fleas)	
1. Sun protection, sunscreens	Continuous for *1* and *2;* as needed for *3*
2. Discontinuation of photosensitizing medications	
3. Topical steroids	
Astemizole, 10 mg q.d.	Constant treatment
and	
Topical steroids	
or	
Ultraviolet light	
Hydrocortisone 2.5% cream and ketoconazole 2% cream applied b.i.d.	Until lesions resolve
Severe: ketoconazole, 200-400 mg PO q.d.	3-4 wk
Maintenance: Hydrocortisone 1% cream and ketoconazole 2% cream applied b.i.d.	Indefinitely
Triamcinolone acetonide 0.1% cream t.i.d.	Indefinitely

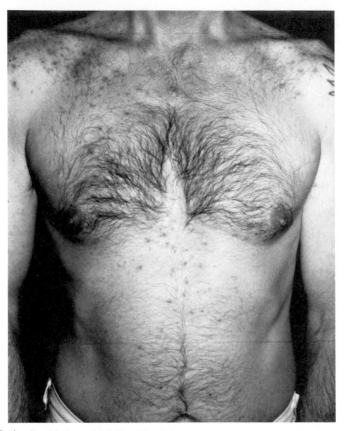

FIGURE 10–1.   Pruritic bacterial folliculitis of the trunk. *Staphylococcus aureus* was cultured from a lesion; the condition cleared with oral antibiotics.

to *S. aureus* alone, as are virtually all suppurative abscesses. All of the above patterns may be accompanied by an associated cellulitis.

The treatment of cutaneous staphylococcal infections is determined by the severity of the infection and the presence of systemic symptoms. Patients with chills, fever, large abscesses, or cellulitis are usually admitted for intravenous therapy. Abscesses should be incised and drained. Localized infection may be treated on an outpatient basis with oral agents once cultures are taken. Patients are reexamined after 3 to 5 days to ensure improvement and to confirm the appropriate antibiotic was chosen. A penicillinase-resistant penicillin or first-generation cephalosporine is the first choice for therapy. Since nasal carriage approaches 50% in these patients, rifampin (600 mg in a single daily dose for at least 5 days) may be added in refractory or relapsing cases. Use of benzoyl peroxide washes or antibacterial soaps may be beneficial to prevent relapse but should be accompanied by vigorous lubrication since dry skin is so common.

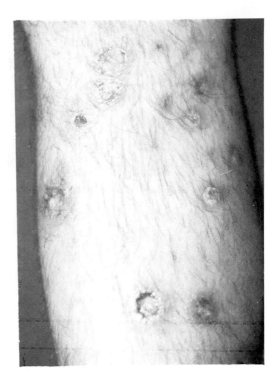

FIGURE 10–2. Ecthyma showing punched-out staphylococcal ulcers of the lower leg.

Bacillary angiomatosis is an uncommon subacute to chronic bacterial infection occurring most commonly in the setting of immune suppression, especially symptomatic HIV disease. The causative organism has been studied by DNA hybridization and membrane lipid analysis and is closely related to the agent causing trench fever, *Rochalimaea quintana*.[13,16] It has a similar degree of homology to *Bartonella bacilliformis* but seems less closely related to it. The bacillary angiomatosis agent is distinct from the closely related bacterium that causes cat-scratch disease.[3] The bacillary angiomatosis agent is extremely difficult to culture,[16] so the diagnosis is usually established by identifying the causative agent in affected tissue histopathologically.

The skin lesions have been the presentation most frequently published and are either friable vascular papules (like granulation tissue), subcutaneous nodules, or cellulitic plaques (Color plate II*A*). They can occur anywhere on the skin and on mucosal surfaces, especially respiratory tract and conjunctiva.

Visceral disease with or without skin lesions is common. Indicators of chronic infection such as fever, night sweats, anemia, or an elevated sedimentation rate are often present. The major forms of visceral disease are involvement of the liver and spleen (peliosis hepatis et splenis),[11] osteolytic bone lesions[1] (Figure 10–3), lymphadenopathy, and bacteremia.[16] Liver disease is the most common visceral disease and is characterized by hepatosplenomegaly, abdominal pain, and elevated liver function tests. Ultrasound may show echogenic lesions, and computerized tomog-

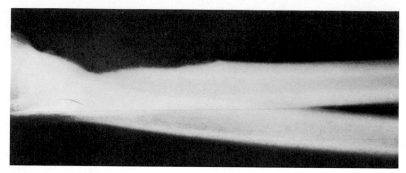

FIGURE 10–3. Osteolytic lesion of the distal radius due to bacillary angiomatosis. It healed totally with 4 months of oral erythromycin.

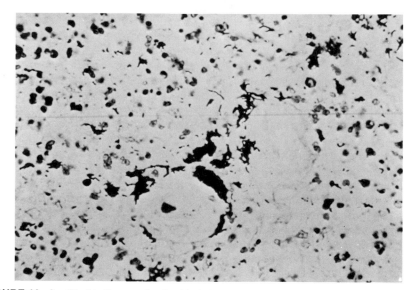

FIGURE 10–4. Warthin-Starry stain of a skin lesion of bacillary angiomatosis demonstrating slender bacilli in a perivascular extracellular location.

raphy demonstrates heterogeneity of the liver parenchyma. Bone lesions occur in approximately 10% of patients and may appear up to a year before other organ involvement. They are seen initially as painful, osteolytic foci, most commonly of the long bones, especially the tibia. *Subacute osteomyelitis in the HIV-infected persons should be considered bacillary angiomatosis until proved otherwise.*

The diagnosis of bacillary angiomatosis should be considered in any HIV-infected person with bacteremia, vascular lesions of the skin, viscera, or bone. A biopsy from any affected tissue should be performed. The pathology of the skin and visceral lesions is that of vascular proliferation, with marked edema and infiltration with many polymorphonuclear leukocytes. This may be initially mistaken for KS or a pyogenic granuloma.

To confirm the diagnosis, the tissue biopsy should be examined with a Warthin-Starry stain or by electron microscopy (Figure 10–4). Often the most direct approach to establish the diagnosis is to seek consultation from a dermatopathologist who has experience with this disease. The University of California at San Francisco (UCSF) and several other centers are actively studying bacillary angiomatosis in an attempt to identify the causative agent and the source of the infection. We would appreciate being contacted at San Francisco General Hospital (415-206-6099) if you know of a case, preferably before treatment is begun.

It is critical to establish this diagnosis since bacillary angiomatosis which is easily treated, can be fatal if untreated. The treatment of choice is erythromycin orally at a dose of 500 mg four times daily. Doxycycline at an oral dose of 100 mg twice daily has also been effective in patients intolerant of erythromycin. The penicillins, cephalosporins, and ciprofloxacin have not been effective in our experience. Although skin lesions usually resolve with 2 to 3 weeks of treatment, a minimum of 6 to 8 weeks of treatment is recommended, even if only cutaneous involvement is found. Visceral disease probably should be treated longer—2 to 4 months. If treated adequately, relapses usually do not occur, and chronic therapy is not required in most cases.

Viral Infections

The herpes viruses are the most common cutaneous viral pathogens, with herpes simplex virus (HSV) and varicella-zoster virus causing the majority of infections (see Chapter 23). **Herpes zoster** commonly occurs during the asymptomatic period of HIV disease.[9] Any person, especially anyone less than 65 years of age, who develops shingles should be queried about risk factors for HIV infection. Usually the course of herpes zoster is uneventful, although persistent postherpetic neuralgia may occur. In patients with more advanced HIV disease, herpes zoster may be very painful, severe, and prolonged. Dissemination may occur but is usually limited to skin. In my experience, disseminated herpetic lesions are almost always due to varicella zoster, not HSV.

Herpes simplex infections occur in the genital, digital, and orofacial areas. Any persistent, nonhealing ulcer in an HIV-infected person must be suspected of being HSV related. It is not unusual for secondary infection of lesions to occur, so cultures may yield *S. aureus* or other pathogens. A viral culture or fluorescent antibody examination should be performed. If its result is negative, a biopsy of the edge of the ulcer should be considered. It is sometimes impossible clinically to diagnose chronic ulcerations in HIV-infected persons, and multiple cultures and skin biopsy may be required.

Molluscum contagiosum is extremely common in patients with symptomatic HIV disease. Lesions are seen as umbilicated, pearly 2- to 5-mm papules on the face and genital area and scattered on the trunk (Figure 10–5). Lesions have a particular predilection for the eyelids. Lesions may number from one to hundreds. Occasional lesions may exceed 1 cm (giant molluscum). Their pearly border and telangiectasias may lead to the misdiagnosis of basal cell carcinoma. Complete eradication is extremely difficult.

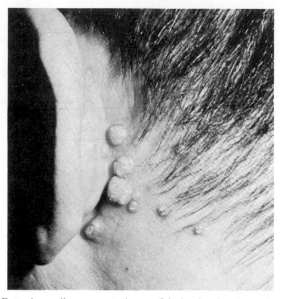

FIGURE 10–5.   Extensive molluscum contagiosum of the head and neck, an almost certain indication of advanced HIV disease with a helper T-cell count of less than 200.

Lesions are usually treated with destructive modalities (cryotherapy with liquid nitrogen, light electrocautery, or curettage). Topical retinoic acid (Retin-A) applied once nightly to the face may slow down the rate of appearance but unless applied to the point of severe irritation does little for established lesions. It cannot be used on the eyelids or genitalia. Disseminated cryptococcosis has mimicked molluscum contagiosum.[5]

HYPERSENSITIVITY DISORDERS

This section discusses those disorders that cause the pruritic eruptions so common in patients with HIV disease. Many of these disorders are poorly characterized, their pathogenesis not understood, and the optimum treatments unknown.[2] Excluding drug reactions, I believe the ability to diagnose half of the pruritic eruptions seen with HIV disease is quite good for our current state of knowledge.

Drug Reactions

It has been long recognized that approximately 50% of persons treated with trimethoprim-sulfamethoxazole (TMP-SMX) for *Pneumocystis* pneumonia will develop a widespread maculopapular eruption[7] (Color plate II*B*). The rash may resolve with continued treatment but often persists or progresses with continuation (see

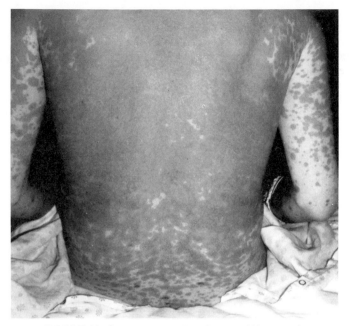

FIGURE 10–6. Drug-induced erythema multiforme major.

Chapter 9). Similar reactions are seen as a result of virtually all the other medications given to HIV-infected persons. Reactions are most common with use of antibiotics, especially the penicillins, and sulfa drugs. Cutaneous reactions are quite rare with use of certain frequently used medications, especially acyclovir and zidovudine. Whether HIV-infected persons have a higher rate of reaction to drugs other than TMP-SMT is unknown. In addition to maculopapular reactions, urticaria, erythema multiforme, and fixed drug eruptions may occur. In some patients the erythema multiforme may be quite severe, appearing as Stevens-Johnson syndrome or toxic epidermal necrolysis (Figure 10–6). These severe reactions are most commonly due to the sulfa drugs and anticonvulsants used to treat central nervous system (CNS) toxoplasmosis or *Pneumocystis* pneumonia.[12] Any HIV-infected person with a widespread eruption should be evaluated carefully for the possibility of its being medication induced.

Insect Bite Reactions

Scabies, flea bites, and mosquito bites can all be extremely florid in a patient with HIV disease. These eruptions present as nonfollicular papules to cellulitic plaques with marked pruritus. The nature of the offending arthropod is determined by the distribution of the eruption and identified biting insects in the patient's environment. In San Francisco fleas are a common cause of lower-leg pruritic papules, nodules, and blisters. In Miami mosquitoes are the most important cause of pruritic papules of the extremities.[10] In all patients the finger webs, genitalia, axillae, and feet should be examined carefully for lesions. When lesions are found in these areas, they should be scraped to search for scabetic mites. Scabies is spread by close personal contact, so the affected person must also be examined for sexually transmitted diseases. Treatment of scabies is by standard methods. A newly released scabicide, 5% permethrin (Elimite, Herbert Laboratories), has been effective in treating the patients who fail lindane treatment. It should be used instead of crotamiton (Eurax) as second-line therapy.

Other insect bite reactions are treated by three steps: (1) *Eliminate the biting insects* from the patient's environment with insecticides; (2) *make the patient less attractive to the insect* by using insect repellents (e.g., Avon's Skin-So-Soft, products containing diethyltoluamide [DEET]), and (3) *block the patient's reaction to the bite* with potent antihistamines taken regularly—not as needed. At least a generous nightly dose should be given (e.g., hydroxyzine, 50 to 75 mg), with additional doses given during the day if it is inadequate. Longer-acting antihistamines may be more beneficial (e.g., terfenadine, astemizole, or doxepin). Persistent pruritic papules are treated with medium- to high-potency topical steroids until they resolve.

Photosensitivity

The presence of HIV disease alone or the medications HIV-infected patients take can lead to cutaneous eruptions predominantly in sun-exposed areas, that is, photodermatitis.[17] These eruptions initially may resemble an enhanced sunburn but may progress or initially appear as pruritic scaly patches. They are frequently excoriated, become thickened, and often are hypopigmented (Figure 10–7). With time the eruptions may extend to unexposed skin. Short-wave ultraviolet irradiation (UVB) is the precipitating spectrum, but longer-wave irradiation (UVA) that comes through window glass may also induce photodermatitis. Photodermatitis is managed by (1) discontinuing potential photosensitizers (e.g., sulfa drugs, NSAIDs), (2) protecting the patient from the sun with sunscreens, hats, and clothing and sun avoidance, and (3) applying a medium- to high-potency topical steroid to the lesions. In my experience this condition is relatively easy to manage if the pattern is recognized. If the condition is allowed to persist, the patient may progress to a state of enhanced photosensitivity that will not respond to these simple measures.

Pruritic Folliculitis

Only approximately one half of HIV-infected persons with pruritic folliculitis have *S. aureus* infection.[6] The cause of the folliculitis in the others is unknown. Usually a skin biopsy is required to rule out other infectious processes (e.g., systemic fungal infections) or to determine the composition of the inflammatory infiltrate. Eosinophilic folliculitis is a chronic, waxing and waning follicular eruption.[15] The primary lesion is an edematous papule, up to 1 cm in size, with a tiny central pustule (Figure 10–8). The lesions are scattered on the trunk, head, and neck.

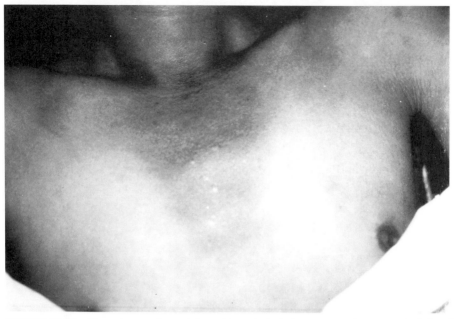

FIGURE 10–7.   Hyperpigmentation and dermatitis exclusively in sun-exposed areas may be induced by certain medications (sulfa drugs, NSAIDs) or may be due to HIV infection alone.

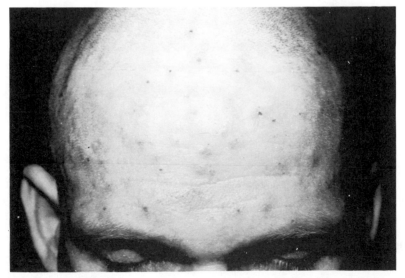

FIGURE 10–8.   Eosinophilic folliculitis of the forehead.

Culture results for bacteria are uniformly negative, and the patients do not respond to antibiotics effective against *S. aureus*. Skin biopsy reveals inflammation containing significant numbers of eosinophils surrounding and involving the hair follicle. No organisms are seen. In my experience chronic use of antihistamines, especially astemizole, and potent topical steroids is partially effective therapy. Phototherapy with UVB may be beneficial.

Papulosquamous Disorders

Three dermatologic disorders characterized by scaling patches and plaques occur more commonly in HIV-infected persons: seborrheic dermatitis, psoriasis, and Reiter's syndrome.[4] These papulosquamous disorders form a spectrum from mild and

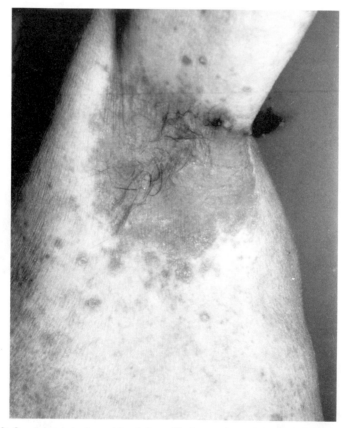

FIGURE 10-9. Seborrheic dermatitis of the axilla in a patient with AIDS. Seborrheic dermatitis commonly is accentuated in the axillae and groin in HIV-infected persons and is distinguished from cutaneous candidiasis by a negative potassium hydroxide scraping. The patient was treated successfully with a mild topical steroid and an imidazole cream mixed together and applied twice daily.

skin only symptoms (seborrheic dermatitis) through moderate or severe but skin only symptoms (psoriasis) to severe with systemic findings (severe psoriasis or Reiter's syndrome).[14] There is considerable overlap, and progression from a mild to a more severe form may occur.

Seborrheic dermatitis is extremely common, affecting to varying degrees a high percentage of persons with symptomatic HIV disease. Lesions are usually located in the hairy areas of the central face, scalp, chest, back, and groin (Figures 10–9 and 10–10). The lesions are mildly erythematous, with a yellowish greasy scale. When limited to the face, lesions are usually asymptomatic, but scalp and trunk lesions are often pruritic. Therapy for the scalp includes the regular use of a dandruff shampoo containing selenium sulfide (e.g., Selsun Blue), zinc pyrithione (e.g., Head and Shoulders, Danex, Zincon), or sulfur and salicylic acid (e.g., Van Seb, Sebulex). In addition, a medium-potency steroid solution (e.g., triamcinolone, 0.1%) may be applied. For facial, trunk, and groin lesions a topical imidazole cream (e.g., ketoconazole, 2%; clotrimazole, 1%) plus a low-potency topical steroid (hydrocortisone, 1% to 2½%) is applied twice daily. For refractory trunk lesions the strength of the topical steroid may be increased. For severe cases use of a 2- to 4-week course of oral ketoconazole (200 to 400 mg daily) may lead to improvement.

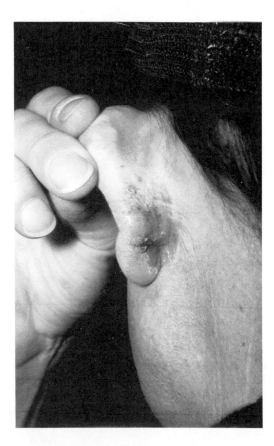

FIGURE 10–10. Seborrheic dermatitis in the retroauricular area. Erosion, weeping, and secondary staphylococcal infection are common in this location.

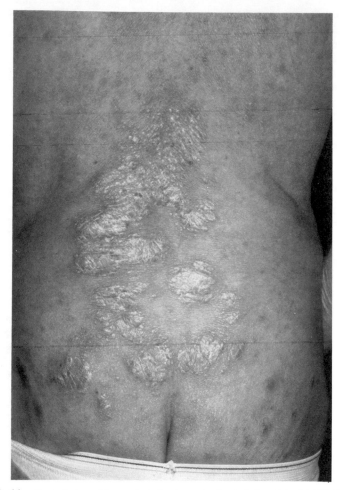

FIGURE 10–11.   Typical plaquelike psoriasis that began in the sixth decade in this HIV-infected man. Pruritus was severe.

Psoriasis often begins after HIV infection, although preexisting psoriasis may also flare after infection. The initial lesions frequently begin like those of seborrheic dermatitis but extend to the axillae and groin and finally involve the elbows, knees, and lumbosacral areas (Figures 10–11 and 10–12). The lesions of psoriasis and seborrheic dermatitis in the axillae and groin are identical. When psoriasis involves the trunk, it tends to form more fixed, less easily treatable lesions with a thicker scale. Psoriasis of the palms and soles often begins as superficial pustules that evolve into hyperkeratotic papules identical to the keratoderma blennorrhagicum of Reiter's syndrome. Arthritis may occur with psoriasis alone or as a part of Reiter's syndrome.

Mild to moderate psoriasis is managed with topical steroids and tar. Patients with severe psoriasis and HIV disease may note a significant improvement of their skin

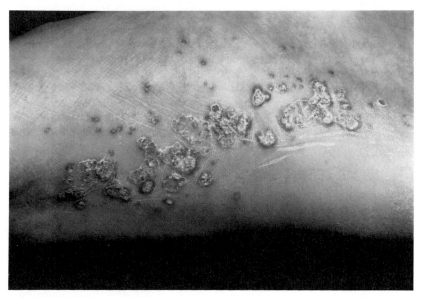

FIGURE 10–12. Pustules evolving into keratotic plaques on the sole. This was the initial manifestation of psoriasis in this HIV-infected person. Although the lesions were identical to those of Reiter's syndrome, this patient had no other characteristic stigmata.

lesions with zidovudine therapy.[8] The use of methotrexate has been associated with rapid immune suppression and death in HIV-infected persons with psoriasis and Reiter's syndrome and should be considered an agent of last resort.[18]

REFERENCES

1. Baron AL, Steinbach LS, LeBoit PE, et al: Osteolytic lesions and bacillary angiomatosis in HIV infection: Radiologic differentiation from AIDS-related Kaposi sarcoma'. Radiology 177:77-81, 1990
2. Berger TG: Evaluation and treatment of pruritus in the HIV-infected patient. In Volberding P, Jacobson MA (eds): AIDS Clinical Review 1989. New York, Marcel Dekker, 1989, pp 205-220
3. Birtles RJ, Harrison TG, Taylor AG: The causative agent of bacillary angiomatosis. N Engl J Med 325:1447, 1991
4. Coldiron BM, Bergstresser PR: Prevalence and clinical spectrum of skin disease in patients infected with human immunodeficiency virus. Arch Dermatol 125:357-361, 1989
5. Concus AP, Helfand RF, Imber MJ, et al: Cutaneous cryptococcosis mimicking molluscum contagiosum in a patient with AIDS. J Infect Dis 158:897-898, 1988
6. Duvic M: Staphylococcal infections and the pruritus of AIDS-related complex. Arch Dermatol 123:1599, 1987
7. Gordin FM, Simon GL, Wofsy CB, et al: Adverse reactions to trimethoprim-sulfamethoxazole in patients with the acquired immunodeficiency syndrome. Ann Intern Med 100:495-498, 1984
8. Kaplan MH, Sadick NS, Wieder J, et al: Antipsoriatic effects of zidovudine in human immunodeficiency virus–associated psoriasis. J Am Acad Dermatol 20:76-82, 1989
9. Melbye M, Grossman RJ, Goedert JJ: Risk of AIDS after herpes zoster. Lancet 1:728-730, 1987
10. Penneys NS, Nayar JK, Bernstein H, et al: Chronic pruritus eruption in patients with acquired

immunodeficiency syndrome associated with increased antibody titers of mosquito salivary gland antigens. J Am Acad Dermatol 21:421-425, 1989

11. Perkocha LA, Geaghan SM, Yen TSB, et al: Clinical and pathological features of bacillary peliosis hepatis in association with human immunodeficiency virus infection. N Engl J Med 323:1581-1586, 1990

12. Porteous DM, Berger TG: Severe cutaneous drug reactions (Stevens-Johnson syndrome and toxic epidermal necrolysis) in human immunodeficiency virus infection. Arch Dermatol 127:740-741, 1991

13. Relman DA, Loutit JS, Schmidt TM, et al: The agent of bacillary angiomatosis. An approach to the identification of uncultured pathogens. N Engl J Med 323:1573-1580, 1990

14. Reveille JD, Conant MA, Duvic M: Human immunodeficiency virus–associated psoriasis, psoriatic arthritis, and Reiter's syndrome: A disease continuum? Arthritis Rheum 33:1574-1578, 1990

15. Rosenthal D, LeBoit PE, Klumpp L, et al: HIV-associated eosinophilic folliculitis: A unique dermatosis associated with advanced HIV infection. Arch Dermatol 127:206-209, 1991

16. Slater LN, Welch DF, Hensel D, et al: A newly recognized fastidious gram-negative pathogen as a cause of fever and bacteremia. N Engl J Med 323:1587-1593, 1990

17. Toback AC, Longley J, Cardullo AC, et al: Severe chronic photosensitivity in association with acquired immunodeficiency syndrome. J Am Acad Dermatol 15:1056-1057, 1986

18. Winchester R, Bernstein DH, Fischer HD, et al: The co-occurrence of Reiter's syndrome and acquired immunodeficiency. Ann Intern Med 106:19-26, 1987

11

ORAL COMPLICATIONS OF HIV INFECTION

JOHN S. GREENSPAN, BSC, BDS, PhD, FRCPath, ScD (hc)
DEBORAH GREENSPAN, BDS, DSc, ScD (hc)
JAMES R. WINKLER, DMD

Oral lesions have been recognized as prominent features of AIDS and HIV infection since the beginning of the epidemic.[29] Some of these changes are reflections of reduced immune function manifested as oral opportunistic conditions, which are often the earliest clinical features of HIV infection. Some, in the presence of known HIV infection, are highly predictive of the ultimate development of the full syndrome, whereas others represent the oral features of AIDS itself. The particular susceptibility of the mouth to HIV disease is a reflection of a wider phenomenon. Oral opportunistic infections occur in a variety of conditions in which the teeming and varied microflora of the mouth take advantage of local and systemic immunologic and metabolic imbalances. They include oral infections in patients with primary immunodeficiency,[62] leukemia,[3] and diabetes,[27] and those resulting from radiation therapy, cancer chemotherapy, and bone marrow suppression.[2,10,16]

Oral lesions seen in association with HIV infection are classified in Table 11–1, and our general approach to the diagnosis and management of oral HIV disease is summarized in Table 11–2. Standardized definitions and diagnostic criteria for these lesions have been proposed.[45,77] In the prospective cohorts of HIV-infected homosexual and bisexual men in San Francisco, hairy leukoplakia is the most common oral lesion (20.4%), and pseudomembranous candidiasis is the next most common (5.8%).[20] Others have shown that a simplified staging system for HIV infection, based on CD4+ cell depletion and oral disease, is more effective than the Walter Reed and other staging classifications.[82]

CANDIDIASIS

The pseudomembranous form of oral candidiasis (thrush) was described in the first group of AIDS patients and is a harbinger of the full-blown syndrome in HIV-seropositive individuals.[59,69] We have shown recently that both oral candidiasis and hairy leukoplakia predict the development of AIDS in HIV-infected patients independently of CD4 counts.[56] However, it is not well recognized that oral candidiasis

161

Table 11–1.   Oral Lesions in HIV Infection

Fungal	**Viral**
Candidiasis	Herpes simplex
Pseudomembranous	Herpes zoster
Erythematous	Cytomegalovirus ulcers
Angular cheilitis	Hairy leukoplakia
Hyperplastic	Warts
Histoplasmosis	**Neoplastic**
Geotrichosis	Kaposi's sarcoma
Cryptococcosis	Non-Hodgkin's lymphoma
Bacterial	Squamous cell carcinoma (?)
HIV-associated gingivitis	**Other**
HIV-associated periodontitis	Recurrent aphthous ulcers
Necrotizing stomatitis	Immune thrombocytopenic purpura
Mycobacterium avium complex	Salivary gland disease
Klebsiella stomatitis	

can take several forms, some of them subtle clinical appearances.[15,41,42,87] The most common form, pseudomembranous candidiasis, presents as removable white plaques on any oral mucosal surface (Figure 11–1). These plaques may be as small as 1 to 2 mm or may be extensive and widespread. They can be wiped off, leaving an erythematous or even bleeding mucosal surface.

The erythematous form (Figure 11–2) is seen as smooth red patches on the hard or soft palate, buccal mucosa, or dorsal surface of the tongue. These lesions may seem insignificant and may be missed unless a thorough oral mucosal examination is performed in good light. Occasionally *Candida* causes hyperkeratosis (candidal leukoplakia). Such white lesions cannot be wiped off but regress with prolonged antifungal therapy. Candidal leukoplakia may be seen on the buccal mucosa, tongue, and hard palate. It can be confused with hairy leukoplakia and other forms of leukoplakia. Distinguishing between them involves the use of smears, histopathologic study, and therapeutic response (see later discussion on hairy leukoplakia).

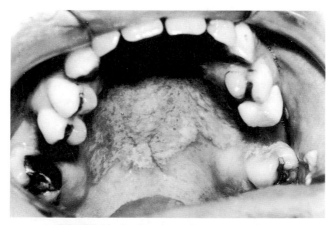

FIGURE 11–1.   Pseudomembranous candidiasis.

Table 11–2. Diagnosis and Management of Oral HIV Disease

CONDITION	DIAGNOSIS	MANAGEMENT
Fungal		
Candidiasis	Clinical appearance KOH preparation Culture	Antifungals
Histoplasmosis Geotrichosis	Biopsy KOH preparation Culture	Systemic therapy Polyene antifungals
Cryptococcosis	Culture Biopsy	Systemic therapy
Bacterial		
HIV-associated gingivitis	Clinical appearance	Plaque removal, chlorhexidine
HIV-associated periodontitis	Clinical appearance	Plaque removal, débridement, povidone-iodine, metronidazole, chlorhexidine
Necrotizing stomatitis	Clinical appearance Culture and biopsy (to exclude other causes) Culture Biopsy	Débridement, povidone-iodine, metronidazole, chlorhexidine
Mycobacterium avium complex	Culture Biopsy	Systemic therapy
Klebsiella stomatitis	Culture	Systemic therapy (based on antibiotic sensitivity testing)
Viral		
Herpes simples	Clinical appearance Immunofluorescence on smears	Most cases are self-limiting Oral acyclovir for prolonged cases (>10 days)
Herpes zoster	Clinical appearance	Oral or intravenous acyclovir
Cytomegalovirus ulcers	Biopsy, immunohistochemistry for CMV	DHPG
Hairy leukoplakia	Clinical appearance Biopsy; in situ hybridization for Epstein-Barr virus	Not routinely treated Oral acyclovir for severe cases
Warts	Clinical appearance Biopsy	Excision
Neoplastic		
Kaposi's sarcoma	Clinical appearance Biopsy	Palliative surgical or laser excision for some bulky or unsightly lesions; radiation therapy; chemotherapy
Non-Hodgkin's lymphoma	Biopsy	Chemotherapy
Squamous cell carcinoma	Biopsy	Excision or radiation therapy or both
Other		
Recurrent aphthous ulcers	History Clinical appearance Biopsy (to exclude other causes)	Topical steroids
Immune thrombocytopenic purpura	Clinical appearance Hematologic workup	
Salivary gland disease	History, clinical appearance, salivary flow measurements Biopsy (to exclude other causes—needle or labial salivary gland biopsy)	Salivary stimulants or change in systemic medication or both Topical fluorides

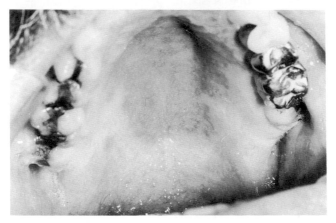

FIGURE 11-2. Erythematous candidiasis.

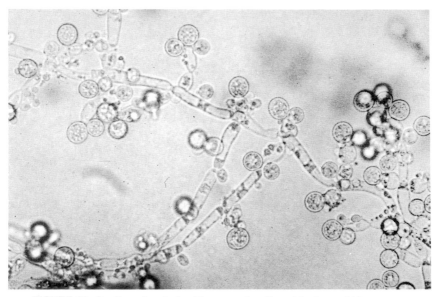

FIGURE 11-3. Potassium hydroxide preparation. Fungal hyphae and blastospores.

Angular cheilitis due to *Candida* infection produces erythema, cracks, and fissures at the corner of the mouth. We have found that erythematous candidiasis is as serious a prognostic indicator of the development of AIDS as pseudomembranous candidiasis.[15]

Diagnosis of oral candidiasis involves potassium hydroxide preparation of a smear from the lesion (Figure 11-3). Culture provides information about the species involved. Biopsy is of use for diagnosing candidal leukoplakia and to aid in distinguishing it from other forms of leukoplakia.

Oral candidiasis in patients with HIV infection usually responds to topical antifungal agents, including nystatin vaginal tablets, 100,000 units three times daily, dissolved slowly in the mouth; nystatin oral pastilles, 200,000 units, one pastille five times daily; or clotrimazole oral tablets, 10 mg, one tablet five times daily. Oral ketoconazole in tablet form, 200 mg once daily, is a systemic antifungal agent that can be used as an alternative. It is effective if absorbed. Fluconazole (Diflucan) is a new systemic antifungal agent. The recommended dose is a 1000-mg tablet, once daily for 9 to 14 days. Antifungal therapy should be maintained for 1 to 2 weeks, and some patients may need maintenance therapy because of frequent relapse. Angular cheilitis usually responds to topical antifungal creams such as nystatin-triamcinolone (Mycolog II), clotrimazole (Mycelex), or ketoconazole (Nizoral).

Occasionally other and unusual oral fungal lesions are seen. They include histoplasmosis,[95] geotrichosis,[50] and cryptococcosis.[24,28,38]

GINGIVITIS AND PERIODONTITIS

Unusual forms of gingivitis and periodontal disease are seen in association with HIV infection. The gingiva may show a fiery red marginal line (Figure 11–4), even in mouths showing absence of significant accumulations of plaque.[48,100,102] The periodontal disease occurs in approximately 30% to 50% of AIDS clinic patients[67] but is rarely seen in asymptomatic HIV-positive individuals.[99] It resembles, in some respects, acute necrotizing ulcerative gingivitis (ANUG) superimposed on rapidly progressive periodontitis (Figure 11–5). Thus there may be halitosis in some cases and a history of rapid onset. There is necrosis of the tips of interdental papillae with the formation of cratered ulcers. However, in contrast to patients with ANUG, these patients complain of spontaneous bleeding and severe, deep-seated pain that is not readily relieved by analgesics. There may be rapid progressive loss of gingival and periodontal soft tissues and extraordinarily rapid destruction of supporting bone.

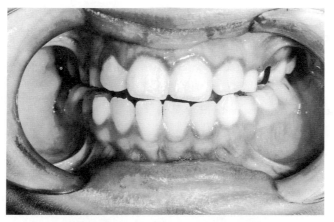

FIGURE 11–4. HIV-associated gingivitis.

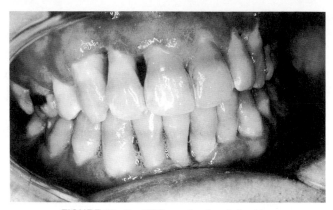

FIGURE 11-5. HIV-associated periodontitis.

Teeth may therefore loosen and even exfoliate. The periodontal disease often demonstrates a severity and a rapid rate of progression that have not been seen by the majority of currently practicing dentists and periodontists. Exposure and even sequestration of bone may occur, producing necrotizing stomatitis lesions[96] similar to the noma seen in severely malnourished persons in World War II and more recently in the developing countries in association with malnutrition and chronic infection such as malaria. The pathologic and microbiologic features of these remarkable periodontal lesions are under investigation.[70,71,105] Current standard therapy for gingivitis and periodontitis is ineffectual. Instead, the therapeutic regimen that is emerging[30,101,102] involves thorough débridement and curettage, followed by application of a combination of topical antiseptics, notably povidone-iodine irrigation (Betadine) followed with chlorhexidine (Peridex) mouthwashes, sometimes supplemented with a 4- to 5-day course of antibiotics such as metronidazole (Flagyl) 250 mg q.i.d., Augmentin 250 mg (1 tab t.i.d.), or clindamycin 300 mg t.i.d. Treatment will fail if thorough local removal of bacteria and diseased hard and soft tissue is not achieved during the initial treatment phase and maintained long-term.

OTHER BACTERIAL LESIONS

A few cases have occurred of oral mucosal lesions associated with unusual bacteria, including *Klebsiella pneumoniae* and *Enterobacter cloacae*.[42] These have been diagnosed using aerobic and anaerobic cultures and have responded to antibiotic therapy based on in vitro sensitivity assays. Oral ulcers caused by *Mycobacterium avium* have also been described.[94]

HERPES SIMPLEX

Oral lesions due to herpes simplex virus (HSV) are a common feature of HIV infection. The condition usually presents as recurrent intraoral lesions with crops of small, painful vesicles that ulcerate. These lesions commonly appear on the palate or gingiva. Smears from the lesions may reveal giant cells, and HSV can be identified using monoclonal antibodies and immunofluorescence.[26] The lesions usually heal, although they may recur. In patients with a history of prolonged bouts (>10 days) of such lesions it may be considered appropriate to treat them with oral acyclovir as soon as symptoms are reported. Usually one 200-mg capsule taken five takes a day is effective. Acyclovir-resistant herpes of the lips and perioral structures has been described. The lesions responded to foscarnet.[66]

HERPES ZOSTER

Both chickenpox and herpes zoster (shingles) have occurred in association with HIV infection.[68,88] In orofacial zoster the vesicles and ulcers follow the distribution of one or more branches of the trigeminal nerve on one side. Facial nerve involvement with facial palsy (Ramsay Hunt syndrome) may also occur. Prodromal symptoms may include pain referred to one or more teeth, which often prove to be vital and noncarious. The ulcers usually heal in 2 to 3 weeks, but pain may persist. Oral acyclovir in doses up to 4 g per day may be used in severe cases, but occasionally patients must be hospitalized to receive intravenous acyclovir therapy.

CYTOMEGALOVIRUS ULCERS

Oral ulcers caused by cytomegalovirus (CMV) occasionally occur.[61] These ulcers can occur on any oral mucosal surface, and diagnosis is made by biopsy and immunohistochemistry. Oral ulcers due to CMV are usually seen in the presence of disseminated disease, but cases have occurred in which the oral ulcer was the first presentation. Whether to treat with DHPG depends on the severity of the viral infection, and full workup is indicated.

HAIRY LEUKOPLAKIA

First seen on the tongue in homosexual men,[37] hairy leukoplakia has since been described in several oral mucosal locations, including the buccal mucosa, soft palate, and floor of mouth and in all risk groups for AIDS.[9,11,20,22,36,43,49,54,60,76,79,81,103] Hairy leukoplakia produces white thickening of the oral mucosa, often with vertical folds or corrugations (Figure 11–6 and Color Plate 1B). The lesions range in size from a few millimeters to involvement of the entire dorsal surface of the tongue. The differential diagnosis includes candidal leukoplakia, smoker's leukoplakia, epithelial dysplasia or oral cancer, white sponge nevus, and the plaque form of lichen planus. Biopsy reveals epithelial hyperplasia with a thickened parakeratin layer showing surface irregularities, projections or "hairs," vacuolated prickle cells, and very little inflammation.[11,36,37,46,47,84] Epstein-Barr virus (EBV) can be identified in vacuolated and other prickle cells and in the superficial layers of the epithelium by using cytochemistry, electron microscopy, Southern blot test, and in situ hybridization.[5,11,36,47,63,72,78,80] For cases in which biopsy is not considered appropriate (e.g., hemophiliacs, children, large-scale epidemiologic studies), we have developed cytospin and filter in situ hybridization techniques.[12] Langerhans' cells are sparse or

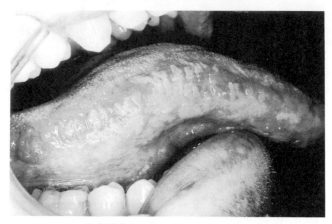

FIGURE 11-6. Hairy leukoplakia.

absent from the lesion.[8] Hairy leukoplakia is not premalignant.[36] Indeed, the keratin profile of the lesions suggests reduced, rather than increased, cell turnover.[97]

Almost all patients with hairy leukoplakia are HIV seropositive, approximately 75% have HIV viremia, and many subsequently develop AIDS (median time, 24 months) and die (median time, 44 months).[39,40] Patients with tiny or extensive lesions show no difference in this tendency.[84] Rare cases have been described in HIV-negative individuals.[18,38,53] Hairy leukoplakia has not been seen on other than oral mucosal surfaces.[51]

Hairy leukoplakia apparently is an EBV-induced benign epithelial thickening. High doses of oral acyclovir appear to reduce the lesion clinically,[6,25,80] and we have shown that the acyclovir pro-drug desciclovir can eliminate both the lesion and the EBV infection present in the epithelial cells.[33] However, these effects are soon reversed after cessation of acyclovir or desciclovir therapy. Hairy leukoplakia may occasionally regress spontaneously, and zidovudine did not appear to increase regression in one recent study.[55]

It is as yet not clear whether hairy leukoplakia is caused by direct infection or reinfection of maturing epithelial cells by EBV from the saliva, by EBV-infected B cells' infiltrating the epithelium, or by latent infection of the basal cell layer.[4,36,73,104] EBV variants, unusual EBV types, and even multiple strains of EBV have been found in the lesion.[75]

WARTS

Oral lesions caused by human papillomavirus (HPV) can present as single or multiple papilliferous warts with multiple white and spikelike projections, as pink cauliflower-like masses (Figure 11-7), as single projections, or as flat lesions resembling focal epithelial hyperplasia.[41,91] In patients with HIV infection we have seen numerous examples of each type. Southern blot hybridization has not revealed (as would be expected) HPV types 6, 11, 16, and 18, which usually are associated with anogenital warts, but HPV type 7, which usually is associated with butcher's warts of the skin, or HPV types 13 and 32, previously associated with focal epithelial

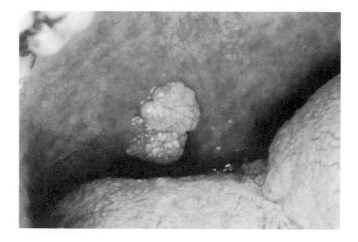

FIGURE 11–7.
Wart on the palate.

hyperplasia.[13,34] Venereal transmission thus seems not involved in these warts. Instead, they may be attributable to activation of latent HPV infection or perhaps autoinfection from skin and face lesions.

If large, extensive, or otherwise troublesome, these oral warts can be removed using surgical or laser excision. In some cases we have seen recurrence after therapy and even extensive spread throughout the mouth.

NEOPLASTIC DISEASE

Kaposi's Sarcoma

Kaposi's sarcoma (KS) in patients with AIDS produces oral lesions in many cases.[14,21,87,89,91] The lesions occur as red or purple macules, papules, or nodules. Occasionally the lesions are the same color as the adjoining normal mucosa. Although frequently asymptomatic, pain may occur because of traumatic ulceration with inflammation and infection. Bulky lesions may be visible or may interfere with speech and mastication. Diagnosis involves biopsy.[31]

Lesions at the gingival margin frequently become inflamed and painful because of plaque accumulation. Excision, by surgical means or by laser, is readily performed and can be repeated if the lesion again produces problems. Local radiation therapy has also been used to reduce the size of such lesions. Oral lesions usually regress when patients receive chemotherapy for aggressive KS, and individual lesions may respond to local injection of vinblastine.[17]

Lymphoma

Although not seen as frequently as with oral KS, oral lesions are a common feature of HIV-associated lymphoma.[58,106,107] A biopsy may prove that poorly defined alveolar swellings or discrete oral masses in individuals who are HIV seropositive are non-Hodgkin's lymphoma.[32] No treatment is provided for the oral lesions separate from the systemic chemotherapy regimen that is usually used in such cases.

Carcinoma

Several cases have been seen of oral squamous cell carcinoma, particularly of the tongue, in young homosexual males.[91] It is not clear whether these lesions are related to HIV infection.

OTHER LESIONS[89,90]

Recurrent aphthous ulcers (RAU) are a common finding in the normal population. There is an impression,[1,20,41,90] not as yet substantiated by prospective studies of incidence, that RAU is more common among HIV-seropositive individuals. These lesions present as recurrent crops of small (1 to 2 mm) to large (1 cm) ulcers on the nonkeratinized oral and oropharyngeal mucosa.[65] They can interfere significantly with speech and swallowing and may present considerable problems in diagnosis. When large and persistent, biopsy may be indicated to exclude lymphoma. The histopathologic features of RAU are those of nonspecific inflammation. Treatment with topical steroids is often effective in reducing pain and accelerating healing. Valuable agents include fluocinonide (Lidex), 0.05% ointment, mixed with equal parts of Orabase applied to the lesion up to six times daily, or clobetasol (Temovate), 0.05% mixed with equal parts of Orabase applied three times daily. These are particularly effective treatments for early lesions. Dexamethasone (Decadron) elixir, 0.5 mg/ml used as a rinse and expectorated, is also helpful, particularly when the location of the lesion makes it difficult for the patient to apply fluocinonide.

Immune thrombocytopenic purpura may produce oral mucosal ecchymoses or small blood-filled lesions.[41] Spontaneous gingival bleeding may occur. Diagnosis by hematologic evaluation is usually straightforward, but, as with any systemic condition presenting as oral lesions, full workup is indicated.

We have seen several cases of parotid enlargement in pediatric AIDS patients[62] (Figure 11–8) and more recently among adults who are HIV seropositive.[23,52,74,84,85]

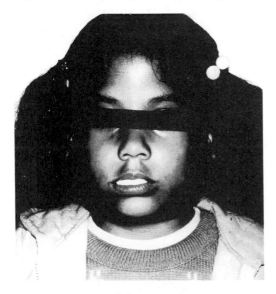

FIGURE 11–8.   Parotid enlargement.

HIV-infected children with parotid enlargement progress less rapidly than those without parotid enlargement.[57] No specific cause for HIV-associated salivary gland disease has been determined, although viral causes are suspected.[83,86] Diagnosis to exclude lymphoma, leukemia, and other causes of salivary gland enlargement may involve labial salivary gland biopsy and major salivary gland needle biopsy. Some of these cases show xerostomia. Furthermore, the latter condition may be seen in association with HIV infection in the absence of salivary gland enlargement. The patient may complain of oral dryness, and there may be signs of xerostomia such as lack of pooled saliva, failure to elicit salivary expression from Stensen's or Wharton's ducts, and obvious mucosal dryness. Tests of salivary function, notably stimulated parotid flow-rate determination, show reduced salivary flow. Some of these cases are attributable to side effects of medications that reduce salivation. In such cases it may be possible to arrange to change the medications or their doses. In other cases stimulation of salivary flow by use of sugarless candy may alleviate some of the discomfort. Topical fluorides and other preventive dentistry approaches are used to reduce the frequency of caries.

SUMMARY

The oral manifestations of HIV infection present as a variety of opportunistic infections, neoplasms, and other lesions. Some of them are common, perhaps the most common, features of HIV disease and are highly predictive of the development of AIDS. Clinicians caring for HIV-infected persons should become familiar with the diagnosis and management of this group of conditions.

The oral lesions of HIV infection present challenges of diagnosis and therapy. They also offer unrivaled opportunities to investigate the epidemiology, cause, pathogenesis, and treatment of mucosal diseases. As the epidemic progresses, it can be expected that further lesions will be observed and that additional rational and effective therapeutic approaches will be developed.

REFERENCES

1. Bach MC, Valenti AJ, Howell DA, Smith TJ: Odynophagia from aphthous ulcers of the pharynx and oesophagus in the acquired immunodeficiency syndrome (AIDS). Ann Intern Med 109:338-339, 1988
2. Barrett AP: Clinical characteristics and mechanisms involved in chemotherapy-induced oral ulceration. Oral Surg 63:424, 1983
3. Barrett AP: Oral changes as initial diagnostic indicators in acute leukemia. J Oral Med 41:234, 1986
4. Becker J, Leser U, Marschall M, et al: Expression of proteins encoded by Epstein-Barr virus trans-activator genes depends on the differentiation of epithelial cells in oral hairy leukoplakia. Proc Natl Acad Sci 88:8332-8336, 1991
5. Belton CM, Eversole LR: Oral hairy leukoplakia: Ultrastructural features. J Oral Pathol 15:493, 1986
6. Brockmeyer NH, Kreuzfelder E, Mertins L, et al: Zidovudine therapy of asymptomatic HIV-1–infected patients and combined zidovudine-acyclovir therapy of HIV-1–infected patients with oral hairy leukoplakia. J Invest Dermatol 92:647, 1989
7. Colebunders R, Mann J, Francis H, et al: Herpes zoster in African patients: A clinical predictor of human immunodeficiency virus infection. J Infect Dis 157:314-318, 1988

8. Daniels TE, Greenspan D, Greenspan JS, et al: Absence of Langerhans' cells in oral hairy leukoplakia, an AIDS-associated lesion. J Invest Dermatol 89:178-182, 1987
9. De Maubeuge J, Ledoux M, Feremans W, et al: Oral "hairy" leukoplakia in an African AIDS patient. J Cutan Pathol 13:235, 1986
10. DePaola LG, Peterson DE, Overholser DJ Jr, et al: Dental care for patients receiving chemotherapy. J Am Dent Assoc 112:198, 1986
11. De Souza YG, Greenspan D, Felton JR, et al: Localization of Epstein-Barr virus DNA in the epithelial cells of oral hairy leukoplakia using in-situ hybridization on tissue sections. N Engl J Med 320:1559-1560, 1989
12. De Souza Y, Freese UK, Greenspan D, Greenspan JS: Diagnosis of EBV infection in hairy leukoplakia using nucleic acid hybridization and noninvasive techniques. J Clin Microbiol 28:2775-2778, 1990
13. de Villiers EM: Prevalence of HPV-7 papillomas in the oral mucosa and facial skin of patients with human immunodeficiency virus. Arch Dermatol 125:1590, 1989
14. Dodd CL, Greenspan D, Greenspan JS: Oral Kaposi's sarcoma in a woman as a first indication of HIV infection. J Am Dent Assoc 122:61-63, 1991
15. Dodd CL, Greenspan D, Katz MH, et al: Oral candidiasis in HIV infection: Pseudomembranous and erythematous candidiasis show similar rates of progression to AIDS. AIDS 5:1339-1343, 1991
16. Dreizen S, McCredie KB, Bodey GP, et al: Quantitative analysis of the oral complications of antileukemia chemotherapy. Oral Surg 62:650, 1986
17. Epstein JB, Scully C: Intralesional vinblastine for oral Kaposi's sarcoma in HIV infection. Lancet 2:1100-1101, 1989
18. Epstein JB, Sherlock CH, Greenspan JS: Hairy leukoplakia-like lesions following bone-marrow transplantation. AIDS 5:101-102, 1991
19. Eversole LR, Jacobsen P, Stone CE, et al: Oral condyloma planus (hairy leukoplakia) among homosexual men: A clinicopathologic study of thirty-six cases. Oral Surg 61:249, 1986
20. Feigal DW, Katz MH, Greenspan D, et al: The prevalence of oral lesions in HIV-infected homosexual and bisexual men: Three San Francisco epidemiology cohorts. AIDS 5:519-525, 1991
21. Ficarra G, Berson AM, Silverman S, et al: Kaposi's sarcoma of the oral cavity: A study of 134 patients with a review of the pathogenesis, epidemiology, clinical aspects, and treatment. Oral Surg Oral Med Oral Pathol 66:543-550, 1988
22. Ficarra G, Barone R, Gaglioti D: Oral hairy leukoplakia among HIV-positive intravenous drug abusers: A clinico-pathologic and ultrastructural study. Oral Surg Oral Med Oral Pathol 65:421-426, 1988
23. Finfer MD, Schinella RA, Rothstein SG, Persky MS: Cystic parotid lesions in patients at risk for the acquired immunodeficiency syndrome. Arch Otolaryngol Head Neck Surg 144:1290-1294, 1988
24. Fowler CB, Nelson JF, Henley DW, Smith BR: Acquired immune deficiency syndrome presenting as a palatal perforation. Oral Surg Oral Med Oral Pathol 67:313-318, 1989
25. Friedman-Kien AE: Viral origin of hairy leukoplakia (letter). Lancet 2:694, 1986
26. Fung JC, Shanley J, Tilton RC: Comparison of herpes-simplex virus–specific DNA probes and monoclonal antibodies. J Clin Microbiol 22:61-63, 1985
27. Glavind L, Lund B, Loe H: The relationship between periodontal state and diabetes duration, insulin dosage and retinal changes. J Periodontol 39:341, 1968
28. Glick M, Cohen SG, Cheney RT, et al: Oral manifestations of disseminated *Cryptococcus neoformans* in a patient with acquired immunodeficiency syndrome. Oral Surg Oral Med Oral Pathol 64:454-459, 1987
29. Gottlieb MS, Schroff R, Schantez HM, et al: *P. pneumoniae* and mucosal candidiasis in previously healthy homosexual men: Evidence of a new acquired cellular immunodeficiency. N Engl J Med 305:1435, 1981
30. Grassi M, Williams CA, Winkler JR, Murray PA: Management of HIV-associated periodontal diseases. In Robertson PB, Greenspan JS (eds): Perspectives on Oral Manifestations of AIDS: Diagnosis and Management of HIV-Associated Infections. Littleton, Mass, PSG, 1988, pp 119-130
31. Green TL, Beckstead JH, Lozada-Nur F, et al: Histopathologic spectrum of oral Kaposi's sarcoma. Oral Surg Oral Med Oral Pathol 58:306-314, 1984
32. Green TL, Eversole LR: Oral lymphomas in HIV-infected patients: Association with Epstein-Barr virus DNA. Oral Surg Oral Med Oral Pathol 67:437-442, 1989
33. Greenspan D, De Souza Y, Conant MA, et al: Efficacy of desciclovir in the treatment of Epstein-Barr virus infection in oral hairy leukoplakia. J Acquir Immune Defic Syndr 3:571-578, 1990

34. Greenspan D, de Villiers EM, Greenspan JS, et al: Unusual HPV types in the oral warts in association with HIV infection. J Oral Pathol 17:482-487, 1988
35. Greenspan D, Greenspan JS: Management of the oral lesions of HIV infection. J Am Dent Assoc 122:26-32, 1991
36. Greenspan D, Greenspan JS: Significance of oral hairy leukoplakia. Oral Surg Oral Med Oral Pathol 73:151-154, 1992.
37. Greenspan D, Greenspan JS, Conant M, et al: Oral "hairy" leucoplakia in male homosexuals: Evidence of association with both papillomavirus and a herpes-group virus. 2:831, 1984
38. Greenspan D, Greenspan JS, De Souza YG, et al: Oral hairy leukoplakia in an HIV-negative renal transplant recipient. J Oral Pathol Med 18:32-34, 1989
39. Greenspan D, Greenspan JS, Hearst NG, et al: Relation of oral hairy leukoplakia to infection with the human immunodeficiency virus and the risk of developing AIDS. J Infect Dis 155:475, 1987
40. Greenspan D, Greenspan JS, Overby G, et al: Risk factors for rapid progression from hairy leukoplakia to AIDS: A nested case-control study. AIDS 4:652-658, 1991
41. Greenspan D, Greenspan JS, Pindborg JJ, Schiodt M: Aids and the Mouth. Copenhagen, Munksgaard, 1990
42. Greenspan D, Greenspan JS, Pindborg JJ, et al: Aids and the Dental Team. Copenhagen, Munksgaard, 1986
43. Greenspan D, Hollander H, Friedman-Kien A, et al: Oral hairy leukoplakia in two women, a hemophiliac and a transfusion recipient (letter). Lancet 2:978, 1986
44. Greenspan JS: Initiatives in oral AIDS research. Oral Surg Oral Med Oral Pathol 73:244-247, 1992
45. Greenspan JS, Barr CE, Sciubba JJ, et al: Oral manifestations of HIV infection: Definitions, diagnostic criteria and principles of therapy. Oral Surg Oral Med Oral Pathol 73:142-144, 1992
46. Greenspan JS, Greenspan D: Oral hairy leukoplakia: Diagnosis and management. Oral Surg Oral Med Oral Pathol 67:396-403, 1989
47. Greenspan JS, Greenspan D, Lennette ET, et al: Replication of Epstein-Barr virus within the epithelial cells of "hairy" leukoplakia, an AIDS-associated lesion. N Engl J Med 313:1564-1571, 1985
48. Greenspan JS, Greenspan D, Winkler JR, et al: Aids—Oral and periodontal changes. In Genco RJ et al (eds): Contemporary Periodontics. St. Louis, CV Mosby Co, 1990
49. Greenspan JS, Mastrucchi T, Leggott P, et al: Hairy leukoplakia in a child. AIDS 2(2):143, 1988
50. Heinic GS, Greenspan D, MacPhail LA, Greenspan JS: Oral *Geotrichum candidum* infection in association with HIV infection: A case report. Oral Surg Oral Med Oral Pathol 1992 (in press)
51. Hollander H, Greenspan D, Stringari S, et al: Hairy leukoplakia and the acquired immunodeficiency syndrome (letter). Ann Intern Med 104:892, 1986
52. Itescu S, Brancato LJ, Buxbaum J, et al: A diffuse infiltrative CD8 lymphocytosis syndrome in human immunodeficiency virus (HIV) infection: A host immune response associated with HLA-DR5. Ann Intern Med 112:3-10, 1990
53. Itin P, Rufli I, Rudlinser R, et al: Oral hairy leukoplakia in a HIV-negative renal transplant patient: A marker for immunosuppression. Dermatologica 17:126-128, 1988
54. Kabani S, Greenspan D, de Souza S, et al: Oral hairy leukoplakia with extensive oral mucosal involvement. Oral Surg Oral Med Oral Pathol 67:411-415, 1989
55. Katz MH, Greenspan D, Heinic GS, et al: Resolution of hairy leukoplakia: An observational trial of zidovudine versus no treatment. 164:1240-1241, 1991
56. Katz MH, Greenspan D, Westenhouse J, et al: Progression to AIDS in HIV-infected homosexual and bisexual men with hairy leukoplakia and oral candidiasis: Results from three San Francisco epidemiologic cohorts. AIDS 6:95-100, 1992
57. Katz MH, Mastrucci MT, Leggott PJ, et al: Prognostic significance of oral lesions in children with perinatally acquired HIV infection. 1992 (submitted for publication)
58. Kaugars GE, Burns JC: Non-Hodgkin's lymphoma of the oral cavity associated with AIDS. Oral Surg Oral Med Oral Pathol 67:433-436, 1989
59. Klein RS, Harris CA, Small CB: Oral candidiasis in high-risk patients as the initial manifestation of the acquired immunodeficiency syndrome. N Engl J Med 311:354, 1984
60. Konrad K: Orale "haarige" Leukoplakie—klinische Fruehmanifestation der HTLV-III–Infektion. Wien Klin Wochenschr 3 (suppl):702, 1986
61. Langford A, Ruf B, Groth A, et al: Cytomegalovirus associated oral ulcerations in HIV-infected patients. (Abstract No. 211). J Dent Res 68:283, 1989; J Oral Pathol Med 19(2):71-76, 1990
62. Leggott PJ, Robertson PB, Greenspan D, et al: Oral manifestation of primary and acquired immunodeficiency diseases in children. Pediatr Dent 9:98, 1987

63. Loning T, Henke RP, Reichart P, Becker J: In situ hybridization to detect Epstein-Barr virus DNA in oral tissues of HIV-infected patients. Virchows Arch [A] 412:127-133, 1987

64. Lynch DP, Naftolin LZ: Oral cryptococcus neoformans infection in AIDS. Oral Surg Oral Med Oral Pathol 64:449-453, 1987

65. MacPhail LA, Greenspan D, Feigal DW, et al: Recurrent aphthous ulcers in association with HIV infection. Oral Surg Oral Med Oral Pathol 71(6):678-683, 1991

66. MacPhail LA, Greenspan D, Schiodt M, et al: Acyclovir-resistant, foscarnet-sensitive oral herpes simplex type 2 lesion in a patient with AIDS. Oral Surg Oral Med Oral Pathol 67:427-432, 1989

67. Masouredis CM, Katz MH, Greenspan D, et al. Prevalence of HIV-associated periodontitis and gingivitis in HIV-infected patients attending an AIDS clinic. J Acquir Immune Defic Syndr 1991 (in press)

68. Melbye M, Grossman RJ, Goedert JJ, et al: Risk of AIDS after herpes zoster. Lancet 1:728-731, 1987

69. Murray HW, Hillan JK, Rubin BY, et al: Patients at risk for AIDS-related opportunistic infections. N Engl J Med 313:1504, 1985

70. Murray PA, Grassi M, Winkler JR: The microbiology of HIV-associated periodontal lesions. J Clin Periodontol 16:636-642, 1989

71. Murray PA, Winkler JR, Sadkowski L, et al: Microbiology of HIV-associated gingivitis and periodontitis. In Robertson PB, Greenspan JS (eds): Perspectives on Oral Manifestations of AIDS: Diagnosis and Management of HIV-Associated Infections. Littleton, Mass, PSG, 1988, pp 105-118

72. Nasemann T, Kimmig W, Schaeg G, et al: Orale "hairy" Leukoplakie-electronenoptische Schenelldiagnostik Durch Negative-Staining-Verfahren. Hautarzt 37:571, 1986

73. Niedobitek G, Young LS, Lau R, et al: Epstein-Barr virus gene expression in oral hairy leukoplakia: Analysis by in situ hybridisation, immunohistology, and immunoblotting. J Virol 1992 (in press)

74. Pahwa S, Kaplan M, Fikrig S, et al: Spectrum of human T-cell lymphotropic virus type III infection in children. JAMA 255:2299, 1986

75. Patton DF, Shirley P, Raab-Traub N, et al: Defective viral DNA in Epstein-Barr virus–associated oral hairy leukoplakia. J Virol 64:397-400, 1990

76. Phelan JA, Saltzman BR, Friedland GH, et al: Oral findings in patients with acquired immunodeficiency syndrome. Oral Surg 64:50, 1987

77. Pindborg JJ: Classification of oral lesions associated with HIV infection. Oral Surg Oral Med Oral Pathol 67:292-295, 1989

78. Rabanus J-P, Greenspan D, Petersen V, et al: Subcellular distribution and life cycle of Epstein-Barr virus in keratinocytes of oral hairy leukoplakia. Am J Pathol 139(1):185-197, 1991

79. Reichart P, Pohle HD, Gelderblom H, et al: Orale Manifestationen bei AIDS. Dtsch Z Mund Kiefer Geschichtschr 9:167, 1985

80. Resnick L, Herbst JHS, Ablashi DV, et al: Regression of oral hairy leukoplakia after orally administered acyclovir therapy. JAMA 259:384-388, 1988

81. Rindum JL, Schiodt M, Pindborg JJ, et al: Oral hairy leukoplakia in three hemophiliacs with human immunodeficiency virus infection. Oral Surg 63:437, 1987

82. Royce RC, Luckmann RS, Fusaro RE, Winkelstein W Jr: The natural history of HIV-1 infection: Staging classifications of disease. AIDS 5:355-364, 1991

83. Schiodt M, Dodd CL, Greenspan D, et al: Natural history of HIV-associated salivary gland disease. 1992 (submitted for publication)

84. Schiodt M, Greenspan D, Daniels TE, Greenspan JS: Clinical and histologic spectrum of oral hairy leukoplakia. Oral Surg Oral Med Oral Pathol 64(6):716-720, 1987

85. Schiodt M, Greenspan D, Daniels TE, et al: Parotid gland enlargement and xerostomia associated with labial sialadenitis in HIV-infected patients. J Autoimmune 2(4):415-425, 1989

86. Schiodt M, Greenspan D, Levy J, et al: Does HIV cause salivary gland disease? AIDS 3:819-822, 1989

87. Schiodt M, Pindborg JJ: Aids and the oral cavity. Epidemiology and clinical oral manifestations of human immune deficiency virus infection: A review. Int J Oral Maxillofac Surg 16:1, 1987

88. Schiodt M, Rindum J, Bygbert I: Chickenpox with oral manifestations in an AIDS patient. Dan Dent J 91:316-319, 1987

89. Scully C, Laskaris G, Pindborg J, et al: Oral manifestations of HIV infection and their management. I. More common lesions. Oral Surg Oral Med Oral Pathol 71:158-166, 1991

90. Scully C, Laskaris G, Pindborg J, et al: Oral manifestations of HIV infection and their management. II. Less common lesions. Oral Surg Oral Med Oral Pathol 71:167-171, 1991

91. Silverman S, Migliorati CA, Lozada-Nur F, et al: Oral findings in people with or at high risk for AIDS: A study of 375 homosexual males. J Am Dent Assoc 112:187, 1986

92. Syrjanen S, Laine P, Happonen RP, Niemela M: Oral hairy leukoplakia is not a specific sign of HIV infection but related to suppression in general. J Oral Pathol Med 18:28-31, 1989

93. Ulirsch RC, Jaffe ES: Sjogren's syndrome-like illness associated with the acquired immunode-ficiency syndrome-related complex. Hum Pathol 18:1063-1068, 1987

94. Volpe F, Schimmer A, Barr C: Oral manifestations of disseminated *Mycobacterium avium intracellulare* in a patient with AIDS. Oral Surg 60:567, 1985

95. Werber JL: Histoplasmosis of the head and neck. Ear Nose Throat J 67:841-845, 1988

96. Williams CA, Winkler JR, Grassi M, Murray PA: HIV-associated periodontitis complicated by necrotizing stomatitis. Oral Surg Oral Med Oral Pathol 69:351-355, 1990

97. Williams DM, Leigh IM, Greenspan D, Greenspan JS: Altered patterns of keratin expression in oral hairy leukoplakia: Prognostic implications. 20:167-171, 1991

98. Winkler JR, Grassi M, Murray PA: Clinical description and etiology of HIV-associated periodontal diseases. In Robertson PB, Greenspan JS (eds): Perspectives on Oral Manifestations of AIDS: Diagnosis and Management of HIV-Associated Infections. Littleton, Mass, PSG, 1988, pp 49-70

99. Winkler JR, Herrera C, Westenhouse J, et al: Periodontal disease in HIV-infected and seronegative homosexual and bisexual men. 1992 (submitted for publication)

100. Winkler JR, Murray PA: Periodontal disease: A potential intraoral expression of AIDS may be rapidly progressive periodontitis. Calif Dent Assoc J 15:20-24, 1987

101. Winkler JR, Murray PA, Grassi M: Clinical evaluation and management of HIV-associated periodontal lesions. J Periodontol 1992 (in press)

102. Winkler JR, Murray PA, Grassi M, Hammerle C: Diagnosis and management of HIV-associated periodontal lesions. J Am Dent Assoc 119(suppl):S25-S34, 1989

103. Wray D, Moody GH, McMillan A: Oral "hairy" leukoplakia associated with human immuno-deficiency virus infection: Report of two cases. Br Dent J 161:338, 1986

104. Young LS, Lau R, Rowe M, et al: Differentiation-associated expression of the Epstein-Barr virus BZLF1 transactivator protein in oral hairy leukoplakia. J Virol 65(6):2868-2874, 1991

105. Zambon JJ, Reynolds HS, Genco RJ: Studies of the subgingival microflora in patients with acquired immunodeficiency syndrome. J Periodontol 61:699-704, 1990

106. Ziegler JL, Beckstead JA, Volberding PA, et al: Non-Hodgkin's lymphoma in 90 homosexual men: Relation to generalized lymphadenopathy and the acquired immunodeficiency syndrome. N Engl J Med 311:565-570, 1984

107. Ziegler JL, Drew WL, Miner RC, et al: Outbreak of Burkitts-like lymphoma in homosexual men. Lancet 2:631-633, 1982

12

GASTROINTESTINAL TRACT MANIFESTATIONS OF AIDS

JOHN P. CELLO, MD

Over the past decade millions of people throughout the world have become infected with the human immunodeficiency virus (HIV). More than 100,000 people have died already from AIDS. The full extent of the pandemic has not yet been elucidated.[3,30] Hardly any organ system in the body is spared the ravages of AIDS. From the very outset of the AIDS epidemic, clinicians everywhere noted a high prevalence of gastrointestinal (GI) signs and symptoms. Some of these manifestations such as weight loss, dysphagia, anorexia, and diarrhea are almost universally found at some point or another in the course of the disease among patients with AIDS. Other GI signs and symptoms such as odynophagia, hemorrhage, jaundice, or abdominal pain are infrequent but important manifestations of AIDS-related conditions. Since most patients with GI manifestations of the illness undergo interventional diagnostic procedures such as endoscopy or sigmoidoscopy, special care and attention must be directed as much toward the use of universal precautions, choice of equipment, supplies, and specimen processing as to disease recognition and diagnosis. I first discuss specific recommendations for specimen processing, then address AIDS-related GI signs and symptoms.

GASTROINTESTINAL "UNIVERSAL BODY SUBSTANCE ISOLATION"

For the interventional evaluation of patients with AIDS-related GI disorders, the practitioner not infrequently is in close contact with body fluids. In dealing with certain conditions such as GI hemorrhage, the potential risks are much greater than usual because of the large volume of contaminated material in the field of evaluation. Not only is the clinician at potential exposure risk, but future patients who might subsequently use the same endoscopic equipment are also. In approaching the evaluation of *all* patients, including those known or suspected of being HIV positive, I strongly recommend practicing universal precautions (Table 12–1) (see Chapter 4).

176

Table 12–1. Guidelines for "Universal Body Substance Isolation"

1. Routinely use high-quality latex gloves (not vinyl) for *all* exposures to body fluids, mucous membranes, and nonintact skin.
2. Change gloves between patients!
3. Wash hands after patient contact.
4. Use gowns, aprons, masks, and goggles or glasses when likely to soil clothing or skin or to splash substance in face or eyes.
5. Be careful with needles; place in puncture-resistant containers.
6. Dispose of soiled articles in leakproof containers.
7. Practice high-level disinfection or sterilization of equipment between patients.

With respect to the last item on the list of universal precautions, it is important to practice high-level disinfection or sterilization of equipment between all patients.[13,15,16,23,32,38,43] Although there are many processes for disinfection of endoscopes, only two procedures will *absolutely* sterilize fiberoptic or video instruments: ethylene oxide gas or peroxyacetic acid immersion. Currently, our facility at San Francisco General Hospital cold sterilizes *every piece* of endoscopy equipment from every patient with the Steris System One (Painsville, Ohio), using automated immersion and all-channel irrigation with peroxyacetic acid. The Steris System allows for *absolute sterilization* of all immersible endoscopic equipment within a 20-minute period of time without resorting to time-consuming ethylene oxide gas sterilization. Although HIV transfection by endoscopy is undocumented and probably unlikely, should clinicians and their present and future patients accept "disinfection" when the technology for "sterilization" is available?

ENDOSCOPY EQUIPMENT SELECTION

In selecting endoscopy equipment for procedures involving AIDS-risk patients, several points should be considered (Table 12–2). First, for examination of esophageal and gastric lesions, I recommend the use of large-channel endoscopes to facilitate passage of large-particle ("jumbo") biopsy forceps or the use of the loop

Table 12–2. Selection of Endoscopy Equipment for Procedures for Patients at Risk for AIDS

Esophageal and Gastric Lesions
1. Use large-channel instruments to facilitate large-forceps or loop cautery biopsies.
2. Use video endoscopes.
3. Use immersible instruments.
Small Bowel Biopsies
1. Use colonoscopes or small bowel endoscopes.
2. Nonendoscopic small bowel biopsies may be difficult to perform in AIDS patients.
Sigmoidoscopy and Colonoscopy
1. Use video colonoscopes and/or immersible instruments.
2. Most AIDS-associated colonic diseases are detected by careful stool analysis and/or sigmoidoscopy alone; pancolonoscopy rarely is needed.

Table 12–3.   Identification of AIDS-Associated Pathogens

DISEASE PATHOGEN	PRINCIPAL DIAGNOSTIC TEST
Candida albicans	Histopathology (H&E stains)
Herpes simplex	Histopathology (H&E, immunofluorescent stains)
Cytomegalovirus (CMV)	Histopathology (H&E, immunofluorescent stains)
Cryptosporidium/Isospora belli	Stool analysis
Entamoeba histolytica	Stool analysis
Mycobacterium avium-intracellulare	Histopathology (H&E, AFB stains)
Microsporidia	Histopathology (H&E stains)
Lymphoma	Histopathology (H&E stains)
Kaposi's sarcoma	Histopathology

H&E, hematoxylin and eosin; AFB, acid-fast bacillus; PAS, periodic acid–Schiff.

cautery technique. The use of *video* endoscopes, if available, is recommended since the proper practice of video endoscopy places the biopsy valve at least 30 cm away from the endoscopist's eyes, nose, and mouth. For lesions in the esophagus or stomach, I recommend the use of immersible instruments and their processing in the peroxyacetic acid Steris System One.

In biopsying small bowel mucosa in search for multiple causes of AIDS-associated diarrhea, I recommend the use of pediatric or adult colonoscopes rather than standard endoscopes to pass well beyond the inferior duodenal angle. I no longer use small bowel biopsy capsule techniques since poor gastric emptying, long duration of intubation needed, and the necessity of obtaining multiple biopsy specimens for special processing render the use of capsule biopsy techniques inappropriate.

Finally, in approaching patients with lower GI tract complaints, the vast majority of AIDS enteric diseases involving the colon and rectum can be detected by careful stool analysis or by sigmoidoscopy alone. I have found that pancolonoscopy is infrequently necessary in diagnosing AIDS-associated lower GI tract conditions. Also, for sigmoidoscopic and colonoscopic evaluation of these patients at risk for AIDS-associated conditions, I again recommend the use of video instruments, which have complete immersibility and cold sterilization capacity.

Special supplies should be available when performing endoscopy or colonoscopy on patients with AIDS-associated conditions (Table 12–3). I use small sterile culture tubes provided with 1 ml of nonbacteriostatic saline solution for the transport of biopsy specimens for microbacteriologic processing. In addition, cold paraformaldehyde fixative should be available for plastic embedding of specimens to facilitate immunohistochemical staining. For small bowel biopsies I recommend the availability of fixatives such as glutaraldehyde or Karnofsky's fixative for preparation of specimens for electron microscopy. Ten percent formaldehyde is routinely used to process specimens for routine histopathology and therefore is always available for specimen fixation.

PRINCIPAL FEATURE	SUPPLEMENTARY DIAGNOSTIC TEST
Tissue-invasive pseudomycelia (PAS or methenamine stains)	Brush cytology
Cowdry type A inclusions	Viral tissue culture
CMV-infected endothelial cells	Viral tissue culture
AFB stain–positive cysts	Small-bowel biopsy
Erythrocytophagous amoeba (use optical micrometer)	Colonic biopsy
Poorly formed granulomata (massive AFB infection of macrophages)	AFB culture
Cysts on small bowel villus surface	Electron microscopy
Malignant lymphocytes	Immunohistochemical stains (B- and T-cell markers)
Vascular "slits," malignant endothelial cells	Special stains (*Ulex europaeus* stain)

AIDS PATHOGEN AND MALIGNANCY DIAGNOSIS

In confirming individual AIDS-associated GI pathogens and malignancies (see Table 12–3), considerable controversy remains about "definitive" diagnostic testing. Studies are needed detailing sensitivity, specificity, and diagnostic efficiency of the various tests. *Candida albicans* can be documented by using histopathology (not cytology) to demonstrate tissue-invasive pseudomycelia; however, promising reports have suggested that transendoscopic, transnasal, or peroral brush cytology may more efficiently and less invasively define *Candida* esophagitis. Serologic testing for *Candida* is not useful.

Herpes simplex virus (HSV) is diagnosed definitively by using histopathology to demonstrate infected cells with classic "Cowdry type A" inclusions. Viral culture is confirmatory for HSV.

Cytomegalovirus (CMV) infection is pervasive among AIDS patients. Its true extent and nature remains undefined. Demonstration of CMV-infected endothelial cells is the hallmark of CMV disease in the immunocompromised patient. Tissue cultures positive for CMV alone are *not* definitive for CMV disease. The yield of CMV by histopathology is enhanced by special immunohistochemical stains.

Cryptosporidiosis and infection with *Isospora belli* are confirmed best by adequate stool analysis. Microsporidia usually require electron microscopic analysis of enteric biopsies for diagnosis. However, occasionally I have diagnosed these infections (i.e., ones caused by cryptosporidia, Microsporidia, and *I. belli*) on the basis of routine enteric biopsies. Finally, *Entamoeba histolytica* is diagnosed best on the basis of stool analysis. However, colonic biopsies can establish the diagnosis in the absence of positive stool results.

For the proper processing of specimens for microbiologic culture and histopathology, special attention should be paid to the last column in Table 12–3. It should be emphasized that this table represents current practice and may change with further clinical studies.

OVERVIEW OF SIGNS AND SYMPTOMS OF HIV INFECTIONS AND MALIGNANCIES

GI abnormalities are commonly encountered in the evaluation and treatment of patients with AIDS. Although some of these GI manifestations (e.g., weight loss, anorexia, and large-volume diarrhea) are often difficult to diagnose and treat specifically, many other manifestations of HIV infection, particularly those in the esophagus, liver, biliary tract, and rectosigmoid, can be expeditiously evaluated, definitively diagnosed, and specifically treated. The most common GI manifestations of HIV infection are reviewed in an organ-related scheme. Emphasis is placed on the diagnosis and management of treatable conditions.

Esophageal Diseases

Dysphagia, odynophagia, and retrosternal esophageal pain (esophagospasm) are common occurrences among patients with acute and chronic HIV infection. In addition, *acute* AIDS esophagitis was reported in eight patients during their initial illness from HIV infection.[31] These patients had dysphagia, odynophagia, and retrosternal pain lasting from 2 to 14 days, with spontaneous resolution thereafter.

The most common esophageal complaint among AIDS patients is dysphagia (difficulty swallowing, with a sensation of food sticking). The most common organism associated with dysphagia is *C. albicans,* with the majority of these patients having both thrush and esophageal candidiasis[40] (Table 12–4). In patients with thrush and esophageal complaints, a course of antifungal therapy, including ketoconazole, 200 mg per day, or fluconazole, 100 mg per day, for 7 to 14 days is indicated (see Chapter 11). Barium contrast radiography may support but not document the diagnosis of esophageal candidiasis; therefore endoscopy need not be performed in AIDS patients with thrush and dysphagia simply to document esophageal involvement unless treatment with ketoconazole or fluconazole fails to produce significant improvement in symptoms.[40] Large, yellow-white plaques throughout the esophagus are usually noted in patients with *Candida* esophagitis, and biopsies or direct cytology brushings should be performed looking for tissue-invasive pseu-

Table 12–4.   Clinical Features of AIDS-Associated Esophagitis

PARAMETER	CANDIDA	CYTOMEGALOVIRUS	HERPES SIMPLEX VIRUS
Thrush	Usual	Occasional	Occasional
Dysphagia	Severe	Moderate	Moderate
Odynophagia	Rare	Moderate	Severe
Esophagospasm	Rare	Moderate	Severe
Localization	Poor	Good	Excellent
Endoscopic feature	Diffuse plaques	Giant shallow ulcers	Deep ulcers
Diagnostic tests	Histology, cytology	Histology	Histology, culture
Therapy	Fluconazole	Ganciclovir	Acyclovir
Response to therapy	Excellent	Fair	Excellent

domycelia. Despite a favorable symptomatic response to current antifungal therapy, esophageal lesions may not completely resolve despite months of therapy.[41]

Pain on swallowing (odynophagia) and retrosternal episodic pain without swallowing (esophagospasm), in addition to dysphagia, are more commonly encountered in patients with herpes esophagitis and CMV esophagitis than in those with *Candida* esophagitis.[39] Although discrete single ulcers have been reported in patients with CMV esophagitis, extremely large (2- to 10-cm long), shallow, superficial ulcerations extending throughout much of the esophagus also have been noted.[39] Indeed, CMV ulcerations may be so extensive and circumferential that virtually no normal mucosa, only infected granulation tissue, is encountered. Although patients with CMV esophagitis may experience an initially favorable response to ganciclovir (DHPG), relapses are common,[18] and ganciclovir maintenance therapy or foscarnet administration is usually needed (see Chapter 23). Oral agents effective against CMV are urgently needed, given the high relapse rate for enteric CMV infection following ganciclovir treatment.

Although sometimes indistinguishable from CMV ulcerations, HSV (type 1 or 2) ulcers are generally fewer, smaller, and deeper than those of CMV. Chronic AIDS-related herpetic esophageal ulcerations are usually deep, clean-based ulcerations, 1 to 2 cm in diameter. These large and deep chronic herpetic ulcerations usually are associated clinically with intense esophagospasm, odynophagia, and dysphagia. Fortunately, the clinical response to acyclovir has been gratifying among patients with HSV esophagitis; however, maintenance therapy is needed (see Chapter 23).

Rarely, primary lymphoma, Kaposi's sarcoma (KS), histoplasmosis (see Chapter 20), or squamous cell carcinoma has been noted in the esophagus among patients with AIDS. On occasion, patients with AIDS have large "geographic" ulcers of the esophagus without any pathogens isolated by histopathology and/or viral cultures. These so-called *idiopathic esophageal ulcerations* look nearly identical to those associated with CMV, and their diagnosis requires careful specimen processing to exclude other disease entities. I routinely have performed repeat endoscopy on these patients with large idiopathic esophageal ulcers but have found no positive identification for CMV or HSV. Anecdotal reports suggest these patients may respond to intralesional steroid injections (by endoscopy) and/or to oral steroid administration. Before treating them with steroids, however, multiple negative biopsy results from at least two endoscopies should be documented.

In addition to these AIDS-specific esophageal diseases, bedridden AIDS and AIDS-related complex (ARC) patients may experience severe esophageal peptic acid reflux, with esophagitis and esophageal ulcerations. Given the multiplicity of possible causes of esophagitis, the distinct possibility of specific therapy, and the relative ease of diagnosis, I strongly recommend performing endoscopy in AIDS patients with esophageal complaints except in those with classic thrush.

Gastric Diseases

Nausea, vomiting, hematemesis, melena, and early satiety occasionally are encountered in evaluating patients with AIDS or ARC.[7,12,34] A thorough investigation is once again indicated since many of these patients will be found to have non–AIDS-related GI diseases[7] (Table 12–5).

**Table 12–5.   Cause of Upper
Gastrointestinal Bleeding in 13
AIDS Patients**

LESION	NUMBER OF PATIENTS
Kaposi's sarcoma	
Gastric	3
Duodenal	1
Lymphoma, gastric	2
Cytomegalovirus	
Esophagitis	1
Gastritis	1
Gastric ulcer	1
Duodenal ulcer	1
Duodenitis	1
Mallory-Weiss tear	1
Variceal bleeding	1

KS is noted frequently on endoscopy in patients with documented cutaneous and/ or nodal KS (see Chapter 25). In one prospective survey of 50 patients with cutaneous and/or nodal KS, 20 (40%) had GI lesions noted on endoscopy and/or flexible sigmoidoscopy.[12,34] Only 7 of 30 (23%) visibly positive endoscopies and/ or sigmoidoscopies could be confirmed histologically, however, probably because of the submucosal location of most KS lesions and the limited depth of biopsy sampling.[12] AIDS-associated KS is rarely symptomatic; however, GI hemorrhage occasionally is encountered.

B-cell non-Hodgkin's lymphomas involving the antrum occasionally are associated with gastric outlet obstruction and/or hemorrhage. Although non-AIDS gastric lymphomas commonly are confined initially to the stomach, AIDS-related gastric lymphomas are more commonly multifocal, with extensive disease throughout the abdomen in addition to gastric involvement. Although smaller lymphoma and KS lesions may go undetected by radiographic techniques and require endoscopy for detection, larger masses commonly are noted radiographically as "target lesions" with central umbilicated ulcerations. Specimens from these lesions should be obtained for biopsy directly by endoscopy.

Hepatobiliary Disease

Abnormal biochemical test results of liver function, right upper quadrant abdominal discomfort, and hepatomegaly increasingly are noted in patients with AIDS or ARC.[2,4,5,9,14,17,20,24,27,35,36] Early and *complete* invasive and noninvasive evaluation of these patients should be undertaken, with particular attention to treatable non– HIV-associated biliary tract disease.

Acalculous cholecystitis, including gangrenous cholecystitis (an entity rarely encountered in young, healthy, ambulatory patients), has been reported in AIDS patients, with the majority of them having CMV and/or *Cryptosporidium* noted on histologic sections.[2,17,24] The pathophysiology of this disease is uncertain; however, several patients have had CMV-infected endothelial cells together with mucosal

Table 12–6.   Hepatic Histology in 85 AIDS Patients

FINDING	BIOPSY (% of total) (N = 26)	AUTOPSY (% of total) (N = 59)	COMBINED (% of total) (N = 85)
Normal	1 (3.8)	9 (15.3)	10 (11.8)
Steatosis	10 (38.5)	26 (44.1)	36 (42.4)
Portal inflammation	14 (53.8)	16 (27.1)	30 (35.3)
Congestion	1 (3.8)	18 (30.5)	19 (22.4)
Granulomata	10 (38.5)	2 (3.4)	12 (14.1)
Focal necrosis	5 (19.2)	5 (8.5)	10 (11.8)
Fibrosis or cirrhosis	4 (15.4)	4 (6.8)	8 (4.7)
Bile stasis	2 (7.7)	3 (5.1)	5 (5.9)
Kupffer cell hyperplasia	3 (11.5)	3 (5.1)	6 (7.1)
Piecemeal necrosis	2 (7.7)	1 (1.7)	3 (1.2)

From Schneiderman DJ, Arenson DM, Cello JP, et al: Hepatology 7:927, 1987.

necrosis and ulceration, suggesting, as with esophagitis, that necrotizing vasculitis is the mechanism of injury.

Hepatic parenchymal disease likewise is common in patients with HIV infection.[4,14,20,27,35] In a retrospective review of hepatic histology, clinical features, and laboratory data in 85 AIDS patients, I noted only one of 26 (3.8%) normal percutaneous liver biopsy specimens and nine of 58 (15%) normal postmortem liver specimens[27] (Table 12–6). Steatosis, portal inflammation, and noncaseating, poorly formed granulomata were the most common histologic abnormalities (Table 12–7). AIDS-specific infections or malignancies were detected in 40% of both biopsy and autopsy groups.

In addition to the high frequency of KS (10 of 26 patients), CMV (10 of 26 patients), and *Mycobacterium avium-intracellulare* (5 of 26 patients), Nakanuma et al.[27] also noted marked depletion of portal tract lymphocytes in livers of AIDS patients. In most instances, however, parenchymal liver disease in patients with

Table 12–7.   AIDS-Specific Hepatic Histologic Features in 85 Patients

FINDING	BIOPSY (% of total) (N = 26)	AUTOPSY (% of total) (N = 59)	COMBINED (% of total) (N = 85)
No pathogens	15 (57.7)	34 (57.6)	49 (57.6)
Mycobacterium avium-intracellulare	8 (30.8)	6 (10.2)	14 (16.5)
Kaposi's sarcoma	0 (0.0)	11 (18.6)	11 (12.9)
Cytomegalovirus	2 (7.7)	6 (10.2)	8 (9.4)
Lymphoma	2 (7.7)	2 (3.4)	4 (4.7)
Cryptococcus	0 (0.0)	2 (3.4)	2 (2.4)
Histoplasma	0 (0.0)	1 (1.7)	1 (1.2)
Coccidioides	0 (0.0)	1 (1.7)	1 (1.2)

From Schneiderman DJ, Arenson DM, Cello JP, et al: Hepatology 7:927, 1987.

AIDS represents a not-unexpected manifestation of a previously diagnosed, widely disseminated disease process, and liver biopsy infrequently documents new AIDS-specific diagnoses. Thus performing a percutaneous liver biopsy is not usually necessary in the majority of patients with abnormal liver function tests.

Obstructive biliary tract disease should, however, be thoroughly and expeditiously evaluated in AIDS patients. We at San Francisco and others have noted profound ultrasound, computed tomography (CT), and endoscopic cholangiographic abnormalities in patients with HIV infection, and the full spectrum of HIV disease manifested in the biliary tree has yet to be elucidated.[2,5,9,17,24,30] Patients with AIDS-associated biliary tract disease often present with fever, pain, and tenderness in the right upper quadrant and dramatic increases in serum alkaline phosphatase (2 to 20 times above upper limits of normal).[9,24,36] Most patients with AIDS-associated biliary tract disease will be noted by ultrasound or CT abdominal scanning techniques to have prominent or dilated intrahepatic or extrahepatic bile ducts, or both, with dilation down to periampullary area, together with marked thickening of the ductal walls.[9] Endoscopic retrograde cholangiopancreatography (ERCP) of 51 AIDS patients by our service at San Francisco General Hospital over the past 6 years demonstrated intrahepatic and extrahepatic sclerosing cholangitis changes (including irregular ductal mucosa) and papillary stenosis in 25 patients, intrahepatic ductal sclerotic changes alone in 6 patients, papillary stenosis alone in 5 patients and high-grade extrahepatic bile duct obstruction in 4 patients (Figures 12–1 to 12–3). Only 11 of 51 AIDS patients studied by ERCP because of pain and markedly elevated

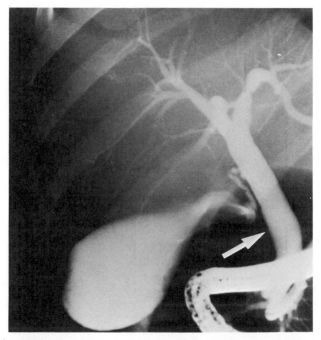

FIGURE 12–1.   AIDS-associated papillary stenosis. Entire biliary tree is filled with contrast. Extrahepatic bile duct *(arrow)* is dilated, as evidenced by comparison to the endoscope (12.5 mm). A sphincterotomy was performed.

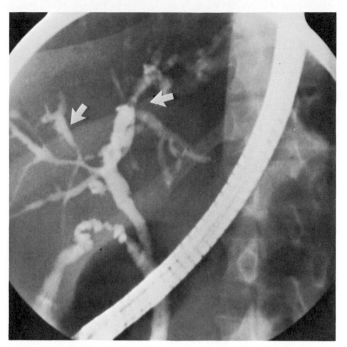

FIGURE 12–2. AIDS-sclerosing cholangitis. Intra- and extrahepatic ducts are markedly irregular. There are focal strictures and irregular dilations of the intrahepatic ducts *(arrows)*.

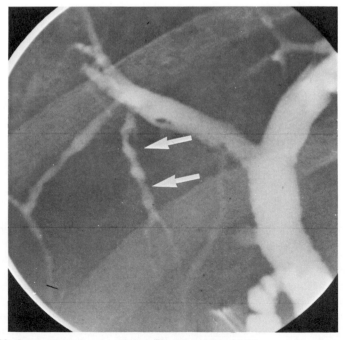

FIGURE 12–3. Intrahepatic sclerosing cholangitis. Intrahepatic ducts are irregular with a beaded appearance *(arrows)*. Extrahepatic ductal mucosa has a serrated appearance.

Table 12–8.   AIDS Cholangiopathy: Clinical Features of 51 Patients Studied at San Francisco General Hospital

FEATURES	ABNORMAL ERCP (n = 40)	NORMAL ERCP (n = 11)	p VALUE
Age (yr)	36 ± 1.2	35.6 ± 3.0	NS
AIDS duration (mo)	10.8 ± 2.2	11.2 ± 2.9	NS
Right upper quandrant pain	35/40 (88%)	8/11 (73%)	NS
Abnormal ultrasound	28/38 (74%)	1/10 (10%)	<0.001
Abnormal computed tomo- graphic scan	12/17 (71%)	0/9 (0)	0.003
Alkaline phosphatase (IU/L)	744 ± 120	700 ± 137	NS
Alanine aminotransferase (IU/L)	95 ± 15	114 ± 30	NS
Bilirubin (mg/dl)	1.4 ± 0.5	2.5 ± 1.4	NS

ERCP, endoscopic retrograde cholangiopancreatography; NS, not significant.

serum alkaline phosphatase levels had normal cholangiograms (Table 12–8). All 20 patients with papillary stenosis *and* abdominal pain underwent ERCP sphincterotomy, with multiple biopsies of the ampulla of Vater. Eighteen of 40 patients (45%) with abnormal cholangiograms had specific AIDS-related pathogens or malignancies in the regions of ductal disease as demonstrated by cholangiography (CMV, 7; *Cryptosporidium,* 5; CMV *and Cryptosporidium,* 1; KS, 1; *M. avium-intracellulare,* 3; lymphoma, 1) (Color Plate II *C*). The pathophysiology of AIDS-associated sclerosing cholangitis and papillary stenosis is uncertain although CMV and/or cryptosporidial ulceration and subsequent fibrotic stricturing of the bile duct have been suggested by our own studies and by limited additional reports. Initial results of a prospective study being conducted at San Francisco General Hospital suggest that more than 10% of asymptomatic AIDS patients have abnormal bile duct morphology.

Small Bowel Disease

Cramping paraumbilical abdominal pain, weight loss, and large-volume diarrhea are common in patients with HIV disease. The majority of AIDS patients with these complaints has specific small bowel infections (Table 12–9).[1,6,8,19,25,29,37,42,45] Certainly routine colonic bacterial pathogens such as *Salmonella* sp., *Shigella* sp., and *Campylobacter* sp., which may be persistent and mimic chronic inflammatory bowel disease, should be excluded by adequate culture techniques. Likewise, routine and atypical parasitic infestation, including that caused by *Giardia lamblia, E. histolytica, Cryptosporidium,* and *I. belli,* must be excluded.[1,8,19,29,37,42,50] In addition to AIDS-associated pathogens, HIV infection of the enterocytes or lamina propria can be associated with abnormal small bowel morphology.[19,42] Limited studies to date have demonstrated the gamut of pathologic findings, ranging from normal small bowel mucosa to subtotal villous atrophy (decreased villous height) and associated crypt changes, consisting largely of decreased mitoses (hypoplasia).[19,42] These changes may represent viral infection of the enterocytes by HIV itself or an unidentified opportunistic viral agent. Small bowel biopsies may be indicated for patients with negative results from evaluations of the stools for specific pathogens.

**Table 12–9.   Infectious Diarrhea in 43
AIDS Patients**

CAUSE	NO.*	PERCENT
Cytomegalovirus	15	20
Mycobacterium avium	10	14
Salmonella sp.	10	14
Cryptosporidium	8	11
Entamoeba histolytica	6	8
Giardia lamblia	4	5
Herpes simplex virus	4	5
Campylobacter jejuni	3	4
Isospora belli	2	3
Clostridium difficile	2	3
Candida sp.	2	3
Strongyloides	2	3
Kaposi's sarcoma	1	1
Other pathogens	5	7
TOTAL	74	

Data from Smith PD, Lane C, Vee J, et al: Ann Intern Med 108:328, 1988; Anthony MA, Brandt LJ, Klein RS, Bernstein LH: Dig Dis Sci 33:1141, 1988.
    *Some with multiple pathogens.

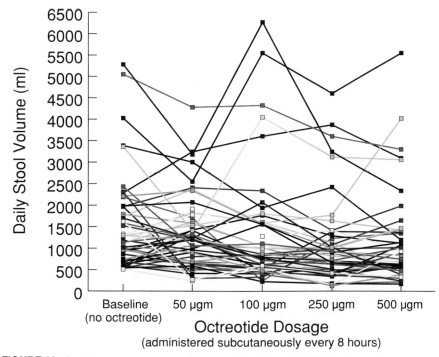

FIGURE 12–4.   Dose response to octreotide among 51 patients with AIDS-related refractory diarrhea. By day 14 of subcutaneous octreotide therapy, mean stool volumes had decreased from 1604 ± 180 ml/day to 1084 ± 162 ml/day ($p < .01$).

Initial studies with octreotide (Sandostatin), a somatostatin analog, suggest that some patients with dehydrating diarrhea respond to it.[6] In our multicenter, open-label clinical trial of octreotide 21 of 51 patients (41%) were partial or complete responders (decrease in daily stool weight to ≤50% baseline or <250 g/day)[6] (Figure 12–4). Baseline laboratory studies (Tables 12–10 and 12–11) demonstrated defects in nutrient absorption, including altered D-xylose, bentiromide, and fat absorption. The latter nutrient absorption was profoundly abnormal (Table 12–11) as evidenced by nearly one quarter of dietary fat appearing as fecal fat in 72-hour collections (nl <7% malabsorption). Responders to subcutaneous octreotide (at dosages ranging from 50 to 500 μg every 8 hours) were significantly less likely to have enteric pathogens than were nonresponders (33% versus 70%, $p < .01$) (Table 12–12). Thus in this study, some patients, particulary those with idiopathic AIDS-associated, large-volume diarrhea, were benefited by octreotide.

Table 12–10.   Laboratory Data*

	DAY 0	DAY 14	DAY 28
Hematocrit (%)	34.1 ± 0.9	32.3 ± 0.9 (n = 50)	34.4 ± 1.3 (n = 29)
White blood count (× 1000)/mm³)	3.5 ± 0.3	3.0 ± 0.2 (n = 50)*	3.3 ± 0.3 (n = 29)
Carotene (μmol/L)	0.87 ± 0.1 (n = 45)	0.79 ± 0.2 (n = 11)	0.70 ± 0.09 (n = 10)
Albumin (g/L)	35 ± 1 (n = 19)	32 ± 2 (n = 19)	35 ± 0.2 (n = 14)
Glucose (mmol/L)	5.2 ± 0.2	5.9 ± 0.4†	5.1 ± 0.2 (n = 31)
D-Xylose (mmol/L)‡	0.63 ± 0.08 (n = 32)	0.52 ± 0.11 (n = 16)	
Bentiromide (%)	45.2 ± 4.1 (n = 20)	59.7 ± 8.2 (n = 9)	
Patient weight (kg)	58.7 ± 1.3	59.1 ± 1.3	59.9 ± 1.4 (n = 29)
Karnofsky score	66 ± 2 (n = 50)	69 ± 2 (n = 50)	76 ± 2* (n = 32)

NOTE: Day 14 (i.e., end of second week of drug) and day 28 (off drug) values not significantly different from day 0 unless indicated.

Normal values: carotene, 1.12-3.72 μmol/L; glucose, 2.22-3.89 mmol/L; D-xylose, >1.67 mmol/L at 2 hr; bentiromide, >57% excretion in 6 hours.

n = 51 unless stated otherwise; all mean values ± S.E.M.

*$p < .01$.

†$p < .001$.

‡After 25-g oral dose; 2-hr serum level.

Table 12–11.   Fat Absorption Balance Studies

PARAMETER	DAY 0	DAY 14	p VALUE
Fat ingested (72 hr; in grams)	282.5 ± 19.3	306.6 ± 23.3	NS
Fecal fat (72 hr; in grams)	53.2 ± 6.7	107.3 ± 18.0	<0.001
Fat malabsorption*	0.22 ± 0.03	0.30 ± 0.04	<0.001

NS, not significant; day 0, baseline; day 14, end of second week of drug administration.

*Calculated as 72-hr fecal fat (g) divided by 72-hr dietary fat intake.

Table 12-12. Octreotide Responders versus Nonresponders at Day 14

PARAMETER	RESPONDERS (n = 21)	NONRESPONDERS (n = 30)	p VALUE
Stool volume (ml)	541 ± 105	1471 ± 245	.002
Stool frequency (per day)	2.54 ± 0.21	5.41 ± .58	<.0001
Hematocrit (%)	35.6 ± 1.7	33.1 ± 0.9	NS
White blood count (× 1000)/mm³	3.5 ± 0.5	3.6 ± 0.3	NS
Carotene (μmol/L)	1.03 ± 0.2 (n = 19)	0.71 ± 0.1 (n = 26)	NS
Glucose (mmol/L)	5.1 ± 0.2	5.3 ± 0.3	NS
D-Xylose (mmol/L)	0.65 ± 0.11 (n = 11)	0.62 ± 0.11 (n = 21)	NS
Fecal fat (72 hr; in grams at day 0)	56.1 ± 10.8	52.9 ± 8.4 (n = 29)	NS
Fecal fat (72 hr; grams at day 14)	96.7 ± 32.7	120 ± 17.5 (n = 27)	p <.05
Bentiromide (%)	48.1 ± 8.1 (n = 8)	43.3 ± 4.6 (n = 12)	NS
Patient weight (kg)	58.7 ± 1.6	58.7 ± 1.9	NS
Karnofsky score	70.7 ± 2.6	63.6 ± 2.6 (n = 29)	NS
Presence of cryptosporidia	5 (24%)	10 (33%)	NS
No pathogens identified	14 (67%)	9 (30%)	<.01

All values ± S.E.M.
NS, not significant.

Colorectal Diseases

Colonic diarrhea usually is associated with frequent *small* volume stools, left lower quadrant or suprapubic cramping, rectal urgency (tenesmus), and proctalgia and dyskesia (painful defecation). On occasion a small amount of bright red blood may be noted. Once again, in the majority of these patients with diarrhea of colonic origin, specific bacterial and parasitic pathogens can and should be easily isolated by careful analysis of the stools alone, including routine bacterial cultures, studies to identify *Clostridium difficile* enterotoxin, and microscopy to identify intestinal parasites. In addition, some patients may have classic herpetic perianal ulcerations, which can be diagnosed by specific viral culture of swabs taken directly from the perianal area.

Among AIDS patients with symptoms of proctitis and/or colonic diarrhea who have *negative* stool evaluations, performing flexible sigmoidoscopy (usually using a 60-cm long, fully immersible instrument) is often useful. CMV proctocolitis has been described as having sigmoidoscopic features suggestive of focal ischemic colitis, that is, submucosal hemorrhages and discrete shallow ulcerations of distal colonic mucosa[25] (see Chapter 23). In addition to causing perianal disease, herpetic ulcerations of the distal colon may be encountered in patients with HSV (type 1 or 2). Once again, obtaining specific biopsy specimens for histology and viral culture is indicated. In those patients with persistent diarrhea, the possibility of *Chlamydia* also should be evaluated by specific culture. Even in the absence of focal or diffuse colonic mucosal changes, biopsy specimens should be taken for histologic evaluation to look for the occasional patient with *Cryptosporidium* whose stools have been negative for this organism.

In addition to HIV-associated pathologic processes, idiopathic inflammatory bowel disease and colorectal neoplasms (including anal cancer) must be carefully excluded, particularly in middle-aged patients with recent diagnosis of AIDS or ARC.

Diarrhea Caused by Protozoa and Parasites

Although many enteric infections in patients with AIDS do respond to specific anti-infective therapy, treatment of protozoan- and parasite-induced disease is poor. Most problematic for both clinicians and patients is cryptosporidiosis. Early studies using spiramycin (especially for treating immunocompetent children) were promising, but more recent clinical trials have been disappointing.[11,26,33,46] Limited early favorable experience with oral bovine transfer factor derived from calves has likewise not been duplicated by follow-up studies.[21] *I. belli* infections do respond to trimethoprim-sulfamethoxazole combination therapy (960 mg, four times daily for 10 days); therefore specific therapy is warranted.[22,28] The importance of Microsporidia in the etiology of AIDS-associated diarrhea has only recently been clarified; thus studies of specific therapies are limited. In one recent study 10 of 13 patients with microsporidiosis treated with metronidazole noted substantial improvement or disappearance of diarrhea.[10] A limited trial of metronidazole for patients with microsporidiosis is probably indicated. In addition to limited successes reported for specific therapies, some benefit can be anticipated from treatment with nonspecific antidiarrheal medications such as loperamide, tincture of opium, and diphenoxylate with atropine.

Peritoneal Disease

On occasion, patients with AIDS or ARC may suddenly develop ascites.[44] Since some HIV-infected patients may have underlying cirrhosis (caused by either alcohol consumption or viral hepatitis), a sizeable percentage of them will have transudative ascites related to their chronic liver disease. Exudative ascites (ascites protein concentration >1.5 to 2.0 g/dl), however, should be thoroughly evaluated in patients with HIV infection. Careful evaluation of the ascites fluid, including performing cytology (sampling large volumes) and acid-fast stains, should be done early to exclude patients with malignancy and tuberculous peritonitis. In patients with new onset of exudative ascites and negative or equivocal evaluations by paracentesis and/or fine-needle aspiration biopsy, I have performed laparoscopic evaluations with directed biopsy of peritoneal implants, noting lymphoma or tuberculosis most frequently.

REFERENCES

1. Antony MA, Brandt LJ, Klein RS, Bernstein LH: Infectious diarrhea in patients with AIDS. Dig Dis Sci 33:1141, 1988
2. Blumberg RS, Kelsey P, Perrone T, et al: Cytomegalovirus—and *Cryptosporidium*-associated acalculous gangrenous cholecystitis. Am J Med 76:1118, 1984
3. Burke DS, Brundage JF, Herbold JR, et al: Human immunodeficiency virus infections among civilian applicants for United States Military Service, October 1985 to March 1986. N Engl J Med 317:131, 1987
4. Caccamo D, Perez NK, Marchevsky A: Primary lymphoma of the liver in the acquired immunodeficiency syndrome. Arch Pathol Lab Med 110:553, 1986
5. Cello JP: Acquired immunodeficiency syndrome cholangiopathy: Spectrum of disease. Am J Med 86:539-546, 1989
6. Cello JP, Grendell JH, Basuk P, et al: Effect of octreotide on refractory AIDS-associated diarrhea. A prospective, multicenter clinical trial. Ann Intern Med 115:705-710, 1991
7. Cello JP, Wilcox CM: Evaluation and treatment of gastrointestinal tract hemorrhage in patients with AIDS. In Friedman SL (ed): Gastrointestinal Manifestations of AIDS. Gastroenterology Clinics of North America. Philadelphia, WB Saunders Co, 1988, pp 639-648
8. DeHovitz JA, Pape JW, Boney M, et al: Clinical manifestations and therapy of *Isospora belli* infection in patients with the acquired immunodeficiency syndrome. N Engl J Med 315:87, 1986
9. Dolmatch BL, Laing FC, Federle MP, et al: AIDS-related cholangitis: Radiographic findings in nine patients. Radiology 163:313, 1987
10. Eeftinck-Schattenkerk JK, van Gool T, van Ketel RJ, et al: Clinical significance of small-intestinal microsporidiosis in HIV-II–infected individuals. Lancet 337:895, 1991
11. Fafard J, Lalonde R: Long-standing symptomatic cryptosporidiosis in a normal man: Clinical response to spiramycin. J Clin Gastroenterol 12:190, 1990
12. Friedman SL, Wright TL, Altman DF: Gastrointestinal Kaposi's sarcoma in patients with acquired immunodeficiency syndrome—Endoscopic and autopsy findings. Gastroenterology 89:102, 1985
13. Gardner JS, Hughes JM: Options for isolation precautions. Ann Intern Med 107:248, 1987
14. Glasgow BJ, Anders K, Layfield LJ, et al: Clinical and pathologic finding of the liver in the acquired immune deficiency syndrome. Am J Clin Pathol 83:582, 1985
15. Henderson DK, Saah AJ, Zak BJ, et al: Risk of nosocomial infection with human T-cell lymphotrophic virus type III/lymphadenopathy-associated virus in a large cohort of intensively exposed health care workers. Ann Intern Med 104:644, 1986
16. Hirsch MS, Wormser GP, Schooley RT, et al: Risk of nosocomial infection with human T-cell lymphotrophic virus III (HTLV-III). N Engl J Med 312:1, 1985
17. Kavin H, Jonas RB, Chowdhury L, et al: Acalculous cholecystitis and cytomegalovirus infection in the acquired immunodeficiency syndrome. Ann Intern Med 104:53, 1986
18. Koretz SH, Collaborative DHPG Treatment Study Group: Treatment of serious cytomegalovirus infections with 9-(1,3 dihydroxy-2-propoxymethyl) guanine in patients with AIDS and other immunodeficiencies. N Engl J Med 314:801, 1986
19. Kotler DP, Gaetz HP, Lange M, et al: Enteropathy associated with the acquired immunodeficiency syndrome. Ann Intern Med 101:421, 1984
20. Lebovics E, Thung SN, Schaffner F, et al: The liver in the acquired immunodeficiency syndrome: A clinical and histologic study. Hepatology 5:293, 1985
21. Louie E, Borkowsky W, Klesius PH, et al: Treatment of cryptosporidiosis with oral bovine transfer factor. Clin Immunol Immunopath 44:329, 1987
22. Lumb R, Hardiman R: *Isospora belli* infection. Med J Aust 155:194, 1991
23. Lynch P, Jackson MM, Cummings J, et al: Rethinking the role of isolation practices in the prevention of nosocomial infections. Ann Intern Med 107:242, 1987
24. Margulis SJ, Honig CL, Soave R, et al: Biliary tract obstruction in the acquired immunodeficiency syndrome. Ann Intern Med 105:207, 1986
25. Meiselman MS, Cello JP, Margaretten W: Cytomegalovirus colitis—Report of the clinical, endoscopic and pathologic findings in two patients with the acquired immune deficiency syndrome. Gastroenterology 88:171, 1985
26. Moskovitz BL, Stanton TL, Kusmierek JJ: Spiramycin therapy for cryptosporidial diarrhea in immunocompromised patients. J Antimicrob Chemother 22(suppl B):189, 1988

27. Nakanuma Y, Liew CT, Peters RL, et al: Pathologic features of the liver in acquired immune deficiency syndrome (AIDS). Liver 6:158, 1986
28. Pape JW, Johnson WD: *Isospora belli* infections. Prog Clin Parasitol 2:119, 1991
29. Pitlik S, Fainstein V, Garza D, et al: Human cryptosporidiosis: Spectrum of disease—Report of six cases and review of the literature. Arch Intern Med 143:2269, 1983
30. Quinn TC, Glasser D, Cannon RO, et al: Human immunodeficiency virus infection among patients attending clinics for sexually transmitted diseases. N Engl J Med 318:197, 1988
31. Rabeneck L, Boyko WJ, McLean DM, et al: Unusual esophageal ulcers containing enveloped virus-like particles in homosexual men. Gastroenterology 90:1882, 1986
32. Raufman JP, Straus EW: Gastrointestinal endoscopy in patients with acquired immune deficiency syndrome: An evaluation of current practices. Gastrointest Endosc 33:76, 1987
33. Saez-Llorens X, Odio CM, Umana MA, Morales MV: Spiramycin vs. placebo for treatment of acute diarrhea caused by cryptosporidium. Pediatr Infect Dis J 8:136, 1989
34. Saltz RK, Kurtz RC, Lightdale CJ, et al: Kaposi's sarcoma—Gastrointestinal involvement correlation with skin findings and immunologic function. Dig Dis Sci 29:817, 1984
35. Schneiderman DJ, Arenson DM, Cello JP, et al: Hepatic disease in patients with acquired immune deficiency syndrome (AIDS). Hepatology 7:925, 1987
36. Schneiderman DJ, Cello JP, Laing FC: Papillary stenosis and sclerosing cholangitis in the acquired immunodeficiency syndrome. Ann Intern Med 106:546, 1987
37. Smith PD, Lane C, Vee J, et al: Intestinal infections in patients with the acquired immunodeficiency syndrome (AIDS). Ann Intern Med 108:328, 1988
38. Spire B, Barre-Sinoussi F, Montagnier L, Cloermann JC: Inactivation of lymphadenopathy associated virus by chemical disinfectants. Lancet 2:899, 1984
39. St. Onge G, Bezahler GH: Giant esophageal ulcer associated with cytomegalovirus. Gastroenterology 83:127, 1982
40. Tavitian A, Raufman JP, Rosenthal LE: Oral candidiasis as a marker for esophageal candidiasis in the acquired immunodeficiency syndrome. Ann Intern Med 104:54, 1986
41. Tavitian A, Raufman JP, Rosenthal LE, et al: Ketoconazole-resistant *Candida* esophagitis in patients with acquired immunodeficiency syndrome. Gastroenterology 90:443, 1986
42. Ullrich R, Zeitz M, Heise W, et al: Small intestinal structure and function in patients infected with human immunodeficiency virus (HIV): Evidence for HIV-induced enteropathy. Ann Intern Med 111:15, 1989
43. Weller IVD, Williams CB, Jeffries DJ, et al: Cleaning and disinfection of equipment for gastrointestinal flexible endoscopy: Interim recommendations of a working party of the British Society of Gastroenterology. Gut 29:1134, 1988
44. Wilcox CM, Forsmark CE, Darragh T, et al: High-protein ascites in patients with the acquired immunodeficiency syndrome. Gastroenterology 100:745, 1991
45. Wolfson JS, Richter JM, Waldron MA, et al: Cryptosporidiosis in immunocompetent patients. N Engl J Med 312:1278, 1985
46. Woolf GM, Townsend M, Guyatt G: Treatment of cryptosporidiosis with spiramycin in AIDS. J Clin Gastroenterol 9:632, 1987

13

MANAGEMENT OF NEUROLOGIC COMPLICATIONS OF HIV-1 INFECTION AND AIDS

JOHN M. WORLEY, DO
RICHARD W. PRICE, MD

Human immunodeficiency virus type 1 (HIV-1) infection, particularly its late phase, the acquired immune deficiency syndrome (AIDS), is complicated by a variety of central nervous system (CNS) and peripheral nervous system (PNS) disorders (for other general reviews, see references 14, 19, 20, 89, and 149). Classification of these disorders according to their underlying pathophysiologic or pathogenetic process provides a rational framework for comprehending and managing the spectrum of conditions to which these patients are susceptible (Table 13–1) and also allows one to deal systematically with new or unusual conditions as they are encountered.

However, in practice the neurologist confronted with a sick patient begins with **neuroanatomic localization.** For this reason in this chapter we classify and discuss the major neurologic disorders according to their predominant pathologic anatomy. An additional important consideration for differential diagnosis relates to the **stage of systemic HIV-1 infection,** reflecting the degree of underlying immunosuppression suffered by the patient at the time of presentation. The underlying immune status exerts a predominating effect on disease vulnerability; hence it strongly influences the probabilities of differential diagnosis. Therefore we discuss the neurologic aspects of early HIV-1 infection separately before dealing with the more common conditions that occur in the late, severely immunocompromised phase of infection.

Our studies of the neurologic complications of AIDS are supported by Public Health Service Grant NS-21703 from the National Institutes of Health.

Table 13–1. Classification of the Neurologic Complications of HIV-1 Infection According to Underlying Pathophysiologic and Pathogenetic Categories

UNDERLYING PROCESS	EXAMPLES
Opportunistic infections	Cerebral toxoplasmosis
	Cryptococcal meningitis
	Progressive multifocal leukoencephalopathy (PML)
Opportunistic neoplasms	Primary central nervous system lymphoma
	Metastatic lymphoma
Metabolic, toxic, and other complications of systemic disease	Hypoxic encephalopathy
	Sepsis
	Stroke
Functional (psychiatric) disorders	Anxiety disorder
	Psychotic depression
Unique conditions (?) related to a primary effect of HIV-1 itself	AIDS dementia complex (vacuolar myelopathy)
	Predominantly sensory polyneuropathy
Autoimmune disorders	Guillain-Barré syndrome
	Chronic inflammatory demyelinating polyneuropathy (CIDP)

NERVOUS SYSTEM INVOLVEMENT EARLY IN HIV-1 INFECTION

Although major clinical attention has focused on the late neurologic sequelae of infection, HIV-1 infection can be accompanied by clinically significant neurologic disorders earlier, including at the time of initial systemic HIV-1 infection. A number of observations also suggest that the CNS is commonly infected by HIV-1 early in the course of systemic infection.

Early Neurologic Complications of Acute HIV-1 Infection

A variety of **CNS disorders** have been described in the period after initial HIV-1 infection[14,18,22,23,37,46,51,68,120,154,165] (see Chapter 5). They may occur from several days to weeks after the seroconversion-related illness that resembles mononucleosis or, less often, in the absence of overt systemic illness. These early neurologic complications may evolve acutely or subacutely and may take the form of focal or diffuse encephalitis or leukoencephalopathy. Meningitis, ataxia, or myelopathy, either alone or together with PNS abnormalities, which include cranial neuropathy, brachial plexopathy, or neuropathy, may be presenting features. These disorders are characteristically monophasic, and most patients appear to recover within a number of weeks, although cognitive deficits may persist in some patients with encephalitis. The cerebrospinal fluid (CSF) usually shows a minor lymphocyte-predominant pleocytosis with a modest rise in protein. Results from using computed tomography (CT) brain scan have been normal, but experience with magnetic resonance imaging (MRI) has not been reported. The electroencephalogram (EEG) may be focally or diffusely slow. Although these early syndromes are apparently uncommon, it is possible their incidence is underappreciated.

Neurologic Complications During "Asymptomatic" Phase of Systemic HIV-1 Infection

More common than these seroconversion-related disorders is the development of demyelinating **neuropathies** during the later asymptomatic or latent phase of HIV-1 infection. These neuropathies resemble Guillain-Barré syndrome or chronic inflammatory demyelinating polyneuropathy (CIDP) seen in other contexts, with the exception that the CSF often exhibits uncharacteristic, albeit mild, pleocytosis.[31,91] The pathophysiology of HIV-1–related demyelinating neuropathies probably parallels that of demyelinating neuropathies in other settings and has an autoimmune basis. Afflicted patients appear to respond favorably to plasmapheresis or corticosteroid administration, although their prognosis may not be as good as that of the non-HIV-1–infected patient.[30] There is some evidence that intravenous immunoglobulin may be also helpful. For the present, plasmapheresis is the generally recommended treatment.

Recently an intriguing multiple sclerosis–like illness has been reported in HIV-1 infected patients in the latent phase of infection.[10,61] The presentation may include remissions and exacerbations, with corticosteroid responsiveness in the presence of preserved CD4+ T-lymphocyte counts. Although these cases may represent the concurrence of two diseases, more likely they relate to an autoimmune process with clinical (and perhaps pathologic) features similar to multiple sclerosis triggered by HIV-1 infection. This illness may involve processes akin to those that underlie immune thrombocytopenic purpura or demyelinating polyneuropathies in this same group of patients.

Asymptomatic HIV-1 Infection of the CNS

Although clinically overt nervous system involvement may occur early in the course of HIV-1 infection, more common is neurologically asymptomatic infection. Studies of CSF in clinically well patients have shown the following: (1) abnormalities of "routine" studies, including cell count, total protein, and immunoglobulin; (2) local, "intra-blood-brain barrier" synthesis of anti-HIV-1 antibody; and (3) isolation of virus.[3,45,56–58,92,96,135,136,161] These abnormalities have been noted in fully functional, asymptomatic patients who have remained well during follow-up care for a year or more. Such "incidental" abnormal levels in cell count, protein, immunoglobulin, oligoclonal bands, and HIV-1 recovery must be taken into account when interpreting CSF results obtained for other diagnostic purposes or in following therapy.

These CSF findings imply that involvement of the nervous system is a part of the ecology of the virus in the human host. They indicate that HIV-1 can be relatively nonpathogenic for the CNS, underscoring the critical question of what leads to the subsequent conversion of this asymptomatic state in some patients to either aseptic meningitis or parenchymal encephalitis.[126,128,129]

LATE NERVOUS SYSTEM INVOLVEMENT BY HIV-1

In the late stages of HIV-1 infection when immune defenses have been severely compromised and systemic complications have begun to accumulate, the nervous system becomes highly susceptible to a wide array of disorders involving all levels of the neuraxis, including meninges, brain, spinal cord, peripheral nerve, and muscle.

Meningitis

Several disorders may involve the leptomeninges in patients with advanced HIV-1 disease (Table 13–2), with symptomatology ranging from mild headache to severe disability with hydrocephalus and cranial nerve palsies. Additionally, a number of conditions can mimic meningitis; for example, parenchymal brain diseases such as toxoplasmosis (see Chapter 21) and primary CNS lymphoma (see Chapter 25) may initially manifest with headache as an important symptom. Nonneurologic disorders may also present with headache as a major or even predominating complaint. We have cared for a number of patients who have been referred for evaluation of headache who very shortly afterward manifested overt *Pneumocystis carinii* pneumonia and whose headache cleared when this condition was specifically treated. In other patients, usually in the transitional or late phases of HIV-1 infection, headache without a clear cause is common and in some patients may be severe. It has been speculated that these headaches are related to systemic production of vasoactive cytokines. Some patients appear to respond to treatment with low-dose tricyclic antidepressants, but this has not been systematically studied.

Among the true meningitides, a syndrome of **aseptic meningitis,** presumably relating to direct HIV-1 infection of the meninges, can occur acutely in the setting of seroconversion as described above, but it is more common in patients with advanced HIV-1 infection.[70,71,149] Hollander and Stringari[71] have segregated the disorder into two types: an acute form and a chronic form. Both occur in the late HIV-1 infection, usually in the transitional phase (200 to 500 CD4 + T lymphocytes/mm³) or, less frequently, in the phase of overt AIDS (<200 CD4 + cells). Both are accompanied by meningeal symptoms (e.g., headache and photophobia), although meningeal signs (e.g., nuchal rigidity) are more characteristic of the acute group. Cranial nerve palsies can also complicate the course, affecting cranial nerves V, VII, and VIII, with "Bell's palsy" sometimes recurring. The CSF shows mild mononuclear pleocytosis, usually with normal or mildly depressed glucose and slightly elevated protein levels. The presumption that this condition is due to direct HIV-1 infection of the meninges relates to two observations: the virus can be isolated

Table 13–2. Meningitides Complicating HIV-1 Infection

Common
Aseptic meningitis (? HIV-1)
Cryptococcal meningitis
Asymptomatic meningeal reaction
Uncommon
Tuberculous meningitis (*Mycobacterium tuberculosis*)
Syphilitic meningitis
Histoplasmosis
Coccidioidomycosis
Lymphomatous meningitis (metastatic)

from the CSF of some, and no other cause has been identified. However, whether HIV-1 infection is the sole or even major cause of the disorder can be questioned, since other causes of aseptic meningitis might be expected to provoke an influx of HIV-1–infected lymphocytes and monocytes into the CSF, thereby increasing the likelihood of viral isolation. Additionally, because of the high prevalence of mild abnormalities in the CSF of HIV-1–infected individuals described earlier, the definition of aseptic meningitis becomes ambiguous in some patients. Difficulties arise when one tries to distinguish clearly HIV-related aseptic meningitis from another cause of headache that coexists with the asymptomatic CSF abnormalities discussed previously.[55] Although the degree of pleocytosis might be used as a guide, presuming that the cellular reaction is involved in the genesis of symptoms, how is the cell count of 5–20/mm^3 in the fluid of a patient with headache interpreted? Further study is needed to clarify this issue. The syndrome itself is benign but may imply a poor prognosis in relation to impending progression to AIDS in some patients. There have been no reports on the effects of antiretroviral therapy on this disorder.

The most important meningeal infection in AIDS patients is caused by *Cryptococcus neoformans,* also the most common CNS fungal infection in these patients[29,40,47,82,115,152,172] (see Chapter 19). This infection usually presents as subacute meningitis or meningoencephalitis with headache, nausea, vomiting, and confusion just as in non-AIDS patients. However, in some patients symptoms can be remarkably mild, and the CSF formula may, likewise, contain few or no cells and little or no perturbation in glucose or protein levels. Hence it is imperative that in such patients cryptococcal antigen be assessed and fungal cultures obtained. An India ink study of the CSF may be helpful to visualize the organism's capsule, especially if the CSF cryptococcal antigen is not immediately available. Of note, the serum cryptococcal antigen is almost always positive, thereby serving as a screen in patients in whom the diagnostic suspicion is low or in whom a lumbar puncture is contraindicated. Therapeutic management[142] of cryptococcal meningitis is considered in Chapter 19.

Tuberculous meningitis is seemingly uncommon in HIV-1–infected patients, and it is not yet certain whether in these patients there is a difference in clinical presentation and response to therapy compared to other settings in which subacute or chronic meningitis manifests with stiff neck, cranial nerve palsies, hydrocephalus, and vascular occlusions[12,167] (see Chapter 18).

Meningeal involvement by syphilis in HIV-1–infected individuals may take the form of acute meningitis or meningovascular syphilis (see Chapter 24). However, there is some evidence suggesting that HIV-1 infection may alter the natural course of neurosyphilis and that meningovascular syphilis may occur both more commonly and earlier in those with HIV-1 infection.[78,80] The full extent to which underlying HIV-1 infection alters the presentation, clinical course, or response to therapy of CNS syphilis is presently unsettled.[11,73,84,108,153] The previously discussed CSF abnormalities common in asymptomatic seropositive patients, including elevated protein and cell counts, render interpretation of such findings in patients with positive syphilis serologies or those undergoing treatment more difficult. Most clinicians now favor more aggressive treatment of new or previously untreated syphilis seropositivity.[93,107,153]

Systemic lymphoma complicating HIV-1 infection may spread secondarily to the CNS, involving the meninges.[85–87,150] Clinical manifestations may be cryptic but usually include cranial nerve palsies, headaches, or increased intracranial pressure (ICP).

Dementia and Diffuse Brain Disease

Affliction of the brain parenchyma in AIDS can be usefully divided into conditions that cause predominantly focal symptomatology and those accompanied by more diffuse dysfunction (Table 13–3). Although there is some overlap in these disorders (e.g., cerebral toxoplasmosis may present with both an "encephalitic" and the more common focal picture), this division is generally valuable as the first step in differential diagnosis. The nonfocal disorders can, in turn, be subdivided into those presenting with parallel impairment of both alertness and cognition and a disorder, the AIDS dementia complex, in which alertness is characteristically spared, but cognition, motor function, and behavior are impaired.

Diffuse Encephalopathies

Diffuse encephalopathies include the metabolic or toxic encephalopathies developing as sequelae to the systemic nonneurologic diseases suffered by AIDS patients such as pneumonias with hypoxia and generalized sepsis. Similarly, various CNS-active drugs may cloud mentation or alertness just as in non-AIDS patients. These effects can occur alone but also may manifest as an exacerbating or unmasking influence on the AIDS dementia complex, resulting in a mixture of the two conditions and exaggerating medication effects. HIV-1–infected patients may also be more sensitive to neuroleptics and thereby manifest parkinsonism or other movement disorders at seemingly low doses.[69]

Certain brain infections also can produce diffuse brain dysfunction. CNS toxoplasmosis, which characteristically causes focal neurologic symptoms and signs, may present as a generalized encephalopathy with clouding of consciousness and diffuse cerebral dysfunction.[62,111] This may be a particularly fulminating illness and relates to the presence of abundant toxoplasmic microabscesses, which may be poorly imaged by CT or MRI scan. Similarly, CNS lymphoma can infiltrate deep structures and impair cognition, alertness, and motor function without prominent focal symptoms or signs.

The clinical importance of CNS cytomegalovirus (CMV) remains imprecisely defined[163] (see Chapter 23). Systemic CMV infection is very common in AIDS patients, and the brain is frequently infected. Pathologically, there is evidence of mild brain infection, marked by scattered microglial nodules with occasional characteristic intranuclear inclusion bodies, or evidence of CMV antigens and/or nucleic

---

**Table 13–3.   Diffuse Brain Disease
Complicating HIV-1 Infection**

With Concomitant Depression of Alertness
Metabolic encephalopathies (alone or as an exacerbating influence)
Toxoplasmosis ("encephalitic" form)
Cytomegalovirus encephalitis
Herpes encephalitis
With Preservation of Alertness
AIDS dementia complex

---

acid in perhaps one quarter of patients dying of AIDS.[2,63,79,106,117,158,163] Clinicopathologic correlation suggests that CMV usually plays only a minor role in causing overt CNS dysfunction.[110] However, it is also clear that a small number of patients can manifest more severe CMV encephalitis, with subacute clouding of consciousness, brain stem signs, or seizures. The clinical diagnosis in such patients is difficult; however, in some of them the presence of ventricular ependymitis, with local signal alteration or contrast enhancement detected by CT or MRI, may aid in the diagnosis of CMV.[59,125] CSF culture results are usually negative except in patients with radiculomyelitis (see below).[106] The effect of gancyclovir or foscarnet on the course of CMV encephalitis has not been adequately assessed.

Encephalitis related to herpes simplex virus types 1 (HSV-1) and 2 (HSV-2) also occurs in AIDS patients and may present as a subacute nonfocal encephalopathy, although the frequency and clinical spectrum need more accurate analysis.[89]

AIDS Dementia Complex

The AIDS dementia complex is characterized by a triad of cognitive, motor, and behavioral dysfunction[110,127,130,134] and is perhaps the most common CNS complication of HIV-1 infection, likely eventually afflicting the majority of AIDS patients in varying degrees. Characteristically, it manifests after patients develop the major opportunistic infections or neoplasms that define systemic AIDS, although patients can also present with this syndrome before these major systemic complications occur.[25,112] However, results of larger cohort studies indicate that this syndrome is uncommon in patients who are systemically well.[76,97,145] On the other hand, once patients develop constitutional symptoms, as many as one third can have equivocal or mild abnormalities by history or neuropsychologic testing.[76] Our own clinical experience suggests that in untreated patients early in the course of systemic AIDS perhaps one third of patients exhibit mild dementia and another quarter may suffer subclinical cognitive loss, which can be documented by careful neurologic history and examination or neuropsychologic examination. In patients with late AIDS the majority exhibit mild-to-severe dementia, and an additional number suffer subclinical AIDS dementia complex. Early and widespread use of zidovudine may have reduced the prevalence of the AIDS dementia complex, as suggested by a study in the Netherlands.[123]

Terminology and Classification

The term *AIDS dementia complex* was introduced to describe a clinical and cohesive constellation of symptoms and signs rather than an established disease entity of uniform etiopathogenesis.[110,127,130,131] Each of the three components was chosen for a reason. *AIDS* was included because the morbidity of the condition is comparable to that of other AIDS-defining complications of HIV-1 infection. *Dementia* was included because of acquired and persistent cognitive decline, marked by prominent mental slowing and inattention. The dementia is characteristically unaccompanied by alterations in the level of alertness. The third component, *complex,* was added because the syndrome also, importantly, includes impaired motor

Table 13–4. Comparison of AIDS Dementia Complex and World Health Organization/American Academy of Neurology (WHO)/(AAN) Classifications

AIDS DEMENTIA COMPLEX CLASSIFICATION	WHO/AAN CLASSIFICATION: HIV-ASSOCIATED COGNITIVE-MOTOR COMPLEX
Stage 0: Normal	
Stage 0.5: Subclinical or Equivocal	No corresponding WHO classification
Minimal or equivocal symptoms	
Mild (soft) neurologic signs	
No impairment of work or activities of daily living (ADL)	
Stage 1: Mild	**HIV-1-Associated Minor Cognitive-Motor Disorder**
Unequivocal intellectual or motor impairment	Symptoms: two of five types in cognitive, motor, behavioral spheres
Able to do all but the more demanding work or ADL	Examination: neurologic or neuropsychologic abnormalities
	Mild impairment of work or ADL
	HIV-Associated Dementia Complex and HIV-Associated Myelopathy
Stage 2: Moderate	MILD
Cannot work or perform demanding ADL	Impaired work and ADL
Capable of self-care	Capable of basic self-care
Ambulatory but may need a single prop	Ambulatory but may need a single prop
Stage 3: Severe	MODERATE
Major intellectual disability	Unable to work or function unassisted
or	*or*
Cannot walk unassisted	Cannot walk unassisted
Stage 4: End Stage	SEVERE
Nearly vegetative	Unable to perform ADL unassisted
Rudimentary cognition	Confined to bed or wheelchair
Para- or quadriplegic	

performance and, at times, behavioral changes. Myelopathy and organic psychosis were encompassed within this term, but neither neuropathy nor "functional" psychiatric disturbance is included.

We have used a staging system for describing the severity of the AIDS dementia complex based on functional and motor status for adult patients.[127,130] It provides a common descriptive vocabulary for both clinical and investigative purposes. Recently the World Health Organization (WHO) and the American Academy of Neurology (AAN) introduced new terminologies with certain useful features that had been omitted from previous classifications.[168,169] The WHO/AAN classification can be translated roughly into the AIDS dementia complex staging scheme (Table 13–4 presents a comparative synopsis of the two schemes).

The WHO/ANN classification introduced the term *HIV-1-associated cognitive-motor complex* to encompass the full constellation of the AIDS dementia complex and added subcategories to refer to patients with predominantly cognitive *(HIV-associated dementia)* or myelopathic *(HIV-1-associated myelopathy)* presentations of sufficient severity to interfere with work or activities of daily living (ADL) (hence severe enough to qualify as stage 2 or greater in AIDS dementia complex staging).

The term *HIV-associated minor cognitive–Motor Disorder* was introduced to designate patients with mild symptoms and signs and only minimal functional impairment of work or ADL (stage 1 AIDS dementia complex). In addition to the advantages of attempting to separate the patients predominantly with myelopathy from those with cognitive changes, this terminology restricts the term *dementia* to a level of cognitive impairment consistent with that used in other formal definitions. It might also simplify reporting this condition as an AIDS-defining disorder if this designation is restricted to a presentation with sufficient functional severity to be termed *HIV-1-associated dementia* or *HIV-1-associated myelopathy*. The requirement for this level of severity (equivalent to stage 2 or greater AIDS dementia complex terminology) is probably both biologically and prognostically consistent with other AIDS-defining conditions. The WHO/AAN classification also does not make the implicit assumption that the disorder is a single disease entity differing only in severity, but allows for the possibility that milder and more severe disease may be a discontinuous process.

Clinical Presentations

The clinical features of the AIDS dementia complex are briefly summarized in Table 13–5. Patients' earliest symptoms usually consist of difficulties with concentration and memory. Those affected begin to lose track of their train of thought or conversation. Many complain of "slowness" in thinking. Complex tasks become more difficult and take longer to complete, whereas memory impairment or difficulty in concentration leads to missed appointments and the need to keep lists. If a patient needs a high level of concentration or organization for his or her occupation or activities at home, the AIDS dementia complex can be recognized early from impaired performance.

Despite these complaints, early in the evolution of the illness bedside mental status testing may be within normal limits, although responses are characteristically slow. As the disease progresses, patients perform poorly on tasks requiring con-

Table 13–5. Major Clinical Manifestations of the AIDS Dementia Complex, a Subcortical Dementia Affecting Cognition, Motor Performance, and Behavior

EARLY	LATE
Cognition	
Inattention	Global dementia
Reduced concentration	
Forgetfulness	
Motor Performance	
Slowed movements	Paraplegia
Clumsiness	
Ataxia	
Behavior	
Apathy	Mutism
Altered personality	
(Agitation)	

centration and attention such as word and digit reversals and serial 7s. With increasing severity, a larger array of mental status tests become abnormal. Slowing remains prominent, and afflicted individuals may appear apathetic, with poor insight and indifference to their illness.

Symptoms of motor dysfunction usually lag behind those of intellectual impairment. When present, complaints include poor balance or incoordination. Patients may drop things more frequently or become slower and less precise with normal hand activities such as eating or writing. Similarly, gait incoordination can result in more frequent tripping or falling or a perceived need to exercise new care in walking. However, even when symptoms are lacking, motor abnormalities can almost always be detected early in the course of the disease. They include slowing of rapid successive and alternating movements of the extremities, impaired ocular smooth pursuits, and saccadic eye movements. Abnormal reflexes may also be present, with generalized hyperreflexia and development of release signs such as snout, glabellar, and, less commonly, grasp responses. As the disease evolves, ataxia and, subsequently, leg weakness limit walking. Patients with early or predominating spastic-ataxic gait usually have vacuolar myelopathy pathologically (see below). Bladder and bowel incontinence is common in the late stages of the disease. At the end stage of the AIDS dementia complex, patients are nearly vegetative, lying in bed with a vacant stare, unable to ambulate and incontinent. However, unless intercurrent illness develops, the level of arousal is usually preserved.

Psychologic depression is surprisingly infrequent in these patients, despite the prominence of psychomotor slowing. Patients appear uninterested and lack initiative but are without dysphoria. In a minority a more agitated organic psychosis may be the presenting or predominant aspect of the illness.[64] Such patients are irritable and hyperactive and may become overtly manic.

In children the disorder has the same general features, although the course may vary somewhat and present in either a progressive or static form.[7,24,50] The progressive form is characterized by the gradual loss of previously acquired motor skills in conjunction with the evolution of motor abnormalities ranging from spastic paraparesis to quadriplegia with pseudobulbar palsy and rigidity. Acquired microcephaly is almost universal.

Table 13–6. Some Comparative Features of Major CNS Processes in AIDS

	CLINICAL FEATURES		
	TEMPORAL PROFILE	LEVEL OF ALERTNESS	FEVER
Cerebral toxoplasmosis	Days	Reduced	Common
Primary CNS lymphoma	Days to weeks	Variable	Absent
Progressive multifocal leuko-encephalopathy	Weeks	Preserved	Absent
AIDS dementia complex	Weeks to months	Preserved	Absent

Neuropsychologic Test Profile.   Formal neuropsychologic studies quantitatively support the clinical findings described above and are helpful in establishing impairment and in serially following the course of disease or response to therapy. In general, the neuropsychologic tests most sensitive to AIDS dementia complex require some or all of the following: performance under time pressure, motor speed, and alternation between two performance rules or stimulus sets.[13,102,145,155]

Neurodiagnostic Studies.   Neuroimaging procedures and CSF examination are essential to the evaluation of AIDS patients with CNS dysfunction. Although most often nonspecific, imaging results are useful as an adjunct to diagnosis of the AIDS dementia complex and, perhaps more importantly, are particularly helpful in excluding the other neurologic conditions complicating AIDS (Table 13–6). Neuroradiologic findings in the AIDS dementia complex include the nearly universal finding of cerebral atrophy. Widened cortical sulci and enlarged ventricles are usually clearly evident by either CT scanning or MRI.[77,110] Additionally, some patients have patchy or diffuse T2-weighted abnormalities on MRI in the hemispheric white matter and, less commonly, the basal ganglia or thalamus.[77,104,124] Children with AIDS-related dementia often have basal ganglia calcification and atrophy.[6]

Examination of the CSF in patients with AIDS dementia complex reveals abnormalities in both "routine" and more specialized tests. However, routine analysis is confounded by the CSF abnormalities described earlier in patients with asymptomatic HIV-1 infection, including HIV-1 isolation from CSF.[67,88,116] The likelihood of detecting HIV-1 p24 core antigen in the CSF increases with AIDS dementia complex severity, although free antigen is still a relatively infrequent finding and thus of low sensitivity diagnostically.[116,122] More recently we have found that the CSF concentrations of β_2-microglobulin and neopterin correlate with both the severity of the AIDS dementia complex and with its response to antiretroviral therapy.[15,16] Although these are nonspecific markers of immune activation, they may prove to have an ancillary role in diagnosis and assessment of therapeutic response.

Neuropathology.   Histologic abnormalities in demented AIDS patients are most prominent in the subcortical structures and can be segregated into three seemingly discontinuous but frequently overlapping sets: (1) gliosis and diffuse white

---

NEURORADIOLOGIC FEATURES

NO. OF LESIONS	TYPE OF LESIONS	LOCATION OF LESIONS
Multiple	Mass effect; spherical ring enhancing	Basal ganglia, cortex
One or few	Mass effect; irregular; weakly enhancing	Periventricular
Multiple	No mass effect; fluffy or diffuse; nonenhancing white matter	White matter, usually subcortical
None, diffuse, or multiple	No mass effect; fluffy or diffuse; cerebral atrophy	Central white matter, basal ganglia

matter pallor, (2) multinucleated-cell encephalitis, and (3) vacuolar myelopathy; a less common additional finding is diffuse or focal spongiform change of the cerebral white matter.[21,109,129,139] The most common of these abnormalities is the central astrocytosis and accompanying diffuse white matter pallor that, in isolation, correlate with milder AIDS dementia complex. Inflammation is characteristically scant, consisting of a few perivascular lymphocytes and brown-pigmented macrophages accompanying the astrocytosis.

Multinucleated cells characteristically are found in patients with more severe clinical disease.[34,39,109] The multinucleated cells usually resemble macrophages and indeed are accompanied by neighboring macrophage and microglial reaction, along with local edema and white matter rarefaction. They are most often concentrated in the white matter and deep grey structures.

Although inflammation with multinucleated cells may also present in the spinal cord, in our experience vacuolar myelopathy is more common.[109,118] The latter pathologically resembles subacute combined degeneration resulting from vitamin B_{12} deficiency, but levels of this vitamin are generally normal in serum. Although there is a general correlation between the incidence of vacuolar myelopathy and the other pathologic abnormalities found in the brain, the myelopathy can occur in the absence of the multinucleated cells. Our own studies suggest that vacuolar myelopathy is independent of productive HIV-1 infection,[138] although others have suggested findings to the contrary.[44]

Etiology and Pathogenesis. Evidence from a growing number of studies supports a primary role for HIV-1 in the AIDS dementia complex, at least in a subset of patients.[36,39,49,54,119,129,157,159] There is also a growing consensus that macrophages and microglia, along with multinucleated cells derived from these two cell types, are the principal participants in productive infection.[53,54,81,101,133,151,157,164] Whether other cell types in the brain, including the native astrocytes, oligodendrocytes, or neurons, are also infected is less clear and requires further investigation. Cell culture studies have demonstrated low-level infection of astrocytic and other neuroectodermal cells and cell lines, involving a non-CD4 virus-cell interaction.[27]

Having said that HIV-1 can be found in the brains of demented individuals, it should be emphasized that this is not an invariant finding. Our own studies have shown that in patients with subclinical or mild AIDS dementia complex (stages 0.5 to 1) the chief pathologic findings are those of astrocytosis and white matter pallor.[34] Even in some patients with more severe (stages 2 and 3) AIDS dementia complex these are the sole histologic findings. Characteristically it is only in the more severely affected patients (stages 2 and greater) that multinucleated cell encephalitis with histologically demonstrable HIV-1 infection is found. Since HIV-1 infection is confined almost exclusively to brains with multinucleated cells, only this group of patients can justifiably be referred to as exhibiting HIV-1 encephalitis. As a consequence of the discrepancy between clinical deficit and both the pathologic and virologic features, indirect pathogenetic processes relating infection and brain injury have been proposed.[41,99,128,129,132,159] These processes may involve virus-coded toxins (e.g., gp120) or cell-coded toxins, particularly cytokines.

Treatment. Several studies have indicated that the AIDS dementia complex responds to zidovudine therapy[121,144,170] (see Chapter 7). Optimum dosing has not been established. A recent placebo-controlled trial involving mild-to-moderate AIDS dementia complex patients suggests improvement in those patients treated with zidovudine.[146] However, the doses used in this trial were higher than those currently recommended for systemic disease. Preliminary reports suggest that the newer nucleoside analog, dideoxyinosine, may also have a salutary effect on this condition, but further studies are needed.[171] The possible role of toxins in the genesis of AIDS dementia complex has also given rise to proposals to attempt to block the effects of these putative intermediaries. For example, the calcium channel blocker nimodipine, which appears to block the neuronal toxicity of HIV-1 gp120 in cell culture,[41] is now being considered for clinical trial.

FOCAL BRAIN DISEASES

A number of focal brain disorders can afflict AIDS patients (Table 13–7). Evaluation of these conditions begins with the recognition of their focal nature along with associated background systemic symptoms and signs (e.g., fever, headache). Investigations include neuroradiologic characterization and often a strategy involving therapeutic trial, followed in some by brain biopsy.

The temporal profile of the onset and evolution of these focal brain disorders is an important aspect of their clinical presentation. Abrupt onset suggests either a vascular cause or seizure. AIDS patients may suffer transient ischemic attacks or even strokes, leaving residual brain injury.[28,48,94] The pathogenesis is often not clear; fortunately most have a benign outcome. Seizures may be related to HIV-1 infection (AIDS dementia complex) or result from the focal opportunistic infections and neoplasms. Careful clinical and neuroimaging investigations are warranted to evaluate for focal diseases.[72,166]

The most common focal disorders characteristically have a subacute onset and evolve over days or, at times, weeks. Of them, cerebral toxoplasmosis characteristically progresses most rapidly (days) and progressive multifocal leukoencephalopathy (PML) most slowly (weeks), whereas primary CNS lymphoma lies somewhere between. A comparison of the major clinical and neuroradiologic features of common CNS processes in patients with AIDS is outlined in Table 13–6. Each may cause similar neurologic deficits, although there usually are differences in the associated findings. Thus a patient with toxoplasmosis commonly presents with a combination of focal deficit and generalized encephalopathy with confusion or clouding of consciousness[111] (see Chapter 21). This contrasts with the patient with

Table 13–7. Focal Brain Diseases Complicating HIV-1 Infection

Acute
Vascular disorders
Seizures*
Subacute
Cerebral toxoplasmosis
Primary central nervous system lymphoma
Progressive multifocal leukoencephalopathy
Tuberculous brain abscess (*Mycobacterium tuberculosis*)
Cryptococcoma
Varicella-zoster virus encephalitis
Herpes encephalitis

*Secondary to focal subacute disorders or to nonfocal processes.

PML, at least at onset, in which focal neurologic deficits are unaccompanied by either diffuse brain dysfunction or evidence of a systemic toxic state.[8,83] The CNS lymphomas, when accompanied by significant mass effect or when deep in the frontal or periventricular region, can cause more global mental dysfunction. Cryptococcoma is usually a complication of cryptococcal meningitis, but when it occurs alone, cryptococcal antigen may be negative in the CSF, making diagnosis difficult.[82]

In approaching patients with focal disease, the use of neuroimaging techniques, particularly CT and more recently MRI, is critical both to confirm the presence of macroscopic focal disease and to determine the nature of the abnormalities. Multiple lesions involving the cortex or deep brain nuclei (thalamus, basal ganglia), with mass effect and surrounded by edema, strongly favor cerebral toxoplasmosis. In most cases toxoplasmic abscesses exhibit ringlike contrast enhancement on CT or MRI scan, but either homogeneous contrast enhancement or nonenhancing hypodense lesions may be noted. Double-dose contrast CT (or preferably MRI) studies may help in defining these lesions more clearly by demonstrating additional spherical lesions characteristic of the disease. Only very rarely will the CT or, more particularly, the MRI scan be normal.[111,113]

Primary CNS lymphomas of B-cell origin are opportunistic neoplasms that complicate the course of AIDS in approximately 5% of patients, although this estimate includes lymphomas noted incidentally at autopsy.[117,150] When symptomatic, patients with primary brain lymphomas present with progressive focal or multifocal neurologic deficits similar to those with toxoplasmosis, although the tempo of disease evolution is usually slower. Neuroradiologic studies are usually sensitive in detecting primary brain lymphomas but do not establish definitive diagnosis. Characteristically these tumors are multicentric but most often show only one or two lesions on CT or MRI. Their location is characteristically deep in the brain and surrounding the ventricles, and they occur most often in the white rather than grey matter. On CT scan they may enhance after contrast administration, but very often such enhancement is either weak or absent, and MRI scanning is more sensitive. However, final diagnosis relies on brain biopsy.

Toxoplasma serology is of additional diagnostic help if the results are appropriately interpreted. Because the disease typically is due to reactivation of the organism, patients with cerebral toxoplasmosis rarely have negative serum IgG antibody titers.[60,111] However, these titers may be low (occasionally an apparently negative titer will be positive when a more concentrated specimen such as a 1:4 dilution is tested) and frequently do not rise during the course of the illness. Thus a positive titer indicates susceptibility, and a negative titer casts doubt on the diagnosis.

In patients with focal disease initial diagnosis is targeted to cerebral toxoplasmosis because of its frequency (5% to 15% of AIDS patients) and response to therapy. In treating patients with cerebral toxoplasmosis and indeed all AIDS patients, the use of **corticosteroids should be avoided when possible.** This is particularly important when considering a therapeutic trial to differentiate between toxoplasmosis and CNS lymphoma. Since the latter may respond symptomatically to corticosteroids alone, clinical or CT improvement on a combination antibiotic-steroid treatment is difficult to interpret. More generally, corticosteroids intensify the impairment of immune defenses in AIDS patients, potentially worsening not only toxoplasmosis but also other systemic opportunistic infections. However, if cerebral edema threatens brain herniation, judicious short-term corticosteroid therapy may be instituted along with appropriate specific therapy and subsequently tapered rapidly once the patient improves.

PML is an opportunistic infection caused by a human papovavirus, JC. It develops in approximately 4% of AIDS patients, and in some it will be their presenting illness. The disease is characterized by selective white matter destruction.[8,83,137] Clinical evolution usually is more protracted than that of either toxoplasmosis or CNS lymphoma, and altered consciousness related to brain swelling is not a feature. Definitive diagnosis is made only by brain biopsy or autopsy, although suspicion is aroused by the clinical history and an examination suggesting more than one cerebral focus, along with a CT scan or MRI demonstrating white matter lesions without mass effect and usually without contrast enhancement. There is no proven effective therapy for the disease. Spontaneous sustained remission of PML in two AIDS patients has recently been reported.[9]

Although unusual, varicella-zoster virus (VZV) and, to a lesser extent, HSV-1 and HSV-2 have been reported as causes of CNS disease in AIDS patients. VZV infections are of three types: (1) multifocal direct brain infection affecting principally the white matter and partially mimicking PML[74,105,141]; (2) cerebral vasculitis, which characteristically occurs with ophthalmic herpes zoster and causes contralateral hemiplegia[42,66]; and (3) myelopathy complicating herpes zoster.[38] Both HSV-1 and HSV-2 have been identified in brains of some AIDS patients,[89] but the clinical correlates of these infections in AIDS patients have not yet been wholly delineated.

MYELOPATHIES

Myelopathies complicating HIV-1–infected individuals can be classified into segmental and diffuse forms (Table 13–8). The segmental forms tend to follow an acute or subacute time course. VZV, toxoplasmosis, and spinal epidural or intradural lymphoma may all give a clinical picture of transverse myelitis.[38,65,98] In addition, CMV polyradiculopathy may also involve the spinal cord in a segmental manner, typically evolving over a number of weeks.[7,103] Combined CMV and HSV infection of the spinal cord has also been described, although antemortem recognition may be exceptionally difficult.[156]

The more slowly progressive vacuolar myelopathy is far more common.[109,118] Usually it is accompanied by varying degrees of cognitive and upper extremity

Table 13–8. Myelopathies Complicating HIV-1 Infection

Acute or Subacute and Segmental Form
TRANSVERSE MYELITIS
Varicella-zoster virus (herpes zoster) myelopathy
Spinal epidural or intradural lymphoma
Toxoplasmosis
WITH POLYRADICULOPATHY
Cytomegalovirus myelopathy
Subacute or Chronic, Progressive, and Diffuse Form
Vacuolar myelopathy
HTLV-I–associated myelopathy (HAM)

affliction; therefore it has been included under the clinical term *AIDS dementia complex* discussed previously. In some patients it occurs in relative isolation or with marked preponderance. These patients exhibit progressive, painless gait disturbance with ataxia and spasticity. Bladder and bowel difficulty usually becomes significant only after considerable gait symptoms appear, and sensory disturbance is less conspicuous unless there is concomitant neuropathy. Patients do not usually manifest a distinct sensory or motor "level" as in patients with transverse myelopathy. Even in those patients with seemingly isolated lower extremity symptoms, examination usually reveals some evidence of disturbance higher in the neuraxis. In typical instances we do not recommend performing myelography; however, although spinal MRI is useful in evaluating AIDS myelopathies, our own attempts to detect vacuolar change using this method have been disappointing.

An additional cause of myelopathy in HIV-1–infected patients relates to coinfection with a second retrovirus, human T-cell lymphotropic virus I (HTLV-I).[1,32,114,140] It relates principally to the convergent epidemiologies of these infections rather than to increased disease susceptibility resulting from immunosuppression and as a result is likely to occur principally in intravenous drug abusers.[17] Clinically the disorder is very similar to vacuolar myelopathy but can be distinguished pathologically. Clinical diagnosis is suspected when positive HTLV-I serology is present. Specific diagnosis may be important since HTLV-I–associated myelopathy (HAM), at least in the non-AIDS patient, may respond to immunosuppressive therapies, including plasmapheresis.[95]

PERIPHERAL NEUROPATHIES

Peripheral neuropathies of several types can complicate the various stages of HIV-1 infection[30,103,148] (Table 13–9). Those occurring in the acute and latent phases of infection have been discussed previously. Neuropathies during the transitional

Table 13–9. Peripheral Neuropathies Complicating HIV-1 Infection

Acute or Seroconversion Phase
Mononeuritides, brachial plexopathy
Acute demyelinating polyneuropathy
Latent ("Asymptomatic") Phase (CD4+ T Lymphocytes >500/mm³)
Acute demyelinating polyneuropathy (Guillain-Barré syndrome)
Chronic inflammatory demyelinating polyneuropathy (CIDP)
Transition Phase (200-500 CD4+ cells)
Herpes zoster neuropathy
Mononeuritis multiplex
Late Phase (<200 CD4+ cells)
Predominantly sensory polyneuropathy
Autonomic neuropathy
Cytomegalovirus polyradiculopathy
Mononeuritis multiplex (severe)
Mononeuropathies associated with aseptic meningitis
Mononeuropathies secondary to lymphomatous meningitis
Nucleoside (ddI, ddC) toxicity

phase include herpes zoster and mononeuritis multiplex. Mononeuritis multiplex is unusual but has been described with HIV-1 infection and may fall into two different settings. One type occurs earlier and has a more benign outcome. The second form occurs later and is more aggressive, leading to progressive paralysis and death in some patients. It has been speculated that the more benign form, which occurs earlier in HIV-1 infection, may relate to an autoimmune vascular lesion.

The later, second form of mononeuritis multiplex pursues a progressive and more malignant course and has been suggested to relate to multifocal CMV infection[143] (see Chapter 23). More clearly related to CMV is a stereotyped ascending polyradiculopathy.[43,52,103] Diagnosis of the latter is aided by finding polymorphonuclear pleocytosis in the CSF. Thickened spinal roots revealed by myelography or MRI scanning have also been reported. Although CMV can be cultured from the spinal fluid of these patients, viral replication and the appearance of cytopathology in culture are too slow to rely on as guides for therapy. Therefore clinical diagnosis should lead to rapid institution of specific antiviral therapy with gancyclovir.[52,103]

The most common neuropathy in AIDS patients is a distal, predominantly sensory and axonal neuropathy.[30,148,149] Characteristically the sensory symptoms far exceed either sensory or motor dysfunction. The prevalence of this disorder is uncertain, but in mild form it probably is very common in late infection. In some patients sensory symptoms with "burning feet" resemble those of severe alcoholic or diabetic neuropathy. Even in patients with the severe form, sensory loss and motor weakness are usually mild, although the painful paresthesias and burning may prevent walking. The pathogenesis of this neuropathy is uncertain; the suspicion that it may relate to direct HIV-1 infection of nerve or dorsal root ganglion has not been clearly documented. Anecdotal experience suggests that it does not generally respond to zidovudine therapy. Treatment therefore relies on symptom management with tricyclics and analgesics.

Of increasing importance are the toxic peripheral neuropathies caused by certain antiretroviral nucleotides, including dideoxyinosine (ddI) and dideoxycytidine (ddC) (see Chapter 7). Both drugs cause axonal neuropathy in a dose-related fashion. Their clinical features are similar to the AIDS-related sensory polyneuropathy that usually begins with foot pain that is described as "aching," "burning," or "bruiselike." Patients may worsen for a few weeks after discontinuation of the drug, a phenomenon known as "coasting." Patients with underlying neuropathies of other types may be more vulnerable to this complication.

Autonomic neuropathy has also been reported in AIDS patients.[33,90] Clinical features range from mild positional hypotension to cardiovascular collapse during invasive procedures such as lung biopsy. In addition, autonomic neuropathy may contribute to chronic diarrhea in HIV-1–infected individuals.[5]

MYOPATHIES

Myopathies can occur at several stages of HIV-1 infection (Table 13–10) but are less common and less well characterized than the neuropathies. A wide range of presentations, ranging from asymptomatic creatine kinase elevation to progressive proximal weakness, is possible.[35,147,148] A polymyositis or dermatomyositis-like illness has been described in AIDS patients, but as with the other myopathies, the

Table 13–10.   Myopathies Complicating HIV-1 Infection

Inflammatory myopathy (polymyositis)
Noninflammatory myopathies
Toxic myopathy (from zidovudine therapy)

pathogenesis is not clear. Viral antigens have been found in the inflammatory lymphoid cells but not in myocytes,[75] and one report has identified multinucleated giant cells in the inflammatory infiltrate.[4]

Zidovudine therapy can also cause myopathy.[100] The clinical and laboratory features of this disorder have not been delineated fully but proximal muscles, especially those of the legs, apparently are affected more often, leading to the term *saggy butt syndrome.* In many of these patients abnormalities of mitochondria are detected in muscle biopsy specimens. Clinical and laboratory improvement may occur after stopping zidovudine therapy.[26]

CONCLUSION

As with other aspects of AIDS, precise neurologic diagnosis is an important exercise since an increasing number of these neurologic disorders can be treated with relief of morbidity or prevention of death. The approach to diagnosis and management of the neurologic complications of HIV-1 infection and AIDS follows that used in general neurologic practice, with the differences relating to the altered probabilities of differential diagnosis in this group of patients whose vulnerabilities to opportunistic and HIV-1–related neurologic disease far overshadow the background incidence of "ordinary" neurologic diseases. With the diagnosis of underlying HIV-1 infection and an understanding of its systemic stage, the neurologic history establishes its temporal profile and usually provides an initial impression of its anatomic localization. The neurologic examination refines this localization and uncovers additional, including asymptomatic, abnormalities. Neuroimaging studies using CT or MRI and, less commonly, myelography or angiography add further precision to anatomic localization and narrow the range of possible underlying pathologic processes. Electrodiagnosis using EEG or evoked potentials can also be helpful in delineating and localizing physiologic dysfunction, and nerve conduction studies and electromyography can similarly refine diagnosis of neuromuscular disease. Examination of CSF provides a direct view of inflammatory reactions in the meninges and can diagnose certain invading organisms or neoplasms. Therapeutic trial and tissue biopsy may be needed for exact diagnosis in some instances. These evaluations, pursued with a background understanding of the spectrum of neurologic disorders affecting these patients, allow accurate neurologic diagnosis in the great majority of patients.

ACKNOWLEDGMENT

We thank Tami Ballew for preparation of this manuscript.

REFERENCES

1. Aboulafia DM, Saxton EH, Koga H, et al: A patient with progressive myelopathy and antibodies to human T-cell leukemia virus type I and human immunodeficiency virus type I in serum and cerebrospinal fluid. Arch Neurol 47:477-479, 1990
2. Anders KH, Guerra WF, Tomiyasu U, et al: The neuropathology of AIDS. Am J Pathol 124(3):537-558, 1986
3. Appleman ME, Marshall DW, Brey RL, et al: Cerebrospinal fluid abnormalities in patients without AIDS who are seropositive for the human immunodeficiency virus. J Infect Dis 158:193-199, 1988
4. Bailey RO, Turok DI, Jaufmann BP, Singh JK: Myositis and acquired immunodeficiency syndrome. Hum Pathol 18:749-751, 1987
5. Batman PA, Miller ARO, Sedgwick PM, Griffin GE: Autonomic denervation in jejunal mucosa of homosexual men infected with HIV. AIDS 5:1247-1252, 1991
6. Belman AL, Lantos G, Horoupian D, et al: Calcification of the basal ganglia in infants and children. Neurology 36:1192-1199, 1986
7. Belman AL, Ultmann MH, Horoupian D, et al: Neurological complications in infants and children with acquired immune deficiency syndrome. Ann Neurol 18:560-566, 1985
8. Berger JR, Kaszovitz B, Post MJ, Dickinson G: Progressive multifocal leukoencephalopathy associated with human immunodeficiency virus infection. Ann Intern Med 107:78-87, 1987
9. Berger JR, Mucke L: Prolonged survival and partial recovery in AIDS-associated PML. Neurology 38:1060-1065, 1988
10. Berger JR, Sheremah WA, Resnick L, et al: Multiple sclerosis-like illness occurring with human immunodeficiency virus infection. Neurology 39:324-329, 1989
11. Berry DC, Hooton TM, Collier AC, Lukehart SA: Neurologic relapse after benzathine penicillin therapy for secondary syphilis in a patient with HIV infection. N Engl J Med 316:1587-1589, 1987
12. Bishburg E, Sunderam G, Reichman LB, Kapila R: Central nervous system tuberculosis with the acquired immunodeficiency syndrome and its related complex. Ann Intern Med 105:210-213, 1986
13. Bornstein RA, Nasrallah HA, Para MF, et al: Rate of CD_4 decline and neuropsychological performance in HIV infection. Arch Neurol 48:704-707, 1991
14. Brew BJ: Medical management of AIDS patients: central and peripheral nervous system abnormalities. Med Clin North Am 76(1):63-81, 1992
15. Brew BJ, Bhalla RB, Fleisher M, et al: Cerebrospinal fluid beta-2 microglobulin in patients infected with human immunodeficiency virus type 1. Neurology 39:830-834, 1989
16. Brew BJ, Bhalla R, Schwartz M, Price RW: CSF Neopterin in HIV-1 infection and as a function of AIDS dementia complex (ADC) severity . Fifth International Conference on AIDS. (Abstract.) Montreal, June 5-9, 1989
17. Brew BJ, Hardy W, Zuckerman E, et al: AIDS-related vacuolar myelopathy is not associated with coinfection by HTLV-1. Ann Neurol 26:679-681, 1989
18. Brew BJ, Perdices M, Darveniza P, et al: The neurological features of early and "latent" human immunodeficiency virus infection. Aust N Z J Med 19:700-705, 1989
19. Brew BJ, Sidtis J, Petito CK, Price RW: The neurological complications of AIDS and human immunodeficiency virus infection. In Plum F (ed): Advances in Contemporary Neurology. Philadelphia, FA Davis Co, pp 1-49, 1988
20. Britton CB, Miller JR: Neurologic complications in acquired immunodeficiency syndrome (AIDS). Neurol Clin 2:315-339, 1984
21. Budka H: Neuropathology of human immunodeficiency virus infection. Brain Pathol 1:163-175, 1991
22. Calabrese LH, Proffitt MR, Levin KH, et al: Acute infection with the human immunodeficiency virus (HIV) associated with acute brachial neuritis and exanthematous rash. Ann Intern Med 107:849-851, 1987
23. Carne CA, Tedder RS, Smith A, et al: Acute encephalopathy coincident with seroconversion for anti–HTLV-III. Lancet 2:1206-1208, 1985
24. Centers for Disease Control: Classification system for human immunodeficiency virus (HIV) infection in children under 13 years of age. MMWR 36:225-236, 1987
25. Centers for Disease Control: Revision of the CDC surveillance case definition for acquired immunodeficiency syndrome. MMWR 36:3S-14S, 1987

26. Chalmers AC, Greco CM, Miller RG: Prognosis in AZT myopathy. Neurology 41:1181-1184, 1991
27. Cheng-Mayer C, Rutka JT, Rosenblum ML, et al: Human immunodeficiency virus can productively infect cultured human glial cells. Proc Natl Acad Sci 84:3526-3530, 1987
28. Cho ES, Sharer LR, Peress NS, Little B: Intimal proliferation of leptomeningeal arteries and brain infarcts in subjects with AIDS. J Neuropathol Exp Neurol 46:385, 1987
29. Chuck SL, Sande MA: Infections with *Cryptococcus neoformans* in the acquired immunodeficiency syndrome. N Engl J Med 321:794-799, 1989
30. Cornblath DR: Treatment of the neuromuscular complications of human immunodeficiency virus infection. Ann Neurol 23:588-591, 1988
31. Cornblath DR, McArthur JC, Kennedy PGE, et al: Inflammatory demyelinating peripheral neuropathies associated with human T-cell lymphotropic virus type III infection. Ann Neurol 21:32-40, 1986
32. Cortes E, Detels R, Aboulafia D, et al: HIV-1, HIV-2, and HTLV-I infection in the high-risk groups in Brazil. N Engl J Med 320:953-958, 1989
33. Craddock C, Pasvol G, Bull R, et al: Cardiorespiratory arrest and autonomic neuropathy in AIDS. Lancet 2(8549):16-18, 1987
34. Cronin KC, Rosenblum M, Brew BJ, Price RW: HIV-1 brain infection: Distribution of infection and clinical correlates. In Fifth International Conference on AIDS. (Abstract.) Montreal, June 5-9, 1989
35. Dalakas MC, Pezeshkpour GH, Gravell M, et al: Polymyositis associated with AIDS retrovirus. JAMA 256:2381-2383, 1986
36. De La Monte SM, Ho DD, Schooley RT, et al: Subacute encephalomyelitis of AIDS and its relation to HTLV-III infection. Neurology 37:562-569, 1987
37. Denning DA, Anderson J, Rudge P, et al: Acute myelopathy associated with primary infection with human immunodeficiency virus. Br Med J 294:143-144, 1987
38. Devinsky O, Cho ES, Petito CK, Price RW: Herpes zoster myelitis. Brain 114:1181-1196, 1991
39. Dickson DW, Mattiace LA, Katsuhiro K, et al: Biology of disease: Microglia in human disease, with an emphasis on acquired immune deficiency syndrome. Lab Invest 64(2):135-156, 1991
40. Dismukes WE: Cryptococcal meningitis in patients with AIDS. J Infect Dis 157:624-628, 1988
41. Dreyer EB, Kaiser AK, Offermann JT, Cipton SA: HIV-1 coat protein neurotoxicity prevented by calcium channel antagonists. Science 248:364-367, 1990
42. Eidelberg D, Sotrel A, Horoupian DS, et al: Thrombotic cerebral vasculopathy associated with herpes zoster. Ann Neurol 19:7-14, 1986
43. Eidelberg D, Sotrel A, Vogel H, et al: Progressive polyradiculopathy in acquired immune deficiency syndrome. Neurology 36:912-916, 1986
44. Eilbott DJ, Peress N, Burger H, et al: Human immunodeficiency virus type 1 in spinal cords of acquired immunodeficiency syndrome patients with myelopathy: Expression and replication in macrophages. Proc Natl Acad Sci U S A 86:3337-3341, 1989
45. Elovaara I, Iivanainen M, Valle SL, et al: CSF protein and cellular profiles in various stages of HIV infection related to neurological manifestations. J Neurol Sci 78:331-342, 1987
46. Elovaara I, Saar P, Valle SL, et al: EEG in early HIV-1 infection is characterized by anterior dysrhythmicity of low maximal amplitude. Clin Electroencephalogr 22(3):131-140, 1991
47. Eng RHK, Bishburg E, Smith SM, et al: Cryptococcal infections in patients with acquired immune deficiency syndrome. Am J Med 81:19-23, 1986
48. Engstrom JW, Lowenstein DH, Bredesen DE: Cerebral infarctions and transient neurologic deficits associated with acquired immunodeficiency syndrome. Am J Med 86:528-532, 1989
49. Epstein LG, Sharer LR, Cho ES, et al: HTLV-III/LAV-like retrovirus particles in the brains of patients with AIDS encephalopathy. AIDS Res 1:447-454, 1985
50. Epstein LG, Sharer LR, Joshi V, et al: Progressive encephalopathy in children with acquired immune deficiency syndrome. Ann Neurol 17:488-496, 1985
51. Fox R, Eldred LJ, Fuchs EJ, et al: Clinical manifestations of acute infection with human immunodeficiency virus in a cohort of gay men. AIDS 1:35-38, 1987
52. Fuller GN, Gill SK, Guilloff RJ, et al: Gancyclovir treatment of lumbosacral polyradiculopathy in AIDS. Lancet 335(8680):48-49, 1990
53. Gabuzda DH, Ho DD, de la Monte SM, et al: Immunohistochemical identification of HTLV-III antigen in brains of patients with AIDS. Ann Neurol 20:289-295, 1986
54. Gartner S, Markovits P, Markovits DM, et al: Virus isolation from an identification of HTLV-III/LAV producing cells in brain tissue from a patient with AIDS. JAMA 256:2365-2371, 1986

55. Goldstein J: Headache and acquired immunodeficiency syndrome. Neurol Clin 8:947-960, 1991
56. Goswami K, Kaye S, Miller R, et al: Intrathecal IgG synthesis and specificity of oligoclonal IgG in patients infected with HIV-1 do not correlate with CNS disease. J Med Virol 33:106-113, 1991
57. Goudsmit J, deWolf F, Paul DA, et al: Expression of human immunodeficiency virus antigen (HIV-Ag) in serum and cerebrospinal fluid during acute and chronic infection. Lancet 2(8500):177-180, 1986
58. Goudsmit J, Wolters EC, Bakker M, et al: Intrathecal synthesis of antibodies to HTLV-III in patients without AIDS or AIDS related complex. Br Med J 292:1231-1234, 1986
59. Grafe MR, Press GA, Berthoty DP, et al: Abnormalities of the brain in AIDS patients: Correlation of postmortem MR findings with neuropathology. AJNR 11:905-911, 1990
60. Grant IH, Gold JWM, Rosenblum M, et al: *Toxoplasma gondii* serology in HIV infected patients: The development of central nervous system toxoplasmosis in AIDS. AIDS 4:519-521, 1990
61. Gray F, Chimelli L, Mohr M, et al: Fulminating multiple sclerosis-like leukoencephalopathy revealing human immunodeficiency virus infection. Neurology 41:105-109, 1991
62. Gray FF, Gherardi R, Wingate E, et al: Diffuse "encephalitic" cerebral toxoplasmosis in AIDS: Report of four cases. J Neurol 236:273-277, 1989
63. Hall WW, Farmer PM, Takahashi H, et al: Pathologic features of virus infection of the central nervous system (CNS) in the acquired immunodeficiency syndrome (AIDS). Acta Pathol Jpn 41:172-181, 1991
64. Harris MJ, Jeste DV, Gleghorn A, Sewell DD: New onset psychosis in HIV infected patients. J Clin Psychiatry 52(9):369-376, 1991
65. Harris TM, Smith RR, Bognanno JR, Edwards MK: Toxoplasmic myelitis in AIDS: Gadolinium-enhanced MR. J Comp Assis Tomogr 14(5):809-811, 1990
66. Hilt DC, Bucholz D, Drumholz A, et al: Herpes zoster ophthalmicus and delayed contralateral hemiparesis caused by cerebral angiitis: Diagnosis and management approaches. Ann Neurol 14:543-553, 1983
67. Ho DD, Rota TR, Schooley RT, et al: Isolation of HTLV-III from cerebrospinal fluid and neural tissues of patients with neurologic syndromes related to the acquired immunodeficiency syndrome. N Engl J Med 313:1493-1497, 1985
68. Ho DD, Sarngadharan MG, Resnick L, et al: Primary human T-lymphotropic virus type III infection. Ann Intern Med 103:880-883, 1985
69. Hollander H, Golden J, Mendelson T, Cortland D: Extrapyramidal symptoms in AIDS patients given low dose metoclopramide or chlorpromazine. Lancet 2(8465):1186, 1985
70. Hollander H, Levy JA: Neurologic abnormalities and recovery of human immunodeficiency virus from cerebrospinal fluid. Ann Intern Med 106:692-695, 1987
71. Hollander H, Stringari S: Human immunodeficiency virus-associated meningitis: Clinical course and correlations. Am J Med 83:813-816, 1987
72. Holtzman DM, Kaku DA, So YT: New onset seizures associated with human immunodeficiency virus infection causation and clinical features in 100 cases. Am J Med 87:173-177, 1989
73. Hook, Edward W III: AIDS commentary. Syphilis and HIV infection. J Infect Dis 160:530-534, 1989
74. Horten B, Price RW, Jimenez D: Multifocal varicella-zoster virus leukoencephalitis temporarily remote from herpes zoster. Ann Neurol 9:251-266, 1981
75. Icca J, Avindra N, Dalakas M: Immunocytochemical and virological characteristics of HIV-associated inflammatory myopathies: Similarities with seronegative polymyositis. Ann Neurol 29:474-481, 1991
76. Janssen RS, Saykin AJ, Cannon L, et al: Neurological and neuropsychological manifestations of HIV-1 infection: Association with AIDS-related complex but not asymptomatic HIV-1 infection. Ann Neurol 26:592-600, 1989
77. Jarvik JG, Hesselink JR, Kennedy C, et al: Acquired immunodeficiency syndrome: Magnetic resonance patterns of brain involvement with pathologic correlation. Arch Neurol 45:731-736, 1988
78. Johns DR, Tierney M, Felsenstein D: Alteration in the natural history of neurosyphilis by concurrent infection with the human immunodeficiency virus. N Engl J Med 316:1569-1572, 1987
79. Kato T, Hirano A, Llena JF, Dembitzer HM: Neuropathology of acquired immunodeficiency syndrome (AIDS) in 53 autopsy cases with particular emphasis on microglial nodules and multinucleated giant cells. Acta Neuropathol 73:287-293, 1987
80. Katz DA, Berger JR: Neurosyphilis in acquired immunodeficiency syndrome. Arch Neurol 46:895-898, 1989

81.   Koenig S, Gendelman HE, Orenstein JM, et al: Detection of AIDS virus in macrophages in brain tissue from AIDS patients with encephalopathy. Science 233:1089-1093, 1986

82.   Kovacs JA, Kovacs AA, Polis M, et al: Cryptococcosis in the acquired immunodeficiency syndrome. Ann Intern Med 103:533-538, 1985

83.   Krupp LB, Lipton RB, Swerdlow ML, et al: Progressive multifocal leukoencephalopathy: Clinical and radiographic features. Ann Neurol 17:344-349, 1985

84.   Lansica M, Lansica DJ, Schmidley JW: Syphilitic polyradiculopathy in an HIV-positive man. Neurology 38:1297-1301, 1988

85.   Levine AM: Epidemiology, clinical characteristics, and management of AIDS related lymphoma. Hematol Oncol Clin North Am 5(2):331-342, 1991

86.   Levine AM, Lourie RO, Sullivan-Halley J, et al: HIV-related lymphoma: Prognostic factors predictive of survival. Blood 72:247A, 1988

87.   Levine AM, Wernz JC, Kaplan L, et al: Low dose chemotherapy with central nervous system prophylaxis and zidovudine maintenance in AIDS-related lymphoma: A multi-institutional trial. Blood 74:897A, 1989

88.   Levy JA, Shimabukuro J, Hollander H, et al: Isolation of AIDS associated retroviruses from cerebrospinal fluid and brain of patients with neurological symptoms. Lancet 2(8454):586-588, 1985

89.   Levy RL, Bredesen DE, Rosenblum ML: Neurological manifestations of the acquired immunodeficiency syndrome (AIDS): Experience at UCSF and review of the literature. J Neurosurg 62:475-492, 1985

90.   Lin-Greenberg A, Taneja-Uppal N: Dysautonomia and infection with the human immunodeficiency virus. Ann Intern Med 106:167, 1987

91.   Lipkin WI, Parry G, Kiprov D, et al: Inflammatory neuropathy in homosexual men with lymphadenopathy. Neurology 35:1479-1483, 1985

92.   Luer W, Poser S, Weber T, et al: Chronic HIV encephalitis-1. Cerebrospinal fluid diagnosis. Klin Wochenschr 66:21-35, 1988

93.   Lukehart S, Hook E, Baker-Zander S, et al: Invasion of the central nervous system by *Treponema pallidum:* Implications for diagnosis and treatment. Ann Intern Med 109:855-862, 1988

94.   Maclean C, Flegg PJ, Kilpatrick DC: Anti-cardiolipin antibodies and HIV infection. Clin Exp Immunol 81:263-266:1990

95.   Matsuo H, Nakamura T, Tsujihata M, et al: Plasmapheresis in treatment of human T-lymphotropic virus type-I associated myelopathy. Lancet 2(8620):1109-1113, 1988

96.   McArthur JC, Cohen BA, Farzadegan H, et al: Cerebrospinal fluid abnormalities in homosexual men with and without neuropsychiatric findings. Ann Neurol 23:534-537, 1988

97.   McArthur JC, Cohen BA, Selnes OA, et al: Low prevalence of neurological and neuropsychological abnormalities in otherwise healthy HIV-1 infected individuals: Results from the Multicenter AIDS Cohort Study. Ann Neurol 26:601-611, 1989

98.   Mehren M, Burns PJ, Mamani F, et al: Toxoplasmic myelitis mimicking intramedullary spinal cord tumor. Neurology 38:1648-1650, 1988

99.   Merrill JE, Chen ISY: HIV-1, macrophages, glial cells and cytokines in AIDS nervous system disease. FASEB J 5:2391-2397, 1991

100. Mhiri C, Baudrimont M, Bonne G, et al: Zidovudine myopathy: A distinctive disorder associated with mitrochondrial dysfunction. Ann Neurol 29:606-614, 1991

101. Michaels J, Price RW, Rosenblum MK: Microglia in the human immunodeficiency virus encephalitis of acquired immune deficiency syndrome: Proliferation, infection and fusion. Acta Neuropathol 76:373-379, 1988

102. Miller EB, Selnes OA, McArthur JC, et al: Neuropsychological performance in HIV-1 infected homosexual men: The Multi-center AIDS Cohort Study (MACS). Neurology 40:197-203, 1990

103. Miller RG, Storey J, Greco C: Ganciclovir in the treatment of progressive AIDS-related polyradiculopathy. Neurology 40:569-574, 1990

104. Moeller AA, Backmund HL: Ventricle brain ratio in the clinical course of HIV infection. Acta Neurol Scand 81:512-515, 1990

105. Morgello S, Block GA, Price RW, et al: Varicella-zoster virus leukoencephalitis and cerebral vasculopathy. Arch Pathol Lab Med 112:173-177, 1988

106. Morgello S, Cho ES, Nielsen S, et al: Cytomegalovirus encephalitis in patients with acquired immunodeficiency syndrome: An autopsy study of 30 cases and a review of the literature. Human Pathol 18:289-297, 1987

107. Musher BM: Editorial on Syphilis in HIV: How much penicillin cures early syphilis? Ann Intern Med 109:849-851, 1988

108. Musher DM, Hamill RJ, Baughn RE: Effect of human immunodeficiency virus (HIV) infection on the course of syphilis and on the response to treatment. Ann Intern Med 113:872-881, 1990

109. Navia BA, Cho ES, Petito CK, et al: The AIDS dementia complex. II. Neuropathology. Ann Neurol 19:525-535, 1986

110. Navia BA, Jordan BD, Price RW: The AIDS dementia complex. I. Clinical features. Ann Neurol 19:517-524, 1986

111. Navia BA, Petito CK, Gold JWM, et al: Cerebral toxoplasmosis complicating the acquired immune deficiency syndrome: Clinical and neuropathological findings in 27 patients. Ann Neurol 19:224-238, 1986

112. Navia BA, Price RW: The acquired immunodeficiency syndrome dementia complex as the presenting or sole manifestation of human immunodeficiency virus infection. Arch Neurol 44:65-69, 1987

113. Nolla-Salas J, Ricart C, D'Olhaberriague L, et al: Hydrocephalus: An unusual CT presentation of cerebral toxoplasmosis in a patient with acquired immunodeficiency syndrome. Eur Neurol 27:130-132, 1987

114. Page JB, Lai S, Chitwodd DD, et al: HTLV I/II seropositivity and death from AIDS among HIV-I seropositive intravenous drug users. Lancet 335(8703):1439-1441, 1990

115. Panther LA, Sande MA: Cryptococcal meningitis in the acquired immunodeficiency syndrome. Semin Respir Infect 5(2):138-145, 1990

116. Paul MO, Brew BJ, Khan A, et al: Detection of HIV-1 in cerebrospinal fluid (CSF): Correlation with presence and severity of the AIDS dementia complex. In Fifth International Conference on AIDS. (Abstract.) Montreal, June 5-9, 1989

117. Petito CK, Cho ES, Lemann W, et al: Neuropathology of acquired immunodeficiency syndrome (AIDS): An autopsy review. J Neuropathol Exp Neurol 45:635-646, 1986

118. Petito CK, Navia BA, Cho ES, et al: Vacuolar myelopathy pathologically resembling subacute combined degeneration in patients with acquired immunodeficiency syndrome. N Engl J Med 312:874-879, 1985

119. Peudenier S, Hery C, Montagnier L, Tardieu M: Human microglial cells: Characterization in cerebral tissue and in primary culture, and study of their susceptibility to HIV-1 infection. Ann Neurol 29:152-161, 1991

120. Piette AM, Tusseau F, Vignon D, et al: Acute neuropathy coincident with seroconversion for anti-LAV/HTLV-III. Lancet 1(8485):852, 1986

121. Pizzo PA, Eddy J, Falloon J, et al: Effect of continuous intravenous infusion of zidovudine (AZT) in children with symptomatic HIV infection. N Engl J Med 319:889-896, 1988

122. Portegies P, Epstein LG, Hung ST, et al: Human immunodeficiency virus type 1 antigen in cerebrospinal fluid. Correlation with clinical neurological status. Arch Neurol 46:261-264, 1989

123. Portegies P, de Gans J, Lange JM, et al: Declining incidence of AIDS dementia complex after introduction of zidovudine treatment. Br Med J 299:819-821, 1989

124. Post MJ, Tate IG, Quencer RM, et al: CT, MR and pathology in HIV encephalitis and meningitis. AJR 151:373-380, 1988

125. Post MJD, Hensley GT, Moskowitz LB, Fischl M: Cytomegalic inclusion virus encephalitis in patients with AIDS: CT, clinical and pathologic correlation. AJR 146:1229-1234, 1986

126. Price RW, Brew B: Infection of the central nervous system by human immunodeficiency virus: Role of the immune system in pathogenesis. Ann NY Acad Sci 540:162-175, 1988

127. Price RW, Brew BJ: The AIDS dementia complex. J Infect Dis 158:1079-1083, 1988

128. Price RW, Brew BJ, Rosenblum M: The AIDs dementia complex and HIV-1 brain infection: A pathogenetic model of virus-immune interaction. In Waksman BH (ed): Immunologic Mechanisms in Neurologic and Psychiatric Disease. New York, Raven Press, 1990, pp 269-290.

129. Price RW, Brew B, Sidtis J, et al: The brain in AIDS: Central nervous system HIV-1 infection and the AIDS dementia complex. Science 239:586-592, 1988

130. Price RW, Sidtis JJ, Brew BJ: AIDS dementia complex and HIV-1 infection: A view from the clinic. Brain Pathol 1:155-162, 1991

131. Price RW, Sidtis JJ, Navia BA: AIDS dementia complex. In Rosenblum ML, Levy RM, Bredesen DE (eds): AIDS and the Nervous System. New York, Raven Press, 1988, pp 203-219

132. Pulliam L, Herndier BG, Tang NM, McGrath MS: Human immunodeficiency virus–infected macrophages produce soluble factors that cause histological and neurochemical alterations in cultured human brains. J Clin Invest 87;503-512, 1991

133. Pumarola-Sune T, Navia BA, Cordon-Cardo C, et al: HIV antigen in the brains of patients with the AIDS dementia complex. Ann Neurol 21:490-496, 1991

134. Reinvang I, Froland SS, Skripeland V: Prevalence of neuropsychological deficit in HIV infection: Incipient signs of AIDS dementia complex in patients with AIDS. Acta Neurol Scand 83(5):289-293, 1985

135. Resnick L, Berger JR, Shapshak P, et al: Early penetration of the blood-brain barrier by HIV. Neurology 38:9-14, 1988

136. Resnick L, DiMarzo-Veronese F, Schupbach J, et al: Intra-blood-brain-barrier synthesis of HTLV-III specific IgG in patients with neurologic symptoms associated with AIDS or AIDS-related complex. N Engl J Med 313:1498-1504, 1985

137. Richardson EP: Progressive multifocal leukoencephalopathy. In Vinken PJ, Bruyn GW (eds): Handbook of Clinical Neurology, vol 9. Amsterdam, Elsevier, 1970, pp 485-499

138. Rosenblum M, Scheck A, Cronin K, et al: Dissociation of AIDS related vacuolar myelopathy and productive HIV-1 infection of the spinal cord. Neurology 39:892-896, 1989

139. Rosenblum MK: Infection of the central nervous system by the human immunodeficiency virus type 1: Morphology and relation to syndromes of progressive encephalopathy and myelopathy in patients with AIDS. Pathol Annu 25:117-169, 1990

140. Rosenblum MK, Brew BJ, Aronow HA, et al: Clinical-pathological features of HTLV-I associated myelopathy (HAM) in AIDS. In Fifth International Conference on AIDS. (Abstract.) Montreal, June 5-9, 1989

141. Ryder JW, Croen K, Kleinschmidt-DeMasters BK, et al: Progressive encephalitis three months after resolution of cutaneous zoster in a patient with AIDS. Ann Neurol 19:182-188, 1986

142. Saag MS, Powderly WG, Cloud GA, et al: Comparison of amphotericin B with fluconazole in the treatment of acute AIDS-associated cryptococcal meningitis. N Engl J Med 326:83-89, 1992

143. Said G, Lacroix C, Chemouilli P, et al: Cytomegalovirus neuropathy in acquired immunodeficiency syndrome: A clinical and pathological study. Ann Neurol 29:139-140, 1991

144. Schmitt FA, Bigleg JW, McKinnis R, et al: Neuropsychological outcome of azidothymidine (AZT) in the treatment of AIDS and AIDS-related complex: A double blind, placebo-controlled trial. N Engl J Med 319:1573-1578, 1988

145. Sidtis J, Price RW: Early HIV-1 infection and the AIDS dementia complex. Neurology 40:323-326, 1990

146. Sidtis JJ, Constantine G, Price RW, et al: Zidovudine treatment of the AIDS dementia complex: Results of a placebo-controlled trial. (submitted for publication)

147. Simpson DM, Bender AN: Human immunodeficiency virus–associated myopathy: Analysis of 11 patients. Ann Neurol 24:79-84, 1988

148. Simpson DM, Wolfe DE: Neuromuscular complications of HIV infection and its treatment. AIDS 5:917-926, 1991

149. Snider WD, Simpson DM, Nielsen S, et al: Neurological complications of acquired immune deficiency syndrome: Analysis of 50 patients. Ann Neurol 14:403-418, 1983

150. So YT, Beckstead JH, Davis RL: Primary central nervous system lymphoma in acquired immune deficiency syndrome: A clinical and pathological study. Ann Neurol 20:566-572, 1986

151. Stoler MH, Eskin TA, Benn S, et al: Human T-cell lymphotropic virus type III infection of the central nervous system—A preliminary in situ analysis. JAMA 256:2360-2364, 1986

152. Sugar AM, Stern JJ, Dupont B: Overview: Treatment of cryptococcal meningitis. Rev Infect Dis 12(suppl 3):S338, 1990

153. Telzak EE, Zweig-Greenberg MS, Harrison J, et al: Syphilis treatment response in HIV infected individuals. AIDS 5:591-595, 1991

154. Tindall B, Cooper DA: Primary HIV infection: Host responses and intervention strategies. AIDS 5:1-14, 1991

155. Tross S, Price RW, Navia BA, et al: Neuropsychological characterization of the AIDS dementia complex: A preliminary report. AIDS 2:81-88, 1988

156. Tucker T, Dix RD, Katzen C, et al: Cytomegalovirus and herpes simplex virus ascending myelitis in a patient with acquired immune deficiency syndrome. Ann Neurol 18:74-79, 1985

157. Vazeux R, Brousse N, Jarry A, et al: AIDS subacute encephalitis: Identification of HIV-infected cells. Am J Pathol 126:403-410, 1987

158. Vinters HV, Kwok MK, Ho HW, et al: Cytomegalovirus in the nervous system of patients with the acquired immunodeficiency syndrome. Brain 112:245-268, 1989

159. Wahl SM, Allen JB, McCartney-Francis N, et al: Macrophage and astrocyte-derived transforming growth factor B as a mediator of central nervous system dysfunction in acquired immune deficiency syndrome. J Exp Med 173:981-991, 1991
160. Watkins B, Dorn HH, Kelly WB, et al: Specific tropism of HIV-1 for microglial cells in primary human brain cultures. Science 249:549-553, 1990
161. Weber T, Freter A, Luer W, et al: The use of recombinant antigens in ELISA procedures for the quantification of intrathecally produced HIV-1 specific antibodies. J Immunol Methods 136:133-137, 1991
162. Wiley CA, Nelson JA: Role of human immunodeficiency virus and cytomegalovirus in AIDS encephalitis. Am J Pathol 133:73-81, 1988
163. Wiley CA, Schrier RD, Denaro FJ, et al: Localization of cytomegalovirus proteins and genome during fulminant central nervous system infection in an AIDS patient. J Neuropathol Exp Neurol 45(2):127-139, 1986
164. Wiley CA, Schrier RD, Nelson JA, et al: Cellular localization of human immunodeficiency virus infection within the brains of acquired immune deficiency syndrome patients. Proc Natl Acad Sci 83:7089-7093, 1986
165. Wiselka MJ, Nicholson KG, Wara SC, Flower AJE: Acute infection with human immunodeficiency virus associated with facial nerve palsy and neuralgia. J Infect 15:189-194, 1987
166. Wong MC, Suite N, Labar DR: Seizures in human immunodeficiency virus infection. Arch Neurol 47:640-642, 1990
167. Woolsey RM, Chambers TJ, Chung HD, McGarry JD: Mycobacterial meningomyelitis associated with human immunodeficiency virus infection. Arch Neurol 45:691-693, 1988
168. Working Group of the American Academy of Neurology AIDS Task Force: Nomenclature and research case definitions for neurologic manifestations of human immunodeficiency virus-type I (HIV-1) infection. Neurology 41:278-285, 1991
169. World Health Organization consultation on the neuropsychiatric aspects of HIV-1 infections. Geneva, January 11-13, 1990. AIDS 4:935-936, 1990
170. Yarchoan R, Berg G, Brouwers P, et al: Response of human immunodeficiency virus associated neurological disease to 3'-azido-3'-deoxythymidine. Lancet 1(8525):132-135, 1987
171. Yarchoan R, Mitsuya H, Thomas RV, et al: In vivo activity against HIV and favorable toxicity profile of 2',3'dideoxyinosine. Science 245:412-415, 1989
172. Zuger A, Louie E, Holzman RS, et al: Cryptococcal disease in patients with the acquired immunodeficiency syndrome. Ann Intern Med 104:234-240, 1986

14

MANAGEMENT OF NEUROPSYCHIATRIC DISORDERS IN HIV-SPECTRUM PATIENTS

JAMES W. DILLEY, MD

Much has been written about the significance of the psychologic and social effects of the AIDS epidemic.[21,30,32] Because of the complexities of these effects on the well-being of those living with HIV, health care providers have had to broaden their usual gaze and carefully consider the psychologic and social milieu of their patients. The use of emotional and social support services is often a mainstay of their care. In addition, supportive services and help in coping with the realities of living with HIV disease are often needed by the patient's family and significant others and those who care for them.[12,39,47] Thus, especially for the front-line practitioner, knowledge about and comfort with the common psychiatric conditions seen in this patient group are critical in successfully caring for HIV-infected patients. Finally, although a discussion of the broader psychosocial implications of the AIDS epidemic would be of interest, the purpose of this chapter is to outline the most common types of psychiatric disorders (Table 14–1) found in the clinical care of patients with HIV disease.[11,14] Although specific diagnostic criteria are not provided, the disorders discussed below are based on criteria from the *Diagnostic and Statistical Manual of Mental Disorders Third Edition, Revised* (DSM-III-R) of the American Psychiatric Association, and recommendations about their management are offered.

ADJUSTMENT DISORDERS

The adjustment disorders are discussed first because they best characterize the psychologic reactions to living with HIV referred most often for psychiatric evaluation. This diagnostic category was most frequently reported in one of the earliest papers documenting psychiatric consultations in hospitalized patients with AIDS and in one of the most recent surveys of patients with HIV-spectrum disease attending an outpatient mental health clinic.[15,35] These reactions, whether dominated

Table 14–1.   Psychiatric Disorders Associated with HIV Infection

Adjustment Disorders
Adjustment disorder with depressed mood
Adjustment disorder with anxious mood
Major Affective Disorders
Major depression
Bereavement
Bipolar disorders
Anxiety Disorders
Generalized anxiety disorder
Organic Mental Disorders
DEMENTIA
HIV-1–associated dementia complex
Dementia associated with opportunistic
  infections and cancers
Infections
Fungal
  Cryptococcal disease
  Candida abscess
Protozoal
  Toxoplasmosis
Bacterial
  Mycobacterium avium-intracellulare
	Organic Mental Disorders *continued*
	Viral
	  Cytomegalovirus
	  Herpes virus
	  Papovavirus (progressive multifocal
	    leukoencephalopathy)
	Cancers
	Primary cerebral lymphoma
	Disseminated Kaposi's sarcoma
	Delirium
	Organic Mood Disorders
	Depressed
	Manic
	Mixed
	Organic Delusional Disorders
	Personality Disorders
	Borderline personality
	Antisocial personality
	Substance Abuse Disorders

primarily by depressive or anxious features, can be brought on by a host of events within the cycle of living with HIV (e.g., a precipitous fall in helper T-cell counts, being placed on disability or curtailing usual work activities, the diagnosis of an opportunistic infection, or the need to change or add additional antiviral medications). The diagnosis of adjustment disorders differs primarily from their major disorder counterparts (major depression and generalized anxiety disorders) only by the severity and duration of symptoms. In either case the individual is believed to have a "maladaptive reaction to a known psychosocial stressor that occurs within three months of the onset of the stressor" *(DSM-III-R)*. A reaction is primarily considered maladaptive when it impairs social or occupational functioning or when the reaction is considered greater than expected. Distinguishing between patients whose symptoms fall within the category of adjustment disorders and those with more serious psychopathology is most important when planning treatment.

Standard treatment for individuals with adjustment disorders may include brief periods of administering antianxiety agents or hypnotics as treatment for temporary insomnia and generally involves referrals for supportive psychotherapy. Primary care providers can also be helpful by scheduling more frequent visits and by making special efforts to reassure and emotionally support the patient. Community referrals can also be helpful as a means of connecting these patients with additional social supports and providing them with a buffer against prolonged social isolation or withdrawal. Furthermore, patients who have recently learned about their HIV infection generally benefit from becoming involved in the community of those living with HIV. This process of becoming involved with others who are coping with their illness can be an important step in an individual's accepting his or her infection and the need to begin to address it.

AFFECTIVE DISORDERS

The cardinal features of affective disorders involve disorders of mood. The most common affective disorder among those with HIV disease is major depression, although as HIV disease becomes more widespread, those with preexisting bipolar disease are being seen more frequently.[2] In both cases the diagnosis is made on the basis of a careful history and the severity and duration of symptoms. These diagnoses are also only made in the absence of known organic causes for depression or mania, a criterion that is often problematic in the evaluation of those with HIV (see the discussion of Organic Mental Disorders).

Major Depression

Evaluating depression in patients with HIV disease is one of the most common tasks requested of psychiatric consultants. Primary care clinicians must maintain a high index of suspicion about the presence of depression in their HIV-spectrum patients and should not hesitate to discuss the possibility of depression with them. At times clinicians fall prey to the notion that the patient's depressive symptoms are "understandable" since he or she is coping with a life-threatening illness and thus downplay the seriousness of symptoms reported. Often this attitude is in response to the patient's wishes: patients frequently will minimize their complaints, wanting to appear to maintain a "fighting" attitude and often expressing feelings of awkwardness or embarrassment that they have been experiencing significant depression. If the physician is pulled into this deception, the patient ultimately suffers because major depression is clearly a treatable illness in patients with HIV disease.[19,24] Major depression is found in as many as 10% to 20% of those with HIV and is the cause of significant morbidity in this patient population.[1,39] Patients will be served best if a referral is made for evaluation whenever a question should arise.

The differential diagnosis of depression is large, and although it is important to be sensitive to the psychologic meanings of the patient's illness and the current psychosocial environment, it is also important to remain aware of the potential contribution of organic factors in assessing patients with HIV. A number of organic disorders can produce symptoms that mimic depression, for example, early HIV-1-associated dementia, metabolic disorders, and medication side effects (e.g., nausea and appetite suppression from trimethoprim-sulfamethoxazole [Septra] therapy). Additionally, the constitutional symptoms of HIV disease itself (e.g., anorexia, weight loss, fatigue) can further cloud the diagnostic picture. However, once major neurologic disorders and medication side effects are ruled out, the distinction between organic mood disorders and the so-called "functional" psychiatric disorders may be less useful in the clinical care of patients.[20] Finally, since the central nervous system (CNS) is affected very early in the course of HIV infection, an absolutely normal CNS may be rare in these patients, perhaps especially so in those with significant psychiatric symptoms.[9,16,26,42] Thus the likelihood of this "blending" of organic and functional factors complicates the diagnostic picture in patients with psychiatric disorders and should be considered the standard in working with this population of patients.

Some clinical tips are helpful in teasing apart these aspects of a patient's presentation. First, a predominantly functional disorder is more likely in patients who have more intact immune function (i.e., those more recently diagnosed and those without other opportunistic infections); those patients who have recently been bereaved (this is especially relevant in caring for HIV patients since many have witnessed an entire network of friends, lovers, and/or family members become ill and die from HIV); those patients with a previous personal or family history of major psychiatric disorder; and those patients for whom a clearly identifiable psychosocial stressor can be identified. Searching for cognitive signs of depression (e.g., feelings of worthlessness, hopelessness, guilt, concerns about being a "bad" person, and suicidal plans) can also be helpful, and the use of formal neuropsychologic testing can help determine the relative proportion of organic versus functional components.

Treatment for patients believed to have major mood disturbances should include psychopharmacologic and/or social interventions and brief, supportive psychotherapy. The use of antidepressant and stimulant medications for these patients is discussed later in this chapter.

Bipolar Disorder

The hallmark characteristics of bipolar disease include discrete periods of an elevated, euphoric, or irritable mood and those characterized by depression. Patients with bipolar disorder and HIV can be managed much as bipolar patients without HIV infection with the exception that if antipsychotic medications are needed, low- or mid-range potency agents should be used (note Psychopharmacology discussion). Also note that secondary manic or hypomanic states have been reported in HIV patients[8,22,45] and have required treatment. Experience has shown that the use of lithium carbonate in this population is well tolerated in the usual dosage ranges (600 to 1500 mg/day). Attempts should be made to maintain blood levels in the usual therapeutic range (0.8 to 1.6 mEq/L) for acutely manic patients; however, determining blood levels may be more useful in ruling out the presence of lithium toxicity than in guiding overall therapeutic decisions, which hinge more on the patient's clinical presentation. In HIV patients, who may develop diarrhea and/or become dehydrated as a consequence of some underlying disease process associated with HIV, the clinician must be careful about the development of lithium toxicity; thus maintenance levels in this group should be kept in the range of 0.4 mEq/L to 0.8 mEq/L. Also, because of the high incidence of neurologic disorders in patients with HIV disease, those with focal neurologic lesions, concomitant HIV-associated dementia, or a history of toxoplasmosis with its risk of seizure might also be treated with carbamazepine (Tegretol), although close monitoring for signs of bone marrow suppression must be an integral part of the treatment plan. Carbamazepine can also be useful in the treatment of those with organic mania (see below). If selected, carbamazepine should be started at 100 mg twice a day, with a gradual increase to a dose of 600 to 1000 mg/day.

ANXIETY DISORDERS

Anxiety disorders are also common among the spectrum of patients living and coping with HIV. The very real threat of living with a chronic, life-threatening illness and the multiple psychosocial stressors with which these patients must contend combine to form a fertile backdrop on which anticipatory anxiety, worry, and fear can grow. Severe anxiety can be both physically painful and psychologically terrifying.

Treatment of anxiety should begin with nonpharmacologic approaches, adding antianxiety agents as needed. Nonpharmacologic approaches include relaxation training and supportive psychotherapy. If these approaches fail, antianxiety agents such as clonazepam (Klonopin), 0.5 mg twice a day, or lorazepam (Ativan), 1 mg twice or three times daily, are suggested initially. Alprazolam (Xanax), diazepam (Valium), and triazolam (Halcion) have also been used successfully, but they also induce depression or have appeared particularly psychologically addicting (e.g., alprazolam, diazepam). Triazolam in particular induces memory impairment (in both young and elderly patients), daytime anxiety, and hyperexcitability; thus their use should be avoided in HIV patients.[23] Patients taking benzodiazepines should be followed closely, and providers should state at the outset that the use of these agents will be short term. Providers should also discuss the possibility of tolerance and psychologic addiction and should establish a time-table for tapering and discontinuing their use. Those patients with histories of previous drug or alcohol dependence pose special problems, and referral to a drug abuse specialist or counselor should be considered. Finally, for those patients in whom HIV-associated dementia is a consideration, the use of benzodiazepines should be avoided since these agents depress cortical function and can produce disinhibition or worsening of dementia.

ORGANIC MENTAL DISORDERS

Clinically apparent CNS or peripheral nervous system disease occurs in at least 30% to 40% of AIDS patients (see Chapter 13). The most common causes of neurologic disease in AIDS patients include infection with HIV itself, other viral and nonviral infections, neoplasms, and cerebrovascular disease.[41]

Because of the neurotropism of HIV, autopsy studies of AIDS patients indicate that 70% to 90% of the brains of these patients show gross and/or microscopic evidence of CNS disease. In fact, several reports have shown that subclinical cognitive impairment due to HIV infection may precede the diagnosis of AIDS in 10% to 25% of patients. Some degree of HIV-associated dementia complex may be present in as many as two thirds of AIDS patients before death.[44] It is clear then that neurologic disease in HIV-infected individuals is a major source of medical

Table 14–2. Common Causes of Organic Mental Disorders in Patients with HIV Disease

HIV-associated dementia complex
Toxoplasmosis
Cryptococcal meningitis
Central nervous system lymphoma
Progressive multifocal leukoencephalopathy

Table 14–3.   Manifestations of AIDS Dementia

EARLY SYMPTOMS	LATE SYMPTOMS
Cognitive	
Memory loss (names, historical details, appointments)	Global dementia
	Confusion
Impaired concentration (loses track of conversation or reading)	Distractibility
	Delayed verbal responses
Mental slowing ("not as quick," less verbal, loss of spontaneity)	
Confusion (time or person)	
Behavioral	
Apathy, withdrawal, "depression"	Vacant stare
Agitation, confusion, hallucinations	Restlessness
	Disinhibition
	Organic psychosis
Motor	
Unsteady gait	Slowing; truncal ataxia
Bilateral leg weakness	Weakness: legs more than arms
Loss of coordination, impaired handwriting	Pyramidal track signs: spasticity, hyperreflexia,
Tremor	tremor

and psychiatric morbidity, and the subsequent development of organic mental disorders should be expected (Table 14–2). In fact, some researchers have suggested that specific difficulties in the dopaminergic system among people with AIDS are responsible for the development of schizophrenia-like organic disorders in this group.[25]

Perhaps the most common of these organic mental disorders develops as a result of the chronic, debilitating encephalitis that is a distinct clinical and neuropathologic syndrome now referred to as *HIV-associated dementia complex*.[50] Clinically, this syndrome is characterized by a triad of cognitive, behavioral, and motor symptoms[31] (Table 14–3). The absolute incidence of this syndrome is unknown, although clinical experience would suggest that it is a common sequela of the disease, particularly in the later stages of the illness. In one study evidence of HIV-associated dementia complex was shown in approximately 70% of autopsied AIDS patients in whom all focal neurologic disease or confounding metabolic encephalopathy had been excluded.[44] Typically the dementia has an insidious onset and progression, although sudden accelerations may occur as may a characteristic waxing and waning of symptoms, which can be initially confusing. Occasionally the dementia has an acute onset and is accompanied by an acute organic psychosis.

The differential diagnosis of cognitive compromise is complex and requires a detailed work-up. The diagnosis of HIV-associated dementia largely depends on the documentation of typical cognitive, behavioral, and motor abnormalities in individuals with AIDS and on performing the neurodiagnostic tests necessary to rule out the other possible CNS disease states. The psychiatric consultant can be helpful in suggesting behavioral management strategies for the cognitively compromised patient and through the use of psychotropic medications. The staff should be taught to understand the importance of helpful interventions such as using orienting cues, clocks, and calendars, to help manage poor short-term memory, and short, simple sentences in communicating with the patient. Recommendations for using medication to control agitation and to reverse altered sleep-wakefulness cycles are also important (see Psychopharmacology discussion). Lastly, understanding and controlling these potentially difficult behavioral problems are extremely important to social workers and discharge planners in arranging for the most appropriate placement for cognitively impaired patients.

PSYCHOTIC SYMPTOMS

Psychotic symptoms may arise in HIV-spectrum patients in multiple contexts, including dementia and delirium. In delirious states treatment is aimed first at correcting the underlying disorder, and AIDS patients are susceptible to multiple potential causes of disordered mentation (Table 14–4).

In assessing an HIV-infected patient with psychotic symptomatology, any history of psychotic illness, drug and alcohol abuse, or early signs of HIV-associated dementia should be assessed. Collateral informants are especially helpful in this circumstance because the patient in this mental state usually is not a very reliable or cooperative historian. Psychiatric consultation should be obtained and the decision made as to whether psychiatric hospitalization is indicated. A primary consideration in this decision is ruling out other possible medical causes for acute mental status changes, which should be undertaken in collaboration with the primary provider.

Treatment for patients with psychotic disorders includes antipsychotic medications and perhaps supportive psychotherapy and social interventions.

Table 14–4.   Potential Causes of Altered Mental States

Alcohol or Drug Withdrawal
Alcohol
Opiates
Sedative hypnotics
Disorders of Fluid, Electrolyte, and Acid-Base Balance
Water intoxification, dehydration, hypernatremia, hypokalemia, hypocalcemia, hypercalcemia, alkalosis, acidosis
Endocrine disorders
Hypoglycemia
Infections
Systemic: bacteremia, septicemia, subacute bacterial endocarditis, pneumonia, *Pneumocystis carinii* pneumonia, cryptococcal pneumonia, herpes zoster, disseminated *Mycobacterium avium-intracellulare*, disseminated candidiasis
Intracranial: cryptococcal meningitis, HIV encephalitis, tuberculous meningitis, toxoplasmosis
Epilepsy
Head trauma
Space-occupying lesions of brain: central nervous system lymphoma, toxoplasmosis, cytomegalovirus infection, abscesses
Blood: anemia
Intoxication
Drugs: antibiotics, anticonvulsants, sedative hypnotics, opiates, phencyclidine, antineoplastic drugs, anticholinergic agents, cocaine
Alcohol
Metabolic Encephalopathies
Hypoxia
Hepatic, renal, pulmonary, pancreatic insufficiency

ORGANIC MOOD DISORDERS

Several cases of secondary depression, hypomania, or frank mania have been reported among people with HIV disease.[13,22,28,45] Of particular note is the group of HIV patients without a history of affective disorder who develop manic episodes during the course of their illness.[9] These patients may develop manic symptoms at various points along the HIV spectrum, and the extent of HIV-related disease progression in these individuals at the time of the manic episode has varied widely.[3] Over a period of weeks to months the affective symptoms typically fade away while the patient becomes progressively demented. A brief case vignette illustrates these points:

> Joe is a 31-year-old homosexual white male brought to the emergency room by two of his friends. They report that Joe, who has had symptoms of HIV disease for at least 2 years, has undergone a radical personality change in the past few weeks. Formerly a rather shy accountant with no history of psychiatric problems, Joe has become increasingly "speedy," irritable, and sexually promiscuous. His friends became particularly worried when they learned he had not slept for several nights and had spent $12,000 on home appliances he did not need. The ER physician notes that Joe has markedly pressured speech, admits to auditory hallucinations, and voices the grandiose delusion that he has become the chief of the United States Health and Welfare Division and has ordered that its entire budget be used for AIDS research. After several weeks of inpatient psychiatric treatment, Joe's euphoria waned and marked symptoms of apathy and confusion predominated.

These disorders generally respond well to standard treatment with the caveats discussed in the section "Psychopharmacology."

FAMILY AND SUPPORT SYSTEM CONFLICTS

One aspect of AIDS that sets it apart from other life-threatening illnesses is the fact that AIDS is most commonly found among members of socially stigmatized groups. This can be a particularly confounding factor in the ability or willingness of the patient's traditional support system to rally to his or her side.

Among many homosexual men who have lived openly homosexual life-styles, for example, it is not uncommon for a nontraditional family to have developed. The patient may have a steady, life-partner relationship that is indistinguishable in tone and form from that of a heterosexual marriage. Alternately, the patient may be without a primary relationship but have a close circle of friends that substitutes for the biologic family. In some cases the biologic parents may be aware of their son's homosexuality, although knowledge of the patient's life-style does not necessarily imply that the family either condones or approves. There may, in fact, be open conflict between the patient's biologic family and his nontraditional family of friends. This outcome is particularly likely when the parents have either not known of their son's homosexuality before his illness or have known but have refused to acknowledge it openly. Conflict can also be expected when families are asked suddenly to become reinvolved with a son or brother toward whom the family has been emotionally distant because of past conflicts over this issue. These parents or siblings are sometimes the most difficult because they often carry a sense of guilt for having rejected their son or brother and now, with his illness, believe they have immediately to compensate for the hard feelings between them over the years. This "unfinished business" can lead to difficulty in negotiating with the patient and his current family because the parents may resent or simply cannot accept the legitimacy of the commitment between their son and his male partner or his friends.

> Stephen is a 33-year-old black homosexual man who has had AIDS for 3 years. Initially diagnosed with Kaposi's sarcoma, Stephen has felt well and has continued to work at his job as a computer programmer. Because his homosexuality has never been acceptable to his middle-class parents, it has remained in large part an issue that was known but never directly discussed. Contact between Stephen and his parents has been minimal for several years, and Stephen decided not to tell his parents about his illness. He is quite open about the fact that he moved to the West Coast some 10 years earlier because he needed to feel free to live an openly homosexual life-style, and he "knows" that his parents would not be supportive of his illness. Joseph is Stephen's partner of 8 years. On returning home from a 3-day business trip, Joseph finds Stephen seriously ill and rushes him to the hospital where Stephen is admitted to the intensive care unit and is placed on a respirator. Because of the grave prognosis, Joseph notifies Stephen's family that Stephen is critically ill with "pneumonia," and the parents arrive the next day. After learning that her son has AIDS and may not recover, Stephen's mother swears at Joseph, saying he has "given" AIDS to Stephen, and turns on him, demanding that he leave the hospital and never return. She insists to the nursing staff that "this man" not be allowed to visit her son and demands to see the hospital administrator. She begins to make plans to have Stephen flown back to the East Coast where she will "be able to take care of him when he gets out of the hospital." Joseph threatens to sue the hospital if attempts are made to prohibit him from seeing his lover. An immediate psychiatric consultation is requested.

Variations on this basic scenario are common, and the potential for emotional crisis that exists in working with people with AIDS results from a combination of medical, psychological, and social factors. When individuals are forced to confront several difficult issues, including homosexuality, long-term estrangement, and unexpected death, simultaneously, the results can be dramatic.

The psychiatric consultant can be helpful in these instances by working individually with both the patient and his or her family. Sometimes resolution can be advanced by the simple, yet important intervention of acknowledging the enormity of conflict and distress each party is feeling. The consultant can serve to defuse the immediacy of the situation and eventually help both appreciate the difficult feelings on each side. Acting as an advocate for the patient, the consultant serves both as a crisis intervention specialist and a mediator to achieve a resolution or at least a compromise that is mutually acceptable to both parties. If no direct communication can be achieved, the consultant can still serve as a liaison between the two sides, conveying information and establishing limits that respect the wishes of both sides as much as possible. After the crisis has passed, the consultant can offer psychologic assistance or referral to the individuals involved. Frequently, families grieving over loved ones with AIDS must suffer alone, sensing that it is unacceptable for them to bring their concerns home to their communities.

PSYCHOPHARMACOLOGY

General Principles

Two general principles should be kept in mind when prescribing psychophar-macologic agents for patients infected with HIV. First, there apparently is nothing particular about HIV infection that precludes the use of commonly used psychotropic medications. These drugs have been used safely in this population for many years, and generally speaking, few problematic drug interactions have occurred in patients receiving antiretroviral drugs and psychotropics. This statement also generally is true for patients receiving prophylactic medications or active treatment for oppor-tunistic disease (Table 14–5). Second, because of the early effects of HIV on the CNS and the increased likelihood that HIV-spectrum patients may have or may develop neurologic dysfunction, psychotropic medications should be used in the lowest doses possible, and changes in medication regimens should be made slowly.

A discussion of commonly used medications follows.

Antidepressants

As mentioned above, medical practitioners may have a bias against the use of antidepressants in HIV patients. The expectation that depression is "normal" if one suffers from AIDS can mistakenly lead to the conclusion that antidepressant therapy is inappropriate even when depressive symptoms are severe. It is also incorrect to assume that in patients who evidence signs of both depression and dementia the presence of the latter absolutely contraindicates treatment for the former. In fact, recent success in the improvement of mild cognitive deficits in patients with symp-tomatic HIV disease with the use of psychostimulants raises the question of whether some of the cognitive symptoms may in part be caused by depression (pseudode-mentia) and at least partially resolve with treatment of depression[18]; even if this is not the case, depressive symptoms are at least potentially treatable, and many patients with AIDS have received significant benefit from antidepressant therapy.

If the patient is acutely medically ill and depressed, waiting a few days before instituting drug treatment is advisable. This delay allows for correction of metabolic abnormalities that may have a profound effect on mood and make treatment with medication more complex or simply less well tolerated.

Once the decision is made to begin treatment with antidepressants, selection of the best agent for an individual patient involves, in part, selecting the agent with the most favorable side effect profile. Since antidepressant medications generally are equally efficacious, unless there is a past history of successful treatment with a particular agent, the clinician should be guided by the drug's side effects. For example, in HIV patients minimizing sedation is often desirable; thus use of drugs with strong anticholinergic side effects such as amitryptiline (Elavil) should be minimized. However, the standard anticholinergic sedation that occurs with some drugs can be useful in treating the agitated and sleepless depressed patient, and these drugs have been used with success in these patients. At the same time, however, the anticholinergic potential for exacerbating cognitive deficits in the cognitively compromised patient and the drying of mucous membranes that may contribute to

Table 14–5. Psychiatric and Neurologic Side Effects of Drugs Used in HIV-Related Treatment

DRUG	SIDE EFFECT
5-Fluorouracil	Cerebellar ataxia
5-Flucytosine	Confusion, headache, sedation
Acyclovir (Zovirax)	Depression, agitation, auditory and visual hallucinations, depersonalization, tearfulness, confusion, hyperesthesia, hyperacusis, insomnia, intrusive thoughts, headache
Amphotericin B	Delirium, peripheral neuropathy, blurred vision, diplopia, weight loss, loss of appetite, headache
Cycloserine	Anxiety, depression, confusion, disorientation, hallucinations, paranoia, loss of appetite, fatigue
Cytosine arabinoside	Peripheral neuropathy, cerebellar ataxia
ddI, ddC	Sensory neuropathies, pancreatitis (with neurologic complications)
Disulfiram/DTC	Peripheral neuropathy
Ethambutol	Headache, dizziness, confusion, visual disturbances
Etoposide (VP-16)	Neuropathy, loss of appetite
Ganciclovir (DHPG)	Irritability, mild euphoria, increased energy
Interferons	Depression, confusion, delirium, memory and psychomotor impairment, fatigue suggestive of frontal lobe changes, reversible impairment of higher cognitive functions, acute encephalitis, chills, myalgias, arthralgias, headache, extrapyramidal symptoms, mania, neurasthenia with catatonia
Interleukin-2	Disorientation, cognitive deterioration
Isoniazid	Depression, agitation, auditory and visual hallucinations, paranoia, peripheral neuropathy, memory impairment
Ketoconazole (Nizoral)	Headache, dizziness, photosensitivity
L-Asparaginase	Reversible encephalopathy
Methotrexate	Headaches, blurred vision, fatigue, photosensitivity, aseptic meningitis, encephalopathy
Pentamadine	Hypoglycemia, tremors, restlessness
Procarbazine	Mania, loss of appetite, headaches, insomnia, nightmares, confusions, malaise
Rifampin	Headache, fatigue, loss of appetite, visual disturbances
Sulfonamides	Headache, neuritis, insomnia, loss of appetite, photosensitivity
Trimethoprim-sulfamethoxazole (Bactrim)	Psychosis, mutism, bizarre mannerisms, depression, loss of appetite, insomnia, apathy, headache, neuritis
Vinblastine	Depression, loss of appetite, headache, neuritis
Vincristine	Hallucinations, headache, neuritis, ataxia, sensory loss, peripheral neuropathy, autonomic and cranial neuropathy
Zidovudine (AZT)	Mania, agitation, headache, insomnia, myositis

Modified from Ostrow DG, Whitaker R: Psychiatric and psychopharmacological problems in HIV-spectrum diseases. Hosp Formulary, December 1991.

the growth of candidiasis throughout the alimentary tract limit the use of these drugs in this population.

For depressed patients with predominant psychomotor slowing, fatigue, and hypersomnia, other, more stimulating antidepressants should be the clinician's first drug of choice. Nortriptyline (Pamelor) and desipramine (Norpramin) are particularly recommended, although many others have been used successfully.[33] Recently the new serotonin-uptake inhibitor fluoxetine (Prozac) has also been used with very good results in these patients. Standard therapy of 20 to 60 mg/day likely will achieve excellent results. Similarly, there is likely a role for the use of the new antidepressant fluvoxamine in the treatment of these patients. When tremulousness, anxiety, or initial insomnia become troublesome, either administering a dose of 20 mg every other day or adding a second serotonin-uptake inhibitor such as trazodone (Desyrel), 50 mg at bedtime, has been helpful. In general, dosing should be modest at first but often must be comparable to doses used in the general population. Finally, tricyclic antidepressants are often helpful in controlling or reducing the pain and discomfort of peripheral neuropathies in these patients.

Stimulants

If tricyclics are refused, ineffective, or contraindicated, the consultant might use methylphenidate or dextroamphetamine for the treatment of depression and/or the palliation of early cognitive deficits.[17,18,43,50] Methylphenidate has been used with some success in patients with both AIDS and symptomatic disease and has led to rapid improvement in depressive symptoms and to increased appetite and improved concentration, attention and memory.[18] Doses typically range from 5 to 40 mg/day. Side effects are generally mild, although anxiety and sleeplessness have been reported. These drugs recently have been proved a well-tolerated treatment, and their use results in little abuse in depressed cancer patients.[17] The clinician contemplating the use of psychostimulants should take into account the patient's drug history and be alert for the possibility of drug-induced psychotic reactions.

Antipsychotics

There are several indications for the use of antipsychotics in this patient population. First, they are useful for decreasing psychotic symptoms in those patients with organic mental disorders. Patients without significant neurologic symptoms or cognitive compromise can tolerate dosages comparable to those tolerated by the general population. However, prophylaxis against extrapyramidal side effects is recommended.[27] Second, these agents can be used to control agitation in demented patients. Dosing should always begin very modestly because these patients are particularly sensitive to drug side effects and may already have neurologic findings that can easily be confused with the development of extrapyramidal symptoms. Third, antipsychotics in modest dosages can be useful in controlling agitation and severe anxiety in severely character-disordered patients.

The choice of antipsychotic agent should be dictated by the side effect profile. Midrange potency agents such as perphenazine (Trilafon) and thiothixene (Navane) may be first drugs of choice rather than the more commonly used high-potency haloperidol. Haloperidol has been associated with neuroleptic malignant syndromes and severe extrapyramidal reactions in some patients with AIDS.[27,38] Initial dosing may begin with perphenazine (2 mg two times daily) or thiothixene (2 to 5 mg/day), with 0.5 to 1 mg of benztropine (Cogentin) twice a day as prophylaxis against the development of extrapyramidal reactions. Upper levels of dosing are dependent on the patient's tolerance, the severity of symptoms, and the emergence of side effects. Chlorpromazine (Thorazine) (25 to 50 mg at bedtime) is also helpful for the control of agitation and sleeplessness and may be especially helpful in patients who have abused benzodiazepines in the past.

Benzodiazepines

Benzodiazepines are widely and often successfully used to lessen anxiety in HIV-spectrum patients (see "Anxiety Disorders"). However, the consultant should be alert for several common mistakes made with their use.

Medically hospitalized patients are frequently prescribed multiple psychoactive drugs, including multiple benzodiazepines (e.g., clonazepam for anxiety, lorazepam for nausea).[33] This increases the likelihood of CNS toxicity. Patients with HIV encephalopathy or other cognitive deficits are at particular risk for side effects such as worsening memory deficits or other cognitive performance, disinhibition, visual hallucinations, and excessive sedation. Benzodiazepines can be used successfully to relieve anxiety and agitation in demented patients who have difficulty tolerating antipsychotics, but these drugs must be used cautiously.

Other Treatments

For patients who develop significant agitation in conjunction with a diagnosis of HIV-associated dementia complex, antipsychotics are the first drug of choice. However, these agents may prove ineffective because of the development of dose-limiting side effects. In these cases the clinician should consider alternative treatments. Lithium carbonate and valproic acid in usual doses has been used successfully in patients presenting with a manic component to their symptoms. Carbamazepine and beta-blockers have also been helpful in controlling agitation.

Psychiatric Sequelae of AIDS Treatments

The nucleoside analogs currently in use as antiretrovirals, zidovudine (azidothymidine [AZT]), and dideoxyinosine (ddI),[36] have been reported to cause anxiety, irritability, racing thoughts and insomnia and frank mania.[29,34] Additionally, this type of reaction has been reported most recently with dideoxycytidine (ddC).[3]

There is also strong evidence of the effectiveness of zidovudine and ddI in the amelioration of symptoms of the AIDS dementia complex,[9,10,46,51] and some have suggested the increased use of zidovudine has resulted in a decrease in the incidence of HIV-associated dementia.[40] However, although some individuals have shown at least temporarily marked improvement, others have shown little or no change, and these patients continue to pose special diagnostic and social service problems.[7]

SUBSTANCE ABUSE DISORDERS

Substance abuse disorders found commonly among people with HIV disease,[48] and the added dimension of their addiction complicates their clinical care. The reader is referred to two reviews for recommendations on the psychiatric treatment of these patients.[4,5]

CONCLUSION

Providing competent psychiatric care for patients with AIDS requires experience and interest in the area. At the same time many of the issues presented here are also present in the care of other chronically or terminally ill patients and should be familiar to the practicing psychiatrist comfortable with the treatment of medically ill patients. However, because of the unique psychosocial and neuropsychiatric ramifications of HIV infection, psychiatric issues comprise an important aspect of care. The clinician should be aware of this element of care; hopefully this review highlights the importance and contribution of the psychiatric consultant as an active member of the AIDS treatment team.

REFERENCES

1. Atkinson JH, Grant I, Kennedy CA, et al: Prevalence of psychiatric disorders among men infected with human immunodeficiency virus: A controlled study. Arch Gen Psychiatry 45:859-864, 1988
2. Baer JW: Study of 60 patients with AIDS or AIDS-related complex requiring psychiatric hospitalization. Am J Psychiatry 146:1285-1288, 1989
3. Barlow I: UCSF AIDS Health Project. San Francisco, 1991
4. Batki SL: Treatment of intravenous drug users with AIDS: The role of methadone maintenance. J Psychoactive Drugs 20:213-216, 1988
5. Batki SL, Sorensen JL, Faltz B, et al: AIDS among drug abusers: Psychiatric aspects of treatment. Hosp Community Psychiatry 39:439-441, 1988
6. Beckett A, Summergrad P, Manschreck T, et al: Symptomatic HIV infection of the CNS in a patient without clinical evidence of immune deficiency. Am J Psychiatry 144(10):1342-1344, 1987
7. Boccellari A, Dilley JW, Shore MD: HIV related cognitive impairment in San Francisco: Associated management and residential placement problems. Hosp Community Psychiatry (in press)
8. Boccellari A, Dilley JW, Shore MD: Neuropsychiatric aspects of AIDS dementia complex: A report on a clinical series. Neurotoxicology 9(3):381-389, 1988
9. Brouwers P, Moss H, Wolters P, et al: Effect of continuous-infusion zidovudine therapy on neuropsychologic functioning in children with symptomatic human immunodeficiency virus infection. J Pediatrics 117(6):980-985, 1990
10. Brunetti AG, Berg G, Di Chiro G, et al: Reversal of brain metabolic abnormalities following treatment of AIDS dementia complex with AZT: A PET-FDG study. J Nucl Med 30(5):581-590, 1989
11. Catalan J: Psychosocial and neuropsychiatric aspects of HIV infection: Review of their extent and implications for psychiatry. J Psychosom Res 32(3):237-248, 1988
12. Cooke M: Learning to care: Health care workers respond to AIDS. FOCUS: A Guide to AIDS Research. UCSF AIDS Health Project 7:1-2, 1987
13. Dauncey K: Mania in the early stages of AIDS. Br J Psychiatry 152:839-842, 1988
14. Dilley JW, Forstein M: Psychosocial aspects of the human immunodeficiency virus (HIV). Rev Psychiatry 9:632-655, 1991
15. Dilley JW, Ochitill HN, Perl M, et al: Findings in psychiatric consultations with patients with AIDS. Am J Psychiatry 85:142-146, 1985
16. Elovaara I, Iivanainen M, Poutiainen E, et al: CSF and serum beta-2-microglobulin in HIV infection related to neurological dysfunction. Acta Neurol Scand 79(2):81-87, 1989
17. Fernandez F, Adams F, Holmes VF, et al: Methylphenidate for depressive disorders in cancer patients. Psychosomatics 28:455, 1987
18. Fernandez F, Adams F, Levy JK, et al: Cognitive impairment in AIDS related complex and its response to psychostimulants. Psychosomatics 29(1):38-46, 1988
19. Fernandez R, Holmes VF, Levy JK, et al: Consultation-liaison psychiatry and HIV-1 related disorders. Hosp Community Psychiatry 40:146-153, 1989

20. Fogel BS: Major depression versus organic mood disorder: A questionable distinction. J Clin Psychiatry 51:2, 53-56, 1990
21. Forstein M: The psychological impact of the acquired immunodeficiency syndrome. Semin Oncol 11:77, 1984
22. Gabel RH, Barnard N, Norkom M, O'Connell RA: AIDS presenting as Mania. Compr Psychiatry 27:251-254, 1986
23. Greenblatt, Harmatz, Shapiro L, et al: Sensitivity to triazolam in the elderly. N Engl J Med 324:169, 1991
24. Hintz S, Kuck J, Peterkin J, et al: Depression in the context of human immunodeficiency virus infection: Implications for treatment. J Clin Psychiatry 51:497-501, 1990
25. Hollander H, Golden J, Mendelson T, Cortland D: Extrapyramidal symptoms in AIDS patients given low-dose metoclopramide or chlorpromazine. Lancet 2:1186, 1987
26. Hollander H, Levy JA: Neurologic abnormalities and recovery of human immunodeficiency virus from cerebrospinal fluid. Ann Intern Med 106:692-695, 1989
27. Hriso E, Kuhn T, Masdeu JC, et al: Extrapyramidal symptoms due to dopamine-blocking agents in patients with AIDS encephalopathy. Am J Psychiatry 148(11):1558-1561, 1991
28. Kermani EJ, Borod JC, Brown PH, Tunnel G: New psychopathological findings in AIDS: Case report. J Clin Psychiatry 46:240-241, 1985
29. Maxwell S, Scheftner WA, Kessler HA, et al: Manic syndrome associated with zidovudine treatment. JAMA 259:3406-3407, 1988
30. Morin SF, Batchelor WF: Responding to the psychological crisis of AIDS. Public Health Rep 99:4, 1984
31. Navia BA, Price RW: Dementia complicating AIDS. Psychiatric Ann 16:3, 1986
32. Nichols SE: Psychological reactions of persons with the acquired immunodeficiency syndrome. Ann Intern Med 103:765, 1985
33. Ochitill, Dilley J, Kohlwes J: Psychotropic drug prescribing for hospitalized patients with acquired immunodeficiency syndrome. Am J Med 90:601-605, 1991
34. O'Dowd MA, McKegney FP: Manic syndrome associated with zidovudine. JAMA 260:3587-3588, 1988
35. O'Dowd MA, Natali C, Orr D, et al: Characteristics of patients attending an HIV-related psychiatric clinic. Hosp Community Psychiatry 42:615-618, 1991
36. Orth JP, Ollivier B, Vinti H, Cassuto JP: Occurrence of acute mania in two AIDS patients during dideoxyinosine treatment at a dose of 750 mg/24h. Seventh International Conference on AIDS. (Abstract No. M.B. 2031.) Florence, Italy, 1991
37. Ostrow DG, Monjan A, Joseph J, et al: HIV-related symptoms and psychological functioning in a cohort of homosexual men. Am J Psychiatry 146:737-742, 1989
38. Perry SW: Organic mental disorders caused by HIV: Update on early diagnosis and treatment. Am J Psychiatry 147(6):696-710, 1990
39. Polon HJ, Hellerstein D, Auchin J: Impact of AIDS-related cases on an inpatient therapeutic milieu. Hosp Community Psychiatry 36:173, 1985
40. Portegies P, de Gans J, Lange JM, et al: Declining incidence of AIDS dementia complex after introduction of zidovudine treatment. Br Med J 299:819-821, 1989
41. Price RW, Brew B, Sidtis J, et al: The brain in AIDS: Central nervous system HIV-1 infection and AIDS dementia complex. Science 239:586-592, 1988
42. Resnick L, Berger JR, Shapshak P, et al: Early penetration of the blood-brain barrier by HIV. Neurology 38(1):9-14, 1988
43. Rosenberg PB, Ahmed I, Hurwitz S: Methylphenydate in depressed medically ill patients. J Clin Psychiatry 52:6, 263-267, 1991
44. Rothenberg R, Woelfel M, Stoneburner R, et al: Survival with the acquired immunodeficiency syndrome: Experience with 5833 cases in New York City. N Engl J Med 311:857, 1984
45. Schmidt U, Miller D: Two cases of hypomania in AIDS. Br J Psychiatry 152:839-842, 1988
46. Schmitt FA, Bigley JW, McKinnis R, et al: Neuropsychological outcome of zidovudine (AZT): Treatment of patients with AIDS and AIDS related complex. N Engl J Med 319:1573-1578, 1988

47. Wachter RM: The impact of the acquired immunodeficiency syndrome on medical residency training. N Engl J Med 314:177, 1986
48. Williams JBW, Rabkin JG, Remien RH, et al: Multidisciplinary baseline assessment of homosexual men with and without human immunodeficiency virus infection. Arch Gen Psychiatry 48:124-130, 1991
49. Woods SW, Tesar GE, Murray GB, et al: Psychostimulant treatment of depressive disorders secondary to medical illness. J Clin Psychiatry 47:12, 1986
50. Working Group of the American Academy of Neuropsychology AIDS Task Force: Robert Janssen, PhD, Division HIV/AIDS, Centers for Disease Control, Atlanta, GA 1991
51. Yarchoan R, Pluda JM, Thomas RV, et al: Long-term toxicity/activity profile of 2',3'-dideoxyinosine in AIDS or AIDS-related complex. Lancet 336:526-529, 1990

15

HEMATOLOGIC MANIFESTATIONS OF HIV INFECTION

JULIE HAMBLETON, MD
DONALD I. ABRAMS, MD

Infection with the human immunodeficiency virus (HIV) is associated with a wide spectrum of hematologic abnormalities. These abnormalities are found in all stages of HIV disease and involve the bone marrow, cellular elements of the peripheral blood, and coagulation pathways. The cause of these abnormalities is multifactorial. A direct suppressive effect of HIV infection, ineffective hematopoiesis, infiltrative disease of the bone marrow, nutritional deficiencies, peripheral consumption secondary to splenomegaly or immune dysregulation, and drug effect all contribute to the variety of hematologic findings in these patients. Many of these abnormalities are clinically significant, whereas others are more of academic interest. Specific abnormalities in the bone marrow, peripheral blood cell lines, and coagulation complex are reviewed here in turn.

BONE MARROW

Hematologic abnormalities in patients with HIV infection are very common.[30] Ineffective hematopoiesis has been described as resulting from direct suppression by HIV infection, infiltrative disease (whether of infectious or neoplastic origin), nutritional deficiencies, and drug effect.

HIV infection alone suppresses normal hematopoiesis.[7,33] Donahue et al.[7] isolated bone marrow progenitors from patients with AIDS and AIDS-related complex (ARC). They found that these progenitor cells were responsive to recombinant human granulocyte-macrophage colony-stimulating factor and recombinant erythropoietin. However, sera taken from patients with antibody to HIV suppressed the in vivo growth of these progenitor cells but did not suppress the in vivo growth of progenitor cells taken from HIV-seronegative controls. Sera from patients with HIV infection and cytopenias did not reveal elevated levels of in vitro colony-stimulating factors (CSFs) or interleukin-1, suggesting that HIV-infected T lymphocytes and monocytes do not produce adequate amounts of cytokines, thus contributing to the cytopenias characteristic of HIV infection.

234

Morphologic Features

The morphologic features of bone marrow findings in patients with AIDS have been described.[1,5,30] Bone marrow biopsies frequently are performed to evaluate peripheral cytopenias or persistent fevers in this patient population. The majority of patients demonstrates normocellular marrow elements. An increased proportion of plasma cells and lymphoid aggregates composed of benign-appearing, well-differentiated lymphocytes has been reported by investigators.[1,5,33] These findings suggest B-cell proliferation related to chronic antigenic stimulation or dysregulation secondary to HIV infection. Increased immunoglobulin production is also often noted.

The myeloid to erythroid (M:E) ratio is generally normal in patients undergoing bone marrow biopsy. Reticulin fiber staining often reveals increased reticulin fibrosis. Abnormalities in maturation with dysmyelopoiesis, megaloblastosis, and hemophagocytosis have also been described, whereas myeloproliferative syndromes and leukemia are not more prevalent in this patient population.[1,33]

Infiltrative disease of the bone marrow commonly contributes to the hematologic abnormalities in these patients. Infectious causes of infiltrative diseases include mycobacterial disease (both *Mycobacterium avium-intracellulare* and *M. tuberculosis*), fungal disease (*Histoplasma, Cryptococcus,* and *Coccidioides*), and rarely parasitic disease (*Pneumocystis* and *Leishmania*). Neoplastic infiltration is due primarily to lymphoma. Infiltration of the bone marrow by *M. avium-intracellulare* usually results in isolated anemia, whereas infiltrative disease of other causes typically manifests as pancytopenia.

Nutritional Effects

Nutritional deficiency has not been well-documented as a direct cause of hematologic abnormalities in HIV-infected patients. Disorders of iron metabolism or iron deficiency and occult vitamin B_{12} deficiency have been described. Folate deficiency, on the other hand, is not more prevalent in this patient population.

Variable reports of increased iron stores to absent iron stores have been published. Most patients have ineffective incorporation of iron into the erythroid cell line, the so-called *anemia of chronic disease*. It leads to normal or increased iron stores noted on Prussian blue iron staining of the bone marrow biopsy. On the other hand, chronic blood loss from the gastrointestinal tract secondary to neoplastic infiltration or invasive infectious enteropathies can lead to an iron-deficient state. In a series of 201 bone marrow biopsies reviewed at San Francisco General Hospital, 75% of the patients had normal iron stores, regardless of their hemoglobin concentration at time of biopsy.

Patients with AIDS have lower serum vitamin B_{12} levels, a condition thought secondary to the presence of altered cobalamin transport proteins[33] or to abnormal absorption of vitamin B_{12}.[13] Given the extent of gastrointestinal dysfunction with chronic diarrhea in this patient population, vitamin B_{12} deficiency from occult malabsorption may contribute to the anemia commonly seen. Harriman et al.[13] described a cohort of 11 men with AIDS or asymptomatic HIV infection. Eight of 11 patients had an abnormal Schilling test result after having been given intrinsic factor and pancrease. Only three patients had a low serum vitamin B_{12} level. Duodenal biopsy specimens revealed chronic inflammation with mononuclear cell infiltration of the lamina propria. Specimens from five of six patients demonstrated HIV in the mononuclear cells.

Perhaps HIV enteropathy involving the terminal ileum where vitamin B_{12} absorption takes place contributes to subclinical malabsorption and occult vitamin B_{12} deficiency, which may, in turn, contribute to the neurologic and hematologic abnormalities seen in patients with HIV-related disease. Although these issues have not been fully delineated, vitamin B_{12} levels should be monitored periodically in this patient population. This may be particularly important in patients being treated with zidovudine in whom concomitant vitamin B_{12} deficiency may potentiate drug-induced anemia.

Diagnostic Utility of Bone Marrow Biopsy

For the most part the marrow changes in HIV-infected patients appear nonspecific and offer little to the clinician as a diagnostic or prognostic tool. There are, however, certain conditions for which performing bone marrow aspiration, culture, and biopsy is indicated.

HIV-infected patients with both non-Hodgkin's and Hodgkin's lymphoma frequently have marrow involvement. Marrow examination is useful not only for staging but also to assess the myeloid reserves before the initiation of cytotoxic therapy. Patients with thrombocytopenia in the absence of anemia or leukopenia warrant bone marrow evaluation to assure adequate megakaryocytes. In rare instances diagnoses other than immune thrombocytopenic purpura such as acute leukemia may be established.

Occasionally a patient has increased constitutional symptoms associated with anemia and/or other cytopenias. In the absence of a revealing workup, bone marrow examination may be indicated to rule out lymphoma or underlying opportunistic infection. Evidence of Kaposi's sarcoma does not characteristically appear in the bone marrow aspirate or biopsy specimen; however, lymphomatous involvement may be found. Granulomatous disease with a positive acid-fast bacillus stain suggests *M. avium-intracellulare* or *M. tuberculosis* infection, although well-formed granulomas may not be apparent.

In a review of 201 bone marrow aspirates and biopsies performed at San Francisco General Hospital, a new AIDS diagnosis was confirmed in less than 15 patients. Most new diagnoses were mycobacterial disease, primarily *M. avium-intracellulare*. In a more recent study Northfelt et al.[28] retrospectively reviewed the medical and laboratory records of patients with known or suspected HIV infection at San Francisco General Hospital who underwent 387 bone marrow biopsy examinations for opportunistic pathogens or lymphoma. Disseminated fungal infections occurred in <5% of patients studied, with bone marrow examination leading to the most rapid and accurate diagnosis. Mycobacterial infection was diagnosed in 16% of patients studied, and bone marrow culture was equally as sensitive for diagnosis of disseminated disease as blood culture (86% versus 77% sensitivity, respectively; $p > .05$). No previously undiagnosed case of lymphoma was found through bone marrow examination for cytopenias and constitutional symptoms, but bone marrow biopsy results were standard for staging lymphoma.

PERIPHERAL CELL LINES

Peripheral cytopenias are common in HIV-infected individuals and are due to either decreased production in the bone marrow or accelerated destruction in the peripheral circulation. In general, the cytopenias increase in frequency as HIV-disease progresses. Zon and Groopman[42] found anemia, granulocytopenia, and thrombocytopenia in 17%, 8%, and 13%, respectively, of asymptomatic HIV-infected individuals. These percentages all increase with advancing HIV disease.

Erythrocyte

Review of the peripheral blood smear in patients with HIV infection often reveals nonspecific abnormalities. Anisopoikilocytosis, often with ovalocytes and rouleau formation, is a common finding.[38] Increased vacuolization of peripheral monocytes has also been described.[38] These changes are not fully understood. Shearing of cells may occur secondary to splenomegaly, and rouleau formation may reflect the hypergammaglobulinemia in these patients.

Anemia is the most common hematologic abnormality noted in patients with HIV disease.[35] In patients with persistent lymphadenopathy the development of anemia often antedates the evolution to overt AIDS. In patients with overt AIDS anemia occurs in 66% to 85%.[33,42] The majority have chronic disease-type anemia, with low reticulocyte counts and low erythropoietin levels.[35] In such states adequate iron stores are demonstrated in the reticuloendothelial system, but the inability to use this stored iron results in ineffective erythropoiesis with normocytic, normochromic anemia. The cause of anemia in these patients is multifactorial and complex. Ineffective erythropoiesis may be a consequence of actual HIV infection of erythroid precursors or result from inappropriate tumor necrosis factor (TNF) release, which is an inhibitor of red blood cell (RBC) production in vitro[8,35] (Table 15–1).

Iron deficiency with microcytic, hypochromic anemia may result from chronic blood loss, which can result from Kaposi's sarcoma or lymphomatous involvement of the gastrointestinal tract. Thrombocytopenia with resultant occult bleeding occasionally leads to iron deficiency.

Infiltrative disease of the bone marrow caused by *M. avium-intracellulare* is a common cause of isolated anemia, usually without concomitant decrement in the other cell lines. Some of the most profound anemias, with hematocrit concentrations in the 15% to 20% range, occur in patients with mycobacterial disease. Similarly, patients with lymphoma may develop profound anemia, often with concomitant cytopenias of the other cell lines.

Antibody-mediated peripheral consumption of RBCs causes anemia but is not commonly seen in this patient population. McGinnis et al.[21] have described the presence of RBC autoantibodies in a cohort of patients with AIDS, ARC, and asymptomatic HIV infection. Forty-three percent of the AIDS patients in their study had a positive direct antiglobulin test (direct Coombs), and other antibodies against various RBC surface antigens were detected. At San Francisco General Hospital an estimated 20% of patients with HIV infection have a positive direct antiglobulin test before their first RBC transfusion.[37] Despite the documentation of erythrocyte autoantibodies, however, frank hemolysis in this patient population is rare.

Table 15–1.   Special Considerations in the Approach to Anemia in the HIV-Infected Individual

---

Microcytosis
Consider involvement of the gastrointestinal tract with Kaposi's sarcoma, lymphoma, or infectious
    enteropathy (especially cytomegalovirus colitis) with resultant iron deficiency secondary to chronic
    blood loss.
Macrocytosis
Consider:
    Vitamin B_{12} or folate deficiency secondary to enteropathy with malabsorption
    Hemolysis with reticulocytosis
        Drugs: dapsone, sulfa
        Autoimmunity
        Thrombotic thrombocytopenic purpura, hemolytic uremic syndrome, or disseminated intravascu-
            lar coagulation or DIC if concomitant thrombocytopenia present
        Zidovudine (AZT) drug therapy
If patient is receiving zidovudine therapy:
    Check erythropoietin level
    If <500 mU/dl, consider recombinant human erythropoietin therapy
    Evaluate vitamin B_{12} level and treat if low
Normocytic Anemia
If hemoglobin level >10 g/dl, patient exhibits no unexplained constitutional symptoms, and no other
    cell lines are involved, the most likely diagnosis is anemia of chronic disease secondary to HIV
    infection. Continued observation is advised.
If hemoglobin <10 g/dl, the patient exhibits unexplained constitutional symptoms, and/or other cell
    lines are involved, consider bone marrow infiltration.
DIFFERENTIAL DIAGNOSIS
    Acid-fast bacillus (AFB): *Mycobacterium avium-intracellulare* or *M. tuberculosis*
    Disseminated fungal disease
        Cryptococcosis
        Histoplasmosis
        Coccidioidomycosis
    Lymphoma
EVALUATION
    Blood culture for *M. avium-intracellulare* and fungus
    Cryptococcal antigen testing
    Giemsa stain of peripheral blood for histoplasmosis
    Purified protein derivative (PPD) and *Coccidioides* skin testing
    Tissue biopsy if clinically indicated
        Lymph node
        Liver
    Bone marrow biopsy
        Plastic sections for neoplasms
        Special stains and culture for AFB and fungi

Brisk anemia has been observed during treatment of AIDS opportunistic infections. Various antibiotics and antivirals have been implicated. Dapsone, frequently
used for treatment of *Pneumocystis carinii* pneumonia, can induce methemoglobinemia or hemolysis in the glucose 6-phosphate-dehydrogenase (G-6-PD)-deficient
individual. Zidovudine antiretroviral therapy results in a transfusion-dependent anemia in approximately 20% of patients.[32] Transfusion of packed RBCs is indicated
for patients who develop symptomatic anemia despite the cause. At present there
is no indication for use of irradiated packed cells.

Leukocytes

HIV infection affects the lymphocyte, neutrophil, and macrophage-monocyte cell lines. Despite the hypergammaglobulinemia noted in these patients, they suffer complications from both defective cellular immunity and dysregulated humoral immunity. The hallmark of HIV infection is the progressive depletion of the CD4+ lymphocytes. This decrement presumably occurs through direct viral invasion of these cells. Early in HIV infection an initial increase in the CD8+ population occurs before a decline in the number of CD4+ cells is noted. Infection of macrophages and monocytes and the triggering of an autoimmune response are two other mechanisms by which lymphocyte depletion can occur. Normally, activated T lymphocytes and monocytes produce cytokines or growth factors necessary for stem cell growth and differentiation. Decreased production of these cytokines results from HIV invasion of these cells. For a current review of the immunopathogenic mechanisms of HIV infection, refer to the review by Fauci et al.[8]

Granulocytopenia independent of drug use is noted in approximately 50% of patients with AIDS. The most common cause probably is ineffective granulopoiesis[15]; however, various investigators have documented the presence of antineutrophilic antibodies as one cause of peripheral neutropenia.[7,19,20,26,33]

Defects in qualitative functions of the monocyte-macrophage and granulocyte line have also been described. Defective polymorphonuclear leukocyte chemotaxis, deficient degranulating responses, inhibition of leukocyte migration, and ineffective killing have all been reported.[25,39] Similarly, monocytes exhibit a marked reduction in chemotaxis in response to stimuli.

Drug-induced neutropenia is common in the HIV-infected individual.[15,32] Medications used to treat infections such as *P. carinii* pneumonia, toxoplasmosis and cytomegaloviral retinitis or colitis cause neutropenia. Similarly, zidovudine is implicated as a cause of neutropenia, often necessitating dose reduction or cessation of therapy. Other dideoxynucleosides used for antiretroviral therapy (e.g., ddC and ddI) have less bone marrow toxicity. The phosphorylation of these compounds (zidovudine, ddC, ddI) by human cells occurs at different rates, leading to variability in marrow toxicity.[15] Table 15-2 lists the more commonly used drugs that can cause neutropenia.

Table 15-2. Drugs Commonly Used in Treating Patients With HIV Infection that Cause Myelosuppression

Antiretroviral dideoxynucleosides (e.g., zidovudine [AZT])
Other antiviral agents (e.g., ganciclovir [DHPG])
Antifungal agents (e.g., flucytosine)
Sulfonamides
Dihydrofolate reductase inhibitors
    Trimetrexate
    Pyrimethamine
    Trimethoprim
Pentamidine
Antineoplastic therapy
Alpha interferon

As for the complications of neutropenia, most documented infections involve gram-negative organisms; however, a retrospective review of community-acquired bacteremia in patients with AIDS revealed that 10 out of 14 patients with neutropenia of varying causes had gram-positive isolates.[17] These findings suggest that antimicrobial therapy for the febrile neutropenic patient with AIDS should include both gram-positive and gram-negative coverage.

HIV-Related Thrombocytopenia

The most common platelet abnormality found in HIV-infected patients is thrombocytopenia. In patients with HIV-related thrombocytopenia, platelet-associated immunoglobulin is present.[16] It has been postulated that patients with platelet-associated IgG who become thrombocytopenic demonstrate the most unencumbered reticuloendothelial system. As patients become more ill, circulating immune complexes and hypergammaglobulinemia block the ability of the spleen to remove antibody-coated platelets from the circulation. At San Francisco General Hospital it has been observed that in thrombocytopenic patients, as they evolve to overt AIDS, the low platelet count spontaneously resolves, supporting this hypothesis.[2]

The presence of circulating immune complexes that precipitate on the platelet surface and lead to destruction through clearance by the reticuloendothelial system has also been described.[16] Patients with HIV-related thrombocytopenia have far higher levels of circulating immune complexes that can be eluted from their platelets than patients with non–HIV-related thrombocytopenia.

Most patients with HIV-related immune thrombocytopenia (ITP) have only minor submucosal bleeding, characterized by petechiae, ecchymoses, and occasional epistaxis. Rare patients have gastrointestinal blood loss. The majority, however, have not demonstrated life-threatening bleeding episodes. Unlike non–AIDS-related immune thrombocytopenia, mild splenomegaly does occur, especially in patients with generalized lymphadenopathy.

Laboratory findings reveal that patients generally have isolated thrombocytopenia, which usually is not accompanied by anemia and leukopenia. Review of the peripheral blood smear reveals a dearth of platelets, with occasional large forms. Bone marrow biopsy may reveal an increased number of megakaryocytes, typical of peripheral platelet consumption. Patients demonstrate the reversal of the helper-to-suppressor T-lymphocyte ratio, which frequently results from increased numbers of the CD8+ suppressor-cytotoxic lymphocyte with relatively well-preserved CD4+ numbers. Patients initially seen with HIV-related thrombocytopenia are at risk to develop overt AIDS because of the underlying retroviral infection, regardless of the therapeutic intervention for their thrombocytopenia. In a natural history study of patients at San Francisco General Hospital the projected 5-year rate for development of an overt AIDS diagnosis was 50%.[2] Normalization of thrombocytopenia often antedates the development of AIDS, much the same way the disappearance of lymphadenopathy in patients with persistent generalized lymphadenopathy may be the harbinger for advancing disease. A group of New York University researchers suggests that thrombocytopenia is an epiphenomenon that imparts no further prognostic significance than the presence of HIV-antibody positivity itself.[16]

Management

Patients with HIV infection, including those being treated with antibiotics for an AIDS-opportunistic infection and those being treated with cytotoxic chemotherapeutic agents for HIV-related malignancies, may also develop thrombocytopenia secondary to a therapeutic intervention. In these patients severe thrombocytopenia should be managed as it is in the non–HIV-infected individual. Medications causing thrombocytopenia should be discontinued, and platelet transfusions should be administered when indicated.

Steroid therapy is the mainstay of treatment of thrombocytopenia in the non–HIV-infected individual with ITP. Its efficacy in patients with HIV-related ITP, however, is variable. Improvement in platelet count is not maintained in most patients as steroid doses are tapered. The overall response to steroid therapy (prednisone, 1 mg/kg/day) is good. However, with an attempt to taper the steroid dose, the platelet count often returns to baseline levels. The risk of further immune suppression in HIV-infected patients with steroid therapy is real. In a series of patients treated at San Francisco General Hospital no cases of AIDS-related opportunistic infection or malignancy resulted as a direct consequence of steroid therapy. However, reactivation of minor opportunistic infections, including herpes, oral candidiasis, and a central nervous system dysphoric syndrome frequently occurred.

Splenectomy has been a successful therapeutic intervention for patients who fail to respond to steroid therapy. At San Francisco General Hospital, 10 out of 15 patients recovered completely after splenectomy.[34] Complications following surgery in patients with HIV-related thrombocytopenia in the absence of overt AIDS have been no greater than in the non–HIV-infected population at large.

Studies using zidovudine in patients with ITP have shown promising results. The Swiss Group for Clinical Studies on AIDS[36] performed a prospective, controlled, double-blind crossover study of the effect of zidovudine on 10 HIV-seropositive patients with thrombocytopenia and no AIDS diagnosis. The patients' platelet counts increased from a mean of 53,000/L to 107,000/L while the patients received zidovudine and were not affected by the placebo. A group of French researchers also found an improvement in HIV-associated thrombocytopenia with the use of zidovudine.[29]

Numerous reports of the success of high-dose intravenous gammaglobulin therapy (400 mg/kg/day for 5 days) have appeared in the literature.[31] These responses have been transient, lasting 2 to 3 weeks. The mechanism probably is transient blockade of the reticuloendothelial system. Consequently, platelets coated with immunoglobulin are not prioritized for clearance. Once the immunoglobulin load clears, thrombocytopenia ensues. The high cost and transient nature of the immunoglobulin therapy make its use limited to situations in which acute bleeding is occurring or as a preoperative intervention for patients undergoing splenectomy when elevation of the platelet count is necessary. Although platelet transfusions generally are contraindicated in patients with thrombocytopenia of immune origin, treatment with intravenous gammaglobulin before transfusion in emergency situations may ensure platelet elevation.

Early reports suggested that the nonandrogenizing testosterone danazol was efficacious in reversing HIV-related thrombocytopenia. No large-scale clinical trial has confirmed these early anecdotal impressions. Six patients treated at San Francisco General Hospital showed no reversal of their thrombocytopenia. Intravenous vincristine and plasmapheresis have been reported anecdotally as efficacious in certain situations; however, the success rate of either does not warrant use as a first-line approach. Other experimental protocols that involve therapy with interferon or anti-CD4 antibody are currently being conducted at San Francisco General Hospital.

Patients with isolated thrombocytopenia in the presence of HIV infection are generally the most healthy in the spectrum of HIV-infected individuals. Clinical bleeding is minimal, and responses to therapeutic interventions have been suboptimal. Thus a viable alternative is to withhold therapeutic intervention and monitor the patient closely. However, zidovudine therapy may be initiated in patients with evidence of CD4+ lymphocyte depletion.

Thrombotic Thrombocytopenic Purpura

Several reports in the literature describe thrombotic thrombocytopenic purpura (TTP) in the HIV-infected population.[18,27] TTP is a relatively rare disease that includes fever, neurologic abnormalities, renal abnormalities, purpura, microangiopathic hemolysis, and thrombocytopenia. The exact pathogenesis of this disease is unknown but seems to arise from vascular injury caused by immune complexes or an endotoxin or from other causes of endothelial injury. The disorder has been associated with increased platelet agglutination and abnormally large circulating von Willebrand factor complexes.

At present it is unclear whether the occurrence of TTP in HIV-infected individuals is related to circulating immune complexes or immunoglobulin dysregulation associated with HIV disease. The mortality rate for this disease is high, as it is in the non–HIV-infected population, and therapy should include use of high-dose steroids, plasma transfusion, and plasmapheresis.

Coagulation Abnormalities

Patients with factor VIII or IX deficiencies and other congenital bleeding disorders have been greatly affected by the HIV epidemic.[10,22] Because of the contamination of pooled factor replacement products, more than 50% of this population has seroconverted after receiving contaminated blood products such as packed RBCs, cryoprecipitate, factor VIII, or factor IX. The risk of seropositivity apparently correlates with having received products from large donor pools as opposed to severity of bleeding disorder or amount or type of product received.[10] Unfortunately, the high price of many recombinant products renders these individuals at continued theoretic risk.

In patients with a variety of disease states such as systemic lupus erythematosus or AIDS, who are intravenous drug users, who receive certain drug therapy (i.e., chlorpromazine), or who have lymphoproliferative malignancies, a circulating inhibitor of coagulation may be noted. This so-called *lupus anticoagulant* is probably an acquired immunoglobulin, either IgG or IgM, that interferes with phospholipid-dependent coagulation assays, resulting in a prolongation of the partial thromboplastin time (PTT). In general, the lupus anticoagulant is an in vitro phenomenon.

Further laboratory testing has revealed abnormal results from a mixing study and an abnormal Russell viper venom time.[4]

Paradoxically, this anticoagulant is associated with increased thrombosis in the non–HIV-infected individual but is not of great clinical significance in the HIV-infected population. Its frequency is greater during HIV-related infections, and it often disappears with treatment of the infection.[33,42] If a patient has a prolonged activated PTT with no history of bleeding, presence of the lupus anticoagulant should be suspected. Invasive procedures may be performed in the presence of the lupus anticoagulant without increasing the bleeding diathesis.[4]

HEMATOLOGIC CONSEQUENCES OF ANTI-HIV THERAPY

Many therapeutic interventions contribute to HIV-related hematologic disorders. Zidovudine, a thymidine analog and the most widely used drug in the care of these patients, greatly affects hematopoiesis. The primary action of zidovudine is termination of reverse-transcriptase DNA synthesis. It may also inhibit DNA polymerases to some extent, thus impairing normal hematopoiesis.[32,33] In a large-scale collaborative study all three hematopoietic cell lines were affected by zidovudine therapy: significant anemia developed in 34% of patients, and blood transfusions were required in 21%; neutropenia developed in 16% of patients; and thrombocytopenia developed in 12%.[32] Advanced HIV disease, pre-existing cytopenias, and low vitamin B_{12} levels were associated with a greater risk of zidovudine-induced hematologic toxicities. Although zidovudine increases the mean corpuscular volume in most patients, bone marrow examination usually reveals hypoplasia, aplasia, or maturation arrest.[9,32,33,40] Overt megaloblastic changes are not always noted.

In general, the myelosuppression seen with zidovudine therapy is reversed by discontinuance of the drug,[32,40] but close observation with monitoring of blood counts is necessary. Ongoing trials have documented the efficacy of lower-dose zidovudine therapy, which results in fewer side effects, and dideoxyinosine (ddI) has been approved as alternative antiretroviral therapy. Other drugs used commonly in treating HIV infections, including ganciclovir (DHPG), foscarnet, sulfa derivatives (used to treat toxoplasmosis or *Pneumocystis* infections), and pentamidine, also cause myelosuppression.

COLONY-STIMULATING FACTORS IN HIV DISEASE

CSFs are becoming increasingly important in the treatment of HIV-related cytopenias. Initially, studies were conducted to address the effect of CSFs on viral replication in hematopoietic cell systems. Theoretically these agents could increase the number of target cells for HIV replication or enhance viral replication within target cells, leading to HIV disease progression.[23] In vitro studies have documented increased viral production in the presence of macrophage-CSF (M-CSF), granulocyte-macrophage CSF (GM-CSF), and interleukin-3, but not with granulocyte-CSF (G-CSF).[15] Clinical studies, however, have revealed favorable data in support of the use of CSFs without alteration of viral expression.[12,23] Increased viral replication may be inhibited by concomitant zidovudine use[12] (Table 15–3).

**Table 15–3.   Colony-Stimulating Factors:
Suggested Guidelines for Use**

Justification for Use
GRANULOCYTE-MACROPHAGE COLONY-STIMULATING FACTOR (GM-CSF)
Chemotherapy (per protocol guidelines)
Patients unable to sustain (ANC) >500 secondary to treatment with other myelosuppressive agents
ERYTHROPOIETIN
Symptomatic anemia while receiving zidovudine with (EPO) level <500
Dosing
GM-CSF
Initial dose, 5 μg/kg/day subcutaneously (SQ)
Titration:
 For neutropenia unresponsive to initial dose after 1 week, increase to 7.5 μg/kg/day
 If unresponsive to 7.5 μg/kg/day after 1 week, increase to 10 μg/kg/day
 If unresponsive to 10 μg/kg/day after 1 week, discontinue GM-CSF therapy
Discontinue therapy for unresponsive neutropenia or ANC >500
Reported side effects: viral-like prodrome, fever, myalgias, and thrombocytopenia (anecdotal); these
 effects occur more frequently with GM-CSF than with granulocyte-CSF (G-CSF)
ERYTHROPOIETIN
Initial dose, 100 μg/kg/day SQ three times each week
Obtain pretreatment EPO level, reticulocyte count, and ferritin level
Follow reticulocyte count
Patient may require iron replacement if reticulocyte count and ferritin level decrease
Injections may be slightly painful

In several trials neutropenic patients with AIDS responded to GM-CSF with a rapid increase in neutrophils and their precursors in conjunction with improved qualitative neutrophil functions,[3,11] and many chemotherapeutic trials now involve the administration of CSFs.

Human recombinant erythropoietin has been administered to HIV-infected patients with anemia secondary to zidovudine therapy. The best response was seen in patients whose intrinsic erythropoietin levels were <500 mU/dl.[23,33] Individual patients with elevated erythropoietin levels may respond to such therapy,[6] but this should be addressed on a case-by-case basis. Clinical trials, which are aimed at limiting the hematologic toxicities of zidovudine, are also being conducted to evaluate the concomitant use of GM-CSF and erythropoietin in conjunction with zidovudine therapy.

REFERENCES

1. Abrams D, Chinn E, Lewis B, et al: Hematologic manifestations in homosexual men with Kaposi's sarcoma. Am J Clin Pathol 81:13-18, 1984
2. Abrams D, Kiprov D, Goedert J: Antibodies to human T lymphotropic virus type III and development of the acquired immunodeficiency syndrome in homosexual men presenting with immune thrombocytopenia. Ann Intern Med 104:47-50, 1986
3. Baldwin C, Gasson J, Quan S, et al: Granulocyte-macrophage colony-stimulating factor enhances neutrophil function in acquired immunodeficiency syndrome patients. Proc Natl Acad Sci 85:2763-2766, 1988
4. Bloom E, Abrams D, Rodgers G: Lupus anticoagulant in the acquired immunodeficiency syndrome. JAMA 256:491-493, 1986
5. Castella A, Croxson T, Mildvan D, et al: The bone marrow in AIDS: A histologic, hematologic, and microbiologic study. Am J Clin Pathol 84:425-432, 1985

6. DaCosta NA, Hultin MB: Effective therapy of human immunodeficiency virus–associated anemia with recombinant human erythropoietin despite high endogenous erythropoietin. Am J Hematol 36:71-72, 1991

7. Donahue R, Johnson M, Zon L, et al: Suppression of in vitro haematopoiesis following human immunodeficiency virus infection. Nature 326:200-203, 1987

8. Fauci AS (moderator), Schnittman SM, Poli G, et al: Immunopathogenic mechanisms in human immunodeficiency virus (HIV) infection. Ann Intern Med 114:678-693, 1991

9. Gill P, Rarick M, Brynes R: Azidothymidine associated with bone marrow failure in the acquired immunodeficiency syndrome. Ann Intern Med 107:502-505, 1987

10. Gjerset GF, Clements MJ, Counts RB, et al: Treatment type and amount influenced human immunodeficiency virus seroprevalence of patients with congenital bleeding disorders. Blood 78:1623-1627, 1991

11. Groopman J, Mitsuyasu R, DeLeo M: Effect of recombinant human granulocyte-macrophage colony-stimulating factor on myelopoiesis in the acquired immunodeficiency syndrome. N Engl J Med 317:593-598, 1987

12. Groopman JE: Management of the hematologic complications of human immunodeficiency virus infection. Rev Infect Dis 12:931-937, 1990

13. Harriman G, Smith P, Horne M, et al: Vitamin B_{12} malabsorption in patients with acquired immunodeficiency syndrome. Arch Intern Med 149:2039-2041, 1989

14. Hirsch M: Azidothymidine. J Infect Dis 157:427-431, 1988

15. Israel DS, Plaisance KI: Neutropenia in patients infected with human immunodeficiency virus. Clin Pharm 10:268-279, 1991

16. Karpatkin S: Immunologic thrombocytopenic purpura in HIV-seropositive homosexuals, narcotic addicts and hemophiliacs. Semin Hematol 25:219-229, 1988

17. Krumholz H, Sande M, Lo B: Community-acquired bacteremia in patients with acquired immunodeficiency syndrome: Clinical presentation, bacteriology, and outcome. Am J Med 86:776-779, 1989

18. Leaf A, Laubenstein L, Raphael B, et al: Thrombotic thrombocytopenic purpura associated with human immunodeficiency virus type 1 infection. Ann Intern Med 109:194-197, 1988

19. Leiderman I, Greenberg M, Adelsberg B, Siegal F: A glycoprotein inhibitor of in vitro granulopoiesis associated with AIDS. Blood 70:1267-1272, 1987

20. McCance-Katz E, Hoecker J, Vitale N: Severe neutropenia associated with anti-neutrophil antibody in a patient with acquired immunodeficiency syndrome-related complex. Pediatr Infect Dis 6:417-418, 1987

21. McGinniss M, Macher A, Rook A, Alter H: Red cell autoantibodies in patients with acquired immune deficiency syndrome. Transfusion 26:405-409, 1986

22. Merigan TC, Amato DA, Balsley J, et al: Placebo-controlled trial to evaluate zidovudine in treatment of human immunodeficiency virus infection in asymptomatic patients with hemophilia. Blood 78:900-906, 1991

23. Miles SA: The use of hematopoietic growth factors in HIV infection and AIDS-related malignancies. Cancer Invest 9:229-238, 1991

24. Molina J, Groopman JE: Bone marrow toxicity of dideoxyinosine (letter). N Engl J Med 321:1478, 1989

25. Murphy P, Lane C, Fauci A, Gallin J: Impairment of neutrophil bactericidal capacity in patients with AIDS. J Infect Dis 158:627-630, 1988

26. Murphy M, Metcalfe P, Waters A, et al: Incidence and mechanism of neutropenia and thrombocytopenia in patients with human immunodeficiency virus infection. Br J Haematol 66:337-340, 1987

27. Nair J, Bellevue R, Bertoni M, Dosik H: Thrombotic thrombocytopenic purpura in patients with the acquired immunodeficiency syndrome–related complex. Ann Intern Med 109:209-212, 1988

28. Northfelt DW, Mayer A, Kaplan LD, et al: The usefulness of diagnostic bone marrow examination in patients with human immunodeficiency virus (HIV) infection. J AIDS 4:659-666, 1991

29. Oksenhendler E, Bierling P, Ferchal F, et al: Zidovudine for thrombocytopenic purpura related to human immunodeficiency virus infection. Ann Intern Med 110:365-368, 1989

30. Perkocha LA, Rodgers GM: Hematologic aspects of human immunodeficiency virus infection: Laboratory and clinical considerations. Am J Hematol 29:94-105, 1988

31. Perret B, Baumgartner C: Workshop on immunoglobulin therapy of lymphoproliferative syndromes, mainly AIDS-related complex, and AIDS. Vox Sang 52:1-14, 1986

32. Richman D, AZT Collaborative Working Group: The toxicity of azidothymidine in the treatment of patients with AIDS and AIDS-related complex. N Engl J Med 317:192-197, 1987

33. Scadden DT, Zon LI, Groopman JE: Pathophysiology and management of HIV-associated hematologic disorders. Blood 74:1455-1463, 1989
34. Schneider P, Abrams D, Rayner A, Hohn D: Immunodeficiency-associated thrombocytopenic purpura: Response to splenectomy. Arch Surg 122:1175-1178, 1987
35. Spivak JL, Barnes DC, Fuchs E, Quinn TC: Serum immunoreactive erythropoietin in HIV-infected patients. JAMA 261:3104-3107, 1989
36. Swiss Group for Clinical Studies on AIDS: Zidovudine for the treatment of thrombocytopenia associated with human immunodeficiency virus. Ann Intern Med 109:718-721, 1988
37. Toy P, Reid M, Burns M: Positive direct antiglobulin test associated with hyperglobulinemia in acquired immunodeficiency syndrome. Am J Hematol 19:145, 1985
38. Treacy M, Lai L, Costello C, Clark A: Peripheral blood and bone marrow abnormalities in patients with HIV related disease. Br J Haematol 65:289-294, 1987
39. Valone F, Payan D, Abrams D, Goetzl E: Defective polymorphonuclear leukocyte chemotaxis in homosexual men with persistent lymph node syndrome. J Infect Dis 150:267-271, 1984
40. Walker R, Parker R, Kovacs J, et al: Anemia and erythropoiesis in patients with the acquired immunodeficiency syndrome and Kaposi sarcoma treated with zidovudine. Ann Intern Med 108:372-376, 1988
41. Yarchoan R, Pluda JM, Perno C, et al: Antiretroviral therapy of human immunodeficiency virus infection: Current strategies and challenges for the future. Blood 78:859-884, 1991
42. Zon L, Groopman J: Hematologic manifestations of the human immune deficiency virus. Semin Hematol 25:208-218, 1988

16

CARDIAC, ENDOCRINE, AND RENAL COMPLICATIONS OF HIV INFECTION

JOHN D. STANSELL, MD

Pulmonary, gastrointestinal, hematologic, and neurologic dysfunction remain the principal, if not sole, manifestations of human immunodeficiency virus (HIV) infection. However, as experience with HIV infection deepens, the pace of the epidemic increases, and longevity improves because of more effective treatment and prophylaxis of opportunistic infections, it becomes clear that no organ system eludes the ravages of HIV. This chapter focuses on the cardiac, endocrine, and renal manifestations of HIV disease. Although still playing a relatively minor role in the clinical course of most HIV-infected patients, abnormalities of these organ systems likely will be encountered by clinicians as the AIDS epidemic further evolves.

CARDIAC DISEASE

Many autopsy studies have documented cardiac involvement in AIDS and AIDS-related conditions.[3,8,17,31,53] Conclusions from these studies differ widely, however, about the prevalence of cardiac disease and the type of cardiac lesion. Early in the epidemic Welsh, Finkbeiner, and Alpers[53] described 11 of 36 patients (31%) with cardiac lesions at necropsy. Similarly, Cammarosano and Lewis[8] found cardiac pathology in 10 of 41 patients (25%) dying of AIDS. Fink et al.[17] described a 73% prevalence of cardiac disease in a small series of AIDS patients. Moreover, Fink et al.[17] were among the first to note the clinical silence of these cardiac abnormalities. Anderson et al.[3] retrospectively evaluated 71 consecutive patients who died of AIDS between 1982 and 1986; 52% demonstrated evidence of cardiac disease at autopsy. Lewis[32] recently described cardiac lesions in 59 of 115 autopsied patients who died from AIDS-related causes. Based on these studies, Anderson and Virmani[2] project that approximately 6% of HIV-infected patients will develop symptomatic heart disease and 1% to 6% ultimately will succumb to cardiac dysfunction.

Findings in these studies included myocarditis, pericarditis, pericardial effusion, ventricular dilatation, nonbacterial, thrombotic endocarditis, metastatic Kaposi's sarcoma (KS), and lymphoma.

Myocarditis

Several observers have noted a high incidence of myocarditis in autopsies of AIDS patients.[3,31] In general, histologic findings include nonspecific interstitial inflammatory infiltrates or interstitial edema. Myocyte necrosis is uncommon. Lafont et al.[31] reviewed 137 consecutive autopsies of AIDS patients and found 56 (41%) with myocarditis. Anderson et al.[3] described similar changes in 52% of 71 patients. A recent review of the literature confirmed autopsy evidence of myocarditis in 184 of 402 AIDS patients (46%).[29] However, only a small percentage of patients with histologic evidence of myocarditis demonstrated signs of ventricular dysfunction before death.

Significantly, myocarditis is not associated with any one or combination of possible causative organisms. Kaul, Fishbein, and Siegel[29] found no specific cause for myocarditis in 80% of 402 autopsied patients. A wide range of organisms was identified in the 15% to 20% of patients in whom a specific cause was found. Opportunists most frequently encountered include *Cryptococcus*,[8,31,33] *Toxoplasma*,[31,39] and mycobacteria.[31,39] Thus the cause of myocarditis in most cases remains unclear.

In the absence of demonstrable organisms, known toxic exposures, or hypersensitivity, Anderson et al,[3] suggest that most patients with AIDS and myocarditis have disease histologically suggestive of viral infection.

The list of **viral** causes of myocarditis in AIDS patients is lengthy. Cytomegalovirus (CMV), coxsackie virus B, and HIV itself have received close attention. Most AIDS patients are infected with CMV. Myocardial tissue, however, rarely shows evidence of CMV inclusions.[8] In short, there is no demonstrated cause-and-effect relationship between CMV and myocardial inflammation. Coxsackie viruses A and B are the most frequent causes of myocarditis in the United States.[46] Dittrich et al.[14] demonstrated rising coxsackie virus B titers in an AIDS patient succumbing to refractory congestive heart failure, and a recent report suggests direct viral infection of myocytes.[47] Finally, HIV itself may damage myocardium either by direct cytolytic infection or by "innocent bystander destruction." The innocent bystander theory, proposed by Ho, Pomerantz, and Kaplan,[25] suggests HIV replication in lymphocytes or macrophages releases enzymes or lymphokines that are toxic to surrounding myocytes. Although several investigators have grown HIV from myocardial biopsies, evidence of direct myocyte infection is scant. A recent abstract reports detection of HIV nucleotide sequences within myocytes using in situ hybridization techniques.[21] The significance of this finding awaits further testing.

No series define optimum workup and treatment of AIDS-related myocarditis. The role of myocardial biopsy, immunosuppressive therapy, or antiviral therapy remains undefined.

Dilated Cardiomyopathy

Investigators have not described isolated right ventricular hypertrophy outside a setting of significant pulmonary disease. Predictably, pulmonary vascular compromise from severe or recurrent infection or interstitial lung disease gives rise to pulmonary hypertension and resulting failure of the right side of the heart.[32]

Many case reports document congestive cardiomyopathy in patients with AIDS.[7,9,11,28] The pathologic hallmark of these cases is biventricular dilatation. Anderson et al.[3] found pathologic features of myocarditis present in all such cases. Thus they postulate congestive cardiomyopathy is the end result of viral infection. Evidence from patients with non-AIDS-associated cardiomyopathy supports this hypothesis. Biopsy specimens from patients with non–AIDS-associated myocarditis and dilated cardiomyopathy have exhibited high viral titers against coxsackie virus B and viral specific RNA sequences. As previously discussed, investigators have cultured HIV from endomyocardial biopsies from patients with congestive cardiomyopathy.[7,14] Speculation arises, however, about the inevitable contamination of myocardial tissue with mononuclear cells.

In addition to infectious causes, nutritional deficiency, cardiotoxins, and immunologic mechanisms can cause dilated cardiomyopathy. Although marked cellular and humoral immune dysfunction defines AIDS, no convincing evidence has emerged implicating autoimmune mechanisms in AIDS-associated heart disease. Similarly, wasting syndrome and cachexia are frequent manifestations of advanced HIV disease. Nevertheless, investigators have failed to show a clear cause-and-effect association between protein-calorie malnutrition, vitamin or trace element deficiency, and AIDS-associated cardiomyopathy. A recent report by Kavanaugh-McHugh et al.[30] presented evidence of decreased ejection fraction and/or ventricular dilatation in four of five pediatric AIDS patients with selenium deficiency. Clarification of the role of nutritional deficiency in patients with AIDS cardiomyopathy awaits further studies.

Drug toxicity is a well-documented source of myocardial damage. Physicians frequently prescribe several categories of drugs in the treatment of patients with HIV disease: antiinfectives, including antifungal and antiviral agents; immune modulators; and chemotherapeutic agents. Although AIDS patients have a high incidence of drug-related adverse reactions, the drugs commonly used in treating opportunistic infections have not shown significant cardiotoxicity. Similarly, the known cardiotoxins—cyclophosphamide, doxorubicin (Adriamycin), bleomycin, and *Vinca* alkaloids—are prominently used in treatment of AIDS-related non-Hodgkin's lymphoma and KS. Investigators, however, describe no increased incidence of cardiac toxicity (L. Kaplan, personal communication). Extensive use of antiviral agents has failed to document significant cardiac side effects. However, a recent case of reversible cardiomyopathy and congestive heart failure due to phosphonoformate was seen at San Francisco General Hospital. The patient, who had no history of cardiac dysfunction, experienced resolution of symptoms after withdrawal of phosphonoformate therapy and recrudescent disease on rechallenge. Similarly, Deyton et al.[13] recently described three patients with AIDS KS who experienced reversible cardiac dysfunction in association with interferon alfa therapy. Endomyocardial biopsy in one patient revealed no inflammatory infiltrate. All three patients showed improved cardiac motion and contractility after withdrawal of interferon-a. Despite widespread use of zidovudine (AZT) since 1987, investigators do not report major cardiac complications (Burroughs, Wellcome Co., personal communication). Similarly, stages I, II, and III clinical testing of dideoxycytidine (ddC) and dideoxyinosine (ddI) do not disclose significant cardiac side effects (Bristol-Meyers and Roche Pharmaceuticals, personal communication). Data on the newer nucleoside analogs, nonnucleoside reverse transcriptase inhibitors, tat inhibitors, and protease inhibitors await clinical testing.

Clinical presentation of AIDS-associated dilated cardiomyopathy is similar to that of dilated cardiomyopathy of any cause. Providers should evaluate by echocardiogram or multiple gated acquisition (MUGA) scan any AIDS patient with progressive breathlessness, edema, auscultory findings of congestive heart failure (CHF), or increased cardiac silhouette. The mainstays of therapy remain afterload reduction, diuretics, and, perhaps, digoxin.

Endocarditis

Autopsies of AIDS patients frequently reveal nonbacterial, thrombotic (marantic) endocarditis. Lesions, found frequently in chronically ill patients and particularly in those patients with malignancy, consist of sterile thrombi. Located on any valve, these lesions may embolize systemically.[8,29,32]

Studies indicate that HIV-seropositive persons have increased skin and nasopharyngeal carriage of *Staphylococcus aureus*. Furthermore, preliminary evidence suggests an increased incidence of staphylococcal endocarditis among HIV-seropositive intravenous drug users. However, HIV-seropositive patients with endocarditis display no altered therapeutic response to antibiotics (H. Chambers, personal communication). Opportunistic organisms have not proved a major cause of endocarditis in AIDS patients, although sparse case reports exist.

Pericardial Disease

Early reports confirmed pericardial effusion, including tamponade, is a major cardiac manifestation of AIDS.[8,17] A recent review of the literature reported 23% (112 of 475) of HIV-infected adult patients with cardiac disease have pericardial effusion. Most of these effusions are sterile[8,39] and are of uncertain clinical significance. Symptomatic pericardial effusion and tamponade are usually infectious.[2] Specific infectious organisms associated with pericarditis and effusion include *Mycobacterium tuberculosis*,[39] *M. avium* complex,[39] and *Cryptococcus*.[8] Since most patients with pericarditis have myocardial inflammation,[1] clinicians should become familiar with this AIDS complication and early pericardiocentesis.

Malignancy

Early in the AIDS epidemic 30% of patients presented with KS. Although KS remains the most common malignancy in patients with AIDS, the incidence of KS has decreased over the ensuing years.

KS has a tendency to metastasize widely to skin, mucosa, lung, lymph nodes, and the gastrointestinal tract. Several investigators have described myocardial or pericardial infiltration with the malignancy.[7,39] Silver et al.[50] found cardiac involvement in five of 18 patients (28%) with widely disseminated disease. All were clinically silent before the patients' deaths.

Concomitant with the declining incidence of KS is a rising incidence of lymphoma. Most often these are high-grade B-cell lymphomas seen as stage IV disease. Although cadiac involvement usually indicates widely metastatic disease, investigators have described primary cardiac lymphoma.[10]

• • •

Autopsy studies clearly document frequent cardiac pathology in patients succumbing to AIDS. Yet, despite more than 200,000 AIDS cases in the United States alone, cardiac complications only rarely have played a major role in AIDS patient management. The clinically silent nature of cardiac involvement in AIDS must give way to a heightened awareness of possible cardiac sources of morbidity and mortality. As prognosis improves, we are likely to confront cardiac manifestations of HIV disease more frequently.

ENDOCRINE DISEASE

Autopsy studies have documented diffuse endocrine pathology in patients with AIDS, usually involving opportunistic organisms or neoplasia.[26,53] Although initially it was believed clinically silent, mounting evidence suggests significant morbidity with HIV-associated endocrine dysfunction. A recent survey of 40 asymptomatic, recently HIV-infected men revealed multiple gonadal, thyroid, and adrenal abnormalities compared to results from seronegative men.[37] The natural history of these endocrinopathies is unknown, but the emergence of endocrine dysfunction early in HIV disease suggests a significant role over the course of HIV-mediated immune decline.[15]

Pituitary Gland

Sano et al.[44] recently reviewed pituitary morphology in 49 autopsied AIDS patients. Six patients (12%) demonstrated direct infectious involvement of the anterior pituitary—five with CMV and one with *Pneumocystis carinii*. In addition, the authors noted two cases (4%) of posterior pituitary infection. Significantly, infection was not associated with an inflammatory response. Moreover, adenomas and nodular hyperplasia were similar to those of age-matched controls. Functional pituitary insufficiency was uncommon. Membrano et al.[36] describe four AIDS patients with adrenal insufficiency and low corticotropin (ACTH). The authors (see below) postulated possible pituitary lesions in AIDS patients based on their findings and blunted 17-deoxysteroid response to sustained ACTH levels. Similarly, inappropriately low gonadotropin levels in the presence of low testosterone levels led Dobs et al.[16] to suggest a hypothalamic-pituitary abnormality in AIDS patients. Opportunistic infections and neoplasms can anatomically and functionally ablate the pituitary; panhypopituitarism due to *Toxoplasma gondii* infection is documented,[38] but similar pathologic findings are likely to occur with cryptococcal or *M. tuberculosis* meningitis or lymphomatous meningitis.

Thyroid Gland

In their evaluation of endocrine changes in early HIV infection, Merenich et al.[37] found no difference in thyroid-stimulating hormone (TSH) or thyroxine (T_4) levels between seropositive patients and controls. However, triiodothyronine (T_3) levels were significantly, but modestly depressed in the seropositive group. Interestingly, the most significant differences occurred in patients with the earliest disease and appeared to normalize with disease progression.

Thyroid function abnormalities in chronic illness ("sick euthyroid syndrome") are common and well documented. This pattern usually is initially seen as a fall in T_3 and a reciprocal rise in reverse T_3 (rT_3). Circulating T_4 may be low to normal. TSH levels usually remain normal. Two recent reports suggest a uniquely different pattern in HIV-related illness. Dobs et al.[16] reported surprisingly normal thyroid function in 70 men with HIV seropositivity, AIDS-related complex (ARC), or AIDS. More recently LoPresti et al.[34] presented evidence suggesting AIDS and ARC patients have high T_3 levels, high T_4 levels, high thyroid-binding globulin, and low rT_3. The rise in thyroid-binding globulin appeared to parallel the advance in HIV infection. The authors speculated that immune dysfunction removed a physiologic check on thyroid hormone metabolism. Sato et al.[45] further speculated that failure to down-regulate enzymes reponsible for conversion of T_4 to T_3 might contribute to the wasting seen in end-stage HIV illness. They further suggested this failure to down-regulate might be secondary to HIV-related cytokine dysregulation. Corroboration awaits further study.

Adrenal Gland

Autopsy studies have consistently found the adrenal the most commonly affected endocrine gland in patients with AIDS. Glasgow et al.[19] surveyed 41 autopsy specimens for evidence of adrenal pathology. Findings included lipid depletion typical of chronic illness, infection with *Cryptococcus* or mycobacteria, and infiltration with KS. Most importantly, CMV adrenalitis, characterized by intranuclear and cytoplasmic inclusions, was the most common infection of the adrenal gland, occurring in 51% of cases. No case showed necrosis involving more than 70% of the adrenal gland, and most showed less than 50% necrosis. Although 32 of the 41 patients showed nonspecific premortem findings consistent with hypocortisolism, only a single patient had documented partial adrenal insufficiency. None had hyperpigmentation. Adrenal gland function usually is not impaired until 80% to 90% of glandular tissue is compromised. Although pathologic involvement of the adrenal gland in AIDS patients is common, clinical adrenal insufficiency is not.

Multiple reports chronicle isolated clinical adrenal insufficiency in advanced disease since the beginning of the HIV epidemic.[20,22,23,51] Merenich et al.[37] found significantly lower baseline and peak ACTH-stimulated serum cortisol levels in patients with early HIV infection compared to levels in a seronegative group. However, both groups had levels within the normal range. In a small series Hilton et al.[24] found normal cortisol reponse to rapid ACTH stimulation in AIDS or ARC patients. Dobs et al.[16] similarly found a normal cortisol rise in response to rapid cosyntropin testing in 92% of HIV-infected men. The 8% with blunted response had no clinical symptoms of hypocortisolism. In the largest study of its kind, Membreno et al.[36] examined adrenal response and reserve in 93 HIV-infected men (74 AIDS patients and 19 ARC patients) compared with 25 normal controls. AIDS patients showed elevated basal cortisol levels compared with levels from unstressed controls. Similar results recently were reported by Villette et al.[52] who found significantly increased cortisol levels in HIV-infected persons compared to levels in seronegative persons no matter the stage of their disease. In contrast, the mean concentrations for ACTH, dehydroepiandrosterone (DHEA), and DHEA-S were significantly lower in the HIV-infected group. Membreno et al.[36] reported that cosyntropin testing revealed 86% of AIDS patients had cortisol levels within 2 standard deviations of mean normal value but only 48% within 1 standard deviation. Although basal 17-deoxysteroid (corticosterone, deoxycorticosterone, 18-hydroxydeoxycorticosterone) levels were normal, they failed to rise normally during acute ACTH testing. ACTH infusion for 3 days confirmed the depressed 17-deoxysteroid response but demonstrated a rise in cortisol to normal level. The plasma ACTH level at 8 AM was normal in 19 AIDS patients, and ARC patients showed basal plasma cortisol levels similar to those of controls. The 19 AIDS patients with ARC, however, responded to consyntropin testing with subnormal rises in cortisol levels similar to those of AIDS patients. In contrast, ARC patients responded to prolonged ACTH stimulation with normal rises in cortisol and 17-deoxysteroid levels. Zona glomerulosa function was normal in both AIDS and ARC patients. These data suggest that AIDS patients have limited adrenal capacity to respond to stress. Membreno et al.[36] and Biglieri[5] recommend administering ACTH stimulation for 3 days to those patients who fail to achieve a plasma cortisol level of 685 nmol/L after consyntropin administration; patients who fail to achieve a concentration of 994 nmol/L after the 3 days should be considered partially adrenal insufficient and should be treated with steroids at times of stress. Biglieri[5] suggests that measurement of 17-deoxysteroid levels after acute ACTH stimulation may help identify those patients with incipient adrenal abnormality. Again, confirmation awaits further study.

Clouding the issue of adrenal function in AIDS and ARC patients is the frequent use of drugs that affect steroidogenesis and steroid metabolism. Ketoconazole, a frequently used antifungal agent, interferes with glucocorticoid, mineralocorticoid, and sex hormone production. Rifampin, widely used in treating mycobacterial disease, is a powerful inducer of hepatic enzymes that metabolize steroids. In the presence of a limited ability to increase steroid production, either drug may precipitate clinical adrenal insufficiency.

Pancreas

Pathologic changes in the pancreas mirror those found in other endocrine tissue. Abnormalities in carbohydrate metabolism most frequently result from administration of pentamidine for *P. carinii* pneumonia. Pentamidine is directly toxic to pancreatic islet cells, producing hypoglycemia through the aberrent release of insulin from injured cells. If injury is sufficiently severe or sustained, development of type I diabetes mellitus and hyperglycemia may result.

Testes

Histologic testicular abnormalities are common in AIDS patients, usually in combination with markedly decreased or absent spermatogenesis. Several studies have documented low testosterone levels in AIDS and ARC patients in association with high levels of luteinizing hormone (LH) or follicle-stimulating hormone (FSH) and normal gonadotropin response to releasing factors.[12,16,52] These data suggest a pattern of primary testicular failure with AIDS and may contribute to the symptoms of decreased libido and impotence seen in patients with advanced immunosuppression. In contrast to the effects in HIV-infected persons with late-stage disease, however, Merenich et al.[37] found elevated levels of total and free testosterone in an asymptomatic cohort. Further, this group of patients had an abnormally robust LH response to gonadotropin-releasing hormone (GnRH) stimulation in the presence of elevated testosterone levels. These data would not support the contention that hypogonadism is an early manifestation of endocrinopathy in HIV-infected persons. As discussed previously, ketoconazole is a powerful inhibitor of androgen production in the testes. In addition, ketoconazole displaces testosterone from sex hormone–binding globulin. Gynecomastia may result.

RENAL DISEASE

Throughout the course of their illness, AIDS patients are at high risk for renal complications. Systemic infection, sepsis, dehydration, hypoxia, and nephrotoxic drugs (Table 16-1) (see Chapter 9) combine to produce disturbances in renal function. Emerging from this background of renal injury, however, is evidence of a HIV-disease–specific nephropathy.[6,18,27,41,42] In 1984 Rao et al.[42] reported on a series of 11 AIDS patients with proteinuria or azotemia. Nine of 11 AIDS patients rapidly

**Table 16–1.   Nephrotoxic Drugs Commonly Used
in AIDS Patients**

Commonly Nephrotoxic
Amphotericin B
Pentamidine
Foscarnet
Aminoglycosides
Radiocontrast dyes
Potentially Nephrotoxic
Trimethoprim-sulfamethoxazole
Pyrimethamine-sulfadiazine
Rifampin
Acyclovir
Nonsteroidal anti-inflammatory drugs
Dapsone

progressed to end-stage renal disease. Renal histology revealed focal and segmental glomerulosclerosis (FSGS) with intraglomerular deposition of IgM and C3 in 10 of 11 cases.

Subsequent studies identified FSGS and mesangial hyperplasia as the glomerular lesions commonly associated with AIDS. FSGS, however, is not specific to AIDS since 20% of adult idiopathic nephrotic syndrome and heroin nephropathy patients also show evidence of FSGS. The association of heroin nephropathy patients with FSGS raises the question of whether intravenous drug use predisposes to renal dysfunction in AIDS patients. Epidemiologic studies that show a disproportionate prevalence of nephropathy among intravenous drug users and autopsy studies of homosexual AIDS patients that fail to document renal pathology support this conclusion.[35,53] Notably, FSGS apparently is a lesion concentrated principally in cities with a high incidence of intravenous drug use.[49] Pardo et al.[41] also found a strong association between a history of drug use, AIDS, and renal disease. This association cannot account for FSGS seen in Haitian AIDS patients with no history of intravenous drug use. Moreover, the clinical course of heroin nephropathy and HIV nephropathy are markedly discordant. Non-HIV-infected patients with heroin nephropathy show slow progression of their disease over months to years and have prolonged survival with hemodialysis. In marked contrast, patients with AIDS nephropathy have rapid progression to end-stage disease over weeks to months and poor prognosis for survival.

Rao, Friedman, and Nicastri[43] reexamined their accumulated data in 1987. Drawing on 750 AIDS cases, they identified 78 with renal disease. Forty-three of 55 patients with massive proteinuria, azotemia, or both progressed to irreversible uremia. All were black, and 55% had a history of intravenous drug use. Thirty-one received maintenance hemodialysis. Despite dialysis, 26 died in less than 3 months, three lived for 3 to 6 months, and two lived for less than 1 year. Death resulted from progressive inanition despite vigorous nutritional support and the presence of opportunistic infections. Eighteen patients who were diagnosed with AIDS after initiation of maintenance dialysis followed a course similar to the preceding one, with a median survival time of less than 1 month. The authors infer that hemodialysis is of no value in prolonging life in patients with AIDS and irreversible uremia. Lending support to this inference is a recent report by Oritz et al.,[40] which found a median survival time of 30 days in AIDS patients receiving dialysis. A recent National Kidney Foundation position paper takes note of the dismal prognosis of patients with AIDS-associated nephropathy but recommends that the decision to use dialysis be evaluated on an individual basis according to the wishes and best interest of the patient.[48] In contrast to their experience with AIDS patients, however, the authors report prolonged survival in seropositive and ARC patients undergoing maintenance dialysis.

A recent letter reports sustained improvement in proteinuria in a patient with HIV-associated focal and segmental glomerulosclerosis through use of zidovudine (AZT).[4] The same letter reports another patient in whom zidovudine therapy resulted in temporary discontinuation of hemodialysis therapy. These intriguing first reports await further study and experience with antiviral therapy.

ACKNOWLEDGEMENT

The author wishes to thank Clint C. Hockenberry for his editorial assistance and technical support.

REFERENCES

1. Acierno L: Cardiac complications in acquired immunodeficiency syndrome (AIDS): A review. J Am Coll Cardiol 13(5):1144-1154, 1989
2. Anderson DW, Virmani R: Emerging patterns of heart disease in human immunodeficiency virus infection. 21(3):253-259, 1990
3. Anderson D. Virmani R, Reilly J, et al: Prevalent myocarditis at necropsy in the acquired immunodeficiency syndrome. J Am Coll Cardiol 11(4):792-799, 1988
4. Babut-Gay M, Echard M: Zidovudine and nephropathy with human immunodeficiency virus (HIV) infection (letter). Ann Intern Med 111(10):856-857, 1989
5. Biglieri E: Adrenocortical function in the acquired immunodeficiency syndrome (AIDS) (medical staff conference). West J Med 148:70-73, 1988
6. Bourgoigine J, Meneses R, Pardo V: The nephropathy related to the acquired immune deficiency syndrome. Adv Nephrol 17:113-126, 1988
7. Calabrese L, Proffitt M, Yen-Lieberman B, et al: Congestive cardiomyopathy and illness related to the acquired immunodeficiency syndrome (AIDS) associated with isolation of retrovirus from myocardium. Ann Intern Med 107(5):691-692, 1987
8. Cammarosano C, Lewis W: Cardiac lesions in acquired immune deficiency syndrome (AIDS). J Am Coll Cardiol 5(3):703-706, 1985
9. Cohen I, Anderson D, Virmani R, et al: Congestive cardiomyopathy in association with the acquired immunodeficiency syndrome. N Engl J Med 315(10):628-630, 1986
10. Constantino A, West T, Gupta M, et al: Primary cardiac lymphoma in a patient with acquired immune deficiency syndrome. 60:2801-2805, 1987
11. Corboy J. Fink L, Miller W: Congestive cardiomyopathy in association with AIDS. 165:139-141, 1987
12. Croxson T, Chapman W, Miller L, et al: Changes in the hypothalamic-pituitary-gonadal axis in human immunodeficiency virus-infected homosexual men. J Clin Endocrinol Metab 68:317-321, 1989
13. Deyton L, Walker R, Kovacs J, et al: Reversible cardiac dysfunction associated with interferon alfa therapy in AIDS patients with Kaposi's sarcoma. N Engl J Med 321(18):1246-1249, 1989
14. Dittrich H, Chow L, Denaro F, et al: Human immunodeficiency virus, coxsackievirus, and cardiomyopathy (letter). Ann Intern Med 108(2):308-309, 1988
15. Dluhy RG: The growing spectrum of HIV-related endocrine abnormalities (editorial). J Clin Endocrinol Metab 70(3):363-365, 1990
16. Dobs A, Dempsey M, Ladenson P, et al: Endocrine disorders in men infected with human immunodeficiency virus. Am J Med 84:611-616, 1988
17. Fink L, Reichek N, St. John, Sutton M: Cardiac abnormalities in acquired immune deficiency syndrome. Am J Cardiol 54:1161-1163, 1984
18. Gardenswartz M, Lerner C, Seligson G, et al: Renal disease in patients with AIDS: A clinicopathologic study. 21(4):197-204, 1984
19. Glasgow B, Steinsapir K, Anders K, et al: Adrenal pathology in the acquired immune deficiency syndrome. J Clin Pathol 84(5):594-597, 1985
20. Greene L, Cole W, Green J, et al: Adrenal insufficiency as a complication of the acquired immunodeficiency syndrome. Ann Intern Med 101(4):497-498, 1984
21. Grody W, Cheng L, Pang M, et al: Direct infection of the heart by the human immunodeficiency virus (HIV). 80(suppl II):II 665, 1989
22. Guenthner E, Rabinowe S, Van Niel A, et al: Primary Addison's disease in a patient with the acquired immunodeficiency syndrome. Ann Intern Med 100(6):847-848, 1984
23. Guy R, Turberg Y, Davidson R, et al: Mineralocorticoid deficiency in the HIV infection. Br Med J 298:496-497, 1989
24. Hilton C, Harrington P, Prasad C, et al: Adrenal insufficiency in the acquired immunodeficiency syndrome. South Med J 81(12):1493-1495, 1988
25. Ho D, Pomerantz R, Kaplan J: Pathogenesis of infection with human immunodeficiency virus. N Engl J Med 317:278-286, 1987
26. Hui A, Koss M, Meyer P: Necropsy findings in acquired immunodeficiency syndrome: A comparison of premortem diagnoses with postmortem findings. 15:670-676, 1984

27. Humphreys M, Schoenfeld P: Renal complications in patients with the acquired immune deficiency syndrome (AIDS) (editorial). Am J Nephrol 7:1-7, 1987
28. Kaminski H, Katzman M, Wiest P, et al: Cardiomyopathy associated with the acquired immune deficiency syndrome. J Acquir Immune Defic Syndr 1:105-110, 1988
29. Kaul S, Fishbein M, Siegel RJ: Cardiac manifestations of acquired immune deficiency syndrome: A 1991 update. Am Heart J 122(2):535-544, 1991
30. Kavanaugh-McHugh A, Rowe S, Benjamin Y, et al: Selenium deficiency and cardiomyopathy in malnourished pediatric AIDS patients (abstract). Fifth International Conference on AIDS. 1989
31. Lafont A, Marche C, Wolff M, et al: Myocarditis in acquired immunodeficiency syndrome (AIDS): Etiology and prognosis (abstract). J Am Coll Cardiol 11(2):196A, 1988
32. Lewis W: AIDS: Cardiac findings from 115 autopies. 32(3):207-215, 1990
33. Lewis W, Cammarosano C: Cryptococcal myocarditis in acquired immune deficiency syndrome. Am J Cardiol 55:1240, 1985
34. LoPresti J, Fried J, Spencer C, et al: Unique alterations of thyroid hormone indices in the acquired immunodeficiency syndrome (AIDS). Ann Intern Med 110(12):970-975, 1989
35. Mazbar SA, Schoenfeld P, Humphreys MH: Renal involvement in patients infected with HIV: Experience at San Francisco General Hospital. 37:1325-1332, 1990
36. Membreno L, Irony I, Dere W, et al: Adrenocortical function in the acquired immunodeficiency syndrome. J Clin Endocrinol Metab 65:482-487, 1987
37. Merenich JA, McDermott M, Asp AA, et al: Evidence of endocrine involvement early in the course of human immunodeficiency virus infection. J Clin Endocrinol Metab 70(3):566-571, 1990
38. Milligan S, Katz M, Craven P, et al: Toxoplasmosis presenting as panhypopituitarism in a patient with the acquired immune deficiency syndrome. Am J Med 77:760-764, 1984
39. Monsuez J, Dinney E, Vittecoq D, et al: AIDS heart disease: Results in 85 patients (abstract). J Am Coll Cardiol 11(2):195A, 1988
40. Ortiz C, Meneses R, Jaffe D, et al: Outcome of patients with human immunodeficiency virus on maintenance hemodialysis. 34:248-253, 1988
41. Pardo V, Meneses R, Ossa L, et al: AIDS-related glomerulopathy: Occurrence in specific risk groups. 31:1167-1173, 1987
42. Rao TK, Fillippone E, Nicastri A, et al: Associated focal and segmental glomerulosclerosis in the acquired immunodeficiency syndrome. N Engl J Med 310(11):669-673, 1984
43. Rao TK, Friedman E, Nicastri A: The types of renal disease in the acquired immunodeficiency syndrome. N Engl J Med 316(17):1062-1067, 1987
44. Sano T, Kovacs K, Scheithauer B, et al: Pituitary pathology in the acquired immunodeficiency syndrome. Arch Pathol Lab Med 113:1066-1070, 1989
45. Sato K, Ozawa M, Demura H, et al: Thyroid function in the acquired immunodeficiency syndrome (AIDS) (letter). Ann Intern Med 111(10):857-858, 1989
46. Savoia MC, Oxman M: Myocarditis, pericarditis and mediastinitis. In Mandell GL (ed): Principles and Practice of Infectious Diseases. New York, Churchill Livingstone, 1990
47. Schimmbeck PL, Schultheiss P, Strauer BE: Identification of a main autoimmunogenic epitope of adenosine nucleotide translocator which cross-reacts with coxsackie B3 virus: Use in diagnosis of myocarditis and dilatiative cardiomyopathy (abstract). 80(suppl II): II 665, 1989
48. Schoenfeld P, Feduska N: Acquired immunodeficiency syndrome and renal disease: Report of the National Kidney Foundation–National Institutes of Health Task Force on AIDS and Kidney Disease. Am J Kidney Dis 16(1):14-25, 1990
49. Seney FD Jr, Burns D, Silva FG: Acquired immunodeficiency syndrome and the kidney. Am J Kidney Dis 16(1):1-13, 1990
50. Silver M, Macher A, Reichert C, et al: Cardiac involvement by Kaposi's sarcoma in acquired immune deficiency syndrome (AIDS). Am J Cardiol 53:983-985, 1984
51. Tapper M, Rotterdam H, Lerner C, et al: Adrenal necrosis in the acquired immunodeficiency syndrome. Ann Intern Med 100(2):239-240, 1984
52. Villette JM, Bourin P, Doinel C, et al: Circadian variations in plasma levels of hypophyseal, adrenocortical and testicular hormones in men infected with human immunodeficiency virus. J Clin Endocrinol Metab 70(3):572-577, 1990
53. Welch K, Finkbeiner W, Alpers C: Autopsy findings in the acquired immune deficiency syndrome. JAMA 252(9):1152-1159, 1984

III

SPECIFIC INFECTIONS AND MALIGNANT CONDITIONS

17

PNEUMOCYSTIS CARINII PNEUMONIA
Current Concepts

PHILIP C. HOPEWELL, MD

Since the recognition of AIDS, *Pneumocystis carinii* pneumonia has been the most frequent AIDS-defining diagnosis in the United States and Europe,[35,57] although the incidence of the disease is decreasing, presumably as a result of antipneumocystis prophylaxis and antiretroviral therapy.[10] Recently there have been several important advances in the understanding of both the biology of *P. carinii* and the disease it causes. This chapter reviews the current concepts concering *P. carinii* pneumonia and highlights more recent information.

MICROBIOLOGIC CHARACTERISTICS OF *P. CARINII*

Since the initial identification of *P. carinii* by Chagas in 1906, there has been controversy about the taxonomy of the organism. Chagas initially considered *P. carinii* a trypanosome. Subsequently it was reclassified by the Delanoes as a parasite.[16] Recently, however, studies of ribosomal RNA of *P. carinii* have shown that, phylogenetically, the organism is most closely related to the Ascomycetes (yeasts); thus *P. carinii* should probably be considered a fungus rather than a parasite.[17,93,100] This reclassification has little clinical relevance but may suggest new therapeutic approaches and culture techniques.

Although a great deal is known about the microbiologic characteristics of *P. carinii*, investigators have been hampered by their inability to culture the organism on cell-free media and to maintain cultures in cell lines. There are at least two important clinical implications of there being no practical means for culturing *P. carinii*. First, to diagnose *P. carinii* pneumonia, there must be a sufficient number of organisms to be detected by microscopic examination of clinical specimens. The

This chapter is modified from Hopewell PC: *Pneumocystis carinii* pneumonia: An update. In Sande MA, Root RK (eds): Treatment of Serious Infections in the 1990s. New York, Churchill Livingstone, 1992, pp 175-204.

threshold for visualization is in the range of 10^4 organisms per milliliter of respiratory secretions; thus the diagnosis cannot be established in the early stages of infection when few organisms are present. Second, testing of the organism for susceptibility to antimicrobial agents cannot be performed in culture systems. For this reason new drugs must be evaluated mainly in animal models.

P. carinii is thought to have a life cycle consisting of three stages: cysts, which are spherical or crescent-shaped forms 5 to 8 μm in diameter; sporozoites or intracystic bodies, found only within the cyst; and trophozoites, found outside the cyst and believed intermediate between the sporozoite and the cyst.[38] Trophozoites are 2 to 5 μm in diameter and have eccentric nuclei and reticular cytoplasm. The different stages have different staining properties. Some stains such as methenamine silver and toluidine blue O are taken up only by the cyst wall; thus only cysts can be identified in preparations stained by these methods. The Giemsa stain is taken up by both the intracystic sporozoites and extracystic trophozoites; cysts are not positively stained and cannot be seen except as negative images within the matrix of a clump of trophozoites. The Gram-Weigert stain also stains sporozoites and trophozoites but not the cyst wall. Newer immunofluorescent stains based on monoclonal antibodies to both cyst wall and trophozoite antigens stain both forms.[47]

EPIDEMIOLOGY

Because *P. carinii* pneumonia does not develop until there has been a marked reduction in host defenses, the disease itself is expressed only in severely immunocompromised patients; thus the epidemiology of *P. carinii* pneumonia largely parallels the epidemiology of immunosuppression.

Until the occurrence of the epidemic of infection with the human immunodeficiency virus type 1 (HIV-1), *P. carinii* pneumonia was an uncommon, sporadic disorder that occurred primarily in patients with leukemia or other recognized causes of impairment of host defenses and in patients who were given immunosuppressive therapy.[8] Because recognition and treatment of disorders of host responsiveness and the ability to identify *P. carinii* mainly were confined to industrialized countries, *P. carinii* pneumonia was reported for the most part only from Western countries. With the epidemic of HIV-1 infection, the incidence and distribution of the disease changed dramatically.

There are data which suggest that, although *P. carinii* apparently is a common organism in the environment, it is not evenly distributed throughout the world.[37] Perhaps the most striking evidence of geographic variation in distribution of *P. carinii* is from the data describing the spectrum of HIV-1 related opportunistic infections in Africa.[18,32,60] Although diseases such as tuberculosis, cryptosporidiosis, and toxoplasmosis are common there, *P. carinii* pneumonia is rare. The reasons for this are not known.

Several studies in the United States have shown that circulating antibodies to *P. carinii* develop in most children by age 2 to 3 years, leading to the conclusion that asymptomatic infection with *P. carinii* is nearly universal, at least in the areas where these studies were conducted.[64,80] In a recent study Peglow et al.[78] used immunoblotting techniques (Western blot) to detect antibodies in sera from different population groups in the United States. In a group of 95 healthy children and adults from Iowa, 86% had immunoglobulin G (IgG) antipneumocystis antibodies detected.

Of children ≤24 months of age, 82% reacted to one or more of the antigens. All healthy adult blood donors from Cincinnati reacted to one or more of the antigens, as did 80% of healthy, HIV-1 seronegative adults from Chicago. Patients with HIV-1 infection but no history of *P. carinii* pneumonia had a lower rate of *P. carinii* antibody positivity, with only 41% of 125 seropositive patients from Cincinnati, Chicago, and New York City showing reactivity to any of the antigens. Of 31 patients with one or more episodes of *P. carinii* pneumonia, 77% had antibodies detected. When followed sequentially, all patients with *P. carinii* pneumonia had antibodies detected at least once. These recent observations support the conclusions from previous serologic studies indicating that infection with *P. carinii* is nearly universal and occurs early in life.

HOST DEFENSES AGAINST *P. CARINII*

Little is known about the mechanisms by which infection with *P. carinii* is contained but the abnormalities in patients in whom *P. carinii* pneumonia develops suggest that both humoral and cell-mediated immunity may be involved. In an extensive review published in 1973 Burke and Good[8] described 53 patients with *P. carinii* pneumonia who had only immunoglobulin abnormalities.

More evidence of a possible role for antibody has been provided recently by Gigliotti and Hughes[29] who demonstrated that a monoclonal antibody directed against a surface antigen of *P. carinii* cysts and trophozoites reduced the intensity of experimental infection when it was given concurrently with an immunosuppressing dose of dexamethasone. These findings support a role for antibodies in containing natural infection. The means by which the antibody produced its effect was not determined, but the authors hypothesized that it may lead to compliment-mediated lysis of the organism or prevention of attachment of the organism to alveolar type 1 cells.

Using mice previously infected with *P. carinii,* Furuta et al.[26] demonstrated both circulating antibody and cell-mediated immune responses after intranasal administration of *P. carinii*. The time course of clearance of the cysts corresponded with the development of cell-mediated immunity rather than humoral antibodies. Moreover, administration of immune serum had no effect in increasing the clearance of cysts from the lungs. These observations were consistent with earlier findings from the same laboratory that in athymic mice with *P. carinii* infection transfer of spleen cells but not immune serum reduced the number of cysts in the lungs.[27] The authors concluded that cell-mediated rather than humoral immunity was the major mechanism by which the infection was contained.

The predominant effect of HIV-1 infection is impairment of cell-mediated immunity resulting from depletion of CD4+ (helper T) lymphocytes. As a consequence, there is a high frequency of infections with organisms that are contained in the normal host by cell-mediated immunity. However, clinical data have shown that *P. carinii* pneumonia in adults rarely develops unless the number of circulating CD4+ cells is fewer than 200/μl.[58]

P. carinii pneumonia can develop in infants who have normal or near-normal numbers of circulating helper T cells. Leibovitz et al.[51] described eight HIV-infected children ranging in age from 3 to 11 months, all but two of whom had CD4+ cell counts >600/μl of blood, who developed *P. carinii* pneumonia.

PATHOGENESIS OF *P. CARINII* PNEUMONIA

Ultrastructural studies have shown that *P. carinii* attaches to type 1 alveolar epithelial cells by close apposition and interdigitation of the cell membranes. Subsequent to attachment, the type 1 cells undergo degeneration. As shown by Limper and Martin[55] attachment of the organism impairs the ability of the alveolar epithelial cells in culture to replicate.

Pottratz and Martin[82] have demonstrated that the attachment of *P. carinii* trophozoites to alveolar epithelium is mediated by fibronectin and that inhibition of fibronectin by specific antibodies decreases the attachment. Presumably attachment is necessary for the development of progressive *P. carinii* infection.

Animal experiments have suggested that decreases in the amount of lung surfactant may play a role in the pathogenesis of *P. carinii* pneumonia. Kernbaum et al.[44] found reduced amounts of phospholipids in bronchoalveolar lavage fluid from rats with *P. carinii* infection. Subsequently, Sheehan et al.[88] not only produced these same findings, but also showed that the reduction in phospholipids was associated with reduced compliance of excised, *P. carinii*–infected lungs.

Injury to alveolar epithelial cells probably accounts for the increases in alveolar-capillary membrane permeability that have been demonstrated in patients. Mason et al.[56] measured the clearance of a radioisotope-labeled aerosol from the lungs of patients with *P. carinii* pneumonia and found that removal was accelerated, indicating increased permeability. Repeat studies showed that as patients improved, the rate of aerosol clearance decreased, a result consistent with a decrease in the permeability. Conversely, patients who failed to improve clinically had either no change or increases in rates of radioaerosol clearance.

In view of these experimental data, the sequence of events in developing *P. carinii* pneumonia could be hypothesized as follows: reduction in cell-mediated and perhaps humoral immunity, leading to a proliferation of organisms within the alveolar space; fibronectin-mediated attachment of *P. carinii* trophozoites to alveolar type 1 cells; injury to and loss from type 1 cells, leading to increased permeability of the alveolar-capillary barrier; subsequent exudation of fluid into the alveolar space; reduction in surfactant content; and intrapulmonary shunting of blood and decreased lung compliance. The result of this sequence of events is hypoxemia, increased work of breathing, and, ultimately, respiratory failure.

DIAGNOSIS

Clinical and Radiographic Presentation

Patients with *P. carinii* pneumonia usually have had nonspecific symptoms such as fever, fatigue, and weight loss for weeks to months before developing respiratory symptoms and often have other HIV-related disorders that indicate severe immunosuppression. The most common presenting symptoms of *P. carinii* pneumonia are fever, nonproductive cough, and progressive shortness of breath. Because zidovudine and aerosol pentamidine prophylaxis decrease the severity of *P. carinii* pneumonia if it does develop, the presenting symptoms may be subtle. Conversely, patients who have not been receiving medical care and who defer seeking medical attention may present with advanced pneumonia and marked symptoms.

The physical examination in patients with *P. carinii* pneumonia is not particularly useful. Examination of the lungs may reveal dry rales, but findings indicative of consolidation are unusual.

Findings caused by extrapulmonary pneumocystosis depend on the site of involvement.[83] In evaluating findings that could be caused by *P. carinii*, appropriate specimens should be obtained to look for the organism. Table 17–1 lists the sites in which extrapulmonary pneumocystosis has been reported.

In patients with *P. carinii* pneumonia chest radiographs most often show diffuse interstitial infiltration involving all portions of the lungs.[33] Several variations may be seen. The infiltration may be heterogenously distributed throughout the lung, or it may be miliary in appearance. Diffuse or focal air-space consolidation may also be noted. In patients who are being given aerosol pentamidine prophylaxis, focal upper lobe infiltrations are relatively common.[62] Cystic changes or pneumatoceles may occur, especially during the healing process, and cavitation within pre-existing nodular lesions has been described. Probably as a result of the cystic or cavitary processes, spontaneous pneumothorax may occur.[33] Pleural effusions and intra-thoracic adenopathy are very uncommon with *P. carinii* pneumonia.

Identification of *P. Carinii*

Although patients with *P. carinii* pneumonia often complain of cough, they rarely spontaneously produce sputum that is suitable for examination, although adequate sputum specimens can be obtained. Data from several institutions indicate that examination of induced sputum is a sensitive and relatively simple means of diagnosis.[3,77,81]

Sputum induced by inhalation of a mist of 3% saline solution produced by an ultrasonic nebulizer is the initial test used to identify *P. carinii* at San Francisco General Hospital. To determine the usefulness of examination of induced sputum, 404 consecutive episodes of HIV-associated lung disease were evaluated with sputum examination as the first potentially definitive study.[74] *P. carinii* was identified in 222 specimens (55%). The sensitivity of sputum for detecting *P. carinii* was 77% and the negative predictive value was 64%. These results indicate the operational value of sputum examination in routine practice and demonstrate that the use of sputum examination provides considerable savings in resources and patient discomfort. Nevertheless, the sensitivity and negative predictive values of sputum examination are such that a negative result cannot be regarded as definitive.

**Table 17–1. Sites of
Extrapulmonary Involvement
with *P. carinii***

Skin	Lymph nodes
External auditory canal	Heart
Meninges	Spleen
Eye	Liver
Pleural space	

Recently the use of both indirect and direct fluorescent antibody stains for *P. carinii* has been evaluated. The initial reports indicate that using these stains will increase the sensitivity of induced sputum.[75,76,102]

Bronchoalveolar lavage and transbronchial lung biopsy are highly sensitive methods for identifying pulmonary infections in patients with AIDS. Stover et al.[92] reported the results of bronchoscopic procedures in 72 patients with AIDS. Both transbronchial biopsy and bronchoalveolar lavage had a high sensitivity (88% and 85%, respectively), and when used together, the sensitivity was 94%. The sensitivity was especially high for *P. carinii* (94%). Similar results were reported by Broaddus et al.,[7] who described the efficacy of bronchoalveolar lavage and transbronchial biopsy in detecting pulmonary pathogens in 276 fiberoptic bronchoscopic examinations performed on 171 patients with known or suspected AIDS. Of 173 pathogens identified during the initial evaluation or in the subsequent month, the initial bronchoscopy detected 166 (96%). Bronchoalveolar lavage and transbronchial biopsy had similar sensitivities of 86% (124 of 145) and 87% (133 of 153), respectively. For *P. carinii,* lavage had an 89% sensitivity, and transbronchial biopsy was 97% sensitive. In patients who had both procedures performed the sensitivity was 100%.

Bronchoalveolar lavage alone has been reported by Golden et al.[30] as having a sensitivity for *P. carinii* of 97%. At the San Francisco General Hospital we have reviewed our experience subsequent to the report by Broaddus et al.[7] and found that only rarely was *P. carinii* identified in transbronchial biopsy specimens when it was not seen in bronchoalveolar lavage fluid. Thus, as a matter of routine in patients with or suspected of having AIDS in whose sputum *P. carinii* is not found, we perform only bronchoalveolar lavage. If that procedure is not diagnostic, the lavage is repeated, and a transbronchial biopsy is performed in an attempt to determine other diagnoses.

It has been suggested by Jules-Elysee et al.[43] that the sensitivity of bronchoalveolar lavage is decreased in patients who have been receiving aerosol pentamidine prophylaxis and that transbronchial biopsy is required more frequently. In patients who had been given aerosol pentamidine, bronchoalveolar lavage had a sensitivity of 62%, compared with 100% in patients who had not been receiving the drug. The sensitivity of transbronchial biopsy was 81% and 84% in the pentamidine and no-pentamidine groups, respectively. Similarly Levine et al.[54] found a significantly decreased sensitivity for induced sputum in patients who had been receiving aerosol pentamidine (64%) versus those who had not been receiving prophylaxis (92%). An analysis of the recent experience at the University of California, San Diego, however, has suggested that using aerosol pentamidine does not decrease the yield of induced sputum examination.[62] In this report induced sputum examination had a sensitivity of 63% in patients who had been receiving aerosol pentamidine and 64% in those who had not received the drug.

In some patients an empiric treatment trial may be used to infer a diagnoses. Generally, however, this method is unsatisfactory, first, because another treatable process may be missed, and second, because such an approach exposes the patient to the risks of therapy, perhaps without benefit. However, in patients with classic clinical features a presumptive diagnosis can be established with a fairly high degree of accuracy by experienced clinicians.[65] This approach may have some applicability in institutions not capable of making diagnoses from induced sputum, but its use does not seem justified when the majority of diagnoses can be established by a noninvasive and relatively inexpensive test. It is not clear that a presumptive diagnosis would result in a substantial reduction in invasive diagnostic procedures in institutions capable of performing induced sputum examinations. Given the inconsistency of the data, it is important that institutions evaluate their results on an ongoing basis to determine the most effective diagnostic strategy based on prevailing local conditions.

TREATMENT

The first line of therapy for *P. carinii* pneumonia remains pentamidine isethionate and trimethoprim-sulfamethoxazole (TMP-SMX). There are, however, several regimens for which there is increasing evidence of efficacy. This section reviews the available therapies, including adjunctive measures such as corticosteroid therapy, and describes the strategies for treatment.

Antipneumocystis Agents

Pentamidine

Pentamidine is an aromatic diamidine that was first used in the 1940s to treat African trypanosomiasis and leishmaniasis. It is active against *Trypanosoma rhodesiense, T. gambiense, Leishmania donovani,* and *P. carinii.*[15]

The mechanism of action of pentamidine on *P. carinii* has not been firmly established. It inhibits dihydrofolate reductase in vitro, although it is not so potent in this regard as other folate antagonists.[97] Pentamidine also interferes with anaerobic glycolysis, inhibits oxidative phosphorylation, and limits nucleic acid and protein synthesis.[5] Data reported more recently indicate that pentamidine inhibits the metabolism of *p*-aminobenzoic acid and the eventual synthesis of dihydrofolate.[46]

The usual dose of pentamidine is 4 mg/kg body weight per day, although Conte et al.[12,13] have reported successful treatment using a dose of 3 mg/kg. Both the 3 and 4 mg/kg doses are based loosely on animal studies and on empiric observations. Because *P. carinii* cannot be maintained in culture, a minimum inhibitory concentration of pentamidine cannot be determined. By measuring the uptake of vital dyes by *P. carinii*, Pesanti[79] showed that a pentamidine concentration of 5 μg/ml was associated with decreased viability after a lag time of 6 hours. This concentration corresponds roughly to the plasma concentrations produced by intramuscular (IM) or intravenous (IV) administration of 4 mg/kg of pentamidine.[14] Because of the tissue tropism of the drug, concentrations in the lung probably are substantially greater than in serum.

Pentamidine is not absorbed from the gastrointestinal tract; thus parenteral administration is necessary. IV administration should be done only when the patient can be observed and the blood pressure measured. The drug should be dissolved in 250 ml of 5% dextrose in water and administered at a constant infusion rate for 1 hour. The dosing interval of 24 hours should be increased for patients with impaired renal function.

The minimum duration of treatment with pentamidine has not been established in a systematic fashion, but in most trials the drug was given for 14 to 21 days. In addition, in patients with AIDS retrospective analysis has suggested that a regimen of 21 days of administration is superior to one of 14 days.[36]

In patients with AIDS most investigators have reported a high frequency of adverse reactions to pentamidine (see Chapter 9). In a prospective study Wharton et al.[101] reported that 14 of 32 (44%) patients given pentamidine had a major adverse reaction that necessitated changing the drug and all patients given the drug had minor adverse reactions. The most frequent major adverse reaction was neutropenia (<1000 polymorphonuclear leukocytes/μL), whereas hyponatremia, abnormal liver function, and azotemia were the most frequent minor reactions. Most reactions in these patients occurred between days 7 and 14 of treatment. Sattler et al.[86] also reported a high frequency of adverse reactions in pentamidine-treated AIDS patients; however, in only one patient was the reaction severe (fatal hypoglycemia), and discontinuation of the drug was not necessary in any patients, at least in part because the threshold for changing therapy was higher than in the study by Wharton and associates.

All but 1 of 20 patients randomly chosen to receive pentamidine were treated successfully in the study by Wharton et al.[101] Similar results in AIDS patients were reported by Klein et al.[45] In the study by Sattler et al.,[86] however, only 61% of patients prospectively chosen at random to receive pentamidine survived.

Conte, Hollander, and Golden[13] and Montgomery et al.[68,70] have reported high rates of successful initial and second-line treatment with no systemic toxicity in pilot studies using aerosol pentamidine in AIDS patients with *P. carinii* pneumonia. In a comparative clinical trial, Montgomery et al.[69] subsequently reported that mild to moderate episodes of *P. carinii* pneumonia responded as well to aerosol pentamidine as to TMP-SMX. Side effects were significantly fewer with aerosol pentamidine, but the rate of improvement was somewhat slower. Conversely, Soo Hoo, Mohsenifar, and Meyer[90] and Conte et al.[12] have reported small comparative trials in which patients treated with aerosol pentamidine responded less well than those treated with the drug given intravenously. Given these conflicting data, the role of aerosol pentamidine as treatment for *P. carinii* pneumonia remains undefined.

Trimethoprim-Sulfamethoxazole

The combination of trimethoprim (TMP) and sulfamethoxazole (SMX) has activity against a wide range of organisms. The two agents act on separate sites to inhibit purine synthesis.[48] Sulfonamides inhibit dihydrofolic synthetase, preventing the conversion of microbial *p*-aminobenzoic acid to dihydrofolic acid. TMP acts on dihydrofolic acid reductase (DHFR), thereby decreasing synthesis of tetrahydrofolic acid.

Both drugs are well absorbed from the gastrointestinal tract. Minimum inhibitory concentrations of TMP and SMX for *P. carinii* have not been determined. In the first report of treatment of patients with TMP-SMX, two different doses were used: 4 to 7 mg/kg/day of TMP with 20 to 35 mg/kg/day of SMX; and 20 mg/kg/day with 100 mg/kg/day of the respective agents.[40] Peak serum concentrations of TMP at the lower dose were approximately 2 μg/ml and at the higher dose were 7 to 10 μg/ml. The peak SMX concentrations were 50 to 60 μg/ml and 80 to 120 μg/ml for the low and high doses, respectively. Two of six patients treated with low doses died, as did two of the 14 patients who received high doses.

Based on this experience, Hughes et al.[39] conducted a prospective randomized study comparing TMP-SMX with pentamidine in immunosuppressed children with *P. carinii* pneumonia, using a dose of 20 mg/kg/day for TMP and 100 mg/kg/day for SMX. Serum levels of both agents were measured 2 hours and 6 hours after oral ingestion of one fourth of the daily dose (5 mg/kg and 25 mg/kg) on days 1, 3, 6, 9, and 12. The concentrations of both drugs tended to remain constant from the third day, although there was moderate variability from day to day. The 2-hour and 6-hour mean concentrations were not substantially different for either drug: for TMP the mean concentrations ranged from approximately 4 to 6.5 μg/ml, and for SMX the range was approximately 115 to 175 μg/ml. Nearly all studies reported since the 1975 paper by Hughes, Feldman, and Sanyal[40] have used these doses. However, Sattler et al.[86] reported no loss of efficacy with a lower dose (approximately 15 mg/kg) of TMP if serum levels were maintained at 5 to 8 μg/ml.

Currently it is recommended that the daily dosage be divided into four doses given at 6-hour intervals. The drug can be given orally, usually in the form of tablets containing 160 mg of TMP and 800 mg of SMX, if there is no condition that would interfere with absorption. For parenteral administration the drug should be diluted in 250 ml of 5% dextrose in water and given over a 30- to 60-minute period at 6-hour intervals. The minimum necessary duration of treatment has not been established. Nearly all published experience, however, has reported using 14 to 21 days of therapy or occasionally more, depending on the clinical course.

As with pentamidine, in patients with AIDS the frequency of significant adverse reactions to TMP-SMX is high. Gordin et al.[34] retrospectively reviewed adverse reactions among AIDS patients who were treated with TMP-SMX and found that 19 of 35 patients treated for more than 2 days were not able to complete a full course of the agent because of adverse reactions. Severe skin rashes, often associated with fever, were the most common reactions. Leukopenia and thrombocytopenia were the next most frequent reasons for discontinuing the drug. Hepatitis occurred in a smaller number. These investigators noted that the adverse reactions nearly always occurred between days 6 and 14 of a planned 21-day course of treatment. (See Chapter 9.)

In the prospective study conducted by Wharton et al.[101] adverse reactions to TMP-SMX were encountered frequently. Of 20 patients allocated to receive the drug, 10 had major adverse reactions necessitating discontinuance of the drugs after a median of 11 days, with nearly all reactions occurring between days 6 and 14. As was noted by Gordin et al.,[34] the most frequent major reactions were severe skin rash (20%), hepatitis (20%), neutropenia (15%), and thrombocytopenia (15%). Minor adverse reactions that did not necessitate discontinuation of the drug were seen in all patients. In addition to lesser degrees of the severe reactions, minor adverse effects included nausea, vomiting, and hyponatremia. Sattler et al.[86] also reported a frequency of adverse effects from TMP-SMX in their prospective study, but these reactions did not necessitate discontinuation of the agent. In part they attributed the lack of severe reactions to dosage reductions based on serum TMP concentrations (as described previously).

Evaluating the success of TMP-SMX in patients with AIDS is difficult because of the high frequency of therapy changes necessitated by adverse reactions. In a retrospective review Haverkos[36] reported a 91% (40 of 44 patients) survival rate in patients who were treated with a full course of the agent. On the other hand, the survival rate was only 31% (11 of 35) in patients who were changed to pentamidine because of a lack of effect of TMP-SMX and 69% in patients changed because of adverse reactions. Overall, 74 of 97 (76%) patients who initially began TMP-SMX therapy survived.

In the patients reported in the National Heart Lung and Blood Institute workshop on the pulmonary complications of AIDS, 88 of 107 (82%) treated with TMP-SMX alone survived.[72] Of 37 patients who failed on TMP-SMX therapy, only 4 (11%) survived, whereas 41 of 41 patients who were changed to pentamidine because of adverse reactions survived.

In the prospective studies by Wharton et al.,[101] Klein et al.,[45] and Sattler et al.,[86] survival rates for patients assigned to receive TMP-SMX were 75% (15 of 20), 63% (22 of 35), and 86% (31 of 36), respectively.

Dapsone

Dapsone (diaminodiphenylsulfone) is a sulfone that has been used nearly exclusively for the treatment of leprosy. By screening a number of agents for antipneumocystis effects, Hughes and Smith[42] found that dapsone was effective in both preventing and treating *P. carinii* pneumonia in the cortisone-treated rat. A dose of 25 mg/kg/day had an effect similar to that of TMP-SMX (50 and 250 mg/kg/day), whereas 5 mg/kg/day had a lesser but still apparent effect.

Based on these experimental results, Leoung et al.[53] conducted an open trial of the combination of dapsone, 100 mg/day, and TMP, 20 mg/kg/day, in treating mild to moderate *P. carinii* pneumonia in patients with AIDS. All of 15 patients recovered, and although 14 of the 15 had minor adverse reactions, it was necessary to discontinue use of the drug in only two patients, both because of rash. The most common minor reactions were nausea and vomiting. Subsequently, investigators from the same institution conducted an open trial of dapsone, 100 mg, without TMP.[66] Treatment with dapsone alone in a dose of 100 mg was associated with treatment failure or lack of improvement in 7 of 18 (39%) patients. There were no adverse effects that required stopping the drug. Based on the results of this study, it was believed that dapsone is probably less effective than standard therapy and that it should not be used alone to treat *P. carinii* pneumonia.

Medina et al.,[61] in a trial comparing TMP-dapsone with TMP-SMX, reported treatment failure in 2 of 29 patients (7%) in each group. Major toxicity occurred in 16 of 29 patients (55%) allocated to TMP-SMX and 9 of 29 (31%) given TMP-dapsone. The adverse effects of TMP-dapsone included skin rash (3 patients), nausea and vomiting (2 patients), and leukopenia, thrombocytopenia, hepatitis, and methemoglobinemia (all 1 patient each). From this study it was concluded that treatment with TMP-dapsone was as effective as that with TMP-SMX and produced fewer adverse reactions in patients with mild to moderately severe *P. carinii* pneumonia.

Clindamycin-Primaquine

The combination of the antibacterial agent, clindamycin, with the DHFR inhibitor, primaquine, has been evaluated in two open studies and in a double-blind trial in which TMP-SMX was the control regimen. Toma[95] reported "cures" in 59 (80%)

of 74 patients who had failed or were intolerant of standard therapy and in 44 (75%) of 59 patients who had not been treated previously. Adverse reactions, predominantly skin rash, occurred in 50% of the patients. Methemoglobinemia was not noted in these patients, perhaps because the dose of primaquine was a 15-mg base instead of the more commonly used 30 mg. These investigators noted that clinical response seemed to occur earlier in the clindamycin-primaquine–treated patients than had been observed in responding patients treated conventionally. In a second open trial Black et al.[4] treated 36 patients who had mild to moderately severe *P. carinii* pneumonia. Of the 36, 28 patients (78%) successfully completed treatment. Although skin rashes occurred frequently, they usually did not necessitate discontinuation of the drug. In all, five (14%) patients required a change in treatment regimen because of adverse reactions.

Ruf, Rohde, and Pohle[85] compared the results of treatment with clindamycin-primaquine in 19 patients to historical control patients treated with TMP-SMX. All patients in both groups were cured, and no patients required discontinuation of clindamycin-primaquine because of adverse reactions. However, all patients developed methemoglobinemia, which, in 7 of the 19, was greater than 10%, with the highest value 19.1%.

In the cited studies clindamycin was given either orally or intravenously. The IV doses ranged from 450 mg (in patients weighing <60 kg) to 900 mg every 6 hours. Oral doses ranged from 300 mg (for patients weighing <60 kg) to 900 mg. Primaquine was given orally in doses of 15 or 30 mg once a day. In addition to the high rates of success and low frequency of adverse reactions, the investigators noted that the rates of response seemed more rapid with clindamycin-primaquine. However, all of the studies involved patients with mild to moderately severe disease and thus adequate systemic oxygen delivery. In patients with marginal oxygenation the amount of methemoglobinemia that has resulted from primaquine administration may cause significant tissue hypoxemia. For this reason methemoglobin concentrations should be measured frequently if oxygenation is impaired.

Specific recommendations for clindamycin-primaquine dosage cannot be made based on the above studies. It appears that either the oral or the IV route is suitable for administration of clindamycin but not for primaquine, which is available only as an oral formulation.

Trimetrexate

Trimetrexate is an antifolate that differs from trimethoprim in that it does not require an active transmembrane transport process to gain entry into cells.[2] It is several thousand times more potent in inhibiting DHFR than TMP and must be administered with leucovorin (preformed tetrahydrofolate) to "rescue" mammalian (host) cells. In an open trial reported by Allegra et al.,[1] 14 of 16 (88%) patients given trimetrexate plus leucovorin as initial treatment for *P. carinii* pneumonia survived, although 4 required additional antipneumocystis agents. Six patients relapsed within 3 months of completion of therapy. In a separate group of 17 patients treated with trimetrexate-leucovorin plus sulfadiazine, survival rate was 77%, and 71% required no other agents. The relapse rate was only 6%. Trimetrexate-leucovorin was also used as "salvage" therapy in 16 patients who were either failing or were intolerant of standard treatment. The survival rate was 69%, no patients required additional agents, and there were no relapses. The major toxicities in all three groups were neutropenia, thrombocytopenia, and increased hepatic enzymes. Trimetrexate dose reductions were required in 19% of the patients.

In a preliminary report by Feinberg et al.[22] 47% of 115 patients who were treated with trimetrexate-leucovorin because of intolerance to conventional therapy survived. Of a second group of 40 patients treated with trimetrexate-leucovorin because of failure to respond to standard agents, only 5 (13%) survived.

566C80

This compound is a hydroxynaphthaquinone that was found active in animal models and, subsequently, in a human trial. In an open trial Falloon, Kovacs, and Hughes[21] treated 34 patients who had mild to moderately severe *P. carinii* pneumonia. Of the 34, 27 (79%) were treated successfully with 566C80 alone. The drug was discontinued in five patients because of lack of response and in four patients because of adverse reactions (two of these patients were considered to have been treated successfully). Three different doses of the drug were used (i.e., 750 mg twice, three times, or four times daily). No differences in outcome were noted. This agent is currently being evaluated in a prospective comparative trial with TMP-SMX.

α-Difluoromethylornithine

α-Difluoromethylornithine (DFMO) inhibits ornithine decarboxylase, thereby decreasing polyamine synthesis. Golden, Sjoerdsma, and Santi[31] used the drug in six AIDS patients who had been treated with standard therapy and had either failed with it or were intolerant of the agents. The dosage was 6 g/m^2 body surface area daily, divided into three doses, given for 8 weeks. All six patients had a successful outcome. Leukopenia and/or thrombocytopenia occurred in five of six patients.

McLees et al.[59] have reported on the results of DFMO therapy in 234 patients with *P. carinii* pneumonia who were said to have failed while receiving standard treatment. The dosage was 400 mg/kg/day given in four doses. The intended duration of IV administration was 14 days, followed by 4 to 6 weeks of oral therapy, 75 mg/kg every 6 hours. These patients were severely ill, with 45% mechanically ventilated. The survival rate was 36% (84 of 234). Reversible thrombocytopenia occurred in 43% and leukopenia in 11%.

Although both studies of DFMO therapy suggest that it might be useful, a prospective comparative evaluation will be necessary to determine the true effectiveness of the agent.

Piritrexim

Piritrexim is another DHFR inhibitor that can be given orally. In a preliminary report of an open study Falloon et al.[20] reported a 77% (10 of 13) success rate in patients given 150 mg/m^2 body surface area twice a day and a 60% (6 of 10) success rate in patients given 250 mg/m^2. Both groups were also given leukovorin.

The drug was discontinued in four patients because of toxicity. Of note was that 7 of 15 patients followed after recovery relapsed within 2 months of completion of therapy.

Treatment Strategies

As a general rule, treatment should be based on a proven diagnosis, especially in institutions having the capability to make diagnoses by examining induced sputum. Because of the high frequency of adverse drug reactions, treatment without a confirmed diagnosis subjects patients to risks that might not be warranted. Moreover, given the rather large number of disorders that comprise the differential diagnosis of lung disease in immunocompromised patients, establishing a precise diagnosis before undertaking treatment is sound practice. This is especially true if administration of corticosteroid treatment is being considered (discussed subsequently).

In patients with mild to moderately severe *P. carinii* pneumonia who can take oral medications, treatment should be initiated with oral TMP, 20 mg/kg/day, and SMX, 100 mg/kg/day. The total dosage can be divided in to two or four doses, although twice-daily administration may not be tolerated because of gastrointestinal upset. If possible, either a TMP or SMX serum concentration should be measured 90 to 120 minutes after administration of the oral or IV dose on day 2 or 3 of therapy. The TMP concentration should range from 5 to 8 μg/ml and SMX concentration from approximately 100 to 120 μg/ml.

Dapsone-TMP apparently is a suitable alternative form of outpatient therapy for patients who do not have severe *P. carinii* pneumonia. Aerosol pentamidine and clindamycin-primaquine are other options for such patients. For patients being treated with dapsone-TMP or clindamycin-primaquine, methemoglobin saturations should be measured at 3- to 5-day intervals.

For patients who are more severely ill or who cannot take oral drugs, TMP-SMX should be given IV in the same doses as for oral administration at 6-hour intervals. Patients who have had adverse reactions to sulfa agents or specifically to TMP-SMX should be started on treatment with pentamidine as should patients who cannot be given the fluid volume required to administer TMP-SMX. The pentamidine dose is 3 to 4 mg/kg/day given IV as a single daily administration. Patients should be monitored for hypotension during and shortly after the infusion.

The usual median time to respond to either agent is approximately 4 to 6 days, and some patients worsen before they begin to improve. Response should be judged by standard indices, including degree of dyspnea, fever, respiratory rate, arterial oxygen tension or oxyhemoglobin saturation determined by pulse oximetry, and chest film. Patients probably should not be considered as treatment failures with either drug until after a minimum of 4 days of therapy. Continued worsening after 4 days or failure to improve after 7 to 10 days is an indication to change therapy, generally from TMP-SMX to pentamidine. The role of trimetrexate in salvage therapy has not yet been established, but current data suggest that it will be useful in this regard. At present, the agent should be reserved for patients who fail both TMP-SMX and pentamidine therapies. Trimetrexate is given IV in a daily dose of 30 to 45 mg/m^2 body surface area and must be given with leucovorin, 20 mg/m^2

orally or IV. Sulfadiazine, 1 g given orally four times a day, seems to decrease the frequency of relapse but does not have a demonstrated role in the initial response.

All patients should be observed carefully for adverse reactions, especially in the second week. At the time treatment is initiated, baseline tests of hepatic and renal function, a complete blood count with a differential count, and a platelet count should be obtained. Blood glucose concentration should be measured in patients being given pentamidine. These tests should be repeated at 3-day intervals at least through day 14 of treatment. Adverse reactions that necessitate changing treatment include neutropenia (<750 polymorphonuclear leukocytes/μl); thrombocytopenia (platelets >40,000 μl); elevation of serum creatinine to >3 mg/dl; increased aspartate or alanine aminotransferase level to more than five times normal; and progressively worsening skin rash, especially if accompanied by mucositis or fever. Hypotension or hypoglycemia produced by pentamidine does not necessarily mean the drug should be discontinued, but special care should be taken in its administration.

The necessary duration of therapy is not well established, but 14 to 21 days are now standard. Assessment of response to therapy should be based on clinical and radiographic grounds. Repeat examinations for *P. carinii* in patients with AIDS who have been successfully treated show *P. carinii* in more than 60%, indicating that this is not a reliable means of determining cure.[89]

P. carinii causes respiratory failure at least in part by increasing the permeability of the alveolar-capillary membrane, which in turn leads to interstitial and, subsequently, alveolar accumulation of fluid. For this reason, in patients with *P. carinii* pneumonia administration of IV fluids should be monitored carefully. Over-vigorous administration of fluids will increase the tendency for pulmonary parenchymal fluid accumulation and will worsen the hypoxemia.

Corticosteroid Therapy

Since early in the AIDS epidemic, anecdotal reports have suggested that patients who receive corticosteroid therapy in addition to antipneumocystis agents had a less severe course than patients treated only with antipneumocystis agents. Recently several prospective controlled studies have documented a beneficial effect of corticosteroid therapy in patients with moderate to severe *P. carinii* pneumonia. Montaner et al.[67] studied a group of patients with *P. carinii* pneumonia and oxyhemoglobin saturation level, measured by pulse oximetry, of 85% to 90% or a decrease in saturation level of 5% with a standard treadmill exercise protocol. Patients were assigned to receive either prednisone, 60 mg/day for 7 days, followed by tapering doses for 14 days, or an identical placebo in addition to antipneumocystis therapy. The major result was that in the steroid treated group only 1 of 18 patients developed early deterioration (defined as at least a 10% decrease in oxyhemoglobin saturation) compared with 8 of 19 placebo-treated patients. The only death in either group occurred in a patient treated with prednisone.

Two subsequent trials also showed a benefit from corticosteroid therapy. Bozzette et al.[6] demonstrated that corticosteroid therapy decreased the frequency of early deterioration in oxygenation and, in addition, had both a short- and intermediate-term mortality benefit. These investigators also showed that administration of corticosteroids as salvage therapy in placebo-treated patients who developed respiratory failure was not effective, as opposed to the finding of Montaner and associates. The benefit of early corticosteroid administration was most evident in patients with more severe impaired oxygenation.

Similarly, Gagnon et al.[28] compared administration of corticosteroids with that of a placebo in more severely ill patients and found both a decreased frequency of respiratory failure and lower mortality in the patients who received corticosteroid therapy.

As an outgrowth of these reports, "consensus" recommendations for the use of corticosteroids in patients with *P. carinii* pneumonia have been published.[94] These recommendations are summarized as follows: (1) corticosteroid therapy should be given to all patients with proven *P. carinii* pneumonia who have an arterial oxygen tension <70 mm Hg; (2) steroid therapy should be started within 72 hours of initiation of antipneumocystis therapy; (3) the dosage should be 40 mg of oral prednisone or the equivalent of methylprednisolone given intravenously twice a day on days 1 through 5, 40 mg given daily on days 6 through 10, and 20 mg given daily on days 11 through 21; and (4) the diagnosis of *P. carinii* should be confirmed rapidly.

COMPLICATIONS

Respiratory Failure

P. carinii produces significant effects on lung function in a large number of patients with the disease. As described earlier, the pathophysiology is essentially that of the adult respiratory distress syndrome, with increased permeability of the alveolar-capillary membrane, leakage of fluid into the alveolar air spaces, and consequent intrapulmonary shunting of blood, causing hypoxemia. The severity of the gas exchange abnormality ranges from none to severe. Generally all that is required to improve arterial oxygenation is administration of supplemental oxygen. Occasionally, however, endotracheal intubation and mechanical ventilation may be necessary. Management of respiratory failure in patients with *P. carinii* pneumonia should follow the same general guidelines as for any patient with acute, diffuse lung injury. Careful attention should be paid to fluid balance, minimizing the potential for overhydration's contributing to the accumulation of extravascular lung water. If mechanical ventilation is necessary, providing relatively large tidal volumes (15 ml/kg body weight) and positive end-expiratory pressure is generally beneficial.

The prognosis for patients who require mechanical ventilation because of respiratory failure caused by *P. carinii* pneumonia has improved substantially in recent years. In the early years of the AIDS epidemic reports indicated a very poor prognosis for such patients.[84,87,98] Mortality rates ranged from 86% to 100%. More recently, however, clinicians from several institutions have described improved outcomes. At San Francisco General Hospital the mortality rate for mechanically ventilated patients with *P. carinii* pneumonia from 1981 through 1985 was 87%, whereas from 1986 through 1988, the morality rate had decreased to 60%.[98,99] The reasons for the decreased mortality rate are not clear. Indicators of the severity of disease were not different in the two periods, and antipneumocystis therapy was identical. More patients in the more recent period were given corticosteroids, although the difference in survival rate between patients with and without steroid therapy was not significant.

Pneumothorax

Patients with current or previous *P. carinii* pneumonia are at increased risk of spontaneous pneumothorax. There are several possible mechanisms by which the pneumothorax may develop. In a patient with acute *P. carinii* pneumonia the lung may rupture as a consequence of actual parenchymal necrosis or formation of pneumatoceles, presumably caused by a check-valve effect in a peripheral airway.[19] Subsequently, with healing and fibrosis, cysts may be formed that can become overdistended and rupture.

Regardless of the mechanism, once a pneumothorax develops, it presents an extremely problematic management issue. If air is rapidly accumulating in the pleural space, a tension pneumothorax may develop. This requires immediate venting of the air to the outside to prevent or reverse the severe cardiorespiratory effects caused by the positive pressure in the affected hemithorax.

Less rapidly developing pneumothoraces also require evacuation. Thus performing tube thoracostomy is almost always required in any patient with a *P. carinii* pneumonia-related spontaneous pneumothorax. Commonly, there is persistent leakage of air through the disruption in the lung into the pleural space (bronchopleural fistula), necessitating long-term chest tube drainage. Various techniques have been used to facilitate closure of the broncopleural fistula. Usually the initial means is simply to maintain full lung inflation (if possible) by application of subatmospheric pressure in the pleural space through the chest tube. Various agents such as tetracycline, bleomycin, or talc can be instilled through the chest tube to incite pleural inflammation and, subsequently, adhesion of the visceral and parietal pleural layers. If this procedure is successful, pleural sclerosis prevents further pneumothoraces. Frequently, however, the attempt at sclerosis is not successful. In this case the options are limited and of unproven value. Attempts may be made to plug the bronchus leading to the fistula, using bronchoscopically guided placement of materials such as a fibrin-thrombin clot. Alternatively, pleuroscopy may be performed and attempts made to seal the leak from the outside using some type of adhesive material. Rarely, thoracotomy and either resection of the abnormal portion of lung or repair of the fistula can be tried.[25] As a final resort, the patient may be discharged with a chest tube in place connected to a one-way valve such as a Heimlich valve.

PREVENTION

Trimethoprim-Sulfamethoxazole

Because of the effectiveness of TMP-SMX in preventing *P. carinii* pneumonia in children with hematologic malignancies, the disease has largely disappeared from this population.[41] Unfortunately, prevention of *P. carinii* pneumonia in patients with AIDS has proved much more problematic. The difficulties result mainly from the high frequency of adverse reactions to TMP-SMX in this group. Fishl, Dickinson, and LaVoie[24] reported both a lower frequency of adverse reactions than previously noted and a significant reduction in the incidence of *P. carinii* pneumonia using TMP-SMX in a dose of 160 mg/800 mg together with 5 mg of folinic acid twice a day. In this study 5 of 30 (16.7%) patients given the drug had adverse effects that necessitated discontinuing the agent, and 50% had minor adverse reactions. Four of the five patients in whom TMP-SMX was discontinued subsequently developed *P. carinii* pneumonia, as did 16 (53%) of 30 patients given placebo. Perhaps the most important observation from this study was that the median survival time in the group given TMP-SMX was 20 months, compared with 11 months in the control group. This observation substantiated that there is a beneficial effect of *P. carinii* prophylaxis on the natural history of HIV infection.

Other investigators have examined the use of lower doses of TMP-SMX in prophylaxis with, in general, efficacy being demonstrated.[50,71,91] In a not-yet-published study conducted by the National Institutes of Health (NIH) AIDS Clinical Trials Group, TMP-SMX (160 mg to 800 mg once a day) was compared with aerosol pentamidine (300 mg once a month) for preventing *P. carinii* pneumonia.[73] Significantly fewer patients develop *P. carinii* pneumonia while receiving TMP-SMX (9.1%) compared with aerosol pentamidine (23.1%). Surprisingly, overall toxicity was no different in the two groups, although more patients in the TMP-SMX group required switching to the other regimen because of toxicity (27% versus 4%).

Aerosol Pentamidine

Leoung, Feigel, and Montgomery,[52] in a prospective, randomized trial of aerosolized pentamidine for prevention of *P. carinii* pneumonia, demonstrated an inverse relationship between the dose of pentamidine and the frequency of *P. carinii* pneumonia. The largest number of cases occurred in patients receiving a pentamidine dose of 30 mg every 2 weeks; patients receiving 150 mg every 2 weeks had an intermediate frequency of the disease; and those given 300 mg once a month had the lowest frequency. Only the difference in frequency of *P. carinii* pneumonia between the 30-mg and the 300-mg doses was statistically significant. The differences between the 30-mg and 150-mg doses and 150-mg and 300-mg doses were not large enough to reach significance. In all three groups the aerosol was generated by a small particle–producing jet nebulizer (mean aerodynamic diameter, 1.6 μm) delivered through a unidirectional breathing circuit that had a small particle filter on the expiration limb of the device (Respigard II, Marquest Co., Englewood, Colorado).

Adverse reactions to inhaled pentamidine aerosol have, in general, been mild. Coughing is common, especially in cigarette smokers, and bronchospasm may occur. These complications can be minimized by pretreatment with an inhaled bronchodilator such as albuterol. A few patients have had hypersensitivity reactions, but in general, even patients who have had adverse reactions to IV pentamidine have not had difficulty with the aerosol.

In the report by Leoung, Feigel, and Montgomery[52] there was no detectable additive toxicity to aerosol pentamidine plus zidovudine, but there was an additive protective effect. Patients who received both agents had greater levels of protection than that provided by either drug alone.

Dapsone

Dapsone used alone apparently is an effective preventive agent for *P. carinii* pneumonia. Metroka, Jacobus, and Lewis[63] have reported substantial protective effects resulting from administration of dapsone, 25 mg four times a day. Adverse reactions occurred in 10% of patients. Likewise Lang et al.[49] found dapsone 50 to 100 mg/day, was effective in preventing *P. carinii* pneumonia and had a low rate of adverse effects. Torres et al.[96] have conducted a prospective randomized trial comparing dapsone, 100 mg twice weekly, with aerosol pentamidine, 100 mg every 2 weeks. No difference in efficacy was detected, and similar rates of adverse reactions were noted.

Dapsone offers the advantage of being very inexpensive and easily administered. However, the cost savings may be offset somewhat by the need to monitor for adverse reactions, especially anemia. Moreover, the possible additive toxic effects of dapsone plus zidovudine have not been determined.

Pyrimethamine-Sulfadoxine

The pyrimethamine and sulfadoxine combination (Fansidar) has been tried in relatively small numbers of patients and seems to decrease the incidence of *P. carinii* pneumonia.[23] However, a major concern has been the propensity of the drug to cause severe adverse reactions, including fatal Stevens-Johnson syndrome. For this reason its use has been limited. Given the better safety and probably at least equal efficacy of other regimens, pyrimethamine-sulfadoxine should not be used as preventive therapy.

Prevention Strategies

Based on available data, the Centers for Disease Control[9] has recommended that prophylaxis for *P. carinii* pneumonia be instituted for any HIV-infected adult who has had a previous episode of *P. carinii* pneumonia, who has fewer than 200 circulating CD4+ lymphocytes/μl peripheral blood, or whose CD4+ cell count is less than 20% of the total lymphocyte count. In infants, because they may develop *P. carinii* pneumonia with CD4+ lymphocyte counts well in excess of 200 cells/μl, it has been suggested that prophylaxis be given simply on the basis of HIV infection.

It is recommended that patients with HIV infection have CD4+ cells measured at 6-month intervals or more frequently if there are HIV-associated conditions such as thrush, which indicate immunocompromise. CD4+ counts may vary considerably over time; thus rigid adherence to the 200 CD4+ cell threshold may miss some patients who are at risk for *P. carinii* infection. Based on the previously cited comparison of TMP-SMX with aerosol pentamidine, prophylaxis should be initiated with TMP-SMX, one double-strength tablet daily. Oral dapsone, 100 mg daily or twice weekly, may be used for patients intolerant of TMP-SMX, and aerosol pentamidine should be administered to those who cannot take either of the oral regimens.

Candidates for prophylaxis with aerosol pentamidine should be evaluated to exclude current active pulmonary diseases, especially tuberculosis. Persons with untreated active pulmonary tuberculosis who are given aerosol pentamidine may pose a particular hazard for spreading the organism.[11] The optimum regimen apparently is 300 mg given once a month, using the Respigard II nebulizer or another nebulizer that generates small particles.

REFERENCES

1. Allegra CJ, Chabner BA, Tuazon CU, et al: Trimetrexate for the treatment of *Pneumocystis carinii* pneumonia in patients with acquired immunodeficiency syndrome. N Engl J Med 317:978, 1987
2. Allegra CJ, Kovacs JA, Drake JC, et al: Activity of antifolates against *Pneumocystis carinii* dehydrofolate reductase and identification of a potent new agent. J Exp Med 165:926, 1987
3. Bigby T, Margolskee D, Curtis J, et al: The usefulness of induced sputum in the diagnosis of *Pneumocystis carinii* pneumonia in patients with the acquired immunodeficiency syndrome. Am Rev Respir Dis 133:515, 1986
4. Black JR, Feinberg J, Murphy RL, et al: Clindamycin and primaquine as primary treatment for mild and moderately severe *Pneumocystis carinii* pneumonia in patients with AIDS. Eur J Clin Microbiol Infect Dis 10:204, 1991
5. Bornstein RS, Yarbro JW: An evaluation of the mechanism of action of pentamidine isethionate. J Surg Oncol 2:393, 1970
6. Bozette SA, Sattler FR, Chiu J, et al: A controlled trial of early adjunctive treatment with corticosteroids for *Pneumocystis carinii* pneumonia in the acquired immunodeficiency syndrome. N Engl J Med 323:1451, 1990
7. Broaddus VC, Dake MD, Stulbarg MS, et al: Bronchoalveolar lavage and transbronchial biopsy for the diagnosis of pulmonary infections in patients with the acquired immunodeficiency syndrome. Ann Intern Med 102:747, 1985
8. Burke BA, Good RA: *Pneumocystis carinii* infection. Medicine 52:23, 1973
9. Centers for Disease Control: Guidelines for prophylaxis against *Pneumocystis carinii* pneumonia for persons infected with human immunodeficiency virus. MMWR 38(S5):1, 1989
10. Centers for Disease Control: HIV/AIDS Surveillance Report, 1991, pp 1-22
11. Centers for Disease Control: *Mycobacterium tuberculosis* transmission in a health clinic — Florida, 1989. MMWR 38:256, 1989
12. Conte JE Jr, Chernoff D, Feigel DW Jr, et al: Intravenous or inhaled pentamidine for treating *Pneumocystis carinii* pneumonia in AIDS. Ann Intern Med 113:203, 1990
13. Conte JE Jr, Hollander H, Golden JA: Inhaled pentamidine or reduced dose intravenous pentamidine for *Pneumocystis carinii* pneumonia. A pilot study. Ann Intern Med 107:495, 1987
14. Conte JE Jr, Upton RA, Phelps RT, et al: Use of a specific and sensitive assay to determine pentamidine pharmacokinetics in patients with AIDS. J Infect Dis 154:923, 1986
15. Drake S, Lampasona V, Nicks HL, et al: Pentamidine isethionate in the treatment of *Pneumocystis carinii* pneumonia. Clin Pharm 4:507, 1985
16. Dutz W: *Pneumocystis carinii* pneumonia. Pathol Ann 5:309, 1970
17. Edman JC, Kovacs JA, Masur H, et al: Ribosomal RHA sequence shows *Pneumocystis carinii* to be a member of the fungi. Nature 334:519, 1988
18. Elvin KM, Lumbwe CM, Luo NP, et al: *Pneumocystis carinii* is not a major cause of pneumonia in HIV-infected patients in Lusaka, Zambia. Trans R Soc Trop Med Hyg 83:553, 1989
19. Eng RHK, Bishburg E, Smith SM: Evidence for destruction of lung tissue during *Pneumocystis carinii* infection. Arch Intern Med 147:746, 1987
20. Falloon J, Kovacs J, Allegra C, et al: A pilot study of piritrexim (PIX) with leucovorin (LCV) for the treatment of *Pneumocystis* pneumonia. Sixth International Conference on AIDS, San Francisco. (Abstract no. ThB399.) 1990
21. Falloon J, Kovacs J, Hughes W: A preliminary evaluation of 566C80 for the treatment of *Pneumocystis carinii* pneumonia in patients with the acquired immunodeficiency syndrome. N Engl J Med 325:1534, 1991
22. Feinberg J, Katy D, McDermott C, et al: Trimetrexate (TMX) salvage therapy of PCP in AIDS patients without any therapeutic options: Interim results of the first AIDS "treatment IND" protocol. Fifth International Conference on AIDS, Montreal. (Abstract TBO 28:201.) 1989

23. Fischl MA, Dickinson GM: Fansidar prophylaxis of *Pneumocystis* pneumonia in the acquired immunodeficiency syndrome (letter). Ann Intern Med 105:629, 1986

24. Fischl MA, Dickinson GM, La Voie L: Safety and efficacy of sulfamethoxazole and trimethoprim chemoprophylaxis for *Pneumocystis carinii* pneumonia in AIDS. JAMA 259:1185, 1988

25. Fleischer AG, McElvaney G, Lawson L, et al: Surgical management of spontaneous pneumothorax in patients with acquired immunodeficiency syndrome. Ann Thorac Surg 45:21, 1988

26. Furuta T, Ueda K, Fujiwara K, Yamanouchi K: Cellular and humoral immune responses of mice subclinically infected with *Pneumocystis carinii*. Infect Immun 47:544, 1985

27. Furuta T, Ueda K, Kyuwa S, Fujiwara K: Effect of T-cell transfer on *Pneumocystis carinii* infection in nude mice. Jpn J Exp Med 54:59, 1984

28. Gagnon S, Boota AM, Fischl MA, et al: Corticosteroids as adjunctive therapy for severe *Pneumocystis carinii* pneumonia in the acquired immunodeficiency syndrome. N Engl J Med 323:1444, 1990

29. Gigliotti F, Hughes WT: Passive immunoprophylaxis with specific monoclonal antibody confers partial protection against *Pneumocystis carinii* pneumonitis in animals. J Clin Invest 81:1666, 1988

30. Golden JA, Hollander H, Stulbarg MS, Gamsu G: Bronchoalveolar lavage as the exclusive diagnostic modality for *Pneumocystis carinii* pneumonia. Chest 90:18, 1986

31. Golden JA, Sjoerdsma A, Santi DV: *Pneumocystis carinii* pneunmonia treated with α-difluoromethylornithine. West J Med 141:613, 1984

32. Goodgame RW: AIDS in Uganda—Clinical and social features. N Engl J Med 323:383, 1990

33. Goodman PC: *Pneumocystis carinii* pneumonia. J Thorac Imaging 6:16, 1991

34. Gordin FM, Simon GL, Wofsy CR, Mills J: Adverse reactions to trimethoprim-sulfamethoxazole in patients with the acquired immunodeficiency syndrome. Ann Intern Med 100:495, 1984

35. Gottlieb MS, Schroff R, Schanker HM, et al: *Pneumocystis carinii* pneumonia and mucosal candidiasis in previously healthy homosexual men. N Engl J Med 305:1425, 1981

36. Haverkos HW: PCP Therapy Project Group. Assessment of therapy for *Pneumocystis carinii* pneumonia. Am J Med 76:501, 1984

37. Hughes WT: Geographic distribution. In Hughes WT: *Pneumocystis carinii* Pneumonitis, vol 1. Boca Raton, Florida, CRC Press, 1987, p 33

38. Hughes WT: The organism. In Hughes WT: *Pneumocystis carinii* Pneumonitis, vol 1. Boca Raton, Florida, CRC Press, 1987, p 9

39. Hughes WT, Feldman S, Chaudhary SC, et al: Comparison of pentamidine isethionate and trimethoprim-sulfamethoxazole in the treatment of *Pneumocystis carinii* pneumonia. J Pediatr 92:285, 1978

40. Hughes WT, Feldman S, Sanyal SK: Treatment of *Pneumocystis carinii* pneumonitis with trimethoprim-sulfamethoxazole. Can Med Assoc J 112:475, 1975

41. Hughes WT, Kuhn S, Chaudhary S, et al: Successful chemoprophylaxis for *Pneumocystis carinii* pneumonitis. N Engl J Med 297:1419, 1977

42. Hughes WT, Smith BL: Efficacy of diaminodiphenylsulfone and other drugs in murine *Pneumocystis carinii* pneumonitis. Antimicrob Agents Chemother 26:436, 1984

43. Jules-Elysee KM, Stover DE, Zaman MB, et al: Aerosolized pentamidine: Effect on diagnosis and presentation of *Pneumocystis carinii* pneumonia. Ann Intern Med 112:750, 1990

44. Kernbaum S, Mosliah J, Alcindor LG, et al: Phospholipase activities in bronchoalveolar lavage fluid in rat *Pneumocystis carinii* pneumonia. Brit J Exp Pathol 64:75, 1983

45. Klein MC, Duncanson FP, Lennox TH, et al: Prospective randomized treatment for *Pneumocystis carinii* (PCP) in AIDS patients. Proc Second Int Conference AIDS 52, 1986

46. Kovacs JA, Allegra CJ, Beaver J, et al: Characterization of de novo folate synthesis in *Pneumocystis carinii* and *Toxoplasma gondii*. Potential utilization for screening therapeutic agents. J Infect Dis 160:312, 1989

47. Kovacs JA, Halpern JL, Swan JC, et al: Identification of antigens and antibodies specific for *Pneumocystis carinii*. J Immunol 140:2023, 1988

48. Kucers A, Bennett NMcK: Trimethoprim and co-trimoxazole. In: The Use of Antibiotics. London, William Heinemann Medical Books, Ltd, 1979, p 687

49. Lang OS, Kessinger JM, Tucker RM, et al: Low dose dapsone prophylaxis of *Pneumocystis carinii* pneumonia. Fifth International Conference on AIDS, Montreal. (Abstract TR05 196.) 1989

50. Larivierre M, Ruskin J: Low dose trimethoprim-sulfamethoxazole (T/S) preventing *Pneumocystis* pneumonia (PP) in AIDS. International Conference on Antimicrobial Agents and Chemotherapy. (Abstract no. 7.) 1990
51. Leibovitz E, Rigaud M, Pollack H, et al: *Pneumocystis carinii* pneumonia in infants infected with the human immunodeficiency virus with more than 4500 CD4 T-lymphocytes per cubic millimeter. N Engl J Med 323:531, 1990
52. Leoung GS, Feigel DW Jr, Montgomery AB: Pentamidine for prophylaxis against *Pneumocystis carinii* pneumonia: The San Francisco community prophylaxis trial. N Engl J Med 323:769, 1990
53. Leoung GS, Mills J, Hopewell PC, et al: Dapsone-trimethoprim for *Pneumocystis carinii* pneumonia in the acquired immunodeficiency syndrome. Ann Intern Med 105:45, 1986
54. Levine SJ, Masur H, Gill VJ, et al: Effect of aerosolized pentamidine prophylaxis on the diagnosis of *Pneumocystis carinii* pneumonia by induced sputum examination in patients infected with the human immunodeficiency virus. Am Rev Respir Dis 144:760, 1991
55. Limper AH, Martin WJ III: *Pneumocystis carinii:* Inhibition of lung cell growth mediated by parasite attachment. J Clin Invest 85:391, 1990
56. Mason GR, Duane GM, Mena I, Effros RM: Accelerated solute clearance in *Pneumocystis carinii* pneumonia. Am Rev Respir Dis 135:864, 1987
57. Masur H, Michelis MA, Greene JB, et al: An outbreak of community acquired *Pneumocystis carinii* pneumonia. N Engl J Med 305:1431, 1981
58. Masur H, Ognibene FP, Yarchoan R, et al: CD4 counts as predictors of opportunistic pneumonias in human immunodeficiency virus (HIV) infection. Ann Intern Med 111:223, 1989
59. McLees BD, Barlow JLR, Kuzma RJ, et al: Successful eflornithine (DFMO) treatment in AIDS patients failing conventional therapy. Am Rev Respir Dis 135:A167, 1987
60. McLeod DT, Neill P, Robertson VJ, et al: Pulmonary diseases in patients infected with the human immunodeficiency virus in Zimbabwe, Central Africa. Trans R Soc Trop Med Hyg 83:694, 1989
61. Medina I, Mills J, Leoung G, et al: Oral therapy for *Pneumocystis carinii* pneumonia in the acquired immunodeficiency syndrome: A controlled trial of trimethoprim-sulfamethoxazole versus trimethoprim-dapsone. N Engl J Med 323:776, 1990
62. Metersky ML, Catanzaro A: Diagnostic approach to *Pneumocystis carinii* pneumonia in the setting of prophylactic aerosolized pentamidine. Chest 100:1345, 1991
63. Metroka CE, Jacobus D, Lewis N: Successful prophylaxis for pneumocystis with dapsone or bactrum. Fifth International Conference on AIDS, Montreal. (Abstract TR04 196.) 1989
64. Meuwissen JHETh, Tauber I, Leeuwenberg ADEM, et al: Parasitologic and serologic observations of infection with *Pneumocystis* in humans. J Infect Dis 136:43, 1977
65. Miller RF, Millar AB, Weller IVD, Semple JSG: Empirical treatment without bronchoscopy for *Pneumocystis carinii* pneumonia in the acquired immunodeficiency syndrome. Thorax 44:559, 1989
66. Mills J, Leoung G, Medina I, et al: Dapsone treatment of *Pneumocystis carinii* pneumonia in the acquired immunodeficiency syndrome. Antimicrob Agent Chemother 32:1057, 1988
67. Montaner JSG, Lawson LM, Levitt N, et al: Corticosteroids prevent early deterioration in patients with moderately severe *Pneumocystis carinii* pneumonia and the acquired immunodeficiency syndrome (AIDS). Ann Intern Med 113:14, 1990
68. Montgomery AB, Debs RJ, Luce JM, et al: Aerosolized pentamidine as a second-line therapy in patients with the acquired immunodeficiency syndrome and *Pneumocystis carinii* pneumonia. Chest 95:747, 1989
69. Montgomery AB, Edison RE, Sattler F, et al: Aerosolized pentamidine vs. trimethoprim-sulfamethoxazole for acute *Pneumocystis carinii* pneumonia (PCP): A randomized double blind trial. Sixth International Conference on AIDS, San Francisco. (Abstract no. ThB395.) 1990
70. Montgomery AB, Luce JM, Turner J, et al: Aerosolized pentamidine as sole therapy for *Pneumocystis carinii* pneumonia in patients with the acquired immunodeficiency syndrome. Lancet 2:480, 1987
71. Moragn A, Graziani A, MacGregor RR: Daily vs. intermittent trimethoprim-sulfamethoxazole for *Pneumocystis carinii* pneumonia prophylaxis. International Conference on Antimicrobial Agents and Chemotherapy. (Abstract no. 856.) 1990
72. Murray JF, Felton CP, Garay S, et al: Pulmonary complications of the acquired immunodeficiency syndrome: Report of a National Heart, Lung and Blood Institute Workshop. N Engl J Med 310:1682, 1984

73. National Institute of Allergy and Infectious Diseases: Note to physicians: Important therapeutic information on prevention of recurrent *Pneumocystis carinii* pneumonia in persons with AIDS. Oct 11, 1991

74. Ng VL, Gartner I, Weymouth LA, et al: The use of mucolysed induced sputum for the identification of pulmonary pathogens associated with human immunodeficiency virus infection. Arch Pathol Lab Med 113:488, 1989

75. Ng VL, Virani NA, Chaisson RE, et al: Rapid detection of *Pneumocystis carinii* using a direct fluorescent monoclonal antibody stain. J Clin Microbiol 28:2228, 1990

76. Ng VL, Yajko DM, McPhaul LW, et al: Evaluation of an indirect fluorescent-antibody stain for detection of *Pneumocystis carinii* in respiratory specimens. J Clin Microbiol 28:975, 1990

77. O'Brien RF, Quinn JL, Myakara BT, et al: Diagnosis of *Pneumocystis carinii* pneumonia by induced sputum in a city with a moderate incidence of AIDS. Chest 95:136, 1989

78. Peglow SL, Smulian AG, Linke MJ, et al: Serologic responses to *Pneumocystis carinii* in health and disease. J Infect Dis 161:296, 1990

79. Pesanti EL: In vitro effects of antiprotozoan drugs and immune serum on *Pneumocystis carinii*. J Infect Dis 141:775, 1980

80. Pifer LL, Hughes WT, Stagno S, Woods D: *Pneumocystis carinii* infection: Evidence for high prevalence in normal and immunosuppressed children. Pediatrics 61:35, 1978

81. Pitchenick AE, Ganjei P, Torres A, et al: Sputum examination for the diagnosis of *Pneumocystis carinii* in the acquired immunodeficiency syndrome. Am Rev Respir Dis 133:226, 1986

82. Pottratz ST, Martin WJ III: Role of fibronectin in *Pneumocystis carinii* attachment to cultured lung cells. J Clin Invest 85:351, 1990

83. Raviglione MC: Extrapulmonary pneumocystosis: The first 50 cases. Rev Infect Dis 12:1127, 1990

84. Rosen MJ, Cucco RA, Teirstein AS: Outcome of intensive care in patients with the acquired immunodeficiency syndrome. J Intensive Care Med 1:55, 1986

85. Ruf B, Rohde I, Pohle HD: Efficacy of clindamycin-primaquine vs. trimethoprim-sulfamethoxazole in primary treatment of *Pneumocystis carinii* pneumonia. Eur J Clin Microbial Infect Dis 10:207, 1991

86. Sattler FR, Cowan R, Nielson DM, Ruskin J: Trimethoprim-sulfamethoxazole compared with pentamidine for treatment of *Pneumocystis carinii* pneumonia in the acquired immunodeficiency syndrome. Ann Intern Med 109:280, 1988

87. Schein RM, Fischl MA, Pitchenik AE, Sprung CL: ICU survival of patients with the acquired immunodeficiency syndrome. Crit Care Med 14:1026, 1986

88. Sheehan PM, Stokes DC, Yeh Y-Y, Hughes WT: Surfactant phospholipids and lavage phospholipase A 2 in experimental *Pneumocystis carinii* pneumonia. Am Rev Respir Dis 134:526, 1986

89. Shelhamer JH, Ognibene FP, Macher AM, et al: Persistence of *Pneumocystis carinii* in lung tissue of acquired immunodeficiency syndrome patients treated for *Pneumocystis* pneumonia. Am Rev Respir Dis 130:1161, 1984

90. Soo Hoo GW, Mohsenifar Z, Meyer RD: Inhaled or intravenous pentamidine therapy for *Pneumocystis carinii* pneumonia in AIDS: A randomized trial. Ann Intern Med 113:199, 1990

91. Stein DS, Terry D, Palte S, Lancaster DJ, Weiner JJ: Thrice weekly dosing of trimethoprim-sulfa (T/S) for primary (1°) and secondary (2°) prophylaxis of *P. carinii* pneumonia. International Conference on Antimicrobial Agents and Chemotherapy. (Abstract no. 854.) 1990

92. Stover DE, White DA, Romano PA, Gellene RA: Diagnosis of pulmonary disease in the acquired immunodeficiency syndrome: Roles of bronchoscopy and bronchoalveolar lavage. Am Rev Respir Dis 131:659, 1984

93. Stringer SL, Hudson K, Blase MA, et al: Sequence from ribosomal RNA of *Pneumocystis carinii* compared to those of four fungi suggests an ascomycetous affinity. J Protozool 36(suppl):14S, 1989

94. The National Institutes of Health—University of California Expert Panel for Corticosteroids as Adjunctive Therapy for *Pneumocystis* Pneumonia: Consensus statement on the use of corticosteroids as adjunctive therapy for *Pneumocystis* pneumonia in the acquired immunodeficiency syndrome. N Engl J Med 323:1500, 1990

95. Toma E: Clindamycin-primaquine for treatment of *Pneumocystis carinii* pneumonia in AIDS. Eur J Clin Microbiol Infect Dis 10:210, 1990

96. Torres R, Thorn M, Ortiz P, et al: Randomized trial of intermittent dapsone versus aerosolized pentamidine for primary and secondary prophylaxis of *Pneumocystis carinii* pneumonia (PCP). Sixth International Conference on AIDS, San Francisco. (Abstract no. ThB407.) 1990

97. Waalkes TP, Makulu DR: Pharmacologic aspects of pentamidine. Dep Health Educ Welfare, Nat Inst Health, Natl Cancer Inst Monogr 43:171, 1976
98. Wachter RM, Luce JM, Turner J, et al: Intensive care of patients with the acquired immunodeficiency syndrome: Outcome and changing patterns of utilization. Am Rev Respir Dis 134:891, 1986
99. Wachter RM, Russi MB, Bloch DA, et al: *Pneumocystis carinii* pneumonia and respiratory failure in AIDS: Improved outcomes and increased use of intensive care units. Am Rev Respir Dis 143:251-256, 1991
100. Watanabe J-I, Hori H, Tanabe K, Nakamura Y: 5 S ribosomal RNA sequence of *Pneumocystis carinii* and its phylogenetic association with rhizopoda/myxomycota/zygomycota group. J Protozool 36(suppl):16S, 1989
101. Wharton JM, Coleman DL, Wofsy CB, et al: Trimethoprim-sulfamethoxazole or pentamidine for *Pneumocystis carinii* pneumonia in the acquired immunodeficiency syndrome. Ann Intern Med 105:37, 1985
102. Wolfson JS, Waldron MA, Sierra LS: Blended comparison of a direct immunofluorescent monoclonal antibody staining method and a Giemsa staining method for identification of *Pneumocystis carinii* in induced sputum and bronchoalveolar lavage specimens of patients infected with human immunodeficiency virus. J Clin Microbiol 28:2136, 1990

18

MYCOBACTERIAL DISEASES

Tuberculosis and Disseminated *Mycobacterium avium* Complex Infection

MARK A. JACOBSON, MD

MYCOBACTERIUM TUBERCULOSIS INFECTION IN AIDS AND ARC

Epidemiology and Pathogenesis

Since the beginning of the AIDS epidemic, an increasing association of *Mycobacterium tuberculosis* infection with AIDS or HIV infection has been noted. Nationwide, by matching the first 53,395 AIDS cases with 144,123 concurrent tuberculosis cases, 3.8% of individuals with AIDS have had tuberculosis, and 1.4% of individuals with tuberculosis have had AIDS.[13]

Between 1978 and 1985 the yearly rate of tuberculosis more than doubled at one New York City hospital. This increase was almost completely attributable to cases among patients with AIDS or AIDS-related complex (ARC).[22] During the same time period the incidence of tuberculosis increased from 15.4/100,000 to 105.5/100,000 among inmates of the New York State prison system, and a majority of inmates with tuberculosis reported in 1985 and 1986 had AIDS or HIV infection.[7] Nationally, from 1980 to 1984 the tuberculosis incidence decreased by 7% each year, but from 1985 to 1987 it increased by 1.4%.[13] In New York, California, Florida, and New Jersey (the states reporting the most cases of AIDS), extrapulmonary tuberculosis increased by 12% to 64%, and tuberculosis among 25 to 44 year olds increased by 14% to 34% from 1985 to 1987.[13] These figures suggest HIV infection is an important factor in the changing epidemiology of tuberculosis.

Tuberculosis has been reported in 2% to 10% of AIDS patients studied in large retrospective series from New York, New Jersey, and Florida.[9,54,55] In San Francisco

12% of 287 consecutive cases of tuberculosis in non-Asian-born males, 15 to 60 years old, also had AIDS.[9] Patients with AIDS and tuberculosis in these series were more likely to be Haitian, black, Hispanic, or intravenous drug users than white and homosexual.[9,54]

Since host resistance to *M. tuberculosis* is mediated by cellular immunity, it is not surprising that tuberculosis has been associated with human immunodeficiency virus (HIV) infection.[10] Epidemiologic data suggest that most cases of AIDS- or ARC-associated tuberculosis represent reactivation of latent *M. tuberculosis* infection acquired in the past rather than progression from recently acquired infection.[49,55] A prospective study of New York City intravenous drug users tested for HIV seropositivity and purified protein derivative (PPD) skin test reactivity demonstrated that, although prevalence and incidence of tuberculosis infection were similar to both HIV-seropositive and HIV-seronegative intravenous drug users, risk of developing **active** tuberculosis was elevated for the HIV-seropositive individuals.[49]

The retrospective studies are remarkably consistent in that tuberculosis preceded the diagnosis of AIDS in half of patients with AIDS-associated tuberculosis and occurred concurrently or following diagnosis of AIDS in the other half.[9,55] However, these retrospective studies, performed by matching tuberculosis and AIDS registries in a given hospital or community, could underestimate the full spectrum of tuberculous disease associated with HIV immune deficiency. A prospective study in Miami addressed this issue by prospectively screening tuberculosis patients for HIV antibody.[46] Of 71 consecutive patients with confirmed tuberculosis, 31% were seropositive for HIV. At the time of tuberculosis diagnosis, only 27% of these HIV-seropositive patients had clinical evidence of AIDS or ARC. In a similarly prospective study in San Francisco, 17 of 60 (28%) non-Asian-born patients 18 to 65 years old and with newly diagnosed tuberculosis were HIV seropositive.[53] Thus the number and incidence of tuberculosis cases related to HIV-induced immunosuppression may be considerably larger than indicated by retrospective studies. In fact, data from Africa suggest that spread of HIV infection has led to a logarithmic increase in tuberculosis rates. In subSaharan African countries 19% to 30% of patients with HIV disease develop tuberculosis, and 15% to 59% of tuberculosis cases are HIV positive.[45]

Clinical Manifestations

Although the pathogenesis of most HIV-associated tuberculosis appears to involve reactivation of latent *M. tuberculosis* infection, the clinical presentation is generally typical of reactivation tuberculosis only for those patients whose immune function is still relatively intact, whereas that of patients with AIDS or ARC is much more typical of progressive primary tuberculosis (Table 18–1). Only one third to one half of AIDS- and ARC-associated tuberculosis is confined to the lungs. The most frequent radiographic manifestations of pulmonary tuberculosis in patients with AIDS and ARC are (1) hilar or mediastinal adenopathy or both and (2) localized infiltrates limited to the middle or lower lung fields.[47] Pulmonary cavitation is rarely seen.[9,49,52] The classic radiographic picture of apical infiltrates in the absence of hilar or mediastinal adenopathy has been reported in less than 10% of AIDS- or ARC-associated cases.[11,49,52]

One half to two thirds of AIDS- and ARC-related tuberculosis involves extra-

Table 18–1. Clinical Features of AIDS- and ARC-Associated Tuberculosis

Radiographic Features of Pulmonary Tuberculosis
Common
  Hilar and/or mediastinal adenopathy
  Localized infiltrate in lower and middle lung fields
Rare
  Cavitation
  Apical infiltrate
Extrapulmonary Sites are Involved in More Than Half of Cases
Sites most likely to be positive: peripheral lymph nodes and bone marrow
Other extrapulmonary sites of infection: blood, bone, urine, joint, liver, spleen, cerebrospinal fluid, skin, gastrointestinal mucosa, ascites
Important unusual syndromes: central nervous system mass lesion (tuberculoma), *Mycobacterium tuberculosis* bacteremia

pulmonary sites (with or without pulmonary involvement).[9,49,52] Peripheral lymph nodes and bone marrow are the extrapulmonary sites most frequently positive for *M. tuberculosis*. Granulomas are observed in approximately 50% of extrapulmonary biopsies but rarely in pulmonary biopsies.[52] Other extrapulmonary sites that have revealed *M. tuberculosis* include urine, blood, bone, joint, cerebrospinal fluid, liver, spleen, skin, gastrointestinal mucosa, and ascites fluid. Two extrapulmonary tuberculosis syndromes described in AIDS and ARC patients are of particular interest: *M. tuberculosis* bacteremia and central nervous system mass lesions. Bacteremia due to *M. tuberculosis*, rarely reported before the AIDS epidemic, has been reported in 26% to 42% of patients with HIV infection who have tuberculosis.[3] Also, central nervous system mass lesions caused by *M. tuberculosis* were reported in a series of eight intravenous drug users with ARC.[6] These mass lesions caused a wide range of clinical manifestations and radiographic appearances on computed tomographic scans of the brain. The diagnosis was confirmed only by brain biopsy.

On the other hand, tuberculosis in patients with otherwise asymptomatic HIV infection usually is clinically similar to tuberculosis in immunocompetent hosts.[10] Chaisson et al.[11] compared clinical findings in 17 HIV-seropositive and 40 HIV-seronegative non-Asian-born men with tuberculosis newly diagnosed at the San Francisco General Hospital TB Clinic. There were no significant differences in PPD reactivity or chest x-ray findings. The median CD4+ lymphocyte count in the HIV-seropositive individuals was 350/µl, substantially higher than that generally observed in individuals with advanced ARC or AIDS. Narciso et al.,[41] in Italy, similarly reported a significant difference in mean CD4+ counts among HIV-infected individuals with miliary tuberculosis (101/µl) and nonmiliary tuberculosis (312/µl).

Diagnosis

Anergy is frequent in patients with AIDS and ARC, and only 10% to 40% of such patients have a positive tuberculin skin test at the time of tuberculosis diagnosis.[9,52] Nevertheless, tuberculin skin tests should be administered when tuberculosis is suspected in an AIDS or ARC patient. However, since false-negative results are common, the absence of skin test reactivity does not rule out the diagnosis.

Individuals with earlier stage HIV disease and tuberculosis are more likely to react to tuberculin antigen. Seventy-nine percent of such patients had a positive PPD result in one study.[11] However, because of the increasing incidence of anergy among HIV-infected individuals, a >5-mm reaction to PPD should be considered evidence of tuberculosis infection.[56]

Appropriate specimens to culture for confirmation of tuberculosis include sputum, urine, blood, lymph node material, bone marrow, and liver. In the presence of pulmonary infiltrates, induced sputum or respiratory secretions obtained by bronchoscopy provide the optimum specimen. In patients with HIV-associated pulmonary tuberculosis, up to half of acid-fast bacteria (AFB) smears of respiratory or extrapulmonary specimens are negative, as later proved by positive culture.[10,37,52] Hence the decision to institute empiric antituberculous therapy often must be made before microbiologic confirmation of the diagnosis.

Therapy

Although tuberculosis is a more rapidly progressive and widely disseminated disease in AIDS and ARC patients than in controls without HIV infection, the response rate of AIDS and ARC patients to antituberculous therapy is generally as favorable as in non-AIDS and non-ARC historical controls. Treatment failures with standard two- to four-day regimens have been uncommon in retrospective series, and drug-resistant strains of *M. tuberculosis* rarely have been isolated (although several recent case clusters have been reported in New York City and Miami).[57] Small et al.[51] recently reviewed results of therapy of 132 AIDS patients treated for tuberculosis. Only 3 (5%) of 58 patients who completed an adequate therapeutic regimen (isoniazid and rifampin for 9 months or isoniazid, rifampin, and pyrazinamide for 6 months) subsequently relapsed during a total of 82.3 patient-years of follow-up. All failures occurred in noncompliant patients. Drug toxicity required modification of the treatment regimen in 18% of patients (three times the percentage of HIV-seronegative individuals in previously reported studies). Although AIDS and ARC patients with tuberculosis had a higher rate of rash and abnormal liver function test results associated with antituberculous therapy compared to non–HIV-infected historical control tuberculosis patients, serious antituberculous drug reactions requiring discontinuation of any effective regimen were rare.

The Centers for Disease Control (CDC) recommend initiating antituberculous chemotherapy whenever AFB are found in a specimen from a patient with HIV infection and clinical evidence of mycobacterial disease.[56] Since it is difficult to distinguish tuberculosis from disseminated *M. avium* complex infection, therapy should continue until culture results are final (usually 6 to 8 weeks). The recommended regimen for adults (Table 18–2) includes isoniazid 300 mg/day, rifampin 600 mg/day (450 mg/day for patients weighing <50 kg), and pyrazinamide 25 mg/kg/day for the first 2 months. Ethambutol 25 mg/kg/day should be added if extrapulmonary tuberculosis or isoniazid resistance is suspected. Subsequently, isoniazid and rifampin alone should be continued. The appropriate duration of treatment for HIV-associated tuberculosis is unknown, but a minimum duration of 9 months or at least 6 months after culture conversion (whichever is longer) seems reasonable. For patients who either cannot tolerate isoniazid or rifampin or have bone or joint disease, therapy probably should continue for 18 months.

Table 18–2. Empiric Regimen for Patients with HIV-Associated Tuberculosis*

First 2 Mo
Isoniazid, 300 mg/day
Rifampin, 600 mg/day†
Pyrazinamide, 25 mg/kg/day
Ethambutol, 25 mg/kg/day, if extrapulmonary disease or isoniazid resistance suspected
Additional 7 Mo or 6 Mo after Cultures Negative
Isoniazid, 300 mg/day
Rifampin, 600 mg/day†

*For use whenever acid-fast bacteria are demonstrated in a specimen from a patient with HIV infection and clinical evidence of mycobacterial disease.
†Use 450 mg/day if weight <50 kg.

Clinicians treating AIDS and ARC patients with isoniazid and rifampin must be aware of pharmacokinetic interactions that can occur between these drugs and the antifungal azoles, ketoconazole and fluconazole (also commonly administered to AIDS and ARC patients for superficial or systemic opportunistic fungal infections), which can lead to subtherapeutic levels of both rifampin and ketoconazole or of fluconazole.[18,35] These drug interactions have been associated with therapeutic failure of antifungal and/or antituberculous treatment.

Although response to antituberculous therapy has been good in retrospective studies, the survival rate among patients with advanced HIV disease and tuberculosis has been poor, similar to that of other AIDS or ARC patients followed for similar periods of time.[51]

Prevention

Since antituberculous prophylactic therapy apparently is effective in HIV-infected populations with *M. tuberculosis* infection, the CDC recommends that all asymptomatic HIV-seropositive individuals be given a skin test with five tuberculin units of PPD and all symptomatic HIV-infected patients should receive both a skin test and a screening chest x-ray examination because of the higher probability of a false-negative skin test result[56] (Table 18–3). Any HIV-infected patient, whatever age, with a tuberculin reaction >5 mm or a history of positive skin test reactivity should receive preventive isoniazid therapy for at least 12 months after sputum cultures have been obtained to exclude active pulmonary tuberculosis.

Table 18–3. Screening for Tuberculosis in HIV-Infected Patients

1. Screening skin test (5 tuberculin units of purified protein derivative) should be administered to all asymptomatic HIV-infected patients; induration >5 mm indicates tuberculous infection.
2. Skin test and chest x-ray examination should be administered to all symptomatic HIV-infected patients.
3. All HIV-infected patients with a positive tuberculin skin test or a history of positive tuberculin skin test should receive prophylactic isoniazid for a minimum of 6 months (sputum mycobacterial cultures should be obtained before instituting isoniazid therapy).

The efficacy of prophylactic isoniazid was highlighted by a prospective study of HIV-infected intravenous drug users in which none of 13 individuals with positive PPD tests who received isoniazid developed tuberculosis during follow-up care as compared to 7 of 36 who did not receive prophylaxis.[49] A shorter course of rifampin plus pyrazinamide is a possible alternative prophylactic regimen for isoniazid-intolerant patients, but the efficacy of this regimen has not been established.[14]

Although risk of developing active tuberculosis is increased by concomitant HIV infection, the risk of spreading tuberculosis to contacts apparently is not greater than that observed with non-HIV-infected tuberculosis cases.[39] However, recent reports of nosocomial transmission of multidrug-resistant tuberculosis to health care workers and HIV-infected patients in the United States emphasize the critical importance of isolating HIV-infected patients with suspected or confirmed tuberculosis until the number of organisms on sequential sputum AFB smears has decreased.[57]

DISSEMINATED *MYCOBACTERIUM AVIUM* COMPLEX INFECTION IN AIDS

Epidemiology and Pathogenesis

The association of disseminated *M. avium* complex (MAC) infection with AIDS was recognized early in the HIV epidemic.[21,38] Disseminated MAC infection has been reported only rarely in patients without AIDS.[25] According to CDC statistics, disseminated MAC was reported in 5.3% of AIDS cases between 1981 and 1987.[26] In a large retrospective series involving 366 AIDS patients, this opportunistic infection was diagnosed during the course of illness in 18% of AIDS patients; however, the attack rate may have been even higher since 53% of 79 autopsies in this series showed evidence of disseminated MAC.[24] Disseminated MAC infection occurs exclusively in patients with very advanced HIV disease, essentially only in patients with CD4 lymphocyte counts $<100/\mu l$.[16,23]

MAC is a ubiquitous soil and water saprophyte. The source of MAC invasion in AIDS patients may be gastrointestinal or respiratory. The presence of large clusters of mycobacteria within macrophages of the small bowel lamina propria suggests the bowel might be the portal of entry. However, respiratory isolation of MAC also frequently precedes disseminated infection, suggesting MAC infection may begin in the lungs as well.[30]

In patients with AIDS the key host defect allowing dissemination of MAC may be macrophage dysfunction. MAC is able to survive within macrophages unless intracellular killing mechanisms (defective in AIDS) are activated. Also, lymphokines present in abnormal levels in patients with AIDS such as tumor necrosis factor, gamma-interferon and interleukin-2 may play an important role in impaired host defense against MAC.

MAC causes high-grade, widely disseminated infection in AIDS patients. Nearly all AIDS patients with invasive MAC infection (as opposed to stool, urinary, or respiratory secretion colonization) have had positive mycobacterial blood cultures.[24] In the majority of those autopsied, MAC also could be isolated from spleen, lymph nodes, liver, lung, adrenals, colon, kidney, and bone marrow. The magnitude of mycobacteremia usually ranges from 10^1 to 10^4 colony-forming units (CFU)/ml of blood.[58] At autopsy, spleen, lymph nodes, and liver have yielded up to 10^{10} CFU/g of tissue.[58] Histopathologic studies of involved organs typically have shown absent or poorly formed granulomas and AFB within macrophages[21] (Color Plate I*D*).

Clinical Manifestations

Since most AIDS patients with disseminated MAC infection have other concomitant infections or neoplasms and since MAC appears to cause little histopathologic evidence of inflammatory response or tissue destruction, the relationship between constitutional symptoms, organ dysfunction, and MAC infection has been uncertain.

Nevertheless, several large retrospective studies strongly suggest a negative effect of disseminated MAC infection on mortality and morbidity in AIDS patients. Horsburgh and Selik[26] compared the survival time of 1101 AIDS patients with disseminated nontuberculous mycobacterial infection (96% of cases due to MAC) to that of 33,808 AIDS patients without disseminated nontuberculous mycobacterial infection. Median survival of patients with an index AIDS diagnosis of disseminated nontuberculous mycobacterial infection was 7.4 months compared with 13.1 or 10.5 months for patients with an index AIDS diagnosis of *Pneumocystis carinii* pneumonia or another AIDS-defining opportunistic infection, respectively. This analysis has been criticized for the passive collection of data, resulting in substantial loss to follow-up.[8]

At San Francisco General Hospital we have examined the association between disseminated MAC infection and survival after index *P. carinii* pneumonia diagnosis.[30] Among 137 consecutive patients in whom a sterile body site cultured for mycobacteria within 3 months of their first AIDS-defining episode of *P. carinii* pneumonia, the median survival time was significantly shorter in those with disseminated MAC infection than in those with negative cultures (107 versus 275 days, $p < .01$) even after controlling for age, absolute lymphocyte count, and hemoglobin concentration. We also have examined the association between disseminated MAC infection and blood transfusion requirements.[32] Between July 1, 1987, and June 30, 1988, blood specimens from 574 patients were submitted to our mycobacteriology laboratory for culture. Among the AIDS and ARC patients transfused during the same time period, patients with a positive blood culture for MAC had a relative risk of 5.23 ($p < .001$) for receiving packed red blood cell (PRBC) transfusions compared to patients whose blood was negative for mycobacterial culture, thus confirming an association between disseminated MAC infection and increased morbidity in AIDS.

Four clinical syndromes, often overlapping, have been associated with disseminated MAC infection. The characteristics of these syndromes are summarized in Table 18–4.

Since 1987 there have been increasing numbers of cases in which AIDS patients receiving antiretroviral therapy with zidovudine (AZT) have developed **localized** visceral or cutaneous MAC abscesses without mycobacteremia.[2,43] Unlike disseminated infection (see below), these lesions have responded remarkably well to drainage and antimycobacterial therapy. These case series have led to speculation that improved immune function resulting from zidovudine therapy was responsible for localization of infection.

Table 18–4.   Clinical Syndromes Associated with Disseminated _M. avium_ Complex Infection in AIDS Patients

Systemic Symptoms
• Fever, malaise, weight loss, often associated with anemia, neutropenia
Gastrointestinal Symptoms
• Chronic diarrhea and abdominal pain (MAC invasion of colon often observed at autopsy)
• Chronic malabsorption (histopathologic changes in small intestine similar to those with Whipple's disease often observed at autopsy)
• Extrabiliary obstructive jaundice secondary to periportal lymphadenopathy

Data from Hawkins, Gold, Whimbey.[24]

Diagnosis

Special blood culture techniques for isolating mycobacteria (e.g., the Bactec system or DuPont isolator) apparently offer the most sensitive method for diagnosing disseminated MAC infection.[62] With these techniques, the sensitivity approaches 100%. Time to culture positivity ranges from 5 to 51 days. Negative blood cultures are uncommon in the presence of positive histology from lymph node, liver, or bone marrow biopsies. However, one advantage to using biopsied specimens is that stains may demonstrate AFB or granuloma weeks before blood cultures turn positive. At one center stool AFB smear and culture positivity correlated well with true MAC bacteremia.[24] However, in other studies stool cultures were positive in only half of mycobacteremias, and only two thirds of positive stools correlated with true disseminated infection. The importance of MAC isolation from sputum is uncertain.

Therapy

MAC is resistant to all standard antituberculous drugs (except ethambutol) at concentrations achievable in plasma. Yet half or more of MAC strains can be inhibited by achievable concentrations of the drugs listed in Table 18–5.[19,20,29,59-62] Unfortunately, drug levels necessary to kill MAC in vitro (minimum bactericidal concentration) have been 8 to > 32 times that of inhibitory levels.[60] Although combinations of antimycobacterial agents have shown in vitro inhibitory synergism, bactericidal synergism has been more difficult to demonstrate.[59,60] In addition, for in vivo killing drugs must penetrate both macrophages and the MAC cell wall. Nevertheless, in animal models of disseminated MAC infection, both single and combination antimycobacterial regimens have reduced mycobacterial colony counts by several logs and improved survival rates.[19,28,34]

In AIDS patients with MAC bloodstream infection, results of uncontrolled, combination antimycobacterial drug trials have been inconclusive. Ansamycin, provided by the CDC under an Investigational New Drug (IND) application, has been given in combination with other antimycobacterial drugs to more than 600 AIDS patients with disseminated MAC infection.[42] Limited follow-up data have shown that eradication of MAC infection was uncommon, and the CDC subsequently terminated this IND program because of lack of evidence of efficacy. Among 13 patients treated at the National Institutes of Health (NIH) with ansamycin and clofazimine, only

**Table 18–5.   Drugs Capable of Inhibiting Most
M. avium Complex Strains at Concentrations
Achievable in Plasma**

Ansamycin (rifabutine)	Clofazimine
Cycloserine	Amikacin
Rifampin	Ciprofloxacin
Ethambutol	Ethionamide
Azithromycin	Clarithromycin
Sparfloxacin	

three had persistently negative results from cultures while receiving therapy, and only one had apparent clinical improvement.[40] Similarly, at Memorial Sloan-Kettering Cancer Center, only three of 15 AIDS patients with disseminated MAC infection had decreased colony forming unit (CFU) counts detected during therapy by sequential cultures.[24]

Several recent uncontrolled clinical trials suggest a more beneficial effect of combination antimycobacterial therapy. Agins et al.[1] reported that five of seven AIDS patients with disseminated MAC infection who were treated with ethambutol, clofazimine, ansamycin, and isoniazid remained abacteremic for 3 to 6 months during which time fever, weight loss, and night sweats resolved. In a California Collaborative Treatment Group study 17 patients who received intravenous amikacin (7.5 mg/kg/day) for 4 weeks and oral ciprofloxacin, ethambutol, and rifampin for 12 weeks had an initial mean 1.5 log decrease in blood mycobacterial counts and a marked reduction in fever and night sweats.[12] Recent preliminary data reported by this same group suggest very similar results were obtained with an all oral regimen of rifampin, ethambutol, ciprofloxacin, and clofazamine, thus casting doubt on the necessity for adding intravenous amikacin.[33] A group of Australian investigators reported that mycobacteremia was cleared in 22 of 25 patients treated with a combination oral regimen of clofazimine, isoniazid, ethambutol, and high-dose rifabutin; 18 of these patients had associated symptomatic improvement.[27]

Given the detrimental effect of this infection on morbidity and survival and the encouraging data from recent controlled trials, it appears that some form of antimycobacterial therapy is indicated for patients with disseminated MAC.[16] Unfortunately, as yet no multicenter controlled trial of therapy for disseminated MAC infection has been done, so the optimum therapeutic regimen is unknown. One reasonable empiric regimen is presented in Table 18–6.

**Table 18–6.   Empiric Regimen for the Treatment
of Disseminated *M. avium* Complex Infection**

Rifampin, 600 mg po qd*
Ethambutol, 15-25 mg/kg po qd
Ciprofloxacin, 750 mg po qd
Clofazimine, 100-200 mg po qd

*Use 450 mg/day if weight <50 kg.

Based on in vitro and in vivo studies, a number of experimental drugs appear to have improved bactericidal activity against MAC. These promising new agents include liposome-encapsulated amikacin and gentamicin, clarithromycin, azithromycin, sparfloxacin, and tumor necrosis factor.[4,5,19,61]

Two of these agents, clarithromycin and azithromycin, are macrolides related to erythromycin and have recently become available outside of clinical trials (i.e., the Food and Drug Adminstration has licensed these agents for the treatment of bacterial upper respiratory infections). Data from a recent, small phase I double-blind cross-over trial of short-term oral clarithromycin monotherapy described a 2 logarithmic decrease in mycobacteremia associated with some symptomatic improvement.[15] Similar results have been reported in a small open-label phase I trial of short-term oral azithromycin.[63] Nevertheless, concern remains about the safety of long-term administration of these agents, which are highly concentrated in body tissues, and about the potential for resistance emerging with chronic antimycobacterial monotherapy.

As mentioned previously, in several small studies of AIDS patients with localized MAC infection, combination antimycobacterial therapy has been quite effective.[2,43]

In HIV-infected patients it may be difficult to distinguish tuberculosis from MAC disease. Therefore an antituberculous regimen should be instituted whenever AFBs are demonstrated in a specimen from a patient with HIV infection and clinical evidence of mycobacterial disease.[56]

ATYPICAL MYCOBACTERIAL INFECTIONS IN AIDS

Disseminated infections caused by *M. kansasii*, *M. gordonae*, *M. fortuitum*, *M. chelonei*, *M. haemophilum*, and *M. xenopi* also have been reported in patients with AIDS.[17,26,36,48] Their clinical presentations generally have been similar to that of MAC infection with pathologic evidence of pulmonary, intestinal, liver, and bone marrow involvement. In vitro sensitivity of isolates to standard antituberculous drugs has been variable.[17,31,48] *M. kansasii* has been the most frequently reported of these other atypical mycobacteria, with disseminated infection present at the time of index AIDS diagnosis in 0.2% of patients.[26] Response to antimycobacterial therapy was poor in one small series of AIDS patients with disseminated *M. kansasii* infection.[50] However, there are reports of complete clinical resolution of pulmonary *M. kansasii* infection in AIDS patients treated with antituberculous therapy.[31,36] Generally, these AIDS-asociated *M. kansasii* isolates have been sensitive to rifampin and ethambutol and resistant to isoniazid. Given the frequent sensitivity of other atypical mycobacteria to one or more standard antituberculous drugs, multidrug therapy tailored to in vitro sensitivities is indicated for AIDS patients with non-MAC atypical mycobacterial infection.

REFERENCES

1. Agins BD, Berman DS, Spicehandler D, et al: Effect of combined therapy with ansamycin, clofazimine, ethambutol, and isoniazid for *Mycobacterium avium* infection in patients with AIDS. J Infect Dis 159:784-787, 1989
2. Barbaro DJ, Orcutt VL, Coldrion BM: *Mycobacterium avium-Mycobacterium intracellulare* in-

fection limited to the skin and lymph nodes in patients with AIDS. Rev Infect Dis 11:625-628, 1989

3. Barnes PF, Bloch AB, Davidson PT, Snider DE: Tuberculosis in patients with human immunodeficiency virus infection. N Engl J Med 324:1644-1650, 1991

4. Bermudez LE, Yau-Young AO, Lin J-P, et al: Treatment of disseminated *Mycobacterium avium* complex infection of beige mice with liposome-encapsulated aminoglycosides. J Infect Dis 161:1262-1268, 1990

5. Bermudez LEM, Young LS: Activities of amikacin, roxithromycin, and azithromycin alone or in combination with tumor necrosis factor against *Mycobacterium avium* complex. Antimicrob Agents Chemother 32:1149-1153, 1988

6. Bishburg E, Sunderam G, Reichman LB, et al: Central nervous system tuberculosis with the acquired immunodeficiency syndrome and its related complex. Ann Intern Med 105:210-213, 1986

7. Braum MM, Truman BI, Maguire B, et al: Increasing incidence of tuberculosis in a prison inmate population. JAMA 261:393-397, 1989

8. Chaisson RE, Hopewell PC: Mycobacteria and AIDS mortality. Am Rev Respir Dis 139:1-3, 1989

9. Chaisson RE, Schecter GF, Theuer CP, et al: Tuberculosis in patients with the acquired immunodeficiency syndrome. Am Rev Respir Dis 136:570-574, 1987

10. Chaisson RE, Slutkin G: Tuberculosis and human immunodeficiency virus infection. J Infect Dis 159:96-100, 1989

11. Chaisson RE, Theurer D, Elias D, et al: HIV seroprevalence in patients with tuberculosis. Presented at Twenty-eighth International Conference on Antimicrobial Agents and Chemotherapy. (Abstract No. 571.) Los Angeles, 1988

12. Chiu J, Nussbaum J, Bozzette S, et al: Treatment of disseminated *Mycobacterium avium* complex infection in AIDS with amikacin, ethambutol, rifampin, and ciprofloxacin. Ann Intern Med 113:358-361, 1990

13. Ciesielski CA, Bloch AB, Dooley SW, Centers for Disease Control—Atlanta: Assessing the impact of human immunodeficiency virus (HIV) on tuberculosis morbidity in the United States. Presented at Twenty-ninth International Conference on Antimicrobial Agents and Chemotherapy. (Abstract No. 269.) Houston, 1989

14. Clermont H, Johnson M, Coberly J, et al: Tolerance of short course TB chemoprophylaxis in HIV-infected individuals. Seventh International Conference on AIDS. (Abstract W.B.2363.) Florence, Italy, 1991

15. Dautzenberg B, Truffot C, Legris S, et al: Activity of clarithromycin against *Mycobacterium avium* infection in patients with the acquired immune deficiency syndrome. Am Rev Respir Dis 144:564-569, 1991

16. Ellner JJ, Goldberger MJ, Parenti DM: *Mycobacterium avium* infection and AIDS: Therapeutic dilemma in rapid evolution. J Infect Dis 163:1326-1335, 1991

17. Eng RHK, Forrester C, Smith SM, et al: *Mycobacterium xenopi* infection in a patient with acquired immunodeficiency syndrome. Chest 86:145-147, 1984

18. Engelhard D, Stutman HR, Marks MI: Interaction of ketoconazole with rifampin and isoniazid. N Engl J Med 311:1681-1683, 1984

19. Fernandes PB, Hardy DJ, McDaniel D, et al: In vitro and in vivo activities of clarithromycin against *Mycobacterium avium*. Antimicrob Agents Chemother 33:1531-1534, 1989

20. Gangadharam PRJ, Kesavalu L, Rao PNR, et al: Activity of amikacin against *Mycobacterium avium* complex under simulated in vivo conditions. Antimicrob Agents Chemother 32:886-889, 1988

21. Greene JB, Sidhu GS, Lewin S, et al: *Mycobacterium avium-intracellulare*: A cause of disseminated life-threatening infection in homosexuals and drug abusers. Ann Intern Med 97:539-546, 1982

22. Handwerger S, Mildvan D, Senie R, McKinley FW: Tuberculosis and the acquired immunodeficiency syndrome at a New York City Hospital: 1978-1985. Chest 91:176-180, 1987

23. Havlik JA, Horsburgh CR, Metchock B, et al: Clinical risk factors for disseminated *Mycobacterium avium* complex infection in persons with HIV infection. Sixth International Conference on AIDS. (Abstract Th.B. 515.) San Francisco, 1990

24. Hawkins CC, Gold JWM, Whimbey E, et al: *Mycobacterium avium* complex infections in patients with the acquired immunodeficiency syndrome. Ann Intern Med 105:184-188, 1986

25. Horsburgh CR, Mason UG, Farhi DC, et al: Disseminated infection with *Mycobacterium avium-intracellulare*. Medicine 64:36-48, 1985

26. Horsburgh CR, Selik RM: The epidemiology of disseminated nontuberculosis mycobacterial infection in the acquired immunodeficiency syndrome (AIDS). Am Rev Respir Dis 139:4-7, 1989

27. Hoy J, Mijch A, Sandland M, et al: Quadruple-drug therapy for *Mycobacterium avium-intracellulare* bacteremia in AIDS patients. J Infect Dis 161:801-805, 1990
28. Inderlied CB, Kolonoski PT, Wu M, et al: Amikacin, ciprofloxacin, and imipenem treatment for disseminated *Mycobacterium avium* complex infection of beige mice. Antimicrob Agents Chemother 33:176-180, 1989
29. Inderlied CB, Kolonoski PT, Wu M, et al: In vitro and in vivo activity of azithromycin (CP 62,993) against the *Mycobacterium avium* complex. J Infect Dis 159:994-997, 1989
30. Jacobson MA, Hopewell PC, Yajko DM, et al: Natural history of disseminated *Mycobacterium avium* complex infection in AIDS. J Infect Dis 164:994-998, 1991
31. Jacobson MA, Isenberg WM: *Mycobacterium kanasii* diffuse pulmonary infection in a patient with acquired immune deficiency syndrome. Am J Clin Pathol 91:236-238, 1989
32. Jacobson MA, Peiperl L, Volberding PA, et al: Red blood cell transfusion therapy for anemia in patients with AIDS and ARC: Incidence associated factors, and outcome. Transfusion 30:133-137, 1990
33. Kemper CA, Chiu J, Meng TC, et al: Microbiologic and clinical response of patients with AIDS and MAC bacteremia to a four oral drug regimen. Thirtieth Interscience Conference on Antimicrobial Agents and Chemotherapy. (Abstract 1267.) Atlanta, 1990
34. Kolonoski PT, Wu M, Petrofsky ML, et al: Combination of amikacin, azithromycin and clofazimine for the treatment of disseminated *Mycobacterium avium* complex infection in beige mice. Presented at Twenty-ninth International Conference on Antimicrobial Agents and Chemotherapy. (Abstract No. 1323.) Houston, 1989
35. Lazar JD, Wilner KD: Drug interactions with fluconazole. Rev Infect Dis 12 (suppl 3):S327-S333, 1990
36. Levine B, Chaisson RE: *Mycobacterium kansasii*: A cause of treatable pulmonary disease associated with advanced human immunodeficiency virus (HIV) infection. Ann Intern Med 114:861-868, 1991
37. Louie E, Rice LB, Holzman RS: Tuberculosis in non-Haitian patients with acquired immunodeficiency syndrome. Chest 90:542-545, 1986
38. Macher AM, Kovacs JA, Gill V, et al: Bacteremia due to *Mycobacterium avium-intracellulare* in the acquired immunodeficiency syndrome. Ann Intern Med 99:782-785, 1983
39. Manoff SB, Cauthen GM, Stoneburner RL: TB patients with AIDS: Are they more likely to spread TB? Presented at the Fourth International Conference on AIDS. (Abstract No. 4621.) Stockholm, 1988
40. Masur H, Tuazon C, Gill V, et al: Effect of combined clofazimine and ansamycin therapy on *Mycobacterium avium-Mycobacterium intracellulare* bacteremia in patients with AIDS. J Infect Dis 155:127-129, 1987
41. Narcisco P, Leoni GC, Sette P, et al: Clinical immunological and prognostic aspects of tuberculosis in HIV patients. Fifth International Conference on AIDS. (Abstract No. Th.B.P.56.) Montreal, 1989
42. O'Brien RJ, Lyle MA, Snider DE: Rifabutin (ansamycin LM 427): A new rifamycin-S derivative for the treatment of mycobacterial diseases. Rev Infect Dis 6:519-530, 1987
43. Packer SJ, Cesario T, Williams JH: *Mycobacterium avium* complex infection presenting as endobronchial lesions in immunosuppressed patients. Ann Intern Med 109:389-393, 1988
44. Perriens J, Karahunga C, Williame JC, et al: Mortality, treatment results and relapse rates of pulmonary tuberculosis in African HIV(+) and HIV(−) patients. Presented at Fifth International Conference on AIDS. (Abstract No. M.B.O.38.) Montreal, 1989
45. Pitchenik AE: Tuberculosis control and the AIDS epidemic in developing countries. Ann Intern Med 113:89-91, 1990
46. Pitchenik AE, Burr J, Suarez M, et al: Human T-cell lymphotropic virus-III (HTLV-III) seropositivity and related disease among 71 consecutive patients in whom tuberculosis was diagnosed. Am Rev Respir Dis 135:875-879, 1987
47. Pitchenik AE, Rubinson HA: The radiographic appearance of tuberculosis in patients with the acquired immune deficiency syndrome (AIDS) and pre-AIDS. Am Rev Respir Dis 131:393-396, 1985
48. Rogers PL, Walker RE, Lane HC, et al: Disseminated *Mycobacterium haemophilum* infection in two patients with the acquired immunodeficiency syndrome. Am J Med 84:640-642, 1988
49. Selwyn PA, Hartel D, Lewis VA, et al: A prospective study of the risk of tuberculosis among intravenous drug users with human immunodeficiency virus infection. N Engl J Med 320:545-550, 1989

50. Sherer R, Sable R, Sonnenberg M, et al: Disseminated infection with *Mycobacterium kansasii* in the acquired immunodeficiency syndrome. Ann Intern Med 105:710-712, 1986
51. Small PM, Schecter GF, Goodman PC, et al: Treatment of tuberculosis in patients with advanced human immunodeficiency virus infection. N Engl J Med 324:289-294, 1991
52. Sunderam G, McDonald RJ, Maniatis T, et al: Tuberculosis as a manifestation of the acquired immunodeficiency syndrome (AIDS). JAMA 256:362-366, 1986
53. Theuer CP, Hopewell PC, Elias D, et al: Human immunodeficiency virus infection in tuberculosis patients. J Infect Dis 162:8-12, 1990
54. Tuberculosis and acquired immunodeficiency syndrome—Florida. MMWR 35:587-590, 1987
55. Tuberculosis and acquired immunodeficiency syndrome—New York. MMWR 36:785-795; 1987
56. Tuberculosis and human immunodeficiency virus infection: Recommendations of the Advisory Committee for the Elimination of Tuberculosis (ACET). MMWR 38:236-250, 1989
57. Uttamchandani R, Reyes R, Dittes S, et al: Nosocomial transmission of multidrug-resistant tuberculosis to health-care workers and HIV-infected patients in an urban hospital—Florida. MMWR 39:718-722, 1990
58. Wong B, Edwards FF, Kiehn TE, et al: Continuous high-grade *Mycobacterium avium-intracellulare* bacteremia in patients with the acquired immune deficiency syndrome. Am J Med 78:35-40, 1985
59. Yajko DM, Kirihara J, Sanders C, et al: Antimicrobial synergism against *Mycobacterium avium* complex strains isolated from patients with acquired immune deficiency syndrome. Antimicrob Agents Chemother 32:1392-1395, 1988
60. Yajko DM, Nassos PS, Hadley WK: Therapeutic implications of inhibition versus killing of *Mycobacterium avium* complex by antimicrobial agents. Antimicrob Agents Chemother 31:117-120, 1987
61. Yajko DM, Sanders CA, Nassos PS, Hadley WK: In vitro susceptibility of *Mycobacterium avium* complex to the new fluoroquinolone sparfloxacin (CI-978; AT-4140) and comparison with ciprofloxacin. Antimicrob Agents Chemother 34:2442-2444, 1990
62. Young LS: *Mycobacterium avium* complex infection. J Infect Dis 157:863-867, 1988
63. Young LS, Wiviott L, Wu M, et al: Azithromycin for treatment of *Mycobacterium avium-intracellulare* complex infection in patients with AIDS. Lancet 338:1107-1109, 1991

19

CRYPTOCOCCAL INFECTION IN AIDS

JOHN D. STANSELL, MD
MERLE A. SANDE, MD

Cryptococcus neoformans and tuberculosis are the major opportunistic infections complicating the HIV epidemic worldwide. Although other pathogens may dominate on individual continents or in specific regions, no other major pathogen poses as great a global threat to those immunocompromised by HIV infection. The first decade of AIDS in the United States saw the incidence of cryptococcal disease swell from a few cases annually to several thousand. The high mortality and morbidity rates associated with cryptococcal infection and the toxicity of traditional therapy have sparked intense interest in new treatment alternatives. A better understanding of the natural history of HIV-mediated immunodepression has seen the emergence of debate about the use and advisability of fungal prophylaxis. This chapter reviews the microbiology, epidemiology, clinical presentation, diagnosis, and treatment of cryptococcal infections in AIDS patients.

MICROBIOLOGY

C. neoformans is an encapsulated, budding, yeast-like fungus. The organism is round to oval and 4 to 6 μm in diameter, making its penetration of the lower respiratory tract easy when inhaled. The yeast reproduces by narrow-based budding, which occasionally is used to distinguish it from the broader-based budding *Candida* species. Surrounding the yeast is the large, characteristic polysaccharide capsule. This unique capsule, composed of unbranched α_{1-3}-linked mannose units, is of variable size and may confer protection from host immune response.[22,27,32] Differences in side chain residues along the polysaccharide backbone, variability in biochemical use of nutrients, and distinct DNA base sequences further delineate four serotypes (A through D) within the *C. neoformans* species.[2,4,47] Serotypes A,D, and the variant AD are similar and classified as *C. neoformans* var. *neoformans*. Similarly, serotypes B and C share common characteristics and are classified as *C. neoformans* var. *gattii*.

In culture *C. neoformans* produces smooth, convex, and yellow or tan colonies. In contrast to most nonpathogenic species of *Cryptococcus, C. neoformans* grows well at 37° C and produces the pigment melanin. This latter characteristic provides the basis for many identification and separation techniques.[17]

EPIDEMIOLOGY

Unlike other fungi causing deep-seated fungal disease in HIV-infected persons, *C. neoformans* is not endemic to any single area but is global in distribution. Serotypes A and D have been isolated throughout the world and are responsible for the vast majority of HIV-related cryptococcal infections. In the United States and Canada fully 90% of infections are caused by serotypes A and D, and 86% of them are serotype A. Serotype D is more common in Europe.[28] The most common ecologic niche of *C. neoformans* var. *neoformans* is soil enriched by bird excrement. High concentrations can be found in pigeon droppings and nesting places. Although the source of a rich media for fungal growth, the pigeon itself is not infected. Less common sources of *C. neoformans* var. *neoformans* growth are fruit skins and juices and unpasteurized milk.[17]

Unlike serotypes A and D, serotypes B and C have a more restricted geographic distribution. *C. neoformans* var. *gattii* usually is found in southern California, Hawaii, Australia, and southeast Asia.[28] Although B and C are much more prevalent in southern California (40% of isolates), almost all cases of HIV-related cryptococcosis are due to A and D.[12] The ecologic niche of serotypes B and C is uncertain, but a recent report suggests a relationship with eucalyptus trees.[19] Serotypes B and C have not been isolated from enriched soil.

Infection likely occurs with inhalation of the unencapsulated aerosolized yeast. However, unlike the endemic fungi *Histoplasma* and *Coccidioides*, no clear-cut exposure-disease association exists. Moreover, no animal-to-human or human-to-human transmission of cryptococcal infection has been documented. It is reported that cryptococcal infections occur more commonly in intravenous drug users, Haitians, and ethnic minorities, with the incidence among blacks twice that among whites.[9,37] Why such a predisposition should exist is unclear, and the possible role of increased exposure has yet to be defined.

Before the AIDS epidemic, cryptococcal infection occurred in small numbers of immunocompromised persons, notably those with lymphoma or diabetes or those who had been treated with chronic steroids. In the AIDS era *Cryptococcus* has become the fourth most common cause of serious infection after *Pneumocystis carinii*, cytomegalovirus, and mycobacterial disease. *Cryptococcus* infection is presently the AIDS-indicator disease in 6% of HIV-infected patients[14] and can be expected to occur in an additional 6% to 8% at some time during their HIV-related illness.[13] Although acquired by the host as an infectious aerosol, only 4% of HIV-infected persons with symptomatic cryptococcal infection were seen initially with fungal pneumonia. In contrast, Chuck and Sande[11] found fully 89% of 106 HIV-infected persons with cryptococcal infection had meningitis. Along with AIDS dementia complex, central nervous system (CNS) toxoplasmosis, CNS lymphoma, and progressive multifocal leukoencephalopathy, cryptococcal meningitis is one of the five leading neurologic complications of AIDS.[31]

CLINICAL PRESENTATION (Table 19–1)

The clinical presentation of cryptococcal disease in AIDS patients is often subtle and nonspecific. A prolonged febrile prodrome, indistinguishable from that accompanying other opportunistic infections, is common. Frequently no localizing signs or symptoms are present to guide the physician toward the diagnosis of cryptococcal disease. In a small series of 26 patients reported by Zuger et al.,[48] duration of symptoms ranged from 1 day to 4 months, with a mean of 31 days. In the largest case series published, Chuck and Sande[11] found that two thirds of 106 patients with cryptococcal disease described fever, headache, and malaise. Similarly, in a more recently published series of 68 patients, Clark et al.[13] described fever and headache in 64% and 57% of patients, respectively. Nausea and vomiting are reported by approximately 50% of patients.[11] Stiff neck and photophobia, classic symptoms of meningeal irritation, are present in less than 20% to 30% of patients.[11,48] Alteration in mental status is recognized in 14% to 28% of cases[11,13,48] and focal neurologic deficits or seizures in less than 10%.[11,13,48]

Although the portal of entry for *C. neoformans* is the lung, pulmonary cryptococcosis is usually clinically silent. Most cases of pulmonary cryptococcal infection are discovered serendipitously, not because of organ specific signs or symptoms. Occasionally, however, pulmonary symptoms dominate the clinical presentation, and progression to respiratory failure and death are not unknown. Chuck and Sande[11] reported that 31% of patients presented with respiratory complaints. Similarly, Clark et al.[13] found cough and dyspnea in 27% of all HIV-infected patients with cryptococcal disease. However, among those patients without CNS involvement, fully two thirds had cough and shortness of breath. In contrast, only 18% of those patients with culture-proven CNS disease had respiratory symptoms. These numbers add weight to the argument that all patients with CNS involvement have or have had antecedent pulmonary infection. A look-back study by Sugar[44] similarly supports a prior spontaneously resolving pneumonia in most patients with cryptococcal meningitis. Thus CNS involvement is in and of itself prima facie evidence of disseminated cryptococcal infection.

Several studies have focused on those AIDS patients with cryptococcal pneumonia.[8,10,46] Of the 31 cumulative reported cases, respiratory symptoms (cough, shortness of breath) were present in more than two thirds. Pleuritic chest pain and productive cough were not uncommon, perhaps distinguishing pulmonary cryptococcosis from more commonly encountered HIV-related opportunistic infections. Despite a predominance of respiratory symptoms in these 31 patients, all the patients had disseminated disease with positive blood or CSF culture results at the time of presentation.

Table 19–1.   Clinical Presentation of Cryptococcal Meningitis in AIDS

Fever (60%-80%)
Headache (>70%)
Stiff neck (20%-30%)
Photophobia (20%)
Nausea, vomiting, malaise (40%-70%)
Altered mental status (19%-28%)
Seizures (4%-8%)

With the exception of CNS and pulmonary involvement, symptomatic crypto-coccal disease is rare. However, isolation of *C. neoformans* from blood, bone marrow, gastrointestinal tract,[6] and genitourinary tract[29] is not uncommon. Persistence of *C. neoformans* in the urinary tract and prostate after adequate therapy for meningitis has suggested a possible sequestrum of infection from which systemic relapse may occur.[29]

The physical signs of cryptococcal infection are similarly nonspecific. Chuck and Sande reported 56% of patients were febrile on examination. Less than one third had nuchal rigidity, and less than 20% had focal neurologic deficits or obvious alteration in mental status. Papilledema is rare in patients with normal sensorium. Lymphadenopathy, oral thrush, and hairy leukoplakia are commonly seen in AIDS patients with opportunistic infections and frequently reported in common with cryptococcosis.[10,46] In patients with pulmonary disease tachypnea and fine rales may be encountered.[8] Occasionally cutaneous lesions mimicking molluscum contagiosum[38] or Kaposi's sarcoma[25] are encountered.

DIAGNOSIS (Table 19–2)

A knowledge of who is at risk of developing opportunistic infections is essential to the workup of any HIV-infected individual. The expression of any infectious disease depends on the virulence of the invading organism and the immune response of the host. Because *C. neoformans* is a pathogen of relatively low virulence, significant impairment in immune response is required for disseminated disease to exist. Masur et al.[33] found that all AIDS patients treated for cryptococcal disease at the National Institutes of Health (NIH) had CD4 counts of $<0.1 \times 10^9/L$ and CD4:CD8 ratios <0.2. Similarly, a recent case series found 82% of 33 patients with cryptococcal meningitis had CD4 counts $<0.050 \times 10^9/L$.[18]

Routine radiographic imaging and blood studies are rarely useful in establishing the diagnosis of cryptococcosis in AIDS patients. Examination of the cerebrospinal fluid (CSF) usually reveals a noninflammatory formula. Detection and measurement of cryptococcal antigen (CRAG) in serum and CSF is the most rapid diagnostic test available; however, the culture of *C. neoformans* from body secretion or tissue remains the "gold standard" diagnostic test.

Table 19–2.   Laboratory Findings of Cryptococcal Meningitis in AIDS

Peripheral Blood Findings
WBC count usually $<4000/mm^3$; range, $1300\text{-}27{,}900/mm^3$
Serum CRAG positive; 99% sensitivity
CSF Findings
High opening pressure in 60%
WBC count low; $<20/mm^3$ in $>60\%$; differential shows lymphocytosis
Glucose normal in $>70\%$
Protein >40 mg/dl in $>50\%$
CRAG positive and lower than serum CRAG; 91% sensitivity
India ink positive in $>70\%$
Abnormal head CT in 29%

Chest Radiography

The most common chest radiographic abnormality in patients with pulmonary cryptococcosis is diffuse or focal interstitial infiltrates.[8,35,43] Occasionally these infiltrates appear somewhat nodular or miliary.[34] Intrathoracic adenopathy is a common finding.[8,10,34] Less often encountered are focal alveolar consolidation,[46] large pulmonary nodules,[10] cavitation,[8,10] or isolated pleural effusion.[8,10,34,46]

Central Nervous System Radiography

Chuck and Sande[11] found abnormal results from computed tomography (CT) of the head in 17 of 58 (29%) patients. Three fifths of noted abnormalities were due to CNS atrophy. In contrast, Clark et al.[13] found 19% of patients with cryptococcosis had abnormal head CT scans, excluding those with atrophy. These investigators found ring-enhancing abscesses, mass lesions, edema, white matter changes, infarcts, and evidence of hemorrhage. A recent retrospective review of CT head scans of 35 patients with intracranial cryptococcal infection revealed 57% with abnormalities. Diffuse atrophy accounted for 34% of the abnormal findings; however, mass lesions, hydrocephalus, and cerebral edema were present in 11%, 9%, and 3%, respectively.[39] These CT findings are neither sensitive nor specific for cryptococcal infection.

Peripheral Blood Studies

Routine blood studies are of little value in diagnosing disease caused by *C. neoformans* in AIDS patients. However, the presence of a specific capsular polysaccharide CRAG provides the basis for a highly sensitive serologic test for invasive cryptococcal disease.[5] False-positive tests occur in the presence of rheumatoid factor or infection with *Trichosporon beigelii*. Interference from rheumatoid factor can be eliminated by pretreatment of serum with reducing agents such as dithiothreitol or protease digestion. Serum CRAG is positive at titers ranging from 1:2 to 1:2,000,000 in 75% to 99% of AIDS patients presenting with cryptococcal meningitis. Similar data are unavailable for patients with isolated extrameningeal cryptococcal infection, but sensitivity likely is equally high.

Serum and CSF CRAG titers almost inevitably increase after initiation of antifungal therapy. Twofold to fourfold increases in CRAG titer are commonly seen and do not indicate a failure of anticryptococcal therapy. CRAG titers often stabilize in the second month of treatment; thereafter, monitoring the serum CRAG may be useful in following the clinical response of patients to therapy. Although it is unusual for a serum CRAG to revert to negative after symptomatic cryptococcal disease, a declining or stable CRAG titer is indicative of quiescent disease. A rising CRAG titer in the presence of adequate antifungal therapy may herald emergence of a resistant organism and recrudescent disease. The significance of a persistently high CRAG titer in common with a negative fungal culture is unknown.

Cerebrospinal Fluid Studies

Routine evaluation of the CSF is rarely useful in establishing the diagnosis of cryptococcal meningitis. Any analysis of abnormal CSF values must be made with the knowledge that HIV infection itself may predispose to CSF abnormalities. Appleman et al.[1] examined CSF from 114 military personnel with HIV infection. Most had intact delayed hypersensitivity and CD4 counts >0.400 × 10⁹/L. Forty percent of these healthy, asymptomatic individuals had one or more CSF abnormalities. Hollander[23] has reported that pleocytosis is quite common among HIV-positive persons at all stages of disease. Similarly, these patients frequently have modest increases in CSF protein.

Two studies have reported CSF opening pressures in excess of 200 mm H_2O in approximately two thirds of patients with cryptococcal meningitis.[11,48] Despite these high pressures, few patients have clinical signs or symptoms of profound hydrocephalus.

The CSF white blood cell (WBC) count is frequently abnormal, usually exhibiting a mild lymphocytosis. Chuck and Sande[11] and Clark et al.[13] found WBC counts of <20/mm³ in 79% and 87%, respectively, of a cumulative 174 patients with cryptococcal disease. One study found 65% of patients had a CSF WBC count of <5/mm³.[26] Personal experience with the AIDS service at San Francisco General Hospital confirms that completely normal CSF cell counts from patients with cryptococcal meningitis are quite common.

CSF glucose and protein levels are of little diagnostic value; as discussed previously, they are neither sensitive nor specific for cryptococcal disease. Two studies have found a glucose concentration <40 mg/dl in 17% and 24% of patients,[11,13] whereas a third, smaller study found 65% of patients had glucose levels <50 mg/dl.[48] Typically, CSF protein levels are quite variable, with elevations >40 to 45 mg/dl reported in 35% to 69% of patients.[11,13,26,48]

Although routine CSF studies are rarely helpful, examination of the CSF for the presence of CRAG, direct visualization of *C. neoformans*, and CSF fungal culture usually establish the diagnosis. Direct examination of the CSF using India ink can provide an immediate presumptive diagnosis of cryptococcal meningitis. Identification of the large carbohydrate capsule and narrow-necked budding yeast in the correct clinical setting is pathognomonic. The largest case series of HIV-related cryptococcal meningitis found three quarters of patients had positive India ink preparations.[11] Although cryptococcal meningitis is easily identifiable with silver, mucicarmine, and periodic acid–Schiff (PAS) stains, Gram's stain of CSF is unreliable.

Detection of CSF CRAG, which is similar to serum CRAG, by latex agglutination or enzyme-linked immunosorbent assay (ELISA) is a highly sensitive test for the presence of *C. neoformans*. Three case studies have reported 100% positivity in patients with culture-proven cryptococcal meningitis.[13,26,48] Of note, Chuck and Sande[11] reported that 8 of 88 patients (9%) with culture-proven cryptococcal meningitis had negative CSF CRAG titers. Although the reasons for this disparity between serum and CSF CRAG sensitivity are unclear, experience at San Francisco General Hospital tends to confirm that patients will have negative CSF serologies yet grow *C. neoformans* in culture. These patients tend to have early, mild disease. Serum CRAG titers usually exceed the titer found in CSF; it is quite rare to have a CSF CRAG titer greater than simultaneous serum titer. Generally, CSF titers run one to two dilutions less than serum titer.

PROGNOSIS

The largest retrospective study of AIDS-associated cryptococcal meningitis found 20% of patients failed to survive acute induction therapy.[11] Despite dramatic changes in the natural history of fungal opportunistic infections wrought by the newer triazoles, little clinical impact has been made on early mortality from severe cryptococcal disease. A recent report described a bimodal survival pattern for persons with AIDS-associated cryptococcal meningitis.[45] Whereas the risk of death was great in the first 6 weeks of treatment, those persons surviving beyond 6 weeks had a good prognosis, with an average survival time of 16 months. Several studies have attempted to delineate those factors that may predict outcome. In their 1986 series Zuger et al.[48] found a 100% mortality rate associated with CSF CRAG titers >1:10,000. A positive India ink test result was associated with a 47% mortality rate. In contrast, a much larger 1989 series found only hyponatremia and culture of *C. neoformans* from an extrameningeal site were adverse prognostic indicators.[11] Other clinical features, including age, prior AIDS diagnosis, symptoms, and results from laboratory and imaging studies, were not associated with differences in survival rates. A recent large AIDS Clinical Trial Group (ACTG)-supported clinical trial (ACTG 059) evaluating amphotericin B versus a triazole as primary therapy for cryptococcal meningitis found three criteria that portended a poor outcome: altered mental status, a CSF CRAG titer >1:1024, and a CSF WBC count <20/mm^3 were adverse clinical predictors.[40,41] Similarly, experience at San Francisco General Hospital would suggest a poor treatment outcome for patients presenting with alteration in mental status or cranial nerve deficits. These markers of disease severity allow the clinician to stage cryptococcal disease into high- and low-risk categories and to offer therapy alternatives based on this staging.

TREATMENT (Table 19–3)

Controversy surrounds the treatment of cryptococcal infection in AIDS patients. The traditional mainstay of therapy is amphotericin B with or without 5-flucytosine (5-FC). However, the toxicity of these drugs has led to the search for equally effective but better tolerated forms of therapy.

Amphotericin B is a member of the polyene macrolide class of antibiotics and possesses broad antifungal activity. Its mechanism of action is due principally to its binding of ergosterol in the membrane of susceptible fungi. Bound to the membrane sterol, amphotericin B alters membrane permeability and allows leakage of electrolytes and cellular components, with resulting cell death. Less than 5% of an oral dose of amphotericin B is adsorbed, making intravenous administration necessary. Amphotericin is primarily bound to β-lipoproteins and is minimally excreted by the kidney. Amphotericin B penetrates tissues poorly, and CSF levels are only 0 to 4% of simultaneous serum levels. However, meningeal levels may exceed CSF levels.[20] Adverse drug reactions are common, and up to 80% of patients experience

Table 19–3.   Management of Suspected Cryptococcal Meningitis

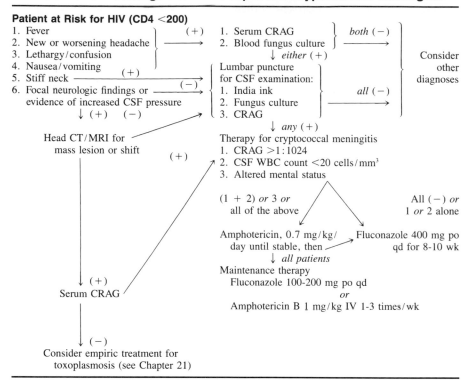

reversible impairment of renal function with amphotericin B administration. In addition, fever, rigors, anemia, thrombophlebitis, headache, myalgias, and arthralgias may accompany amphotericin B administration. Studies of liposomal encapsulated or lipid complexed amphotericin suggest that this pharmaceutical manipulation significantly decreases toxicity and allows more rapid drug administration.[16,21,42] The impact this result will have on treatment of cryptococcal disease awaits further clinical testing.

The total dose and length of amphotericin B therapy are uncertain given variations in patient response to treatment. Dosing usually ranges from 0.5 to 0.8 mg/kg/ day. Current ACTG protocols call for the administration of amphotericin B at 0.7 mg/kg/day. There is no advantage to dose escalation with amphotericin B; rather, patients should receive full dosage immediately. Use of a 1-mg test dose is traditional but offers no distinct advantage over simply slowly administering the first full amphotericin B dose. Intrathecal administration of amphotericin B causes a severe inflammatory reaction of the meninges and offers no therapeutic advantage over intravenous dosing.

5-FC is a fluorinated pyrimidine related to 5-fluorouracil (5-FU), a commonly used antineoplastic agent. In fact, within susceptible fungi, 5-FC is deaminated to 5-FU, undergoes further metabolism, and inhibits thymidylate synthetase. Fungal DNA synthesis is thus impaired. Mammalian cells do not convert 5-FC to 5-FU, which is the basis for the drug's selective antifungal action. 5-FC is administered orally and is 100% absorbed from the gastrointestinal tract. Its half-life is 3 to 6 hours, and the drug is excreted principally by the kidney. 5-FC readily crosses into the CSF and reaches concentrations 65% to 90% of simultaneous serum concentrations. Bone marrow suppression is the principal toxicity and may be accentuated in patients with renal insufficiency. Other untoward effects include rash, nausea, vomiting, enterocolitis, and hepatitis.[3] Because of the rapid emergence of resistance when used as a single agent, 5-FC should always be used in concert with another antifungal agent.

Chuck found a 79% survival rate after 6 weeks of therapy using 1.5 g of amphotericin B. The addition of 5-FC amphotericin B therapy did not improve the cumulative survival rate compared to that of amphotericin B alone. However, combined treatment with 5-FC was associated with significantly increased toxicity, which required stopping the administration of 5-FC in 53% of patients. Similarly, Clark et al.[13] found 58% of 5-FC-treated patients developed adverse drug reactions that necessitated discontinuation of the drug. A prospective, double-blind clinical trial (ACTG 159) comparing administration of amphotericin B alone to administration of amphotericin B plus 5-FC for AIDS-associated cryptococcal meningitis is now accruing.

Ketoconazole is an imidazole antifungal agent metabolized by the liver. It requires an acid environment for absorption and penetrates the CSF poorly. Gastrointestinal intolerance, hepatic dysfunction, and alteration in steroidogenesis are the major toxicities. Ketoconazole is not an effective primary treatment and is clearly inferior to fluconazole for maintenance therapy. This drug should play no role in the treatment of cryptococcal disease.

Itraconazole, an investigational triazole, is structurally similar to ketoconazole. Oral absorption requires gastric acidity and can be enhanced by taking the drug with food. Itraconazole is 99% protein bound and undergoes extensive liver metabolism. It is minimally excreted by the kidney and has a serum half-life of 20 to 30 hours. CSF penetration is negligible. Despite this inability to penetrate the blood-brain barrier, animal studies showed 70% of mice with cryptococcal meningitis were cured. Based on these data, Denning et al.[15] treated 47 AIDS patients with cryptococcal meningitis. Of 47 who received less than 14 days of therapy, 11 were considered unevaluable. Of 36 (64%) evaluable patients, 23 had complete responses (clinical resolution and negative cultures), 8 (22%) had a partial response, and 5 (14%) failed therapy. Based on these encouraging data, a large, multicentered, prospective clinical trial (ACTG 159) comparing fluconazole and itraconazole is now accruing. Itraconazole is generally well tolerated, with nausea and mild elevation in liver enzymes the most common adverse drug reactions.

Fluconazole, a triazole, has pharmacologic properties strikingly different from those of ketoconazole and itraconazole. Fluconazole is water soluble and almost completely absorbed from the gastrointestinal tract, independent of gastric acidity. Renal excretion accounts for over 90% of elimination, and elimination half-life is approximately 25 hours. Fluconazole has good penetration into the CSF, achieving concentrations 60% to 80% that of serum concentration. Unlike ketoconazole, fluconazole does not inhibit steroidogenesis.[3] Side effects are minimal, with mild nausea the most common. Several studies comparing the efficacy of fluconazole to amphotericin B with or without 5-FC are complete or ongoing. Additionally, the combination of fluconazole with 5-FC has yielded encouraging preliminary results but awaits further confirmatory clinical testing.[24]

Larsen, Leal, and Chan[30] recently reported on a small series of AIDS patients with cryptococcal meningitis who were treated with either fluconazole 400 mg/day or amphotericin B >0.3 mg/kg/day with 5-FC 100 mg/kg/day. Of the 14 patients randomly assigned to receive fluconazole, 5 (36%) were cured, 1 (7%) improved, and 8 (57%) failed. This contrasted with results from the amphotericin B–5-FC group in which 5 (57%) were cured, 2 improved, and none failed. Moreover, 4 patients in the fluconazole group died versus none in the amphotericin B group. Although generally well matched, the amphotericin B–treated group had almost twofold higher CD4 counts at the time of study entry. A possible confounding effect cannot be completely discounted.

A larger, prospective study by the National Institute of Allergy and Infectious Diseases (NIAID) Mycoses Study Group and the ACTG has completed accrual and analysis.[41] The trial studied 194 AIDS patients with cryptococcal meningitis. Patients received either amphotericin B >0.3 mg/kg/day or fluconazole 200 mg/kg/day as primary therapy. Randomization was on a 2:1 basis, with two patients enrolled in the fluconazole group for each patient receiving amphotericin B. There were no significant differences between the patient groups at enrollment. Successful treatment was defined as clinical improvement and two negative CSF cultures at least 1 week apart. Failure was defined as "quiescent" disease (clinical improvement but persistent culture positivity), disease progression, toxicity, or death. Of the amphotericin B and fluconazole treatment groups, 40% and 34%, respectively, were successfully treated. When patients with quiescent disease were combined with those successfully treated, the numbers rose to 67% and 60%. Differences in treatment outcome were not statistically significant. Mortality due to progressive disease was 17% overall, with 14% of the amphotericin B and 18% of the fluconazole group succumbing to cryptococcal disease. However, amphotericin B consistently led to more rapid clearance of fungemia and conversion of CSF cultures from positive to negative among successfully treated patients (16 days for amphotericin B versus 30 days for fluconazole). Moreover, early deaths (<2 weeks of therapy) occurred more frequently within the fluconazole-treated group. When subjected to multivariate analysis, three factors emerged as predictive of adverse early outcome: abnormal mental status (obtundation or lethargy), a CSF CRAG titer >1:1024, and a CSF WBC count of <20 cells/mm^3. Based on these findings, the authors propose that patients be stratified into high- and low-risk categories. The mortality rate among low-risk patients treated with amphotericin B or fluconazole was 2.6% and 4.9%, respectively. In contrast, the mortality rate among the high-risk group was 33% for amphotericin B–treated patients and 40% for fluconazole-treated patients. Although optimum therapy is not defined by this study, the trend toward early deterioration and death among high-risk patients in the fluconazole-treated group clearly indicates there is no treatment advantage to triazole therapy for these patients. Currently our recommendation for persons with cryptococcal disease who fall within this high-risk category or have significant pulmonary symptoms is that they receive amphotericin B with or without 5-FC for 2 weeks or until clinically stable. Persons not within the high-risk group probably can be safely started on fluconazole from the outset of treatment (see Table 19–3).

Controversy envelops the treatment of symptomatic increased intracranial pressure due to *C. neoformans* infection. As stated previously, most patients present with abnormally elevated opening pressures (>180 mm CSF). Fortunately, few of these patients have clinical symptoms of hydrocephalus. The contribution of increased intracranial pressure to the early mortality rate discussed previously is unclear.[15] It is clear, however, that those persons who do have symptomatic intracranial hypertension benefit from a reduction in pressure. If noncommunicating hydrocephalus is present on radiographic imaging, performing a shunt procedure should be considered. If communicating hydrocephalus is documented, repeated daily lumbar puncture with removal of 15 to 30 ml of CSF may provide an adequate opportunity for antifungal drugs to exert their effect. If repeated taps fail to reduce intracranial pressure or if symptoms of hydrocephalus persist, inhibition of CSF production using acetazolamide 250 mg four times daily can be attempted. If hydrocephalus is severe and conservative management is deemed inappropriate or has failed, a trial of high-dose corticosteroids should be used. However, given the risk for further dissemination of fungal disease and possible interaction with antifungal drugs, corticosteroids should be used with caution in attempting to control symptomatic hydrocephalus.

MAINTENANCE THERAPY

Many studies have made it clear that chronic administration of antifungal agents is necessary for disease-free survival of the AIDS patient. The optimum maintenance therapy is only now being defined.

In one retrospective study patients receiving either weekly amphotericin B or daily ketoconazole had significantly prolonged survival time (280 and 238 days, respectively) when compared to those receiving no maintenance therapy (141 days).[11] Zuger et al.[48] found a 100% disease-free survival rate at 24 weeks in patients maintained on a regimen of weekly amphotericin B versus a 42% rate for those receiving no maintenance therapy. Clark et al.[13] reported relapses in two of 27 patients receiving weekly amphotericin B maintenance therapy versus three of six patients receiving no maintenance therapy.[13] Finally, a recently published double-blind, placebo-controlled trial of fluconazole 100 to 200 mg/day maintenance therapy after acute therapy for cryptococcal meningitis found 10 of 27 (37%) assigned to placebo versus 1 of 34 (3%) assigned to fluconazole developed recurrent cryptococcal disease at a mean follow-up period of 125 days.[7]

In contrast to the primary therapy studies, comparison trials of fluconazole and amphotericin B as maintenance therapy have documented the superiority of the triazole. The recently completed ACTG 026 trial compared the administration of fluconazole 200 mg/day with that of amphotericin B 1 mg/kg/week in 189 patients with cryptococcal meningitis after they had received primary therapy with a minimum of 15 mg/kg of amphotericin B with or without 5-FC. Patients were followed for a mean of 286 days, with over 90% of patients followed for more than 1 year. Discontinuation of the study was recommended by the Data Safety Monitoring Board after early significant results. The rate of clinical relapse for patients receiving amphotericin B 1 mg/kg/week was 18% versus 2% for those receiving fluconazole 200 mg/day. An additional 15% of the amphotericin B–treated group and 6% of the fluconazole-treated group had drug-related toxicities that necessitated drug discontinuation. Thus the overall rates of failure for the two drugs were 33% and 8%, respectively. The average time to relapse with amphotericin B was 140 days versus 279 days for fluconazole. The rate of disease-free survival at 1 year was 70% for the amphotericin B–treated group and 98% for the fluconazole-treated group. Finally, the incidence of bacterial infection was 35% in the amphotericin B group and 17% in the triazole group, presumably reflecting the increased risk associated with chronic intravenous access.[40]

Based on the above data, we recommend that all patients who complete induction therapy for cryptococcal meningitis begin fluconazole 200 mg/day for lifelong maintenance therapy (see Table 9–3).

Studies evaluating the usefulness of itraconazole for cryptococcal meningitis maintenance therapy are now accruing and await analysis.

FUNGAL PROPHYLAXIS?

The topic of prophylaxis against deep-seated fungal infections stirs immediate debate among those who care for AIDS patients. A recent report by Nightingale et al.[36] compared 289 patients with CD4 counts <68/mm³ who were treated with fluconazole 100 mg/day for prophylaxis and 366 historical controls who were not treated prophylactically. The groups were followed 106 and 168 patient-years, respectively. One cryptococcal infection occurred in the fluconazole group at 3 weeks of treatment compared with 20 infections in the control group (14 cryptococcus and 6 histoplasmosis). Other reports cite the emergence of resistant strains of *Candida* and *C. neoformans* with chronic triazole use. Ultimately, we must await the results of large-scale clinical trials such as ACTG 981 to determine whether fungal prophylaxis should be widely used.

SUMMARY

Cryptococcosis is a common, life-threatening disease in HIV-infected patients worldwide. Routine laboratory tests are of little value, and diagnosis depends on isolation of the organism from body secretions or tissue. Amphotericin B remains the treatment of choice for severe disease, but its toxicities and difficult administration make alternative, equally effective therapy a major goal of investigation. The role of triazoles in acute therapy is now being defined. Triazoles are superior to amphotericin B for maintenance therapy and significantly prolong disease-free survival time.

REFERENCES

1. Appleman ME, Marshall D, Brey RL, et al: Cerebrospinal fluid abnormalities in patients without AIDS who are seropositive for the human immunodeficiency virus. J Infect Dis 158:193-198, 1988
2. Aulakh HS, Straus S, Kwon-Chung KJ: Genetic relatedness of *Filobasidiella neoformans (Cryptococcus neoformans)* and *Filobasidiella bacillispora (Cryptococcus bacillispora)* as determined by deoxyribonucleic acid base composition and sequence homology studies. J Syst Bacteriol 31:97-103, 1981
3. Bennett JE: Antifungal agents. In Mandell GL (ed): Principles and Practice of Infectious Diseases. New York, Churchill Livingstone, 1990

4. Bennett JE, Kwon-Chung K, Theodore TS: Biochemical differences between serotypes of *Cryptococcus neoformans*. 16:167-174, 1978
5. Bloomfield N, Gordon M, Elmendorf D Jr: Detection of *Cryptococcus neoformans* antigen in body fluids by latex particle agglutination. Proc Soc Exp Biol Med 114:64-67, 1963
6. Bonacini M, Nussbaum J, Ahluwalia C: Gastrointestinal, hepatic, and pancreatic involvement with *Cryptococcus neoformans* in AIDS. J Clin Gastroenterol 12:295-297, 1990
7. Bozzette SA, Larsen R, Chiu J, et al: A placebo-controlled trial of maintenance therapy with fluconazole after treatment of cryptococcal meningitis in the acquired immunodeficiency syndrome. N Engl J Med 324:580-584, 1991
8. Cameron ML, Bartless J, Gallis HA, et al: Manifestations of pulmonary cryptococcosis in patients with acquired immunodeficiency syndrome. Rev Infect Dis 13:64-67, 1991
9. Chaisson RE, Volberding P: Clinical manifestations of HIV infection. In Mandell GL (ed): Principles and Practice of Infectious Diseases. New York, Churchill Livingstone, 1990
10. Chechani V, Kamholz S: Pulmonary manifestations of disseminated cryptococcosis in patients with AIDS. 98:1060-1066, 1989
11. Chuck SL, Sande M: Infections with *Cryptococcus neoformans* in the acquired immunodeficiency syndrome. N Engl J Med 321:794-799, 1989
12. Clancy M, Fleischmann J, Howard DH, et al: Isolation of *Cryptococcus neoformans gattii* from a patient with AIDS in Southern California. J Infect Dis 161:809, 1990
13. Clark RA, Greer D, Atkinson W, et al: Spectrum of *Cryptococcus neoformans* infection in 68 patients infected with human immunodeficiency virus. Rev Infect Dis 12:768-777, 1990
14. Centers for Disease Control: HIV/AIDS Surveillance Report, 1991
15. Denning DW, Armstrong R, Lewis BH, et al: Elevated cerebrospinal fluid pressures in patients with cryptococcal meningitis and acquired immunodeficiency syndrome. Am J Med 91:267-272, 1991
16. DeWit S, Rossi C, Duchateau J, et al: Safety, tolerance and immunomodulatory effect of amphotericin B lipid complex (ABLC) in HIV infected subjects. Thirty-first Interscience Conference on Antimicrobial Agents and Chemotherapy. 1991
17. Diamond RD: *Cryptococcus neoformans*. In Mandel GL (ed): Principles and Practice of Infectious Diseases. New York, Churchill Livingstone, 1990
18. Douglas W, Pietroski N, Buckley M, et al: Incidence of cryptococcal meningitis in HIV+ patients with low CD4 cells. Seventh International Conference on AIDS. 1991
19. Ellis DH, Pfeiffer T: Natural habitat of *Cryptococcus neoformans* var. *gattii*. J Clin Microbiol 28:1642-1644, 1990
20. Gallis H, Drew RH, Pickard WW: Amphotericin B: 30 years of clinical experience. Rev Infect Dis 12:308-329, 1990
21. Graybill JR, Sharkey P, Vincent D, et al: Amphotericin B lipid complex (ABLC) in treatment of cryptococcal meningitis in patients with AIDS. Thirty-first Interscience Conference on Antimicrobial Agents and Chemotherapy. 1991
22. Henderson DK, Kan V, Bennett JE: Tolerance to cryptococcal polysaccharide in cured cyptococcosis patients: Failure of antibody secretion in vitro. Clin Exp Immunol 65:639-646, 1986
23. Hollander H: Cerebrospinal fluid normalities and abnormalities in individuals infected with human immunodeficiency virus. J Infect Dis 158:855-888, 1988
24. Jones BE, Larsen R, Bozzette S, et al: A phase II trial of fluconazole plus flucytosine for cryptococcal meningitis. Seventh International Conference on AIDS. 1991
25. Jones C, Orengo I, Rosen T, et al: Cutaneous cryptococcosis simulating Kaposi's sarcoma in the acquired immunodeficiency syndrome. 45:163-167, 1990
26. Kovacs JA, Kovacs A, Polis M, et al: Cryptococcosis in the acquired immunodeficiency syndrome. Ann Intern Med 103:533-538, 1985
27. Kozel TR, Hermerath C: Binding of cryptococcal polysaccharide to *Cryptococcus neoformans*. Infect Immun 43:879-886, 1984
28. Kwon-Chung KJ, Bennett J: Epidemiologic differences between the two varieties of *Cryptococcus neoformans*. Am J Epidemiol 120:123-130, 1984
29. Larsen RA, Bozzette S, McCutchan JA, et al: Persistent *Cryptococcus neoformans* infection of the prostate after successful treatment of meningitis. Ann Intern Med 111:125-128, 1989
30. Larsen RA, Leal M, Chan LS: Fluconazole compared to amphotericin B plus flucytosine for the treatment of cryptococcal meningitis: A prospective study. Ann Intern Med 113:183-187, 1990
31. Levy RM, Janssen R, Bush TJ: Neuroepidemiology of acquired immunodeficiency syndrome. J Acquir Immune Defic Syndr 1:31-40, 1988

32. Macher A, Bennett J, Gadek J, et al: Complement depletion in cryptococcal sepsis. J Immunol 120:1686-1690, 1978
33. Masur H, Ogniben F, Yarchoan R, et al: CD4 counts as predictors of opportunistic pneumonias in human immunodeficiency virus (HIV) infection. Ann Intern Med 111:223-231, 1989
34. Miller WT Jr, Edelman J, Miller WT: Cryptococcal pulmonary infection in patients with AIDS: Radiographic appearance. 175:725-728, 1990
35. Murray J, Mills J: State of the art: Pulmonary infectious complications of human immunodeficiency virus infection. Parts I and II. Am Rev Respir Dis 141:1356-1372, 1582-1598, 1990
36. Nightingale S, Peterson D, Loss S, et al: Fluconazole prophylaxis of disseminated fungal infections in HIV+ patients. Seventh International Conference on AIDS. 1991
37. Panther LA, Sande M: Cryptococcal meningitis in the acquired immunodeficiency syndrome. 5:138-145, 1990
38. Picon L, Vaillant L, Duong T, et al: Cutaneous cryptococcosis resembling molluscum contagiosum: A first manifestation of AIDS. Acta Derm Venereol (Stockh) 69:365-367, 1989
39. Popovich MJ, Arthur R, Helmer E: CT of intracranial cryptococcosis. Am J Radiol 154:603-606, 1990
40. Powderly W, Saag M, Cloud G, et al: Fluconazole versus amphotericin B as maintenance therapy for prevention of relapse of AIDS-associated cryptococcal meningitis. Thirtieth Interscience Conference on Antimicrobial Agents and Chemotherapy. 1990
41. Saag MS, Powderly W, Cloud GA, et al: Comparison of amphotericin B with fluconazole in the treatment of acute AIDS-associated cryptococcal meningitis. N Engl J Med 326:83-89, 1992
42. Schurmann D, de Matos Marques B, Grunewald T, et al: Safety and efficacy of liposomal amphotericin B in treating AIDS-associated disseminated cryptococcosis. J Infect Dis 164:620-622, 1991
43. Stansell JD: Fungal disease in HIV-infected persons: Cryptococcosis, histoplasmosis, and coccidioidomycosis. J Thorac Imaging 6:28-35, 1991
44. Sugar AM: Overview: Cryptococcosis in the patient with AIDS. 114:153-157, 1991
45. Waskin H, Ingram C, Cameron M, et al: Survival trends and cryptococcal meningitis. Seventh International Conference on AIDS. 1991
46. Wasser L, Talavera W: Pulmonary cryptococcosis in AIDS. 92:692-695, 1987
47. Wilson DE, Bennett J, Bailey JW: Serologic grouping of *Cryptococcus neoformans*. Proc Soc Exp Biol Med 127:820-823, 1968
48. Zuger A, Louie E, Hozman RS, et al: Cryptococcal disease in patients with the acquired immunodeficiency syndrome: Diagnostic features and outcome of treatment. Ann Intern Med 104:234-240, 1986

20

ENDEMIC MYCOSES IN HIV INFECTION

GEORGE A. SAROSI, MD

The endemic mycoses—histoplasmosis, coccidioidomycosis, blastomycosis, and paracoccidioidomycosis—follow well-delineated geographic patterns. A fifth rather uncommon endemic mycoses that seldom leads to systemic disease, sporotrichosis, appears more cosmopolitan.

All of these fungal organisms share one important common feature: the inhaled infectious particles cannot be killed by neutrophils once they convert to their tissue phase in the alveoli.[48] In contrast, inhaled hyphal elements of many other commonly occurring fungi are easily killed by neutrophils. Any nonimmune host is susceptible to infection by these fungi, and this infection ultimately must be controlled by specific T-cell–mediated immunity, since nonspecific, nonimmune phagocytosis cannot destroy the invading organisms. Although normal hosts recover from their primary infections uneventfully (unless inhalation of a massive aerosol produces respiratory failure), patients with inherited or acquired T-cell deficiency will progress to uncontrolled and widely disseminated disease. Therefore infection by the human immunodeficiency virus (HIV) predisposes to the disseminated form of these fungal infections.[1]

All of the endemic mycoses share certain important clinical features:

1. All of the fungi in question are soil organisms—their natural habitat is soil heavily fertilized by animal or bird droppings, providing an ample supply of organic nitrogen.[5] Growth of the fungi in nature occurs in the mycelial form, and sporulation occurs under favorable climatic conditions, usually at readily definable periods during the year.

2. Human (or other mammalian) exposure occurs by inhalation of the infecting spores. This usually occurs when sporulating mycelia are disrupted and an infective aerosol is produced.

3. In four of the endemic mycoses, histoplasmosis, coccidioidomycosis, blastomycosis, and paracoccidioidomycosis, the primary portal of entry is the lung. In the vast majority of cases of sporotrichosis, the primary portal of entry is in the skin. Only in extremely rare instances will sporotrichosis enter the human host through the lung. The primary pulmonary infection in all is usually self-limited; the vast majority of immunologically intact persons who are able to mount a specific T-cell–mediated immunity will recover spontaneously, and treatment usually is not

needed. The exception to this rule is when the infected person encounters an inordinately high infective aerosol. In this patient life-threatening illness develops, largely because of the development of interference with normal gas exchange.

4. All five of these organisms are dimorphic. Although their growth is in the hyphal form in nature, they propagate in the infected host by other mechanisms. In all instances the inhaled infectious particles can be destroyed easily by roving neutrophils—the fungus, to evade killing by these neutrophils, will convert at tissue temperatures to its pathogenic form. Four of the five fungi—*Histoplasma capsulatum, Blastomyces dermatitidis, Paracoccidioides brasiliensis,* and *Sporothrix schenckii*—convert to a yeast; *Coccidioides immitis* converts to the giant spherule. This ability of the endemic fungi to convert to a tissue-invasive phase has enabled the organisms to propagate themselves successfully in human and other mammalian tissues because once they convert to the tissue phase, they cannot be destroyed by nonimmune means.[4]

5. Except in extremely rare instances in which inoculation occurs from a mucosal surface to another mucosal surface, there is no person-to-person spread. Thus infected individuals are not infectious to other humans, and isolation is not warranted.

6. Although in healthy individuals spontaneous recovery is the rule, in an individual with defective cell-mediated immunity (e.g., in a patient with advanced HIV infection) there is rapid and progressive dissemination outside the lungs, leading to unchecked progressive disease, which is highly lethal when left untreated.

HISTOPLASMOSIS

The main endemic areas for histoplasmosis are the central and south-central states of the United States. The disease also extends north to the Canadian provinces of Ontario and Quebec, sparing only New England. Westward, the endemic area extends all the way across south Texas and is actually coendemic with coccidioidomycosis in the region of San Antonio, Texas.[9]

For all practical purposes, the primary infection is always a pulmonary infection. In an immunologically intact, nonimmune host inhalation of the arthroconidia leads to rapid conversion to the yeast phase. These yeasts are phagocytosed by cells of the reticuloendothelial system where they continue to multiply. The organisms disseminate throughout the body, usually inside reticuloendothelial cells, and reach their target organs within these cells. With the advent of specific T-cell–mediated immunity, usually 2 to 3 weeks after the original infection, the now "armed" macrophages are able to kill the infecting yeast. This usually brings to a close the acute infection, and the only residual effect of an acute bout of histoplasmosis is the presence of a presumably lifelong immunity from second exogenous infection. In endemic areas these previously infected individuals frequently can be identified by the presence of multiple, discrete calcifications viewed on chest radiographs, both in the parenchyma and hilar nodes. These calcifications can be recognized in the liver and spleen as well. Thus in normal hosts during the preimmune phase of the infection, the organism widely disseminates throughout the body, but progression does not occur because of the development of specific T-cell–mediated immunity.[16]

In patients with defective T-cell–mediated immunity this disseminated infection cannot be brought under control and progression occurs. This progressive form of the disease is referred to as *progressive disseminated histoplasmosis (PDH)*.[10]

PDH is an uncommon manifestation of the infection in immunologically normal hosts. In a large community-wide outbreak of histoplasmosis in Mason City, Iowa, in 1962, the incidence of PDH was 0.12:1000.[16] In a more recent outbreak in Indianapolis the incidence of PDH increased fourfold to 0.46:1000, most likely as a result of the increased number of immunocompromised individuals who live in the community.[21] It was during the investigation of this outbreak that the immunosuppressed state was recognized as the single most important predictor of the development of PDH after the primary infection.[23]

Therefore it is not surprising that HIV infection and AIDS should predispose to the development of PDH. Although PDH was mentioned in one of the first publications dealing with opportunistic infections in AIDS,[2] it was not considered an AIDS-defining illness until 1987,[1] probably because the HIV outbreak involved both the East and West Coasts, areas not normally associated with histoplasmosis. As early as 1983, however, it was noted that PDH in endemic areas occurred most frequently in immunocompromised patients.[13]

Because of the rapid spread of the HIV epidemic, which included the U.S. Midwest, an increasing number of patients with PDH complicating HIV infection have been recognized. A recent publication, in summarizing the total experience, found more than 230 cases.[17]

Clinical Presentation

In the majority of the patients PDH in HIV-infected individuals is a febrile and wasting illness in which up to one half of the involved patients do not have symptoms referable to the respiratory system.[12] Although shortness of breath has been noted in many, respiratory symptoms are surprisingly scant, even in the presence of a markedly abnormal chest radiograph. Physical examination is usually not specific. Only rarely are there any cutaneous ulcers, and lymphadenopathy is not a prominent feature. Hepatosplenomegaly occurs in up to one third of the patients, and evidence of recent weight loss is readily seen. A number of patients have a clinical picture reminiscent of that of septic shock in which the tempo of the illness is extremely rapid.

Routine laboratory evaluation to determine the presence of PDH is seldom helpful. Although anemia, leukopenia, and thrombocytopenia are common, these conditions in patients with PDH are not significantly different from those in other febrile HIV-infected patients; evidence of disseminated intravascular coagulation is frequently seen, especially in patients presenting with the septic shock–like picture.

The admission chest radiograph is variable. When the radiograph appears abnormal, diffuse pulmonary involvement is the most frequent abnormality and is present in approximately half of the patients. This diffuse abnormality has been variably described as either interstitial or reticulonodular (see Chapter 26). In my experience the chest radiograph usually shows interstitial disease, with small, 1- to 2-mm nodules interspersed. In occasional patients focal radiographic abnormalities such as hilar adenopathy, small peripheral nodules, or pleural effusion are noted. However, up to one third of the patients will have a clear chest radiograph at the time of presentation. In the majority of these individuals the chest radiograph will become abnormal during the course of their illness, even though they receive treatment.[17]

Diagnosis

Standard Serodiagnostic Studies

Results from standard serodiagnostic studies are usually positive in patients with PDH and HIV infection. Immunodiffusion test results for the M-precipitant band are usually positive, whereas results from the more specific test for the H-precipitant band are seldom so. Results from the standard complement-fixing serologic test are positive in approximately three fourths of the patients. Taken together, immunodiffusion and complement-fixing test results are positive in approximately 80% of the patients.[21] The main problem with serodiagnostic tests is that they take a long time to become positive; thus in the case of the critically ill patient they are seldom timely enough. Use of the recently developed histoplasma polysaccharide antigen (HPA), as reported by Wheat et al.,[21,22] apparently is an excellent method for diagnosis. Unfortunately, this test is available only through Wheat's laboratory. Thus it also is seldom timely.

Histopathologic and Cultural Recognition of Organism

The "gold standard" for the diagnosis of PDH requires either cultural recovery of the fungus or visualization of the organism in histopathologic material. Recent data show that use of the blood culture, using the lysis-centrifugation system (DuPont Isolater, Wilmington, Delaware), is highly effective. In carefully done studies, in approximately 90% of the patients the blood culture yielded the fungus (Color Plate II*D*).[21]

In my hands the most rapid and most reliable diagnostic test has been evaluation of the bone marrow.[3] Examination of the bone marrow, stained with either one of the many variations of the silver stain or with periodic acid-Schiff (PAS) technique, usually reveals the organisms inside macrophages. Because the PAS stain preserves morphologic detail better, I recommend its use over the silver stain with which loss of morphologic detail tends to occur. Respiratory secretions are also productive sites for recovery of the organism, and bronchoalveolar lavage and transbronchial biopsy both offer excellent ways to obtain the diagnostic material.[15]

Whenever skin or mucocutaneous ulcers are present, a specimen should be obtained for biopsy. These lesions represent a readily available source for the fungus, and they should not be missed.

Treatment

Amphotericin B is still the best treatment for PDH in HIV-infected individuals (see Chapter 19). Although many different ways of administration have been proposed, my goal is to administer amphotericin B rapidly. I begin with a 20-mg infusion, and if I encounter no significant difficulties, later that day an additional 30 mg is infused. Beginning on day 2, 50 mg of amphotericin B is infused daily until the patient has either stabilized or the development of rapidly rising creatinine concentration forces reduction and less frequent administration of the dose. The goal of amphotericin B treatment is to reach a 1- to 2-gm cumulative dose as rapidly as the patient and his renal function can tolerate and then switch to suppressive therapy. The most successful method of suppression has been to deliver approximately 2 g of amphotericin B, followed by administration of 50 to 80 mg of amphotericin B given weekly or every other week. Use of this method has resulted in excellent survival statistics with virtually no relapses.[14,17] Recent trials have shown that itraconazole, a not-yet-available triazole, is extremely successful as suppressive therapy following the initial course of amphotericin B. In this yet-to-be published study, 200 to 400 mg of itraconazole given once a day was highly effective therapy, with no relapses during the first 6 months of the study.[20]

Early during the HIV outbreak the orally available azole, ketoconazole, was used on a number of patients. Examination of the published evidence indicates that ketoconazole as primary therapy for PDH is not effective. Similarly, ketoconazole has also been used as suppressive therapy—in that capacity ketoconazole has also failed and should not be used.[17,21]

COCCIDIOIDOMYCOSIS

C. immitis exists in the United States from western Texas to the coast of California, to latitudes not exceeding 40 degrees and altitudes less than 3500 feet. It is also common in the adjacent provinces of Mexico. The interesting epidemiologic observation is that the majority of primary infections occur after the end of the brief rainy season in the involved areas.

Infection by the fungus follows inhalation of the infecting particles. After these particles lodge in the alveoli, conversion to the giant spherule phase occurs. Macrophage ingestion of the organisms then takes place, and until the development of specific T-cell–mediated immunity, the fungus is not destroyed. In patients with normal T-cell–mediated immunity, similar to what occurs in such patients with histoplasmosis, with the advent of T-cell–mediated immunity, the organisms are destroyed and the patient recovers. In patients with inadequate T-cell–mediated immunity, on the other hand, active and progressive coccidioidomycosis, both inside and outside the lung, will develop. Evidence for the key role of the T-cell–mediated immunity is the recognition of the development of severe coccidioidomycosis in patients receiving cancer chemotherapy, among recipients of solid organ transplants, and in patients receiving chronic glucocorticoid therapy.[6] Thus it was anticipated that severe coccidioidomycosis would complicate the course of the HIV infection.

Epidemiology

Although several patients with coccidioidomycosis complicating HIV infection have been reported from outside the endemic area, they probably represent incubation of the illness following departure from the endemic zone. Alternatively, it is conceivable that these individuals developed their disease as a result of endogenous reactivation when T-cell function waned.

Recent carefully collected data from the endemic area, however, show that the greatest risk for acquisition of the disease is residency in the endemic area. In addition, a CD4 lymphocyte count <250 is a significant risk factor, as is the presence of anergy to skin tests.[7] It is unclear whether the development of severe coccidioidomycosis in this population in the endemic area is the result of a rapidly spreading primary infection or whether it is secondary to endogenous reactivation.

Clinical Manifestations

A number of different clinical manifestations of coccidioidomycosis in HIV-infected patients have been noted. In patients with a near-normal CD4 count the manifestations of the disease are indistinguishable from those in immunologically competent hosts. These patients usually do not develop extensive dissemination or severe disease, and spontaneous recovery has been noted.[7]

On the other hand, a characteristic illness has been recognized in patients whose HIV infection has progressed and whose CD4 counts are <250. In a recent published series from the University of Arizona, approximately 40% of these patients had this characteristic clinical picture.[7,19] In my hospital the majority of the patients with severe coccidioidomycosis fall in this category. These patients usually present with severe shortness of breath, fever, and anorexia. This history, plus their physical examination, shows these patients are similar to those with a much more common pulmonary infection, *Pneumocystis carinii* pneumonia.

The chest radiograph reveals a picture that is similar but in many subtle ways distinct from that seen in patients with *P. carinii* pneumonia (see Chapter 26). Characteristically, the chest film shows larger nodules, diffusely present throughout all lung fields and not quite as interstitial in appearance. Nevertheless, occasionally serious mistakes have been made when the presenting chest radiograph of a patient with coccidioidomycosis was misinterpreted as showing *Pneumocystis* pneumonia. Frequently these patients are hypoxemic and in need of intensive care. A number of such patients initially thought to have *P. carinii* pneumonia were started on antipneumocystic therapy and high-dose glucocorticoid treatment, with occasional near-disastrous results.

Routine laboratory examination is seldom helpful, and usually there is no distinguishing feature to enable differentiation of coccidioidomycosis from other anticipated pulmonary infections.

Diagnosis

Serodiagnosis

The standard immunologic tests are quite helpful in evaluating patients with suspected coccidioidomycosis. Nevertheless, their results may be negative in the presence of rapidly progressive disease. Results from the standardized tests for measuring IgM antibody (tube precipitant and/or latex agglutination) are frequently negative, but the absence of IgM antibodies cannot be used to rule out coccidioidomycosis. Complement-fixing testing for IgG response usually has positive results sometime during active coccidioidomycosis and can be used for diagnosis.[7] In a significant number of cases seen by me, complement-fixing tests could not be performed because of the anticomplementary nature of the serum.

Histopathologic Evaluation

Although coccidioidomycosis is frequently recognized in examination of spontaneously expectorated sputum or from material obtained by bronchoalveolar lavage, these test results are less reliable in HIV-infected patients. Neither the standard 20% potassium hydroxide digest nor the Papanicolaou preparations are positive in many of the patients.

Our approach has been to pursue the diagnosis aggressively; if necessary, we use repeated bronchoscopic examination and bronchoalveolar lavage. We routinely use the Papanicolaou stain (Color Plate II*E*) and obtain appropriate cultures. In the event that repeated examinations fail to yield the diagnosis, moving rapidly to biopsy of lung tissue should be considered.

Treatment

Although no systemic evaluation of any treatment modality has been performed, most investigators in the endemic areas believe that amphotericin B should be used in most acutely ill patients. The drug usually is delivered rapidly in a method similar to that outlined under "Histoplasmosis." What is unclear, however, is how much amphotericin B to administer or for how long. What emerged from my experience is that amphotericin B should be given to tolerance (that of both the patient and the doctor)[7,19]; after that I recommend the use of fluconazole in 400 mg/day doses for the duration of the patient's life.[8] I attempt to reach doses of at least 1½ to 2½ g of amphotericin B before switching to fluconazole.

Fluconazole apparently is highly useful also in the treatment of meningeal dissemination in HIV-infected patients. Meningeal disease may also be treated with both systemic and intracisternal use of amphotericin B. Many physicians practicing in the endemic areas are using fluconazole as primary therapy, with apparent success in some cases. My experience has been limited in the use of fluconazole for primary therapy, and until further data emerges, it cannot be recommended in the treatment of the acutely ill patient.

REFERENCES

1. Centers for Disease Control: Revision of the CDC surveillance case definition of acquired immunodeficiency syndrome. JAMA 258:1143-1154, 1987
2. Centers for Disease Control: Update on acquired immunodeficiency syndrome (AIDS) among patients with hemophilia A. MMWR 31:644-652, 1981
3. Davies SF, McKenna RW, Sarosi GA: Trephine biopsy of the bone marrow in disseminated histoplasmosis. Am J Med 67:617-622, 1979
4. Davies SF, Sarosi GA: Pulmonary mycoses. In Bone R, Dantzker D, George R, et al (eds): Comprehensive Textbook of Pulmonary Medicine. Chicago, Mosby–Year Book (in press)

5. Davies SF, Sarosi GA: Treatment of fungal infections. In Kelley WN (ed): Textbook of Internal Medicine, vol 2, ed 2. Philadelphia, JB Lippincott Co, 1992, pp 1650-1653
6. Deresinski SC, Stevens DA: Coccidioidomycosis in compromised hosts. Experience at Stanford University Hospital. Medicine 54:377-395, 1974
7. Fish DG, Ampel NM, Galgiani JN, et al: Coccidioidomycosis during human immunodeficiency virus infection. A review of 77 patients. Medicine 69:384-391, 1990
8. Galgiani JN: Fluconazole, a new antifungal agent (editorial). Ann Intern Med 113:177-179, 1990
9. Goodwin RA Jr, DesPres RM: State of the art: Histoplasmosis. Am Rev Respir Dis 117:929-956, 1978
10. Goodwin RA Jr, Shapiro JL, Thurman GH, et al: Disseminated histoplasmosis: Clinical and pathologic correlations. Medicine 59:1-32, 1980
11. Johnson PC, Hamill RJ, Sarosi GA: Clinical review: Progressive disseminated histoplasmosis in the AIDS patient. Semin Respir Infect 4:139-146, 1989
12. Johnson PC, Khardori N, Najjar AF, et al: Progressive disseminated histoplasmosis in patients with acquired immunodeficiency syndrome. Am J Med 85:152-158, 1988
13. Jones PG, Cohen RL, Batts DH, Silva J Jr: Disseminated histoplasmosis, invasive pulmonary aspergillosis, and other opportunistic infections in a homosexual patient with acquired immune deficiency syndrome. Sex Transm Dis 10:202-204, 1983
14. McKinsey DS, Gupta MR, Riddler SA, et al: Long-term amphotericin B therapy for disseminated histoplasmosis in patients with the acquired immunodeficiency syndrome (AIDS). Ann Intern Med 111:655-659, 1989
15. Salzman SH, Smith RL, Aranda CP: Histoplasmosis in patients at risk for the acquired immunodeficiency syndrome in a nonendemic setting. Chest 93:916-921, 1988
16. Sarosi GA, Davies SF: Fungal infections. In Murray JF, Nadel JA (eds): Textbook of Respiratory Medicine. New York, WB Saunders Co, 1988, pp 917-949
17. Sarosi GA, Johnson PC: Disseminated histoplasmosis in HIV infected patients. Clin Infect Dis 14(suppl 1):S60-S67, 1992
18. Schaffner A, Davis CE, Schaffner T, et al: In vitro susceptibility of fungi to killing by neutrophil granulocytes discriminates between primary pathogenicity and opportunism. J Clin Invest 78:511-524, 1986
19. Spitz BL, Thomas AR, Sarosi GA, Kelly PC: Coccidioidomycosis (CI) in HIV infected patients. Am Rev Respir Dis 143(suppl):A720, 1991
20. Wheat LJ: Mycoses Study Group, Study No. 14. Pilot study to determine the feasibility of itraconazole for suppression of relapse of disseminated histoplasmosis in patients with acquired immunodeficiency syndrome. In Dismukes WE (principal investigator): Twelfth Annual Mycoses Study Group Meeting. Bethesda, Maryland, Nov 15 and 16, 1990, pp 134-137
21. Wheat LF, Connolly-Stringfield PA, Baker RL, et al: Disseminated histoplasmosis in the acquired immune deficiency syndrome: Clinical findings, diagnosis and treatment, and review of the literature. Medicine 69:361-374, 1990
22. Wheat LJ, Kohler RB, Tewari RP: Diagnosis of disseminated histoplasmosis by detection of *Histoplasma capsulatum* antigen in serum and urine specimens. N Engl J Med 314:83-88, 1986
23. Wheat LJ, Slama TG, Norton JA, et al: Risk factors for disseminated or fatal histoplasmosis. Analysis of a large urban outbreak. Ann Intern Med 96:159-163, 1982

21

AIDS-ASSOCIATED TOXOPLASMOSIS

DENNIS M. ISRAELSKI, MD
JACK S. REMINGTON, MD

Toxoplasma gondii is among the most prevalent causes of latent infection of the central nervous system (CNS) throughout the world. Although a complete review of the biology of *Toxoplasma* is beyond the scope of this chapter, it is important to understand that *Toxoplasma* is a protozoan that exists in three forms: proliferative (tachyzoite), tissue cyst, and oocyst. Felines are the definitive host and reservoir for sporozoite production (oocysts), but only tachyzoites and cysts are found in an incidental host (e.g., mammals). Each of these forms is potentially infectious for humans.[162] After an acute infection, cysts of *T. gondii* persist in the CNS and in multiple extraneural tissues. Although normal human hosts have immunity sufficient to maintain infection in a quiescent state, immunocompromised individuals may be at risk for reactivation and dissemination of chronic (latent) infection.[62,64] Defective cellular immunity in patients with AIDS results in loss of the primary arm of host defense against this parasite. Infection with HIV may lead to depletion of helper-inducer (CD4) T-cell lymphocyte and macrophage dysfunction and predispose to reactivation and dissemination of latent *Toxoplasma* infection.[57] Reactivation of latent infection in patients with AIDS may lead to clinically apparent disease (toxoplasmosis), which usually is initially seen as life-threatening encephalitis. Thus patients with AIDS who have been infected previously with *Toxoplasma* are at considerable risk for development of CNS toxoplasmosis.

Toxoplasmic encephalitis was observed early in the AIDS epidemic[79,123] and currently is recognized as a major cause of opportunistic infection of the CNS and the most frequent cause of focal intracerebral lesions in patients with AIDS.[116,137,156,174,192] Because AIDS patients in the United States who develop toxoplasmic encephalitis are almost always chronically infected with the protozoan,[121] patients with AIDS (or even individuals without AIDS who have antibody to HIV and who are known also to have antibodies to *T. gondii*) should be considered at significant risk for development of toxoplasmic encephalitis from the outset. Recently published data have demonstrated that 20% to 47% of AIDS patients who are seropositive for *T. gondii* will ultimately develop toxoplasmic encephali-

The work discussed in this chapter was supported in part from grants AI04717 and AI30230 from the National Institutes of Health, Bethesda, Maryland.

tis.[10,73,129,195] Seroprevalence varies between geographic locales and even within subpopulations of the same locale.[61,120,122,162,196] Studies performed in our laboratory have found a prevalence of *Toxoplasma* antibodies among HIV-positive adults of 8% to 16% in major urban areas of the United States. The prevalence is higher (≥25%) among certain ethnic groups.

Because of the increasing incidence of HIV infection in women of childbearing years, we predict that the incidence of infants congenitally infected with HIV and *Toxoplasma* will increase.[132,135,145] A prospective case-controlled study sponsored by the National Institute of Allergy and Infectious Diseases (NIAID) Division of AIDS Treatment Research Program is currently underway to determine whether infants born to women infected with HIV are at increased risk of congenital toxoplasmosis.

The high risk of toxoplasmosis in patients with AIDS makes it essential that physicians caring for such patients understand how to diagnose and manage toxoplasmosis.

CLINICAL PRESENTATION

In the United States AIDS patients who develop toxoplasmic encephalitis generally do so after the diagnosis of AIDS has been made.[123,141,169,194] In areas where seroprevalence of *T. gondii* infection is high, toxoplasmic encephalitis frequently is the initial manifestation of AIDS.[32,34,110,152,159,195] Of the patients with indicator diseases for AIDS reported to the Centers for Disease Control (CDC) in Atlanta in 1989, only 5% had toxoplasmic encephalitis.[23] These figures considerably underestimate the prevalence of CNS toxoplasmosis in patients with AIDS since the vast majority of cases in the United States are presumptively diagnosed after the diagnosis of AIDS has already been made; therefore these cases are not reported to the CDC. Whether the prevalence of toxoplasmosis in AIDS patients will be altered by the advent of aggressive primary and secondary prophylaxis of *Pneumocystis carinii* pneumonia has not been determined.[103] A number of retrospective studies show promising results but require confirmation in carefully controlled prospective trials.

When taking a medical history, it is important to note the geographic origin or residence and dietary habits of the patient since these factors will reflect the relative risk of acquired *Toxoplasma* infection. *T. gondii* is a ubiquitous organism and causes infection throughout most of the developing world. When infected beef, lamb, or pork is consumed raw or undercooked, as is customary in certain cultures, infection with *Toxoplasma* can result. Owing largely to their eating habits, 50% to 75% of the adult populations of Germany and France have serologic evidence of *Toxoplasma* infection.[32,48]

Independent of category of risk for acquisition of HIV infection, AIDS-associated toxoplasmosis in the United States occurs significantly more often in Hispanic than in white patients.[19] In addition, a recent study found the frequency of toxoplasmosis is significantly higher in poor Mexican patients with AIDS compared to counterparts with a higher socioeconomic status.[98]

A review of the literature indicates that AIDS patients with toxoplasmic encephalitis may or may not have fever or complain of headache.[35,41,80,110,115,141,159,176] Altered mental status, manifested by confusion, lethargy, delusional behavior, frank psychosis, global cognitive impairment, anomia, or coma may be present initially in as many as 60% of patients.[35,41,80,110,141,152] Seizures are the cause of their seeking medical attention in approximately one third of AIDS patients with toxoplasmic encephalitis.[41,80,110,115,141,152] Focal neurologic deficits are evident on neurologic examination in approximately 60%.[41,110,141,152] Although hemiparesis is the most common focal neurologic finding, patients may have evidence of aphasia, ataxia, visual field loss, cranial nerve palsies, dysmetria, hemichorea-hemiballismus, tremor, parkinsonism, akathisia, or focal dystonia.[17,18,104,141,183] In addition, infection of the spinal cord with *Toxoplasma* has been described in cases of transverse myelitis and conus medullaris syndrome.[78,83,101,131,150] A rapidly fatal, panencephalitis form of diffuse cerebral toxoplasmosis has also been described; unfortunately, computed tomography (CT) of the head was unrevealing in these cases.[74]

Ocular toxoplasmosis usually presents as a focal necrotizing retinochoroiditis, which may be associated with vasculitis, papillitis, and vitritis.[12,65] Ocular involvement may precede or accompany CNS disease.[66,87,151,190] Ophthalmologic examination may reveal uniocular[151] or bilateral,[190] focal or diffuse[87] necrosis (white or yellow-white lesions) and hemorrhage.[13] In contrast to the immunocompetent host with toxoplasmic retinochoroiditis in whom gross and histopathologic examination will usually reveal marked inflammation, in patients with AIDS-associated toxoplasmic chorioretinitis there frequently is only scant retinal inflammation.[87] Thus the features of toxoplasmic retinochoroiditis commonly observed in the immunocompetent host may be absent when occurring in patients with AIDS. Toxoplasmic optic neuritis has also been described.[65]

Endocrinopathies secondary to the syndrome of inappropriate antidiuretic hormone secretion (SIADH) or panhypopituitarism may be the primary manifestation or a later complication of CNS toxoplasmosis.[56,75,133] The lung is the second most common major organ involved in AIDS-associated toxoplasmosis.[47] Toxoplasmic pneumonitis has been increasingly recognized as a cause of pulmonary infiltrates in patients with AIDS[21,46,47,147] and should be considered in the appropriate clinical setting, especially in patients receiving aerosolized pentamidine for prophylaxis against *P. carinii* pneumonia and who present with symptoms and signs referable to the lung.[53,103,147] Autopsy series and case reports[67,84,127,138,164,186] indicate that pathology caused by replication of *T. gondii* outside of the CNS is common and should be considered in the differential diagnosis of unexplained disorders of the skin,[84] heart,[72,127,138,164] peritoneum,[95] stomach,[173] pancreas,[127] colon,[127] pituitary and adrenal glands,[75,133] and testes.[38,143]

AIDS patients with CNS toxoplasmosis are characteristically anergic and have a history of oral candidiasis and depressed numbers of CD4 T lymphocytes.[39,134,159,161,176] In two studies the median number of CD4 T lymphocytes in AIDS patients with acute toxoplasmic encephalitis was $\leq 60/mm^3$,[41,129] with approximately 80% of patients having a CD4 count $<100/mm^3$.[50,129]

Abnormalities in routine clinical laboratory tests are too nonspecific to be of diagnostic use. Commonly, AIDS patients are receiving antimicrobial agents that can cause hematopoietic, hepatic, or renal abnormalities. Hyponatremia may occur from SIADH, presumably as a result of intracerebral mass lesions.[56] A case of toxoplasmic encephalitis with laboratory abnormalities of the hypothalamic-anterior pituitary-adrenal axis has been described.[133] CSF may be normal or reveal mild pleocytosis (predominantly lymphocytes and monocytes) and an elevated protein level, whereas the glucose content is usually normal.[56,141,189,194] Results from magnetic resonance imaging (MRI) or CT studies are almost always abnormal and may be highly suggestive of toxoplasmic encephalitis.

DIAGNOSIS

At present, the definitive diagnosis of toxoplasmic encephalitis can be made only by demonstration of the organism in brain tissue (Table 21–1). Although the morbidity associated with obtaining a brain biopsy is less than that which would accrue from an erroneous diagnosis,[28] neurosurgery is often deferred since many AIDS patients with neurologic syndromes frequently present with inaccessible intracerebral lesions. The desire to avoid brain biopsy has resulted in the almost universal practice of initiating empiric anti-*Toxoplasma* therapy in AIDS patients who have characteristic findings on neuroradiologic imaging studies. In this setting alternative causes should be sought when the patient fails to respond clinically or radiographically; brain biopsy is frequently the only alternative in this situation.

Serology

Toxoplasmic encephalitis in patients with AIDS in the United States almost always represents reactivation of chronic (latent) infection; therefore the presence of IgG *Toxoplasma* antibodies in an AIDS patient must be regarded as a marker for the potential development of toxoplasmosis. If the serologic status of an AIDS patient with suspected toxoplasmic encephalitis is unknown, determination of IgG antibody status should be performed.

Although almost all AIDS patients with toxoplasmic encephalitis have detectable IgG *Toxoplasma* antibodies in their serum, published series have reported a 0% to 3% seronegativity rate.[48,152,179] Although the prevalence of *Toxoplasma* infection has not been shown as higher in HIV-infected individuals than in uninfected individuals[48] (D.M. Israelski et al., manuscript in preparation), recent data demonstrate that

**Table 21–1. Methods for Definitive or Presumptive
Diagnosis of Toxoplasmic Encephalitis
in Patients with AIDS**

Brain biopsy
    Histopathologic evaluation
    Immunoperoxidase staining
    Isolation study
Demonstration of *Toxoplasma* in cerebrospinal fluid (CSF) (Wright-Giemsa stain)
Isolation of *Toxoplasma* from body fluid (blood, CSF)
Computed tomography (CT) and magnetic resonance imaging (MRI)
Antigen detection in body fluid (serum, CSF, urine)
Serology (including titer in agglutination assay, IgG, IgM*)
Intrathecal production of *Toxoplasma*-specific antibodies
Polymerase chain reaction (PCR) of CSF and blood

CSF, cerebrospinal fluid.
*Useful mainly in areas of high seroprevalence.

among *Toxoplasma*-infected individuals, those with HIV infection have significantly higher titers of *Toxoplasma* antibodies than do individuals without HIV infection.[48] In some studies significantly more elevated antibody titers have been observed in AIDS patients with toxoplasmosis compared to those with latent *Toxoplasma* infection.[48,73,152] Although a single determination of IgG antibody titer measured by standard techniques cannot be used to distinguish latent from active infection, we observed, by using a modification of the whole cell agglutination method, that the magnitude of antibody titer to formalin-fixed *Toxoplasma* antigen had a high predictive value for the diagnosis of toxoplasmic encephalitis.[179]

When cerebrospinal fluid (CSF) is available, measurement of intrathecal production of antibody to *T. gondii* may serve as a useful ancillary test.[148,158] A similar investigation has demonstrated little use for antibody load in the diagnosis of ocular toxoplasmosis in AIDS.[25]

IgM *Toxoplasma* antibodies, routinely measured to diagnose acute toxoplasmosis in non-AIDS patients, are rarely demonstrable in AIDS patients with toxoplasmic encephalitis when measured by standard assays.[48,73] The specificity of the IgM immunosorbent agglutination assay (ISAGA) in AIDS patients is unclear.[88,89] IgA *Toxoplasma* antibodies are rarely elevated in AIDS patients with acute toxoplasmic encephalitis.[177]

Isolation Studies

Isolation of *Toxoplasma* from body fluids or, in the appropriate clinical setting, from tissue obtained from a patient with AIDS should be considered diagnostic of active infection. Because isolation of the organism may not be evident for 6 days to 6 weeks after mice or tissue cultures are inoculated, the results are often not helpful in initial management of the patient. Nevertheless, isolation of the organism may obviate future need for brain biopsy.

The epidemic of toxoplasmic encephalitis in patients with AIDS has renewed the interest in methods for in vitro isolation of the organism.[85] *Toxoplasma* readily forms plaques in tissue cultures of human foreskin fibroblasts (Figure 21–1) and most other cultured cells. The plaques, when stained with Wright-Giemsa and examined microscopically, are seen to consist of necrotic and heavily infected cells and numerous extracellular tachyzoites. As few as three organisms can cause plaque formation in a semiconfluent human fibroblast monolayer as early as 4 days after inoculation,[45] although this result varies with the virulence of the strain of *T. gondii*.

In a recently reported therapeutic trial *Toxoplasma* was isolated from the blood of four (14%) of 28 patients in whom an attempt at isolation was made just before initiation of treatment.[41] In contrast, a group of French investigators recently reported isolation of *T. gondii* from the blood of each of 12 patients with toxoplasmosis who were studied before initiation of treatment.[182] This unusual result requires confirmation. *Toxoplasma* may also be isolated from bronchoalveolar lavage fluid in patients with toxoplasmic pneumonitis as early as 48 hours after tissue culture inoculation.[46]

Any diagnostic microbiology or virology laboratory that can inoculate the buffy coat of blood or bronchoalveolar fluid into tissue culture has the capacity to isolate *T. gondii* from patients with active infection.[46,171]

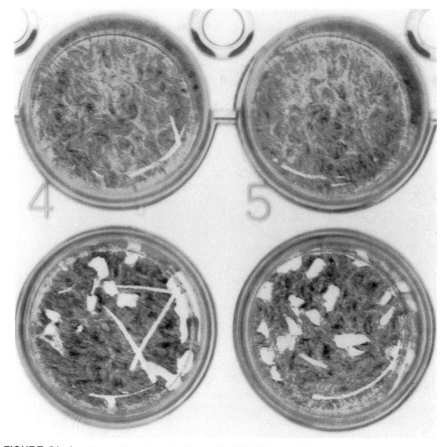

FIGURE 21–1. Plaque formation by *T. gondii;* 100 RH strain *Toxoplasma* were inoculated onto semiconfluent monolayers of human foreskin fibroblasts. Plaques *(bottom row)* were observed at 96 hours. Top row shows uninfected (control) monolayers.

Antigen and DNA Detection

Reliable methods for detection of antigens of *T. gondii* in body fluids of patients with AIDS have not yet been developed. Enzyme-linked immunosorbent assay (ELISA) has been used to detect low concentrations of *Toxoplasma* antigen in serum, amniotic fluid, and CSF of non-AIDS patients with acute toxoplasmosis.[7] In preliminary studies using a modification of this ELISA technique, *Toxoplasma* antigens were detected in urine samples from five of 20 patients with AIDS-associated toxoplasmic encephalitis.[92] The polymerase chain reaction (PCR) test has been used successfully to detect nucleic acids of *T. gondii* in brain tissue and CSF of patients with toxoplasmosis[14,90,187] (S. Parmley et al., manuscript in preparation).

Neuroradiologic Studies

Toxoplasmic encephalitis is the most common cause of focal intracerebral lesions in patients with AIDS (Table 21–2). Imaging studies of the brain have become indispensable for diagnosis and management of these patients.[117] Typically, multiple, bilateral, hypodense, enhancing mass lesions are found on computed tomography (CT) scan[51,56,141,155] (Figure 21–2). Lesions have a predilection for, but are not limited to, the basal ganglia and hemispheric corticomedullary junction.[15,51,56,155] A significant degree of enhancement of intracerebral lesions is generally present on CT scan.[15,51,56,71,110,141,155,156] Toxoplasma abscesses may, however, fail to enhance or be solitary and located anywhere in the brain.[29,30,42,106]

Masses demonstrated by the more sensitive magnetic resonance imaging (MRI) may be absent on CT scan,[106,118] whereas the converse apparently is not true. In a review of 82 AIDS patients with focal neurologic symptoms a CT scan was as good as an MRI scan in detecting focal brain lesions (70% versus 74%). However, in 111 AIDS patients with nonfocal neurologic symptoms only 22% had CT scans that revealed focal lesions, compared to 42% found by MRI studies. As in CT scans, lesions found on MRI scans of AIDS patients with toxoplasmic encephalitis are frequently bilateral and located in the basal ganglia or cerebral corticomedullary junction.[106,157] Deep lesions, which generally range from 1 to 3 cm in diameter, may show central patterns of both low and high signal intensity, suggestive of necrosis.[42] Unlike CT scans, MRI scans usually reveal multiple lesions.[29,30,106,157] In fact, a single lesion seen on an MRI scan should alert the clinician to other possible causes for the focal neuroradiologic findings (e.g., lymphoma, fungal abscesses, tuberculoma, or Kaposi's sarcoma).[30]

As with results of CT scans, no MRI finding can be considered pathognomonic for toxoplasmic encephalitis. Although primary CNS lymphoma cannot be distinguished from toxoplasmosis solely on the basis of neuroradiologic criteria, progress is being made in the characterization of these two disorders by CT scan and MRI.

Table 21–2. Histopathologic Diagnosis in AIDS Patients with Focal Lesions on Computerized Tomography

DIAGNOSIS	PATIENTS (%)
Toxoplasmosis	50-70
Primary central nervous system lymphoma	10-25
Progressive multifocal leukoencephalopathy	10-22
Nondiagnostic	10
Candida albicans abscess	3
Cryptococcoma	2
Kaposi's sarcoma	2
Mycobacterium tuberculosis abscess	1
Herpes simplex virus type 2	1

Modified from De La Paz RL, Enzman D: Neuroradiology of acquired immunodeficiency syndrome. In Rosenblum ML et al (eds): AIDS and the Nervous System. New York, Raven Press, 1988, p 123.

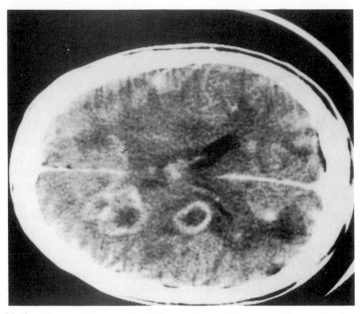

FIGURE 21–2.   Computed tomography (CT) scan of an AIDS patient with toxoplasmic encephalitis. Multiple, hypodense, ring-enhancing lesions were seen.

In a recent study the most reliable distinguishing features of lymphoma from toxoplasmosis in AIDS patients was the presence of hyperattenuation on nonenhanced CT scans and subependymal location on either CT or MRI.[49] The neuroradiologic response of toxoplasmic encephalitis to specific treatment is seen on CT as a reduction in mass effect, number and extent of lesions, and enhancement.[42] Although the time to resolution of lesions may vary from 20 days to 6 months, the vast majority of patients who respond clinically will show radiologic improvement (>50%) by the third week of treatment (personal communication, B. Luft to D. Israelski). The response of abnormalities on MRI scan to specific therapy also varies with the location and complexity of the mass lesion. Peripheral lesions of uniform signal intensity on MRI scan frequently resolve after 3 to 5 weeks of therapy, whereas deeper lesions with complex central signal patterns, consistent with necrosis, take longer to resolve and leave residual lesion(s) at the site of necrosis.[42]

Histopathology

As alluded to previously, despite highly suggestive neuroradiologic studies, definitive diagnosis of toxoplasmic encephalitis often requires demonstration of the organism on histopathologic sections of brain tissue obtained at biopsy. Needle brain biopsy or aspiration is limited by lack of specificity and sensitivity of the procedure to make a definitive diagnosis since size of the specimen may be too small or there may be sampling error.[189] Some evidence demonstrates the superiority of open excisional biopsy compared to needle biopsy in making the histopathologic diagnosis of toxoplasmic encephalitis.[189] Moreover, the observation of abnormal lymphocytes in areas of involvement demonstrated by needle biopsy or aspiration not infrequently has led to the erroneous diagnosis of cerebral lymphoma.

The response of the brain to *Toxoplasma* infection can vary from a granulomatous reaction with gliosis and microglial nodule formation to a severe focal or generalized necrotizing encephalitis.[56,124,141,155] Granulomatous lesions with a cellular infiltrate of abnormal lymphocytes, plasma cells, neutrophils, and monocytes may enlarge and develop central regions of necrosis.[56,124,141,155] Perivascular and intimal inflammatory cell infiltrates can lead to fibrosis or necrosis, which can result in hemorrhage[193] or thrombosis, accounting for the neurologic signs and symptoms of the patient. Based on recent histopathologic studies, it has been suggested that the invasion and multiplication of *Toxoplasma* in the cerebral vascular walls causes focal fibrotic hyperplasia, which leads to an obliterative vasculitis and discrete coagulative necrosis in the CNS.[43,91]

The presence of numerous *Toxoplasma* tachyzoites or cysts surrounded by an inflammatory reaction is diagnostic.[162] Tachyzoites, when observed, are usually found within the inflammatory reaction surrounding areas of necrosis (Figure 21–3). Cysts or free organisms not demonstrable on routine histopathologic examination can be identified using the peroxidase-antiperoxidase method to stain *Toxoplasma* antigens and organisms in brain tissue.[36,189] This method is significantly more sensitive and no less specific in making the diagnosis of toxoplasmic encephalitis than is direct visualization of the organisms in association with cerebral inflammation and necrosis.[36,110] A rapid, sensitive, and specific method for diagnosis

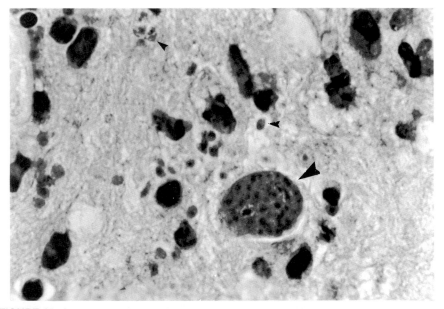

FIGURE 21–3.   Hematoxylin-eosin stain of brain section from AIDS patient demonstrating necrosis and presence of *T. gondii* cysts *(broad arrowhead)* and extracellular tachyzoite forms *(narrow arrowheads)*.

of toxoplasmic encephalitis by electron microscopy has been described.[24] Thus when routine histopathologic studies fail to provide a definitive diagnosis, appropriately fixed brain tissue should be stained by the immunoperoxidase technique or analyzed by electron microscopy in an attempt to identify *T. gondii* antigens or organisms.

Wright-Giemsa–stained touch preparations should be made as immediately as is feasible from tissue obtained at brain biopsy. This can be rapidly accomplished in the clinical laboratory in which stains of blood smears are performed. If organisms are demonstrated, potentially life-saving therapy can be initiated promptly. Similarly, when cerebrospinal fluid (CSF) can be safely obtained, Wright-Giemsa stain of a cytocentrifuge preparation of CSF may reveal the presence of tachyzoites.[44]

Differential Diagnosis

In AIDS patients with focal abnormalities on neurologic examination, multiple enhancing lesions on CT scan and a positive *Toxoplasma* antibody titer strongly suggest the diagnosis of toxoplasmic encephalitis. Regardless of results of *Toxoplasma* serology, the differential diagnosis for individuals with nonfocal symptoms and one or two lesions on CT scan includes, in addition to CNS toxoplasmosis, lymphoma, fungal abscess, mycobacterial or cytomegaloviral disease, and Kaposi's sarcoma. Since therapy is available for each of these disorders, brain biopsy for histopathologic diagnosis may become necessary for successful management of the patient. The characteristic appearance of progressive multifocal leukoencephalopathy (PML) on neuroimaging studies often permits differentiation of this disorder from other causes of intracerebral mass lesions.

Skin testing for anergy and quantitation of T-lymphocyte subsets are recommended during routine outpatient evaluation of the HIV-infected patient. Results of these tests may help gauge suspicion for the presence of an AIDS-related opportunistic CNS process.[134,161] Thus patients capable of delayed-type hypersensitivity reactions to common antigens or who are without severely depressed CD4 cell counts may suffer from conditions unassociated with HIV infection such as bacterial abscesses, primary or metastatic brain tumors, neurocysticercosis, arteriovenous malformations, or multiple sclerosis.

MANAGEMENT

General Principles

Since toxoplasmic encephalitis generally reflects reactivation of a latent infection, we believe the serum of all individuals with HIV infection should be tested for *Toxoplasma*-specific IgG antibody. Patients with positive titers are at risk for development of toxoplasmic encephalitis, and the results of the serology should be clearly available in the chart in case a patient presents with signs referable to the CNS (Figure 21–4).

Head CT scan has been the standard initial test for evaluation of AIDS patients suspected of having CNS toxoplasmosis. In patients with neurologic abnormalities and a negative CT scan on presentation, an MRI scan should be obtained. Patients with only one lesion on CT scan should undergo MRI to attempt to determine if

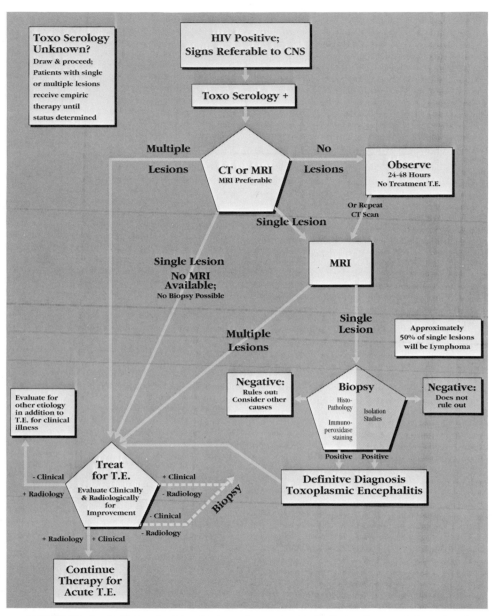

FIGURE 21–4. Guidelines for the evaluation and management of patients with suspected toxoplasmic encephalitis. (From Opportunistic Infections in AIDS, University of Texas Health Science Center, Houston, June, 1991.)

more than a single lesion is present. In patients with nonfocal neurologic abnormalities MRI is the preferred initial evaluation. Since a single lesion on MRI is uncharacteristic of *Toxoplasma* infection and more than 50% of these lesions are lymphomas,[29,30] early biopsy of the involved area should be considered; expedient and aggressive evaluation of AIDS patients with CNS mass lesions allows earlier use of specific therapies and averts use of erroneous and potentially toxic treatment regimens.

AIDS patients with multiple focal lesions visible on neuroimaging studies should begin therapy for presumptive toxoplasmic encephalitis. The presence of multiple simultaneous intracranial lesions is a common feature of CNS dysfunction in AIDS patients.[115] Focal intracranial lesions caused by *Toxoplasma* may occur in association with cerebral lymphoma[119] or *Mycobacterium tuberculosis*.[156] In patients with concurrent focal and diffuse CNS disease, toxoplasmosis has also been found in association with cytomegalovirus (CMV) encephalitis and cryptococcal meningitis.[20,156]

Diffuse toxoplasmic encephalitis may be underdiagnosed and should be suspected when a patient with severe CD4− cell depletion and positive *Toxoplasma* serology presents with unexplained fever and neurologic disease.[102] When diagnostic investigations fail to disclose a specific cause in these cases, a trial of empiric anti-*Toxoplasma* treatment should be considered.

The majority of patients who respond to treatment for toxoplasmosis exhibits clinical improvement within 14 days after initiation of therapy. Repeat neuroradiologic study by the same modality as originally selected should be performed 2 to 4 weeks after the initiation of therapy in patients who demonstrate a satisfactory clinical response (or earlier if response is poor). Lesions should have diminished in size and possibly in number. Change in degree of enhancement is, however, too nonspecific to be of value in the assessment of therapeutic response.[52] Progression of clinical or radiologic abnormalities after 1 week or lack of improvement after 10 days of treatment should raise the possibility of alternative or multiple causes. Patients with extraneurologic toxoplasmosis should be evaluated for CNS disease since most will have intracerebral involvement as well.[111,127]

Corticosteroids are frequently required for the management of patients with intracranial hypertension caused by the mass effect from *Toxoplasma* abscesses. Whether corticosteroids affect the outcome in AIDS patients with toxoplasmic encephalitis is unknown. At present, therefore, AIDS patients with toxoplasmic encephalitis should receive additional immunosuppression by corticosteroids only when it is neurologically contraindicated to withhold their adminstration. We believe whenever corticosteroids are used, the course of administration should be as brief as possible.

Whether administration of anticonvulsant agents is necessary for prevention of seizures has not been determined, although one retrospective study has shown a negative correlation between survival and treatment with anticonvulsant medications in patients with AIDS-associated toxoplasmic encephalitis.[35] Whether this finding represents a true drug effect or it is that more seriously ill patients receive anticonvulsant agents is unknown. As a guideline, patients with seizures at presentation should receive anticonvulsant agents, at least during primary treatment of the acute encephalitis.

It is important to distinguish between two forms of therapy for toxoplasmic encephalitis in patients with AIDS: primary therapy and maintenance therapy (Table 21–3). Primary therapy is administered during what is considered the acute neu-

Table 21–3. Guidelines for Specific Therapy of Toxoplasmic Encephalitis in Patients with AIDS

DRUG	DOSE, INTERVAL, ROUTE
Primary Therapy*	
Pyrimethamine (Daraprim)†	200 mg loading dose then 50-75 mg daily P.O.‡
Folinic acid (leucovorin)§	10-50 mg daily
plus	
Sulfadiazine or trisulfapyrimidines‖	4-6 g/day P.O.
alternative	
Clindamycin	600 mg q6h P.O. or IV¶
Chronic Maintenance Therapy**	
Pyrimethamine	25-50 mg/day P.O.
Folinic acid (leucovorin)	10-20 mg/day
plus	
Sulfadiazine or trisulfapyrimidines	2 g/day P.O.
alternative††	
Clindamycin††	300 mg q6h P.O.

*Primary therapy should be continued until there is complete resolution or marked improvement in clinical and neuroradiologic abnormalities. Such response usually requires at least 4 weeks of treatment; as a guideline we recommend 6 weeks of primary therapy.

†Patients should have complete blood counts (CBC) with white blood cell differential performed at least once weekly.

‡This dose level was agreed on by a special panel of experts meeting in Rome in June 1991.[163] Some investigators prefer 75-100 mg/day in hope of achieving uniformly high blood levels (see text) and because of the variability of sensitivity of different strains of *T. gondii*.

§Folinic acid may be incrementally adjusted to as high as 50 mg daily, if needed, to attempt to ameliorate pyrimethamine-induced bone marrow toxicity. Folinic acid should be administered in two to four divided daily doses and may be given parenterally if poor absorption is suspected.

‖If a sensitivity reaction to sulfadiazine occurs, the patient may not have a cross-reaction when a trisulfapyridimine preparation that does not contain sulfadiazine is substituted. When mild or moderate untoward reactions to a sulfonamide occur and the severity of the disease is significant, it is reasonable either to continue sulfadiazine or to change to trisulfapyrimidines (all preparations of trisulfapyrimidines available in the United States in 1990 contain sulfadiazine in addition to sulfamethazine and sulfamerazine). If toxoplasmic encephalitis is not clinically severe, it may be reasonable to continue pyrimethamine and to wait (i.e., 24-48 hr) for the presumed drug reaction to decrease and then to substitute the alternative sulfonamide preparation. Oral desensitization with sulfadiazine has been successful in such settings.[181]

¶Clindamycin may be used as an alternative primary therapy in combination with pyrimethamine in any patient who has a severe reaction to sulfonamides.

**The relapsing nature of toxoplasmic encephalitis makes lifelong chronic maintenance therapy necessary for secondary prophylaxis against recrudescence of disease.

††We await results of definitive studies of the efficacy of trimethoprim-sulfamethoxazole, pyrimethamine-sulfadoxine (Fansidar), or pyrimethamine plus dapsone before making any specific recommendations for their use in secondary prophylaxis of toxoplasmic encephalitis.

‡‡Clindamycin may be used as alternative suppression therapy when sulfonamides cannot be tolerated. We suggest use of clindamycin in combination with pyrimethamine whenever possible. It should be noted that *Pneumocystis carinii* pneumonia has been well described in patients compliant with this regimen.

rologic disease. Maintenance therapy is administered after an adequate clinical and neuroradiologic response has been observed. Maintenance therapy should be continued for life since the rate of relapse is prohibitively high when treatment is discontinued.

Remarkable variability in susceptibility of different *Toxoplasma* strains to different antimicrobial agents[2,4] and the potential for development of drug resistance may complicate the medical management of AIDS-associated toxoplasmosis.

Primary Therapy

At present it is standard practice to administer the combination of pyrimethamine and sulfadiazine (or trisulfapyrimidines). This combination sequentially blocks folic acid metabolism of the proliferative form of the organism and is synergistic against *T. gondii* both in vitro[37] and in vivo.[54,55] There is no general agreement about the exact dosages of pyrimethamine and sulfonamides to use for the treatment of acute encephalitis.[35,70,125,152,191]

Pyrimethamine, a potent dihydrofolate reductase inhibitor, is the cornerstone of current treatment of AIDS-associated toxoplasmic encephalitis. The half-life of pyrimethamine varies from 20 to 175 hours.[191] Serum concentrations of pyrimethamine in individuals treated with the same dose of drug have great variability.[22,108,191] This variability may in part reflect erratic absorbtion of pyrimethamine in patients with AIDS-associated enteropathies. Although serum concentrations cannot be predicted for a given dose[108,191] or even for a given patient on a given day, serum concentrations of pyrimethamine significantly increase with increasing dose.[108] A recent study noted several patients with AIDS-associated CNS toxoplasmosis who were treated daily with 25 or 50 mg of pyrimethamine had peak or trough serum concentrations lower than or barely exceeding the concentration of pyrimethamine required in vitro for toxoplasmacidal activity.[96,108,126] In contrast, all patients who were treated daily with 100 mg of pyrimethamine had peak and trough serum concentrations well above the minimum concentration required in vitro for toxoplasmacidal activity.[108] When CSF penetration of pyrimethamine was studied in small numbers of patients with AIDS[191] and meningeal leukemia,[68,178] the CSF concentration of drug was between 10% and 25% of the serum concentration. Whether pyrimethamine is present and active in abscess cavities in the brain is not known. Recent data, however, suggest that pyrimethamine may be concentrated in the brain.[109]

Because it is not possible to predict serum or brain concentrations of pyrimethamine in patients with AIDS and toxoplasmic encephalitis, we recommend using the synergistic combination of pyrimethamine plus sulfadiazine (or trisulfapyrimidines) for the management of acute encephalitis (see Table 21–3). Despite small retrospective studies that suggest efficacy,[16,82,175] trimethoprim-sulfamethoxazole cannot, at present, be recommended for acute therapy of toxoplasmic encephalitis since the activity of this combination against *Toxoplasma* is significantly inferior to that of the combination of pyrimethamine and sulfadiazine both in vitro and in animal models of toxoplasmosis.[58,76]

Standard therapy is limited by the high incidence of toxicity associated with both drugs in combination. The most notable toxicity of pyrimethamine is dose-related bone marrow suppression resulting in thrombocytopenia, granulocytopenia, or megaloblastic anemia.[100,139,140] At doses of 75 to 100 mg/day hematologic abnormalities should be anticipated but may be difficult to disassociate from those associated with HIV infection per se. Complete blood counts of patients receiving pyrimethamine should be monitored frequently for the development of drug-associated bone marrow toxicity.

Folinic acid (leucovorin calcium) may prevent or be used to treat patients with marrow toxicity caused by pyrimethamine[100,162] and is not antagonistic to the activity of pyrimethamine or sulfadiazine against *T. gondii.*[63] The oral dose of folinic acid administered to these patients is usually 10 to 20 mg/day in divided doses[144] (see Table 21–3). If hematologic abnormalities develop and malabsorbtion of the folinic acid is suspected, folinic acid may be administered parenterally. Some investigators increase folinic acid up to 50 mg per day for suspected pyrimethamine-associated hematologic toxicity.[110] Few data suggest that higher doses prevent progression of or reverse the hematologic toxicities. Folic acid must not be used since it will inhibit the antitoxoplasma activity of pyrimethamine.[63] Although 65% to 90% of patients with toxoplasmic encephalitis will have an initial favorable response to pyrimethamine plus sulfadiazine therapy,[41,110,141] untoward reactions, most frequently rash,[41] to this combination may limit duration of therapy. Studies reveal that as many as 40% of AIDS patients who receive sulfadiazine and pyrimethamine for toxoplasmic encephalitis manifest signs of toxicity sufficiently severe to prompt discontinuation of the drug(s) during the primary phase of treatment.[77,80,110]

It is likely that sulfonamide is discontinued prematurely in many cases in which, with continuation, lessening or disappearance of the rash would occur. Recent data suggest that the majority of patients with AIDS who experience sulfonamide-associated cutaneous reactions can be successfully desensitized to these agents.[181,184] Crystal-induced nephrotoxicity is another well-recognized adverse reaction to sulfadiazine.[136,149,172] The substantial toxicities associated with standard anti-*Toxoplasma* treatment underscore the urgent need to develop safe and effective alternative drug regimens.

In the search for such regimens, most studies have evaluated the safety and efficacy of a nonsulfonamide agent in combination with pyrimethamine.[40,59,99,107] Whether toxoplasmic encephalitis can be effectively treated solely with pyrimethamine deserves further investigation.

Two prospective controlled studies of the regimens have shown clear efficacy of pyrimethamine plus clindamycin and no significant differences in clinical outcome when compared to pyrimethamine plus sulfadiazine.[41,99] Gastrointestinal disturbance was associated more often with clindamycin plus pyrimethamine, whereas hematologic toxicity was more commonly observed in patients treated with sulfonamide plus pyrimethamine.[41,99] Thus clindamycin may be regarded as an effective alternative to sulfadiazine (when used in combination with pyrimethamine) in the treatment of acute toxoplasmic encephalitis. A panel of experts recently recommended the administration of 600 mg orally (or intravenously) every 6 hours.[163]

The National Institutes of Health (NIH) AIDS Clinical Trials Group (ACTG) recently completed a multicentered study of oral clindamycin in combination with pyrimethamine for primary therapy of toxoplasmic encephalitis in patients with AIDS. Further data about the safety and efficacy of oral clindamycin at 2.4 g/day will be available after the results of this prospective trial have been analyzed.

Investigational Agents

Spiramycin, which has long been used for prevention of transplacental transmission of *T. gondii,* has been reported as ineffective for prevention, treatment, or suppression of toxoplasmic encephalitis.[114] Although spiramycin's use with pyrimethamine and sulfadiazine has not been critically evaluated, at present there is no justification for the use of the three drugs in primary or maintenance therapy of patients with toxoplasmic encephalitis.[166]

The new macrolide-azalide antibiotics azithromycin,[2,9] roxithromycin,[26,86] and clarithromycin[27] were effective in a murine model of toxoplasmosis. Recently a clinical trial with clarithromycin plus pyrimethamine demonstrated efficacy comparable to that of the standard regimen.[59] Prospective noncomparative, dose-escalation studies to evaluate the safety and efficacy of azithromycin are ongoing through the ACTG. Results of carefully controlled prospective clinical trials are needed before the new macrolide-azalide antibiotics can be routinely recommended for the treatment of acute toxoplasmic encephalitis.

Like pyrimethamine, trimetrexate inhibits *Toxoplasma* dihydrofolate reductase but far more potently.[105] Unfortunately, the high incidence of reported relapse of patients with biopsy-proven toxoplasmic encephalitis who were receiving trimetrexate suggests that this drug, when used alone, has only transient activity against this disorder.[154]

A series of experiments in our laboratories has revealed remarkable activity of 566C80, an hydroxynaphthoquinone, against the tachyzoite and cyst (bradyzoite) forms both in vitro and in vivo.[3,4] In a small noncomparative, "salvage" study recently completed at the NIH, 566C80 was found safe and effective.[128] Further data about the safety and efficacy of 566C80 for treatment of AIDS-associated toxoplasmosis will be available after analysis of a Burrough's Wellcome–sponsored multicentered trial.

Other drugs that have been active against the parasite in experimental systems include dapsone,[1] minocycline,[26] and the purine analog aprinocid.[125] Recent studies in our laboratory revealed remarkable in vivo synergy when minocycline was added to clarithromycin[6] and when sulfadiazine or pyrimethamine was added to azithromycin[5] (F.G. Araujo et al., manuscript in preparation). Clinical studies are needed to determine if there is a role for these compounds and combinations in treatment or prevention of toxoplasmosis in AIDS patients.

Because AIDS patients, with their profound defect in cellular immunity, are so susceptible to uncontrolled infection with *Toxoplasma,* there is much interest in the possibility of immunologic reconstitution of these patients through the use of biologic response modifiers. Of particular interest is interferon-γ, which is a known major mediator of host resistance to *T. gondii.*[180] Recombinant interferon-γ (rIFN-γ) can activate monocyte-derived macrophages of AIDS patients to kill *T. gondii* and has significant activity in animal models of toxoplasmosis.[130] Further, in murine models of toxoplasmic encephalitis significant enhancement of antimicrobial activity was observed when either roxithromycin, azithromycin, pyrimethamine, or clindamycin was combined with rIFN-γ.[8,86,94] In view of the important immunologic role of rIFN-γ, future clinical trials should be designed to determine whether the use of antiretroviral agents in combination with rIFN-γ can be used to improve outcome and tolerance to specific anti-*Toxoplasma* therapy. Other biologic response modifiers such as rIFN-β[168] and recombinant interleukin-2[170] also had anti-*Toxoplasma* activity in experimental models but have not been used to treat AIDS-associated toxoplasmosis.

Maintenance Treatment (Secondary Prophylaxis)

The unique pathogenesis of toxoplasmic encephalitis in patients with AIDS requires that intensive therapy be followed by a lifelong suppressive regimen. Whereas the combination of pyrimethamine plus sulfadiazine is highly active against the proliferative form, neither it nor any of the currently used drugs is effective against the cyst form. Relapse of patients with toxoplasmic encephalitis after withdrawal of therapy has been attributed to the cyst form, and its incidence may approach 100%. After discontinuation of specific therapy, the presence of *Toxoplasma* cysts or cells that contain viable forms that have failed to respond to therapy may lead to recrudescence of a necrotizing encephalitis. The CT or MRI scans of patients who relapse often demonstrate mass lesions in the same location as at initial presentation.[188] Thus it is essential that AIDS patients who complete a primary course and who have achieved a favorable clinical and radiologic response to therapy for toxoplasmic encephalitis be maintained on lifelong anti-*Toxoplasma* agents.

Unfortunately, lack of published data from prospective controlled clinical studies has resulted in treatment recommendations based mainly on analysis of accumulated anecdotal reports and small retrospective analyses. In one such study 20 (57%) of 36 patients who had been treated for biopsy-proven toxoplasmic encephalitis had enough lesions of toxoplasmic encephalitis at autopsy for its inclusion as the cause of death.[80]

In a prospective study by Leport et al.[110] 31 of 35 (89%) AIDS patients with toxoplasmic encephalitis had either a complete (n = 10) or partial (n = 21) response to 4 to 6 weeks of primary therapy; 24 who responded to primary therapy were followed for a mean duration of 8 months (range, 2.5 to 28 months) while receiving lower doses of pyrimethamine and sulfadiazine for maintenance treatment. Six (25%) of these patients had 10 relapses, both clinically and by CT scan; of the 10 episodes of relapse, seven occurred within 5 to 7 weeks of discontinuation of primary therapy. Reinitiation of combination therapy at higher doses led to complete resolution of signs and symptoms in eight (80%) of the episodes and partial response in one patient, but the other patient died of the relapse before therapy could be reinitiated. Four of the six patients that relapsed died; three of the deaths were unrelated to toxoplasmic encephalitis as judged by autopsy or by having had clinical response to therapy. Nevertheless, even when postmorten examination of brains of patients who had been treated until death failed to disclose cerebral toxoplasmosis, most had immunoperoxidase stains positive for *T. gondii*. The reported persistence of the proliferative form of *T. gondii* after chronic maintenance treatment and the high relapse rate of toxoplasmic encephalitis in AIDS patients after discontinuation of therapy underscores the necessity for lifelong suppression.

After successful primary therapy, drug dosages are generally decreased for lifelong maintenance therapy (see Table 21–3). Although the most satisfactory regimen for suppression is unknown, most investigators favor the daily use of pyrimethamine with sulfadiazine. Study patients given clindamycin alone or in combination with pyrimethamine have been followed for too brief a duration or are too few in number to permit evaluation of efficacy for maintenance therapy. Failures have occurred in substantial numbers of these patients.[112,152] Some failures likely were due to non-compliance,[188] further confounding interpretation of the data. To use clindamycin for maintenance therapy, at least 1200 mg should be administered daily in divided doses in combination with pyrimethamine.[163] It should be noted, however, that patients have developed *P. carinii* pneumonia while on this maintenance treatment regimen.[69,112]

Relapses have been observed when pyrimethamine is used alone[60,152] or when a regimen is taken less frequently than daily.[110] Studies are needed to clarify how frequently relapses are due to a failure of the drug regimen and how often to lack of compliance on the part of the patient. Potential for pharmacokinetic interactions between maintenance anti-*Toxoplasma* agents and a variety of other drugs used by the patient with AIDS should be investigated. In addition, as in the provocative results reported by Pedrol et al.,[152] further controlled clinical trials should be performed to determine whether advantage can be taken of the long half-life of pyrimethamine to define an effective and convenient maintenance regimen.

Pyrimethamine-sulfadoxine (Fansidar) may be effective as a biweekly regimen for chronic suppression of toxoplasmic encephalitis, but we are aware of a number of relapses in patients receiving this regimen.[11] Given the long half-life of sulfadoxine and reports of associated death(s) and life-threatening Stevens-Johnson syndrome and toxic epidermal necrolysis,[160] we and other physicians have been reluctant to prescribe this fixed drug combination to patients with AIDS. Pyrimethamine plus dapsone should be evaluated further in clinical trials for maintenance treatment. Whether pyrimethamine plus dapsone or even trimethoprim-sulfamethoxazole alone has efficacy as secondary prophylaxis of toxoplasmosis should be evaluated prospectively.

When patients are placed on maintenance therapy for toxoplasmic encephalitis, we and others[33] recommend that zidovudine be added to the medical regimen. Thereafter complete blood counts with white blood count differentials should be obtained at sufficiently frequent intervals to detect adverse drug reactions and allow for timely modifications of dosages of drugs. Close attention to results of hematologic studies may avert significant complications of drug therapy and increase the ability of patients to withstand a chronic regimen in addition to specific antiviral treatment.

Prevention (Primary Prophylaxis)

Serologic testing for *Toxoplasma* antibodies will distinguish those HIV-infected individuals who are at risk for reactivation of infection from those at risk for acquisition of newly acquired infection. All patients who are seronegative for *Toxoplasma* antibodies and who have evidence of deficient cellular immunity, especially those seronegative for *Toxoplasma* antibodies, should be educated about appropriate precautions to take to prevent acquisition of *Toxoplasma* infection (Table 21–4).

Whether chemoprophylaxis of patients with chronic *Toxoplasma* infection and HIV infection who have severely depressed CD4 cells can prevent the development of toxoplasmic encephalitis is an important issue to resolve. Using decision model analysis, it has been suggested that among AIDS patients with positive *Toxoplasma*

Table 21–4.   Methods for Preventing Toxoplasmosis in Patients with HIV Infection

Individuals should take the following precautions:

Cook meat to ≥66° C; smoke it or cure it in brine.
Avoid touching mucous membranes of mouth and eyes while handling raw meat.
Wash hands thoroughly after handling raw meat.
Wash kitchen surfaces that come into contact with raw meat.
Wash fruits and vegetables before consumption.
Prevent access of flies, cockroaches, etc., to fruits and vegetables.
Avoid contact with materials that are potentially contaminated with cat feces (e.g., cat litter boxes) or wear gloves when handling such materials or when gardening.
Disinfect cat litter box for 5 minutes with nearly boiling water.

serology, the benefits of long-term primary prophylaxis outweigh the risks (of therapy) unless the prophylactic regimen used is both toxic and ineffective.[165]

Uncontrolled, nonrandomized experience with trimethoprim-sulfamethoxazole[81,142,146,167] and dapsone plus pyrimethamine[31,185] suggests that these drug combinations may be effective in prevention of toxoplasmosis. However, critical to such a conclusion will be results of appropriately designed studies. Similarly, in another uncontrolled study biweekly administration of pyrimethamine, 25 mg, and sulfadoxine, 500 mg (Fansidar), used for secondary prophylaxis of *P. carinii* pneumonia was highly effective as primary prophylaxis of toxoplasmosis (personal communication, B. Ruf to J.S. Remington).

Recently it was necessary to modify a randomized, multicenter, placebo-controlled trial comparing pyrimethamine to clindamycin in HIV-infected patients seropositive for *Toxoplasma* antibodies and with fewer than 200 CD4 cells because of the unacceptable rate of clindamycin-associated diarrhea.[97]

SUMMARY

AIDS-associated toxoplasmosis is almost always observed in patients with a chronic (latent) infection with *T. gondii* who are in the advanced stages of their HIV infection. Therefore patients who from outset of their HIV infection or AIDS are known to have antibodies to *T. gondii* should be considered at risk for development of toxoplasmosis. Routine serologic tests cannot distinguish active from latent infection, and a small number of patients with toxoplasmosis are seronegative. Toxoplasmic encephalitis is recognized as a major CNS complication in patients with AIDS and is the most frequent cause of focal intracerebral lesions in these patients. Neuroradiologic studies may be highly suggestive of toxoplasmic encephalitis, but at present the definitive diagnosis can be made only by demonstration of *Toxoplasma* in brain tissue. The unique pathogenesis of toxoplasmic encephalitis in patients with AIDS makes necessary intensive primary therapy followed by a lifelong maintenance regimen. We recommend pyrimethamine plus sulfadiazine for the treatment of acute disease. Clindamycin plus pyrimethamine should be used in those patients who cannot tolerate sulfonamides. Treatment should be continued until complete resolution or marked improvement of clinical and neuroradiologic abnormalities is observed. Thereafter the dose of drugs may be reduced for chronic maintenance against relapse of encephalitis. Because most patients will respond to primary therapy, those who fail to improve clinically within 14 days should be evaluated for additional or alternative causes for their intracerebral pathology. This evaluation will often necessitate brain biopsy.

REFERENCES

1. Allegra CJ, Boarna D, Kovacs JA, et al: Interaction of sulfonamide and sulfone compounds with *Toxoplasma gondii* dihyropteroate synthase. J Clin Invest 85:371-379, 1990
2. Araujo FG, Guptil DR, Remington JS: Azithromycin, a macrolide antibiotic with potent activity against *Toxoplasma gondii*. Antimicrob Agents Chemother 32:755-757, 1988
3. Araujo FG, Huskinson-Mark J, Gutteridge WE, Remington JS: In vitro and in vivo activities of the hydroxynaphthoquinone 566C80 against the cyst form of *Toxoplasma gondii*. Antimicrob Agents Chemother (in press)
4. Araujo FG, Huskinson J, Remington JS: Remarkable in vitro and in vivo activities of the hydroxynaphthoquinone 566C80 against tachyzoites and tissue cysts of *Toxoplasma gondii*. Antimicrob Agents Chemother 35:293-299, 1991
5. Araujo FG, Lin T, Remington JS: The combination of sulfadiazine and azithromycin is synergistic for treatment of toxoplasmosis in mice. Eur J Clin Microbiol Infect Dis (in press)
6. Araujo FG, Prokocimer P, Remington JS: Clarithromycin-minocycline is synergistic in a murine model of toxoplasmosis (letter). J Infect Dis (in press)
7. Araujo FG, Remington JS: Antigenemia in recently acquired acute toxoplasmosis. J Infect Dis 141:144-150, 1980
8. Araujo FG, Remington JS: Synergistic activity of azithromycin and gamma interferon in murine toxoplasmosis. Antimicrob Agents Chemother 35:1672-1673, 1991
9. Araujo FG, Shepard RM, Remington JS: In vivo activity of the macrolide antibiotics azithromycin, roxithromycin and spiramycin against *Toxoplasma gondii*. Eur J Clin Microbiol Infect Dis 10:519-524, 1991
10. Aspöck H, Hassl A: Parasitic infections in HIV patients in Austria: First results of a long-term study. Zentralbl Bakteriol 272:540-546, 1990
11. Balzer T, Rolfs A, Hoffken G, et al: The value of pyrimethamine/sulfadoxin (Fansidar) in the prevention of CNS-toxoplasmosis in AIDS patients. Presented at Fifth International Conference on AIDS. (Abstract No. WBP33.) Montreal, June 1989
12. Bottoni F, Gonnella P, Autelitano A, Orzalesi N: Diffuse necrotizing retinochoroiditis in a child with AIDS and toxoplasmic encephalitis. Graefes Arch Clin Exp Ophthalmol 228:36-39, 1990
13. Boyer DS: Discussion of paper by Holland et al: Acquired immunodeficiency syndrome; Ocular manifestations. Ophthalmology 90:872-873, 1983
14. Burg JL, Grover CM, Pouletty P, Boothroyd JC: Direct and sensitive detection of a pathogenic protozoan, *Toxoplasma gondii*, by polymerase chain reaction. J Clin Microbiol 27:1787-1792, 1989
15. Bursztyn EM, Lee BCP, Bauman J: CT of acquired immunodeficiency syndrome. AJNR 5:711-714, 1984
16. Canessa A, Del Bono V, De Leo P, et al: Cotrimoxazole treatment of *Toxoplasma* encephalitis in AIDS patients. Presented at Sixth International Conference on AIDS. (Abstract No. ThB477.) San Francisco, June 1990
17. Carrazana E, Rossitch E Jr, Martinez J: Unilateral "akathisia" in a patient with AIDS and a toxoplasmosis subthalamic abscess. Neurology 39:349-350, 1989
18. Carrazana E, Rossitch E Jr, Samuels MA: Parkinsonian symptoms in a patient with AIDS and cerebral toxoplasmosis. J Neurol Neurosurg Psychiatry 52:1445-1446, 1989
19. Castro KG, Selik RM, Jaffe HW, et al: Frequency of opportunistic diseases in AIDS patients by race/ethnicity and HIV transmission categories—United States. Presented at Twenty-eighth Interscience Conference on Antimicrobial Agents and Chemotherapy. (Abstract No. 570.) Los Angeles, October 1988
20. Catania S, Nobili C, Trinchieri V, et al: Cryptococcal meningitis and *Toxoplasma* encephalitis in an AIDS patient. Acta Neurol (Napoli) 12:82-84, 1990

21. Catterall JR, Hofflin JM, Remington JS: Pulmonary toxoplasmosis. Am Rev Respir Dis 133:704-705, 1986
22. Cavallito JC, Nichol CA, Brenckman WD Jr, et al: Lipid-soluble inhibitors of dihydrofolate reductase. I. Kinetics, tissue distribution and extent of metabolism of pyrimethamine, metroprine, and etoprine in the rat, dog, and man. Drug Metab Dispos 6:329-337, 1978
23. Centers for Disease Control: HIV/AIDS surveillance (year-end edition). January 1990
24. Cerezo L, Alvarez M, Price G: Electron microscopic diagnosis of cerebral toxoplasmosis. J Neurosurg 630:470-472, 1985
25. Chakroun M, Meyohas MC, Pelosse B, et al: Emergence de la toxoplasme oculaire au cours du SIDA. Ann Med Interne (Paris) 141:472-474, 1990
26. Chang HR, Comte R, Piguet PF, et al: Activity of minocycline against *Toxoplasma gondii* infection in mice. J Antimicrob Chemother 27:639-645, 1991
27. Chang HR, Perchere JC: In vitro effects of four macrolides roxithromycin, spiramycin, azithromycin (CP-62,93) and A-56268 on *Toxoplasma gondii*. Antimicrob Agents Chemother 32:524-529, 1988
28. Cimino C, Lipton R, Williams A, et al: The evaluation of patients with human immunodeficiency virus–related disorders and brain mass lesions. Arch Intern Med 151:1381-1384, 1991
29. Ciricillo S, Rosenblum ML: Use of CT and MR imaging to distinguish intracranial lesions and to define the need for biopsy in AIDS patients. J Neurosurg 73:720-724, 1990
30. Ciricillo SF, Rosenblum ML: Imaging of solitary lesions in AIDS. J Neurosurg 74:1029, 1991
31. Clotet B, Sirera G, Romeu J, et al: Twice-weekly dapsone-pyrimethamine for preventing PCP and cerebral toxoplasmosis (letter). AIDS 5:601-602, 1991
32. Clumeck N: Some aspects of the epidemiology of toxoplasmosis and pnemocystis in AIDS in Europe. Eur J Clin Microbiol Infect Dis 10:177-178, 1991
33. Clumeck N, De Wit S, Hermans P, et al: The benefit of zidovudine on the long-term survival of AIDS patients with CNS toxoplasmosis. Presented at Twenty-eighth Interscience Conference on Antimicrobial Agents and Chemotherapy. (Abstract No. 1474.) Los Angeles, October 1988
34. Clumeck N, Sonnet J, Taelman H, et al: Acquired immunodeficiency syndrome in African patients. N Engl J Med 310:492, 1984
35. Cohn JA, McMeeking A, Cohen W, et al: Evaluation of the policy of empiric treatment of suspected *Toxoplasma* encephalitis in patients with acquired immunodeficiency syndrome. Am J Med 86:521-527, 1989
36. Conley FK, Jenkins KA, Remington JS: *Toxoplasma gondii* infection of the central nervous systems. Use of the peroxidase-antiperoxidase method to demonstrate *Toxoplasma* in formalin fixed, paraffin embedded tissue sections. Hum Pathol 12:690-698, 1981
37. Cook MK, Jacobs L: In vitro investigations on the action of pyrimethamine against *Toxoplasma gondii*. J Parasitol 44:280-288, 1958
38. Crider SR, Horstman WG, Massy GS: Toxoplasma orchitis: Report of a case and a review of the literature. Am J Med 85:421-424, 1988
39. Crowe SM, Carlin JB, Stewart KI, et al: Predictive value of CD4 lymphocyte numbers for the development of opportunistic infections and malignancies in HIV-infected persons. J Acquir Immune Defic Syndr 4:770-776, 1991
40. Dannemann BR, Israelski DM, Remington JS: Treatment of toxoplasmic encephalitis and intravenous clindamycin. Arch Intern Med 148:2477-2482, 1988
41. Dannemann BR, McCutchan JA, Israelski DM, et al: Treatment of toxoplasmic encephalitis in patients with AIDS: A randomized trial comparing pyrimethamine plus clindamycin to pyrimethamine plus sulfonamides. Ann Intern Med 116:33-43, 1992
42. De La Paz RL, Enzman D: Neuroradiology of acquired immunodeficiency syndrome. In Rosenblum ML et al (eds): AIDS and the Nervous System. New York, Raven Press, 1988
43. De La Torre R, Gorraez M: Toxoplasma-induced occlusive hypertrophic arteritis as the cause of discrete coagulative necrosis in the central nervous system. Hum Pathol 20:604, 1989
44. Dement SH, Cox MC, Grupta PK: Diagnosis of central nervous system *Toxoplasma gondii* from the cerebrospinal fluid in a patient with AIDS. Diagn Cytopathol 3:148-151, 1987
45. Derouin F, Mazeron MC, Garin YJF: Comparative study of tissue culture and mouse inoculation methods for demonstration of *Toxoplasma gondii*. J Clin Microbiol 25:1597-1600, 1987
46. Derouin F, Sarafti C, Beauvais B, et al: Laboratory diagnosis of pulmonary toxoplasmosis in patients with acquired immunodeficiency syndrome. J Clin Microbiol 27:1661-1663, 1989
47. Derouin F, Sarfati C, Beauvais B, et al: Prevalence of pulmonary toxoplasmosis in HIV-infected patients (letter). AIDS 4:1036, 1990

48. Derouin F, Thulliez P, Garin YJF: Value and limitations of toxoplasmosis serology in HIV patients. Pathol Biol (Paris) 39:255-159, 1991

49. Dina T: Primary central nervous system lymphoma versus toxoplasmosis in AIDS. Radiology 179:823-828, 1991

50. Eliaszewicz M, Lecomte I, De Sa M, et al: Relation between decreasing serial CD4 lymphocyte count and outcome of toxoplasmosis in AIDS patients: A basis for primary prophylaxis. Presented at Sixth International Conference on AIDS. (Abstract No. ThB481.) San Francisco, June 1990

51. Elkin CM, Leon E, Grenell SL, et al: Intracranial lesions in the acquired immunodeficiency syndrome: Radiological (CT) features. JAMA 253:393-396, 1985

52. Enzman DR: Imaging of Infections and Inflammations of the Central Nervous System: Computed Tomography, Ultrasound and Nuclear Magnetic Resonance. New York, Raven Press, 1984

53. Evans TG, Schwartzman JD: Pulmonary toxoplasmosis. Semin Respir Infect 6:51-57, 1991

54. Eyles DE, Coleman N: Synergistic effect of sulfadiazine and daraprim against experimental toxoplasmosis in the mouse. Antibiot Chemother 3:483-490, 1953

55. Eyles DE, Coleman N: An evaluation of the curative effects of pyrimethamine and sulfadiazine alone and in combination on experimental mouse toxoplasmosis. Antibiot Chemother 5:529-539, 1955

56. Farkash AE, MacCabbee PJ, Sher JH: Central nervous system toxoplasmosis in AIDS: A clinical-pathological-radiological review of 12 cases. J Neurol Neurosurg Psychiatry 49:744-748, 1986

57. Fauci AS: The human immunodeficiency virus: Infectivity and mechanisms of pathogenesis. Science 239:617-622, 1988

58. Feldman HA: Effects of trimethoprim and sulfisoxazole alone and in combination on murine toxoplasmosis. J Infect Dis 128S:774, 1973

59. Fernandez-Martin J, Leport C, Morlat P, et al: Pyrimethamine-clarithromycin combination for therapy of acute *Toxoplasma* encephalitis in patients with AIDS. Antimicrob Agents Chemother 35:2049-2052, 1991

60. Foppa CU, Bini T, Gregis G, et al: A retrospective study of primary and maintenance therapy of toxoplasmic encephalitis with oral clindamycin and pyrimethamine. Eur J Clin Microbiol Infect Dis 10:187-189, 1991

61. Frappier-Davignon L, Walker M, Adrien A, et al: Anti-HIV antibodies and other serological and immunological parameters among normal Haitians in Montreal. J Acquir Immune Defic Syndr 3:166-172, 1990

62. Frenkel JK: Effect of cortisone, total body irradiation and nitrogen mustard on chronic latent toxoplasmosis. Am J Pathol 33:618, 1957

63. Frenkel JK, Hitchings GH: Relative reversal by vitamins (*p*-aminobenzoic, folic and folinic acids) of the effects of sulfadiazine and pyrimethamine on *Toxoplasma,* mouse and man. Antibiot Chemother 7:630-638, 1957

64. Frenkel JK, Nelson BM, Arias-Stella J: Immunosuppression and toxoplasmic encephalitis. Hum Pathol 6:97, 1975

65. Friedman D: Neuro-ophthalmic manifestations of human immunodeficiency virus infection. Neurol Clin 9:55-72, 1991

66. Gagliuso DJ, Teich SA, Friedman AH, Orellana J: Ocular toxoplasmosis in AIDS patients. Trans Am Ophthalmol Soc 88:63-86, 1990

67. Garcia LW, Hemphill RB, Marasco WA, Ciano PS: Acquired immunodeficiency syndrome with disseminated toxoplasmosis presenting as an acute pulmonary and gastrointestinal illness. Arch Pathol Lab Med 115:459-463, 1991

68. Geils GF, Scott CW Jr, Baugh CM, Butterworth CE Jr: Treatment of meningeal leukemia with pyrimethamine. Blood 38:131-137, 1971

69. Girard PM, Lepretre A, Detruchis P, et al: Failure of pyrimethamine-clindamycin combination for prophylaxis of *Pneumocystis carinii* pneumonia. Lancet 1:1459, 1989

70. Glatt AE, Chirgwin K, Landesman SH: Treatment of infections associated with human immunodeficiency virus. N Engl J Med 318:1439-1448, 1988

71. Goldstein J, Dickson D, Moser F, et al: Primary central nervous system lymphoma in acquired immunodeficiency syndrome. Cancer 67:2756-2765, 1991

72. Grange F, Kinney EL, Monsuez JJ, et al: Successful therapy for *Toxoplasma gondii* myocarditis in acquired immunodeficiency syndrome. Am Heart J 120:443-444, 1990

73. Grant IH, Gold JMW, Rosenblum M, et al: *Toxoplasma gondii* serology in HIV-infected patients: The development of central nervous system toxoplasmosis in AIDS. AIDS 4:519-521, 1990

74. Gray F, Gherard R, Wingate E, et al: Diffuse "encephalitic" cerebral toxoplasmosis in AIDS. Report of four cases. J Neurol 236:273-274, 1989
75. Groll A, Schneider M, et al: Morphology and clinical significance of AIDS-related lesions in the adrenal and pituitary. Dtsch Med Wochenschr 115:483-488, 1990
76. Grossman PL, Remington JS: The effect of trimethoprim and sulfamethoxazole on *Toxoplasma gondii* in vitro and in vivo. Am J Trop Med Hyg 28:445-455, 1979
77. Guichard A, Zamora L, Caumes E, et al: Cutaneous side effects: A major problem in the treatment of toxoplasmosis encephalitis. Presented at Seventh International Conference on AIDS. (Abstract No. MB2188.) Florence, June 1991
78. Harris TM, Smith RR, Bognanno JR, Edwards MK: Toxoplasmic myelitis in AIDS: Gadolinium-enhanced MR. J Comput Assist Tomogr 14:809-811, 1990
79. Hauser WE, Luft BJ, Conley BK, et al: Central nervous system toxoplasmosis in homosexual and heterosexual adults. N Engl J Med 307:498-499, 1982
80. Haverkos HW: Assessment of therapy for *Toxoplasma* encephalitis. Am J Med 82:907, 1987
81. Heald A, Renold C, Gabriel V, et al: Maintenance treatment after cerebral toxoplasmosis protects against *Pneumocystis carinii* pneumonia (PCP). Presented at Seventh International Conference on AIDS. (Abstract No. WB2218.) Florence, June 1991
82. Herrera G, Villalta O, Visona K, et al: Trimethoprim-sulfamethoxazole treatment of *Toxoplasma* encephalitis in AIDS patients. Presented at Seventh International Conference on AIDS. (Abstract No. WB2321.) Florence, June 1991
83. Herskovitz S, Siegel SE, Schneider AT, et al: Spinal cord toxoplasmosis in AIDS. Neurology 39:1552-1553, 1989
84. Hirschmann JV, Chu AC: Skin lesions with disseminated toxoplasmosis in a patient with the acquired immunodeficiency syndrome (letter). Arch Dermatol 124:1446-1447, 1988
85. Hofflin JM, Remington JS: Tissue culture isolation of *Toxoplasma* from blood of a patient with AIDS. Arch Intern Med 145:925-926, 1985
86. Hofflin JM, Remington JS: In vivo synergism of roxithromycin (RU965) and interferon against *Toxoplasma gondii*. Antimicrob Agents Chemother 31:346-348, 1987
87. Holland GN, Engstrom RE Jr, Glasgow BJ, et al: Ocular toxoplasmosis in patients with the acquired immunodeficiency syndrome. Am J Ophthalmol 106:653-667, 1988
88. Holliman RE: Clinical and diagnostic findings in 20 patients with toxoplasmosis and the acquired immune deficiency syndrome. J Med Microbiol 35:1-4, 1991
89. Holliman RE, Johnson JD, Gillespie SH, et al: New methods in the diagnosis and management of cerebral toxoplasmosis associated with the acquired immune deficiency syndrome. J Infect Dis 22:281-285, 1991
90. Holliman RE, Johnson JD, Savva D: Diagnosis of cerebral toxoplasmosis in association with AIDS using polymerase chain reaction. Scand J Infect Dis 22:243-244, 1990
91. Huang TE, Chou SM: Occlusive hypertrophic arteritis as the cause of discrete necrosis in CNS toxoplasmosis in AIDS. Hum Pathol 19:1210-1214, 1988
92. Huskinson J, Stepick-Biek P, Remington JS: Detection of antigens in urine during acute toxoplasmosis. J Clin Microbiol 27:1099-1101, 1989
93. Israelski DM, Byers E, Dannemann BR, et al: Prevalence of infection with *Toxoplasma gondii* in a cohort of homosexual men. Presented at Thirtieth Interscience Conference on Antimicrobial Agents and Chemotherapy. (Abstract No. 1155.) Atlanta, October 1990
94. Israelski DM, Remington JS: Activity of γ interferon in combination with pyrimethamine or clindamycin in treatment of murine toxoplasmosis. Eur J Clin Microbiol Infect Dis 9:358-360, 1990
95. Israelski DM, Skowren G, Leventhal JP, et al: *Toxoplasma* peritonitis in a patient with AIDS. Arch Intern Med 148:1655-1657, 1988
96. Israelski DM, Tom C, Remington JS: Zidovudine antagonizes the action of pyrimethamine in experimental infection with *Toxoplasma gondii*. Antimicrob Agents Chemother 33:30-34, 1989
97. Jacobson MA, Besch CL, Child C, et al: Randomized study of clindamycin (C) or pyrimethamine (P). Prophylaxis for toxoplasmic HIV disease. Presented at Thirty-first Interscience Conference on Antimicrobial Agents and Chemotherapy. (Abstract No. 298.) Chicago, September-October 1991
98. Jessurun J, Angeles-Angeles A, Gasman N: Comparative demographic and autopsy findings in AIDS in two Mexican populations. J Acquir Immune Defic Syndr 3:579-583, 1990
99. Katlama C: Evaluation of the efficacy and safety of clindamycin plus pyrimethamine for induction and maintenance therapy of toxoplasmic encephalitis in AIDS. Eur J Clin Microbiol Infect Dis 10:189-191, 1991

100. Kaufman HE, Geisler PH: The hematologic toxicity of pyrimethamine (Daraprim) in man. Arch Ophthalmol 64:140-146, 1960
101. Kayser C, Campbell R, Sartoriuous C, Bartlett M: Toxoplasmosis of the conus medullaris in a patient with hemophilia A-associated AIDS. J Neurosurg 73:951-953, 1990
102. Khuong MA, Matheron S, Marche C, et al: Diffuse toxoplasmic encephalitis without abscess in AIDS patients. Presented at Thirtieth Interscience Conference on Antimicrobial Agents and Chemotherapy. (Abstract No. 1157.) Atlanta, October 1990
103. Koeppen S, Gruenewald T, Ruf B, et al: Aerolsolized pentamidine vs. Fansidar in the primary and secondary prophylaxis of *Pneumocystis carinii* pneumonia. Presented at Seventh International Conference on AIDS. (Abstract No. WB2212.) Florence, June 1991
104. Koppel B, Daras M: "Rubrual" tremor due to midbrain toxoplasmosis abscess. Mov Disord 5:254-256, 1990
105. Kovacs JA, Allergra CJ, Chabner BA, et al: Potent effect of trimetrexate, a lipid-soluble antifolate, on *Toxoplasma gondii*. J Infect Dis 155:1027-1032, 1987
106. Kupfer M, Zee CS, Colletti PM, et al: MRI evaluation of AIDS-related encephalopathy: Toxoplasmosis vs. lymphoma. MRI 8:51-57, 1990
107. Leport C, Bastuju-Garin S, Perronne C, et al: An open study of the pyrimethamine-clindamycin combination in AIDS patients with brain toxoplasmosis. J Infect Dis 160:577-578, 1989
108. Leport C, Meulemans A, Dameron, et al: Levels of pyrimethamine in serum of AIDS patients treated for toxoplasmic encephalitis. Presented at Fourth European Congress of Clinical Microbiology. (Abstract No. 843.) Nice, April 1989
109. Leport C, Meulemans A, Robine D, et al: Penetration of pyrimethamine into human brain tissue after a single dose administration. Presented at Twenty-ninth Interscience Conference on Antimicrobial Agents and Chemotherapy. (Abstract No. 248.) Houston, September 1989
110. Leport C, Raffi F, Katlama C, et al: Treatment of central nervous system toxoplasmosis with pyrimethamine/sulfadiazine combination in 35 patients with acquired immunodeficiency syndrome. Am J Med 84:94-100, 1988
111. Leport C, Remington JS: Toxoplasma and AIDS. La Presse Medicale (in press)
112. Leport C, Tournerie C, Raguin G, et al: Long-term follow-up of patients with AIDS on maintenance therapy for toxoplasmosis. Eur J Clin Microbiol 160:312-320, 1989
113. Leport C, Tournerie C, Raguin G, et al: Long-term follow-up of patients with AIDS on maintenance therapy for toxoplasmosis. Eur J Clin Microbiol Infect Dis 10:191-193, 1991
114. Leport C, Vilde JL, Katlama C, et al: Failure of spiramycin to prevent neurotoxoplasmosis in immunosuppressed patients. JAMA 255:2290, 1987
115. Levy RM, Bredesen DE: Central nervous system dysfunction in acquired immunodeficiency syndrome. J Acquir Immune Defic Syndr 1:41-64, 1988
116. Levy RM, Bredesen DE, Rosenblum ML: Neurological manifestations of AIDS: Experience in UCSF and review of the literature. J Neurosurg 62:475-495, 1985
117. Levy RM, Breit R, Russell R, Dal Canto MC: MRI-guided stereotaxic brain biopsy in neurologically symptomatic AIDS patients. J Acquir Immune Defic Syndr 4:254-260, 1991
118. Levy RM, Mills CM, Posin JP, et al: The efficacy and clinical impact of brain imaging in neurological symptomatic AIDS patients: A prospective CT/MRI study. J Acquir Immune Defic Syndr 3:461-471, 1990
119. Levy RM, Rosenbloom S, Perrett LV: Neuroradiological findings in AIDS: A review of 200 cases. AJNR 7:833-839, 1986
120. Liesnard C, VanVooren JP, Farber CM: Risk of cerebral toxoplasmosis according to toxoplasmosis seroprevalence in African and European HIV seropositive patients and recommendations for cerebral toxoplasmosis primary prevention. Presented at Sixth International Conference on AIDS. (Abstract No. FB426.) San Francisco, June 1990
121. Luft BJ, Brooks RG, Conley FK, et al: Toxoplasmic encephalitis in patients with AIDS. JAMA 252:913, 1984
122. Luft BJ, Castro KG: An overview of the problem of toxoplasmosis and pneumocystosis in AIDS in the USA: Implication for future therapeutic trials. Eur J Clin Microbiol Infect Dis 10:178-181, 1991
123. Luft BJ, Conley FK, Remington JS: Outbreak of central nervous system toxoplasmosis in Western Europe and North America. Lancet 1:781-784, 1983
124. Luft BJ, Remington JS: Toxoplasmosis of the central nervous system. In Remington JS, Swartz MN (eds): Current Topics in Infectious Disease, vol 6. New York, McGraw-Hill Book Co, 1985

125. Luft BJ, Remington JS: Toxoplasmic encephalitis. J Infect Dis 157:1-6, 1988
126. Mack DG, McLeod R: New micromethod to study the effect of antimicrobial agents on *Toxoplasma gondii:* Comparison of sulfadoxine and sulfadiazine individually and in combination pyrimethamine and study of clindamycin, metronidazole and cyclosporin A. Antimicrob Agents Chemother 26:26-30, 1984
127. Marche C, Mayorga R, Trophilme D, et al: Pathological study of extraneurological toxoplasmosis (ENT) in AIDS. Presented at Fourth International Conference on AIDS. (Abstract No. 7074.) Stockholm, June 1988
128. Masur H, O'Neill D, Feuerstein I, et al: 566C80 is effective as salvage treatment for *Toxoplasma* encephalitis. Presented at Seventh International Conference on AIDS. (Abstract No. WB31.) Florence, June 1991
129. Matheron S, Dournon E, Garakhanian S, et al: Prevalence of toxoplasmosis in 365 AIDS and ARC patients before and during zidovudine treatment. Presented at Sixth International Conference on AIDS. (Abstract No. ThB476.) San Francisco, June 1990
130. McCabe RE, Luft BJ, Remington JS: Effect of murine interferon gamma on murine toxoplasmosis. J Infect Dis 150:961-962, 1984
131. Mehren M, Burns PJ, Mamani MD, et al: Toxoplasmic myelitis mimicking intramedullary cord tumor. Neurology 38:1648-1650, 1988
132. Miller M, Remington JS: Toxoplasmosis in infants and children with HIV infection or AIDS. In Pizzo PA, Wilfert CM (eds): Pediatric AIDS: The Challenge of HIV Infection in Infants, Children, and Adolescents. Baltimore, Williams & Wilkins Co, 1990
133. Milligan SA, Katz MS, Craven PC: Toxoplasmosis presenting as panhypopituitarism in a patient with AIDS. Am J Med 77:760-764, 1984
134. Miro JM, Buira E, Mallolas J, et al: Relation between CD4 T lymphocyte counts, tuberculosis, other opportunistic infections or Kaposi's sarcoma in Spanish AIDS patients. Presented at Seventh International Conference on AIDS. (Abstract No. MB2347.) Florence, June 1991
135. Mitchell CD, Erlich SS, Mastrucci MT, et al: Congenital toxoplasmosis occurring in infants perinatally infected with human immunodeficiency virus 1. Pediatr Infect Dis J 9:512-518, 1990
136. Molina JM, Belenfant X, Doco-Lecompte T, et al: Sulfadiazine-induced crystalluria in AIDS patients with *Toxoplasma* encephalitis. AIDS 5:587-589, 1991
137. Moller A, Backmund H: CT findings in different stages of HIV infection: A prospective study. J Neurol 237:94-97, 1990
138. Moskowitz L, Hensley GT, Chan JC, Adams: Immediate cause of death in AIDS. Arch Pathol Lab Med 109:735-738, 1985
139. Myatt AV, Coatney GR, Hernandez T, et al: A further study of the toxicity of pyrimethamine (Daraprim) in man. Am J Trop Med 2:1000-1001, 1953
140. Myatt AV, Hernandez T, Coatney GR: Studies in human malaria. Am J Trop Med 2:788-795, 1953
141. Navia BA, Petito CK, Gold JWM, et al: Cerebral toxoplasmosis complicating AIDS: Clinical and neuropathological findings in 27 patients. Ann Neurol 19:224-238, 1986
142. Nicholas P, Pierone G, Lin J, et al: Trimethoprim-sulfamethoxazole in the prevention of cerebral toxoplasmosis. Presented at Sixth International Conference on AIDS. (Abstract No. ThB482.) San Francisco, June 1990
143. Nistal M, Santana A, Paniaqua R, Palacios J: Testicular toxoplasmosis in two men with AIDS. Arch Pathol Lab Med 110:746, 1986
144. Nixon PF, Bertino JR: Effective absorption and utilization of oral formyl-tetrahydrofolate in man. N Engl J Med 186:175-179, 1972
145. O'Donohoe JM, Brueton MJ, Holliman RE: Concurrent congenital human immunodeficiency virus infection and toxoplasmosis. Pediatr Infect Dis J 8:627-628, 1991
146. O'Farrell N, Bradbeer C, Fitt S, et al: Cerebral toxoplasmosis and cotrimoxazole prophylaxis. Lancet 337:986, 1991
147. Oksenhendler E, Cadranel J, Sarfati C, et al: *Toxoplasma gondii* pneumonia in patients with the acquired immunodeficiency syndrome. Am J Med 88, 1990
148. Orefice G, Carrieri PB, De Marinis T, et al: Use of the intrathecal synthesis of anti*Toxoplasma* antibodies in the diagnostic assessment and in the follow-up of AIDS patients with cerebral toxoplasmosis. Acta Neurol (Napoli) 12:79-81, 1990
149. Oster S, Hutchison F, McCabe R: Resolution of acute renal failure in toxoplasmic encephalitis despite continuance of sulfadiazine. Rev Infect Dis 12:618-620, 1990

150. Overhage JM, Griest A, Brown DR: Conus medullaris syndrome resulting from *Toxoplasma gondii* infection in a patient with the acquired immunodeficiency syndrome. Am J Med 89:814-815, 1990

151. Parke DW, Font RL: Diffuse toxoplasmic retinochoroiditis in a patient with AIDS. Arch Ophthalmol 104:571-575, 1986

152. Pedrol E, Gonzalez-Clemente J, Gatell JM, et al: Central nervous system toxoplasmosis in AIDS patients: Efficacy of an intermittent maintenance therapy. AIDS 4:511-517, 1990

153. Pohle H, Koeppen S, Gruenewald T, et al: Cerebral toxoplasmosis: An impending risk in patients on sole aerosolized pentamidine prophylaxis. Presented at Seventh International Conference on AIDS. (Abstract No. WB2189.) Florence, June 1991

154. Polis MA, Masur H, Tuazon C, et al: Salvage therapy of trimetrexate-leucovorin for treatment of cerebral toxoplasmosis in AIDS patients. Clin Res 37:437A, 1989

155. Post MJD, Chan JC, Hensley GT, et al: *Toxoplasma* encephalitis in Haitian adults with AIDS: A clinical-pathologic-CT correlation. AJNR 140:861-868, 1983

156. Post MJD, Kursunoglu SJ, Hensley GT, et al: Cranial CT in AIDS: Spectrum of disease and optimal contrast enhancement technique. AJNR 6:743-754, 1984

157. Post MJD, Sheldon JJ, Hensley GT, et al: Central nervous system disease in AIDS: Prospective correlation using CT, MRI and pathologic studies. Radiology 158:141-148, 1986

158. Potasman I, Resnick L, Luft BJ, Remington JS: Intrathecal production of antibodies against *Toxoplasma gondii* in patients with toxoplasmic encephalitis and AIDS. Ann Intern Med 108:49-51, 1988

159. Ragnaud JM, Beylot J, Lacut JY, et al: Toxoplasmic encephalitis in 73 AIDS patients (Bordeaux, France 1985-1989). Presented at Seventh International Conference on AIDS. (Abstract No. MB2090.) Florence, June 1991

160. Raviglione MC et al: Fatal toxic epidermal necrolysis during prophylaxis with pyrimethamine and sulfadoxine in a human immunodeficiency virus-infected person. Arch Intern Med 148:2683-2685, 1988

161. Redfield RR, Wright DC, Tramont EC: The Walter Reed staging classification for HTLV-II/LAV infection. N Engl J Med 314:131-132, 1986

162. Remington JS, Desmonts G: Toxoplasmosis. In Remington JS, Klein JO (eds): Infectious Diseases of the Fetus and Newborn Infant. Philadelphia, WB Saunders Co, 1990

163. Remington JS, Vilde J: Clindamycin for *Toxoplasma* encephalitis in AIDS. Lancet 338:1142-1143, 1991

164. Roldan EO, Moskowitz L, Hensley GT: Pathology of the heart in AIDS. Arch Pathol Lab Med 111:943-946, 1987

165. Rose D: Prevention of *Toxoplasma* activation among immunocompromised patients: A decision analysis. Presented at Sixth International Conference on AIDS. (Abstract No. ThB484.) San Francisco, June 1990

166. Ruf B, Pohle HD: Role of clindamycin in the treatment of acute toxoplasmosis of the central nervous system. Eur J Clin Microbiol Infect Dis 10:183-186, 1991

167. Ruskin J, LaRiviere M: Low-dose co-trimoxazole for prevention of *Pneumocystis carinii* pneumonia in human immunodeficiency virus disease. Lancet 337:468-471, 1991

168. Schmitz JL, Carlin JM, Borden EC, et al: Beta interferon inhibits *Toxoplasma gondii* growth in human monocyte-derived macrophages. Infect Immun 57:3254-3256, 1989

169. Selik RM, Starcher ET, Curran JW: Opportunistic diseases reported in AIDS patients: Frequencies, associations, and trends. J Acquir Immune Defic Syndr 1:175-182, 1987

170. Sharma SD, Hofflin JM, Remington JS: In vivo recombinant interleukin 2 administration enhances survival against a lethal challenge with *Toxoplasma gondii*. J Immunol 135:4160-4163, 1985

171. Shepp DH, Hackman RC, Conley FK, et al: *Toxoplasma gondii* reactivation identified by detection of parasitemia in tissue culture. Ann Intern Med 103:218-221, 1985

172. Simon DI, Brosius FC, Rothstein DM: Sulfadiazine crystalluria revisited. Arch Intern Med 150:2379-2384, 1990

173. Smart PE, Weinfeld A, Thompson NE, Defortuna SM: Toxoplasmosis of the stomach: A cause of antral narrowing. Radiology 174:369-370, 1990

174. Snider WD, Simpson DM, et al: Neurological complications of AIDS: Analysis of 50 patients. Ann Neurol 14:403, 1983

175. Solbreux P, Sonnet J, Zech F: A retrospective study about the use of contrimoxazole as diagnostic support and treatment of suspected cerebral toxoplasmosis in AIDS. Acta Clin Belg 45:85-96, 1990

176. Speirs G, Mijch A, Lucas CR, et al: Central nervous system toxoplasmosis in AIDS patients: A clinical, pathological, serological and radiological review of 39 cases. Presented at Seventh International Conference on AIDS. (Abstract No. MB2017.) Florence, June 1991

177. Stepick BP, Thulliez P, Araujo FG, Remington JS: IgA antibodies for diagnosis of acute congenital and acquired toxoplasmosis. J Infect Dis 162:270-273, 1990

178. Stickney DR, Simmons WS, De Angelis RL, et al: Pharmacokinetics of pyrimethamine (PRM) and 2,4-diamino-5-(3′,4′-dichlorophenyl)-6-methylpyrimide (DMP) relevant to meningeal leukemia. Proc Am Assoc Cancer Res 14:52, 1973

179. Suzuki Y, Israelski DM, Dannemann BR, et al: Diagnosis of toxoplasmic encephalitis in patients with AIDS by using a new serologic method. J Clin Microbiol 26:2541-2543, 1988

180. Suzuki Y, Orellana MA, Schreiber RD, et al: Interferon-γ: The major mediator of resistance against *Toxoplasma gondii*. Science 240:516-518, 1988

181. Tenant-Flowers M, Boyle M, Carey D, et al: Sulphadiazine desensitization in patients with AIDS and cerebral toxoplasmosis. AIDS 5:311-315, 1991

182. Tirard V, Niel G, Rosenheim M, et al: Diagnosis of toxoplasmosis in patients with AIDS by isolation of the parasite from the blood (letter). N Engl J Med 324:634, 1991

183. Tolge C, Factor S: Focal dystonia secondary to cerebral toxoplasmosis in a patient with AIDS. Mov Disord 6:69-72, 1991

184. Torgovnick J: Desensitization to sulfonamides in patients with HIV infection. Am J Med 88:548-549, 1990

185. Torres R, Thorn M, Barr M, et al: Dapsone prophylaxis for toxoplasmosis and *Pneumocystis carinii* pneumonia. Presented at Seventh International Conference on AIDS. (Abstract No. WB2248.) Florence, June 1991

186. Tschirhart D, Klatt EC: Disseminated toxoplasmosis in the acquired immunodeficiency syndrome. Arch Pathol Lab Med 112:1237-1241, 1988

187. Van de Ven E, Melchers W, Galama J, et al: Identification of *Toxoplasma gondii* infections by BI gene amplification. J Clin Microbiol 19:2120-2124, 1991

188. Walckenaer G, Leport C, Longuet P, et al: Relapses of brain toxoplasmosis in 15 AIDS patients. Presented at Thirty-first Interscience Conference on Antimicrobial Agents Chemotherapy. (Abstract No. 251.) Chicago, 1991

189. Wanke C, Tuazon CU, Kovacs A, et al: *Toxoplasma* encephalitis in patients with acquired immune deficiency syndrome. Am J Trop Med Hyg 36:509-516, 1987

190. Weiss A, Margo CE, Ledford DK, et al: Toxoplasmic retinochoroiditis as a initial manifestation of AIDS. Am J Opthalmol 101:248-249, 1986

191. Weiss LM, Harris C, Berger M, et al: Pyrimethamine concentrations in serum and cerebrospinal fluid during treatment of acute *Toxoplasma* encephalitis in patients with AIDS. J Infect Dis 157:580-583, 1988

192. Whelan MA, Kricheff II, Handler M, et al: AIDS: Cerebral computed tomographic manifestations. Radiology 149:477, 1983

193. Wijdicks EFM, Borleffs JCC, Hoepelman AIM, Jansen GH: Fatal disseminated hemorrhagic toxoplasmic encephalitis as the initial manifestation of AIDS. Ann Neurol 29:683-686, 1991

194. Wong B, Gold JWM, Brown AE, et al: Central nervous system toxoplasmosis in homosexual men and parenteral drug abusers. Ann Intern Med 100:36-42, 1984

195. Zangerle R, Allerberger F, Pohl P, et al: High risk of developing toxoplasmic encephalitis in AIDS patients seropositive to *Toxoplasma gondii*. Med Microbiol Immunol 180:59-66, 1991

196. Zumla A, Savva D, Wheeler RB, et al: *Toxoplasma* serology in Zambian and Ugandan patients infected with the human immunodeficiency virus. Trans R Soc Trop Hyg 85:227-229, 1991

22

BACTERIAL INFECTIONS IN HIV DISEASE

RICHARD E. CHAISSON, MD

Although many serious infections in patients with HIV infection are due to protozoa, fungi, or viruses, bacterial infections are also important pathogens in this population. Disseminated atypical mycobacterial infections were recognized early in the epidemic,[13] and a growing list of bacterial complications of AIDS has been observed over time (Table 22–1). The incidence of serious infections with *Streptococcus pneumoniae, Haemophilus influenzae,* and *Salmonella* species is increased in HIV-infected or AIDS patients compared to control populations.[7,49] These infections are characterized by atypical presentations, high rates of bacteremia, and frequent relapses despite appropriate therapy. It has recently been observed that other bacterial infections, including sinusitis, gram-positive and gram-negative bacteremia, and bacillary angiomatosis, occur more often in HIV-infected patients than in normal hosts. This chapter reviews the pathophysiology, epidemiology, clinical features, and management of bacterial infections in persons with HIV-infection and AIDS.

PATHOPHYSIOLOGY

A number of bacterial pathogens are able to evade host defense mechanisms in HIV-infected individuals. Table 22–2 lists the derangements in immune function that are associated with pyogenic infections in HIV-infected persons. T-cell abnormalities, primarily of the CD4+ lymphocytes, result in infection and disease caused by a number of bacterial agents that require intact cell-mediated immunity (CMI) for control. Quantitative loss of CD4+ cells, impairment in clonal proliferation of CD4+ cells, and a decline in the production of interferon-γ all contribute to infections with organisms that require a CMI response.[5,28] Mycobacteria, *Salmonella* sp., *Shigella* sp., and *Listeria monocytogenes* are thought to cause disease in AIDS patients because of impaired cellular immunity.

Derangements of cellular immunity recently have been demonstrated in the gut of patients with AIDS and AIDS-related complex (ARC).[46] The intestinal mucosa of patients infected with HIV has abnormally low numbers of T cells, especially CD4+ cells, and reversal of the CD4+:CD8+ ratio. Generalized increases in

346

Table 22–1. HIV-Related Bacterial Infections

Pneumonia	**Meningitis**
Streptococcus pneumoniae	*Listeria monocytogenes*
Haemophilus influenzae	**Disseminated Infection**
Moraxella catarrhalis	*Salmonella*
Group A streptococci	*Staphylococcus aureus*
Pseudomonas aeruginosa	*R. quintana*
Klebsiella pneumoniae	*S. Pneumoniae*
Staphylococcus aureus	*P. aeruginosa*
Rhodococcus equii	*Escherichia coli*
(Legionella pneumophila)	Other Enterobacteriaceae
Gastroenteritis	**Sinusitis**
Shigella flexneri	*S. pneumoniae*
Salmonella species	*P. aeruginosa*
Campylobacter jejuni	Staphylococci
Campylobacter fennelliae	Anaerobes
Campylobacter cinaedi	
Clostridium difficile toxin	
Skin Infections	
Rochalimaea quintana	
Staphylococci	
Streptococci	

Table 22–2. Factors Associated with Bacterial Infections in Persons with HIV

T-Cell Defects	**Macrophage Defects**
Loss of CD4+ lymphocytes	Decreased bacterial killing
Decreased interleukin-2 production	Decreased phagocytosis
Decreased interferon-γ production	**Granulocyte Defects**
? Impaired cytotoxic T-lymphocyte function	Drug-induced neutropenia
B-Cell Defects	Impaired chemotaxis (?)
Spontaneous proliferation	Impaired bacterial killing (?)
Polyclonal gammopathy	
Impaired response to de novo antigens	
Loss of memory Immunoglobulins	

mucosal mononuclear cells and CD8+ lymphocytes are also seen.[46] Alterations in the production of mucosal IgA have been reported in AIDS and HIV-seropositive patients. These defects in cellular and humoral immunity in the gut of patients with advanced HIV disease may explain both the increased incidence of enteric infections and the high rate of their systemic spread, for local defenses are unable to contain pathogens and prevent access to the bloodstream.

A number of B-cell abnormalities have been described in association with HIV infection and AIDS, and they are associated with infectious complications with bacteria that require intact humoral immunity for control.[1,24,27,37] HIV infection frequently results in spontaneous B-cell proliferation, with a nonspecific polyclonal increase in IgG secretion.[28] Coinfection with Epstein-Barr virus or cytomegalovirus may potentiate this effect. The polyclonal gammopathy of AIDS often is associated with increases in circulating immune complexes, which may have a variety of clinical consequences.[5]

The most serious change in humoral immunity seen in patients with AIDS is a lack of response to a variety of de novo antigenic stimuli.[1,27,37] Paradoxically, in spite of generalized increases in immunoglobulin synthesis, the HIV-infected individual may be unable to mount a humoral immune response to new antigens from infectious agents such as encapsulated bacteria. The relatively greater incidence of infections with encapsulated organisms seen in children with HIV infection may be the result of lack of differentiated B cells producing specific antibodies to these agents, whereas adults with previous exposure presumably are more likely to maintain effective antibodies to these pathogens.[3,36]

Impairment of macrophage function may also result in infections with pyogenic bacteria in AIDS patients.[5] HIV directly infects monocytes and macrophages, resulting in qualitative functional defects. Moreover, decreased production of interferon-γ by T cells is associated with diminished phagocytic and bacteriocidal activity of macrophages. Loss of phagocytic function by macrophages, coupled with B-cell defects, is probably a factor in the high incidence of bacteremic pyogenic infections in patients with advanced HIV disease.

Granulocytes from patients with HIV infection may show decreased chemotaxis, impaired phagocytosis, and reduced bacterial killing.[11] Moreover, an increasing frequency of granulocytopenia is being seen in persons with HIV infection because of the use of myelotoxic drugs. In particular, the antiviral agents zidovudine[45] and ganciclovir cause severe reductions in granulocytes and may result in opportunistic infection with *Staphylococcus aureus, Pseudomonas aeruginosa, Klebsiella pneumoniae, Escherichia coli,* and other Enterobacteriaciae. Antitumor therapy for Kaposi's sarcoma is often associated with granulocytopenia, and myelosuppression secondary to severe mycobacterial disease is not uncommon in AIDS patients. Although the degree of granulocytopenia is frequently less severe than that seen in patients with malignancies treated with antitumor regimens, the relative granulocytopenia apparently is associated with an increased risk of pyogenic infections. Whether the use of recombinant colony-stimulating factors will reduce the incidence of bacterial infections in patients receiving myelosuppressive drugs is not known.

EPIDEMIOLOGY AND CLINICAL PRESENTATION

Bacterial Pneumonia

Pneumonia caused by pyogenic bacteria has been noted in patients with AIDS since early in the epidemic[32] (Table 22–3). Simberkoff et al.[50] in 1984 reported on four cases of community-acquired pneumococcal pneumonia, two with bacteremia, in AIDS patients from New York. An additional patient had hospital-acquired pneumococcal pneumonia despite having received pneumococcal vaccine against the specific serotype of *S. pneumoniae* that caused his illness.

Polsky et al.[39] found that 10% of pneumonias in AIDS patients at Memorial Sloan-Kettering Cancer Center were due to community-acquired bacteria, with an annual attack rate of 17.9 per 1000 AIDS patients. Eight of 18 episodes were due to pneumococcus, and another eight were caused by *H. influenzae.* Four of 13 patients had recurrences 2 to 6 months after the initial episode. Antibody titers

**Table 22–3.   Incidence of Bacterial Pneumonias in
Patients with HIV Infection or AIDS**

AUTHORS	POPULATION	NO. CASES/ TOTAL PATIENTS
Simberkoff et al.[50]	Hospitalized AIDS patients	5
Polsky et al.[39]	Hospitalized AIDS patients	13/336
Gerberding et al.[15]	Hospitalized AIDS patients	22
Witt et al.[58]	Hospitalized AIDS patients	21/59
Selwyn et al.[49]	Intravenous drug users	14/159*

*Seronegative control rate, 6/277 (p <.05).

failed to rise appropriately after infection with the pneumococcus in the three patients tested. Gerberding, Krieger, and Sande[15] in San Francisco described 17 patients with AIDS or ARC who had pneumonia caused by encapsulated organisms, including 10 who had relapses after receiving appropriate therapy. Seventy-five percent of episodes were bacteremic. Witt, Craven, and McCabe[58] recently have reported community-acquired pneumonias in 21 of 59 AIDS and ARC patients from Boston City Hospital. The prevalence of pneumonia was higher among intravenous (IV) drug users and Caribbean-born heterosexuals (58% and 53%, respectively) than in homosexual or bisexual men (14%). One third of the patients had recurrent bacterial pneumonia despite appropriate therapy. Agents responsible for infection included the pneumococcus, *H. influenzae,* other *Haemophilus* species, *Moraxella catarrhalis,* group B streptococci, *S. aureus, Legionella,* and *Mycoplasma pneumoniae.* Schlamm and Yancovitz[48] found a high rate of *H. influenzae* pneumonia in young adults with AIDS, ARC, or risk factors for HIV infection.

In a 12-month prospective study of HIV infection in IV drug users by Selwyn et al.[49] 14 of 159 (9%) HIV-seropositive patients developed bacterial pneumonias, primarily caused by *H. influenzae* and pneumococcus, compared to six of 277 (2%) seronegative controls (p <0.05). Data from the death registry in New York City show a more than twelvefold increase in mortality rate from community-acquired pneumonias in IV drug users between 1978 and 1986, probably the result of HIV-induced immunosuppression.[53] A recent study of community-acquired pneumonia at Johns Hopkins Hospital showed that 42% of hospitalized patients with pneumococcal infection were HIV seropositive.[31] In addition, of known HIV-seropositive patients admitted with an undiagnosed, community-acquired pneumonia, 38% had bacterial pneumonia (19% pneumococcal) compared to 22% with *Pneumocystis carinii* pneumonia.

Bacteremia with a variety of organisms, some associated with pneumonias, has been reported in AIDS patients from several institutions.[12,15,50,57,58] In a study of 10 San Francisco hospitals Redd et al.[43] found that 25% of patients with pneumococcal bacteremia had symptomatic HIV infection. The incidence of pneumococcal bacteremia in AIDS patients, 9.4 cases per 1000 persons per year, was 100-fold higher than previously reported. Yamaguchi, Charache, and Chaisson,[60] at Johns Hopkins Hospital, Baltimore, Maryland, observed a 46% prevalence of bacteremia in HIV-seropositive patients with pneumococcal pneumonia. The incidence of pneumococcal bacteremia at the hospital increased eightfold from 1985 to 1989, primarily as a result of HIV infection in the community.

The presentation of bacterial pneumonias in AIDS patients is similar to that seen in nonimmunosuppressed hosts and differs from the typical presentation of *P. carinii* pneumonia.[26] The onset of symptoms is often abrupt, and the duration of symptoms is generally only several days.[15,58] Fever, productive cough, and dyspnea are characteristic, and pleuritic chest pain was present in 69% of patients in one series.[15] Localized findings such as rales, bronchial breath sounds, egophany, and dullness to percussion on physical examination are common. Laboratory studies usually show a relative leukocytosis, with an increased number of band forms, elevated sedimentation rate, and arterial hypoxemia. Chest radiographs are almost always abnormal, with focal lobar or segmental consolidation more common than diffuse infiltrates (Figure 22–1A). *H. influenzae* may be associated more often with diffuse infiltrates than *S. pneumoniae,* with more than one quarter of *H. influenzae* pneumonias causing diffuse, bilateral infiltrates.[39] Gram's stain of the sputum reveals many neutrophils, and organisms suggestive of the causative agent may be seen. Sputum culture results are usually positive, and blood culture results are positive in 40% to 80% of cases.

Differential diagnosis includes other opportunistic infections, particularly *P. carinii* pneumonia. Patients presenting with symptoms consistent with a bacterial pneumonia whose chest x-ray studies show focal consolidation should have sputum Gram's stain and cultures of sputum and blood performed and should receive empiric antimicrobial therapy. In patients for whom a definitive diagnosis is not made or in those who fail to respond to therapy, diagnostic evaluation for pneumocystosis should be performed (Figure 22–1B). In several series up to 10% of HIV-infected patients with pyogenic pneumonia presented with concomitant *P. carinii* pneumonia.

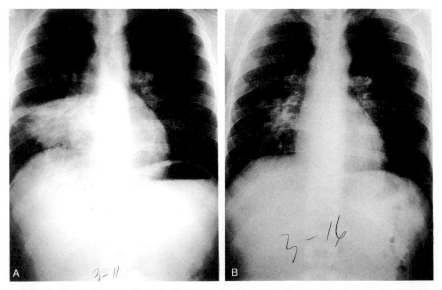

FIGURE 22–1. **A,** Chest radiograph of a homosexual man with fever, productive cough, and pleuritic chest pain. Sputum and blood cultures produced *Streptococcus pneumoniae*. **B,** Five days later the focal infiltrate is resolving, but symptoms persist. Giemsa-stained induced sputum revealed *Pneumocystis carinii*.

Patients with diffuse pulmonary infiltrates are less likely to have bacterial pneumonias than those with focal infiltrates. Nevertheless, sputum induction for *P. carinii* examination and/or bronchoalveolar lavage specimens should be stained and cultured for pyogenic pathogens, particularly if purulence is noted.

Empiric treatment of suspected bacterial pneumonia should include coverage for the most common pathogens. Trimethoprim-sulfamethoxazole is an excellent agent, providing activity against the pneumococcus, *H. influenzae*, *M. catarrhalis*, and *P. carinii*. Patients allergic to sulfa can be empirically treated with a second-generation cephalosporin, ampicillin-clavulanate, or a semisynthetic penicillin and an aminoglycoside. Broad-spectrum agents such as third-generation cephalosporins and imipenem are not usually indicated.

Enteric Pathogens

Multiple case reports of nontyphoidal salmonellosis in patients with AIDS have been published.[4,14,16,22,33,40,55] Case series from Jacobs et al.[22] and Glaser et al.[16] include high rates of *Salmonella* bacteremia and frequent relapses despite appropriate antimicrobial therapy. Occurrence of salmonellosis before the diagnosis of AIDS was noted in a substantial proportion of cases.

Celum et al.[7] found the incidence of salmonellosis in San Francisco AIDS patients was twentyfold greater than that in age- and sex-matched controls. Using population-based disease registries for both AIDS and *Salmonella,* these investigators found a significantly higher prevalence of bacteremia in AIDS patients than in controls (45% versus 9%) and noted that one third of *Salmonella* infections occurred before the diagnosis of AIDS. An association between salmonellosis and raw milk consumption was seen.

Sexually transmitted enteric infections with *Shigella* sp., *Campylobacter jejuni*, *C. cinaedi*, and *C. fennelliae* were previously prevalent in homosexual men and are associated with risk of HIV infection.[30,41,42] Clinical experience with patients with HIV disease suggests that infections with *Shigella* sp. and *Campylobacter sp.* are more resistant to therapy and tend to recur after treatment with appropriate agents.[10] Bacteremia, particularly with *Campylobacter* sp., is not unusual, although comparative studies with immunocompetent controls have not been reported.[34]

Antibiotic-associated colitis (pseudomembranous colitis), caused by the toxin of *Clostridium difficile,* is a growing problem in patients with HIV infection who receive prolonged courses of antibiotic treatment. A recent retrospective study by Harrison and Bartlett[20] at Johns Hopkins Hospital found that 3.3% of patients hospitalized on an AIDS ward had *C. difficile* toxin identified in their stool, a percentage significantly greater than in other patient populations. More than one third of cases were acquired in the hospital, and the majority of patients had received ampicillin, clindamycin,or a cephalosporin before developing symptoms. Fatal pseudomembranous colitis was reported in four of 26 patients (15%).

Diarrhea is a common complaint in AIDS patients and is associated with a host of organisms in addition to bacteria (Table 22–4) (see Chapter 12). Salmonellosis in AIDS and ARC patients initially is seen as diarrhea in more than one half of cases, whereas up to 45% is manifested by a febrile illness without colitis. When diarrhea is present, it is usually severe and may be associated with cramping, bloating, and nausea. Tenesmus and rectal pain are rare and suggest proctitis caused

Table 22–4. Causes of Diarrhea in AIDS Patients

ENTEROCOLITIS	PROCTITIS
Entamoeba histolytica	*Neisseria gonorrhoeae*
Giardia lamblia	*Chlamydia trachomatis*
Cryptosporidium	Herpes simplex virus
Shigella flexneri	*Treponema pallidum*
Campylobacter jejuni	
Salmonella sp.	
Cytomegalovirus	
Microsporidia	
Clostridium difficile toxin	
Mycobacterium avium- complex	
Isospora belli	

by herpes simplex virus, *Neisseria gonorrhoeae, Chlamydia,* or syphilis. Fever is present in the majority of patients with salmonellosis. Blood counts and blood chemistries are nonspecific. Stool examination may show fecal leukocytes, but the sensitivity of this test in AIDS patients with salmonellosis is not established. Cultures of stool and blood establish the diagnosis. *Shigella* and *Campylobacter* are usually associated with severe, often bloody, diarrhea, cramping, nausea, and fever. Fecal leukocytes are generally present, and cultures reveal the organism.

Asymptomatic enteric infections, previously reported in sexually active homosexual men, are also prevalent in patients with AIDS. Laughon et al.[29] found that 39% of 28 AIDS patients without diarrhea harbored pathogenic organisms in stool. Fifty-five percent of AIDS patients with diarrhea were found to have an infectious cause. *Shigella* and *Campylobacter* accounted for one quarter of the symptomatic infections (Table 22–5).

Table 22–5. Bacterial and Other Enteric Infections in AIDS Patients with and without Diarrhea

	NO. POSITIVE/NO. CULTURED (% Positive)	
	AIDS AND DIARRHEA (n = 49)	AIDS AND NO DIARRHEA (n = 28)
Shigella sp.	2/41 (5)	0/20
Campylobacter sp.	5/47 (11)	2/24 (8)
Chlamydia trachomatis	5/44 (11)	2/16 (12.5)
Vibrio parahaemolyticus	2/47 (4)	0/26
Clostridium difficile toxin	3/42 (7)	0/19
Cryptosporidium	7/45 (16)	0/19
Giardia lamblia	2/45 (4)	1/19 (5)
Isospora belli	1/45 (2)	0/19
Herpes simplex virus	7/38 (18)	
Any agent	28/49 (57)	11/28 (39)

Modified from Laughon BE, Druckman DA, Vernon A, et al: Prevalence of enteric pathogens in homosexual men with and without acquired immunodeficiency syndrome. Gastroenterology 94:984-993, 1988.

Evaluation of the patient with HIV infection and diarrhea should include a careful history and physical examination and an orderly laboratory workup (see Chapter 12). The cause of diarrhea in up to 50% of patients is established after a stool bacterial culture, *C. difficile* toxin assay, and stool examination for ova and parasites. Stool should also be examined for *Cryptosporidium*. When no diagnosis is established with these tests and diarrhea persists, both upper and lower endoscopy may be performed to allow inspection and biopsy for cytomegalovirus, *Mycobacterium avium*–complex, and microsporidia. The diagnosis in 50% of AIDS patients with chronic diarrhea is established by complete endoscopy.[19] The remaining patients are presumed to have an idiopathic, HIV-associated enteropathy.

Therapy for enteric pathogens should be directed against a specific organism. Empiric therapy for presumed bacterial enterocolitis requires agents active against *Salmonella, Shigella,* and *Campylobacter.* Therapy with the quinolones norfloxacin and ciprofloxacin is usually adequate to treat these organisms. *Salmonella* may be treated with ampicillin, chloramphenicol, trimethoprim-sulfamethoxazole, or a cepholosporin, depending on antimicrobial sensitivities. Although nonimmunocompromised hosts are generally not treated for salmonellosis, therapy is always indicated in immunocompromised, HIV-infected patients. The duration of treatment for bacteremia should be at least 10 to 14 days; AIDS patients with enteritis should receive 1 to 2 weeks of therapy. Judicious use of antimotility agents such as loperamide may decrease symptoms. *C. difficile* colitis can be treated with oral metronidazole or oral vancomycin, with vancomycin preferred for more severe cases. Hospitalization is frequently necessary for administration of IV hydration and management of electrolyte disturbances. Surgery is reserved for life-threatening disease.

AIDS patients apparently are uniquely susceptible to recurrent episodes of *Salmonella* bacteremia. Patients typically present with fever and chills, usually without evidence of the septic shock syndrome (hypotension and progressive metabolic acidosis). All blood cultures are usually positive for nontyphoidal strains of *Salmonella*. Therapy with conventional antibiotics such as ampicillin and trimethoprim-sulfamethoxazole results in disappearance of symptoms and resolution of bacteremia. However, once antibiotics are discontinued, relapse of bacteremia is common. Jacobson et al.[23] reported therapeutic success with ciprofloxacin, 750 mg twice daily by mouth, both as initial therapy (with clearing of bacteremia) and as suppressive treatment. It has recently been suggested that zidovudine, which has significant activity against gram-negative organisms, may prevent the occurrence or recurrence of *Salmonella* bacteremia in patients with HIV infection.[47]

Other Bacteremias

In addition to the bacteremias associated with pulmonary and enteric infections, patients with HIV infection have a high incidence of community-acquired and catheter-related bacteremia. Staphylococcal bacteremia is particularly prevalent in patients with central venous catheters. In a review of published studies of catheter-related infections in patients with HIV disease, Northfelt and Polsky[35] found that the incidence of bacteremia was 0.23 cases per 100 catheter days. This rate is substantially higher than rates reported in other patient populations with central venous catheters. Several reasons that patients with HIV may experience more infections include more frequent manipulation of catheters, granulocytopenia associated with ganciclovir therapy, or injection of illicit drugs into catheters. A small study of prophylactic antibiotics for patients with HIV infection and central venous catheters found no benefit from vancomycin administration at the time of catheter placement.[2]

Gram-negative bacteremia is also frequently seen in patients with advanced HIV disease. Yamaguchi and Chaisson[59] reported that 5% of patients hospitalized on the Johns Hopkins AIDS ward had gram-negative bacteremia. The most common isolate was *P. aeruginosa,* followed by *E. coli, Salmonella, Klebsiella,* and others. One third of patients had indwelling catheters, one third had no identified source of infection, and the remainder had respiratory, gastrointestinal, or genitourinary sources of bacteremia. Neutropenia was an uncommon finding, with only 15% of patients ever having a total neutrophil count $<1500/mm^3$. The mortality rate was 38%, indicating that prompt evaluation and aggressive treatment of HIV-infected patients with possible gram-negative bacteremia is essential.

Sinusitis

Sinusitis is a recently recognized complication of HIV infection. Godofsky et al.[17] recently identified 72 patients with HIV infection and sinusitis, documented radiographically and clinically. Microbiologic assessment of patients was very limited, but *P. aeruginosa, H. influenzae,* and the pneumococcus were all isolated from sinus aspirates. Patients presented clinically with fever, headache, congestion, and cough. Multiple sinuses were involved in 72% of patients, and the degree of sinus opacification radiographically was extensive in the majority of patients. Results of treatment were initially successful in most patients, but chronic sinusitis developed in 64% of patients. Chronic disease was significantly more likely to occur in patients with CD4 cells counts $<200/mm^3$.

Patients with HIV and sinusitis should undergo a diagnostic sinus aspiration if possible before the initiation of antimicrobial therapy. Empiric therapy with a second-generation cephalosporin and an agent active against anaerobes (e.g., clindamycin) is appropriate. If *Pseudomonas* is identified or if patients fail to respond to empiric therapy, an antipseudomonal agent should be added. Adjunctive therapy with decongestants and anti-inflammatory agents is essential. Chronic suppressive antibiotic therapy may be required.

Bacillary Angiomatosis

Bacillary angiomatosis is a newly identified syndrome prevalent in patients with HIV infection that may resemble cutaneous Kaposi's sarcoma[9,52] (see Chapter 10). Bacillary angiomatosis manifests clinically with raised, friable, erythematous subcutaneous nodules and lymphadenopathy in patients with HIV, a presentation similar to that of cat scratch disease.[25] In addition to causing cutaneous disease, bacillary angiomatosis has been seen in association with disseminated disease, including hepatitis and osteomyelitis. Recent studies using the polymerase chain reaction and other sophisticated molecular techniques have identified the causative organism to be an alpha purple bacterium closely related to the *Rickettsia*-like organism *Rochalimaea quintana*.[38,44] Although this organism is closely related to the cat scratch bacillus, clinical evidence suggests that it is not the same. The bacillary angiomatosis bacillus has been identified in cutaneous, osseus, hepatic, and blood specimens from patients with symptomatic disease, and the organism is the causative agent of peliosis, a cystic hepatic infection. Diagnosis of bacillary angiomatosis requires biopsy of affected tissues and staining with Warthin-Starry silver stain or immunoperoxidase, using cat scratch bacillus antiserum. Treatment of bacillary angiomatosis is with erythromycin or doxycycline for at least 4 weeks. Several failures of ciprofloxacin in treating HIV-associated bacillary angiomatosis have been described recently.[54]

PREVENTION

The use of preventive measures for the control of bacterial infections in AIDS patients may reduce the incidence of disease. Three approaches—hygienic measures, prophylactic antibiotics, and immunotherapy—can be used in selected settings. Hygienic control is particularly important for prevention of enteric infections. Avoidance of oral-anal sexual contact reduces the transmission of pathogenic organisms. *Salmonella* infections in AIDS patients have been linked to raw milk, snake powders, pet turtles, and domestic turkeys.[7,55,56] Patients with HIV infection should avoid unsanitary water supplies, particularly in developing countries. Appropriate infection control precautions should be used in the care of patients with enteric infections. Strict infection control measures should also be taught to patients who are receiving chronic therapy through indwelling central venous catheters.

Antibiotic prophylaxis with trimethoprim-sulfamethoxazole is recommended for children with AIDS and adults who are at risk for *P. carinii* pneumonia[8] (see Chapter 17). Unfortunately, the incidence of adverse reactions to this agent limits its use in this population.[18] Limited evidence suggests that AIDS patients receiving trimethoprim-sulfamethoxazole for *P. carinii* prophylaxis have a lower incidence of serious bacterial infections than patients receiving aerosol pentamidine. Prophylactic penicillin may be appropriate for AIDS patients who have had relapses of pneumococcal disease, although the efficacy of this therapy is not established.

Passive immunotherapy with immune globulin can reduce the incidence of bacterial infections in children with ARC or AIDS, and a monthly immunoglobulin injection is indicated for children with symptomatic HIV infection.[6] The use of immunoglobulin in adults is not routinely recommended.

Active immunization with polyvalent pneumococcal vaccine is probably not effective in the majority of symptomatic HIV-infected patients[1,39,50] (see Chapter 6). Responses to pneumococcal vaccine are suboptimum in the majority of AIDS and ARC patients, although HIV seropositive individuals with more than 450 CD4 + cells/μl appear to respond as well as uninfected controls.[21] Immunization with protein-conjugated–*H. influenzae* type b capsular vaccine is recommended for all HIV-infected children in accordance with childhood immunization guidelines. A recent study of adults with varying stages of HIV infection demonstrated that response to a protein-conjugated–*H. influenzae* type vaccine was significantly better than that to a polysaccharide vaccine in all patients except those with AIDS, whose median CD4 lymphocyte count was 64/mm³.[51] This study also confirmed that patients with higher CD4 cell counts responded better to vaccination. Efforts are now underway to develop a protein-conjugated pneumococcal vaccine that would be more immunogenic in patients with or without HIV infection.

REFERENCES

1. Ammann AS, Schiffman G, Abrams D, et al: B-cell immunodeficiency in acquired immune deficiency syndrome. JAMA 251:1447-1449, 1984
2. Battan R, Raviglione MC, D'Amore T, et al: Vancomycin prophylaxis for long term central venous catheter infections in AIDS patients. Sixth International Conference on AIDS. (Abstract 531:524.) San Francisco, 1990
3. Bernstein LJ, Krieger BZ, Novick B, et al: Bacterial infection in the acquired immunodeficiency syndrome of children. Pediatr Infect Dis 4:472-475, 1985
4. Bottone EJ, Wormser GP, Duncanson FP: Nontyphoidal *Salmonella* bacteremia as an early infection in acquired immunodeficiency syndrome. Diagn Microbiol Infect Dis 2:247-250, 1984
5. Bowen DL, Lane HC, Fauci AS: Immunopathogenesis of the acquired immunodeficiency syndrome. Ann Intern Med 103:704-709, 1985
6. Calvelli TA, Rubinstein AR: Intravenous gamma-globulin in infant acquired immunodeficiency syndrome. Pediatr Infect Dis 5(suppl 3):S207-210, 1985
7. Celum CL, Chaisson RE, Rutherford GW, et al: Incidence of salmonellosis in patients with AIDS. J Infect Dis 156:998-1002, 1987
8. Centers for Disease Control: Guidelines for prophylaxis against *Pneumocystis carinii* pneumonia for persons infected with human immunodeficiency virus. MMWR 38(suppl 5):1-9, 1989
9. Cockerell CJ, Whitlow MA, Webster GF, Friedman-Kien AE: Epithelioid angiomatosis: A distinct vascular disorder in patients with the acquired immunodeficiency syndrome or AIDS-related complex. Lancet 2:654-656, 1987
10. Dworkin B, Wormser GP, Abdoo RH, et al: Persistence of multiply antibiotic-resistant *Campylobacter jejuni* in a patient with acquired immune deficiency syndrome. Am J Med 5:965-970, 1986
11. Ellis M, Gupta S, Galant S, et al: Impaired neutrophil function in patients with AIDS or AIDS-related complex: A comprehensive evaluation. J Infect Dis 158:1268-1276, 1988
12. Eng RH, Bishburg E, Smith SM, et al: Bacteremia and fungemia in patients with acquired immune deficiency syndrome. Am J Clin Pathol 1:105-107, 1986
13. Fainstein V, Bolivar R, Mavligit G, et al: Disseminated infection due to *Mycobacterium avium-intracellulare* in a homosexual man with Kaposi's sarcoma. Ann Intern Med 97:539-546, 1982
14. Fischl MA, Dickinson GM, Sinave C, et al: *Salmonella* bacteremia as manifestation of acquired immunodeficiency syndrome. Arch Intern Med 146:113-115, 1986
15. Gerberding JL, Krieger J, Sande MA: Recurrent bacteremic infection with *S. pneumoniae* in patients with AIDS virus (AV) infection. Program and Abstracts of Twenty-sixth Interscience Conference on Antimicrobial Agents and Chemotherapy. American Society for Microbiology. (Abstract 443.) 1986
16. Glaser JB, Morton-Kute L, Berger SR, et al: *Salmonella typhimurium* bacterium associated with the acquired immunodeficiency syndrome. Ann Intern Med 102:189-193, 1985
17. Godofsky E, Zinreich J, Armstrong M, et al: Sinusitis in HIV positive patients. Program and Abstracts of Thirty-first Interscience Conference on Antimicrobial Agents and Chemotherapy. American Society for Microbiology. (Abstract 557.) 1991
18. Gordin FM, Simon GL, Wofsy CB, Mills J: Adverse reactions to trimethoprim-sulfamethoxazole in patients with the acquired immunodeficiency syndrome. Ann Intern Med 100:495-499, 1984
19. Greenson JK, Belitsos P, Yardley JH, Bartlett JG: AIDS enteropathy: Occult enteric infections and duodenal mucosal alterations in chronic diarrhea. Ann Intern Med 114:366-372, 1991
20. Harrison KS, Bartlett JG: *Clostridium difficile* diarrhea in AIDS patients. Program and Abstracts of the Thirty-first Interscience Conference on Antimicrobial Agents and Chemotherapy. American Society for Microbiology. (Abstract 547.) 1991
21. Huang K-L, Ruben FL, Rinaldo CR, et al: Antibody responses after influenza and pneumococcal immunization in HIV-infected homosexual men. JAMA 257:2047-2050, 1987

22. Jacobs JL, Gold JWM, Murray HW, et al: Salmonella infections in patients with the acquired immunodeficiency syndrome. Ann Intern Med 102:186-188,1985
23. Jacobson MA, Hahn SM, Gerberding JL, et al: Ciprofloxacin for *Salmonella* bacteremia in the acquired immunodeficiency syndrome (AIDS). Ann Intern Med 110:1027-1029, 1989
24. Katz IR, Krown SE, Safai B, et al: Antigen-specific and polyclonal B-cell responses in patients with acquired immunodeficiency disease syndrome. Clin Immunol Immunopathol 39:359-367, 1986
25. Koehler JE, LeBoit PE, Egbert BM, Berger TG: Cutaneous vascular lesions and disseminated cat-scratch disease in patients with the acquired immunodeficiency syndrome (AIDS) and AIDS-related complex. Ann Intern Med 109:449-455, 1988
26. Kovacs JA, Hiemenz JW, Macher AM, et al: *Pneumocystis carinii* pneumonia: A comparison between patients with the acquired immunodeficiency syndrome and patients with other immunodeficiencies. Ann Intern Med 100:663-671, 1984
27. Lane HC, Depper JM, Green WC, et al: Qualitative analysis of immune function in patients with the acquired immunodeficiency syndrome: Evidence for a selective defect in soluble antigen recognition. N Engl J Med 313:79-84, 1985
28. Lane HC, Masur H, Edgar LC, et al: Abnormalities of B-cell activation and immunoregulation in patients with the acquired immunodeficiency syndrome. N Engl J Med 309:453-458, 1983
29. Laughon BE, Druckman DA, Vernon A, et al: Prevalence of enteric pathogens in homosexual men with and without acquired immunodeficiency syndrome. Gastroenterology 94:984-993, 1988
30. Moss AR, Osmond D, Bacchetti P, et al: Risk factors for AIDS and HIV seropositivity in homosexual men. Am J Epidemiol 125:1035-1047, 1987
31. Mundy L, Autwater P, Burton A, et al: Etiology of community acquired pneumonia (CAP): HIV + vs HIV − patients. Programs and Abstracts of Thirty-first Interscience Conference on Antimicrobial Agents and Chemotherapy. American Society for Microbiology. (Abstract 569.) 1991
32. Murray JF, Felton CP, Garay SM, et al: Pulmonary complications of the acquired immunodeficiency syndrome: Report of a National Heart, Lung and Blood Institute Workshop. N Engl J Med 310:1682-1688, 1984
33. Nadelman RB, Mathur-Wagh U, Yancovitz SR, Mildvan D: *Salmonella* bacteremia associated with the acquired immunodeficiency syndrome (AIDS). Arch Intern Med 145:1968-1971, 1985
34. Ng VL, Hadley WK, Fennell CL, et al: Successive bacteremias with *"Campylobacter cinaedi"* and *"Campylobacter fenneliae"* in a bisexual male. J Clin Microbiol 25:2008-2009, 1987
35. Northfelt D, Polsky B: Bacteremia in patients with HIV infection. In Volberding P, Jacobson MA (eds): AIDS Clinical Review 1991. New York, Marcel Dekker, 1991
36. Oleske J, Minnefor A, Cooper R Jr, et al: Immune deficiency syndrome in children. JAMA 249:2345-2349, 1983
37. Pahwa SG, Quilop MTJ, Lange M, et al: Defective B-lymphocyte function in homosexual men in relation to the acquired immunodeficiency syndrome. Ann Intern Med 101:757-763, 1984
38. Perkocha LA, Geaghan SM, Benedict Yen TS, et al: Clinical and pathological features of bacillary peliosis hepatitis in association with human immunodeficiency virus. N Engl J Med 323:1581-1586, 1990
39. Polsky B, Gold JWM, Whimbey E, et al: Bacterial pneumonia in patients with the acquired immunodeficiency syndrome. Ann Intern Med 104:38-41, 1986
40. Profeta S, Forrester C, Eng RHK, et al: *Salmonella* infections in patients with the acquired immunodeficiency syndrome. Arch Intern Med 145:670-672, 1985
41. Quinn TC, Goodell SE, Fennell C, et al: Infections with *Campylobacter jejuni* and *Campylobacter*-like organisms in homosexual men. Ann Intern Med 101:187-192, 1984
42. Quinn TC, Stamm WE, Goodell SE, et al: The polymicrobial origin of intestinal infections in homosexual men. N Engl J Med 309:576-582, 1983
43. Redd SC, Rutherford GW III, Sande MA, et al: The role of human immunodeficiency virus infection in pneumococcal bacteremia in San Francisco residents. J Infect Dis 162:1012-1017, 1990
44. Relman DA, Loutit JS, Schmidt TM, et al: The agent of bacillary angiomatosis: An approach to the identification of uncultured pathogens. N Engl J Med 323:1573-1580, 1990
45. Richman DD, Fischl MA, Grieco MH, et al: The toxicity of azidothymidine (AZT) in the treatment of patients with AIDS and AIDS-related complex: A double-blind, placebo-controlled trial. N Engl J Med 317:192-197, 1987
46. Rogers VD, Kagnoff MF. Gastrointestinal manifestations of the acquired immune deficiency syndrome. West J Med 146:57-67, 1987
47. Salmon D, Detruchis P, Leport C, et al: Efficacy of zidovudine in preventing relapses of *Salmonella* bacteremia in AIDS. J Infect Dis 163:415-416, 1991

48. Schlamm HT, Yancovitz SR: *Haemophilus influenzae* pneumonia in young adults with AIDS, ARC, or risk of AIDS. Am J Med 86:11-14, 1989

49. Selwyn PA, Feingold AR, Hartel D, et al: Increased risk of bacterial pneumonia in HIV-infected drug users without AIDS. AIDS 2:267-272, 1988

50. Simberkoff MS, El Sadr W, Schiffman G, Raha JJ Jr: *Streptococcus pneumoniae* infections and bacteremia in patients with acquired immunodeficiency syndrome, with report of pneumococcal vaccine failure. Am Rev Respir Dis 130:1174-1176, 1984

51. Steinhoff MC, Aeurbach B, Nelson KE, et al: Effect of HIV infection on the antibody responses of adult men to *Haemophilus influenzae* type b vaccines. N Engl J Med 325:1837-1842, 1991

52. Stoler MH, Bonfiglio TA, Steigbigel RT, Pereira M: An atypical subcutaneous infection associated with acquired immune deficiency syndrome. Am J Clin Pathol 80:714-718,1983

53. Stoneburner RL, Des Jarlais DC, Benezra D, et al: A larger spectrum of severe HIV-1–related disease in intravenous drug users in New York City. Science 242:916-919, 1988

54. Tappero JW, Koehler JE: Cat scratch disease and bacillary angiomatosis. JAMA 266:1938-1939, 1991

55. Tauxe RV, Rigau-Perez JG, Wells JG, Blake PA: Turtle-associated salmonellosis in Puerto Rico: Hazards of the global turtle trade. JAMA 254:237-239, 1985

56. Weber J: Gastrointestinal disease in AIDS. Clin Immun All 6:519-541, 1986

57. Whimbey E, Gold JWM, Polsky B, et al: Bacteremia and fungemia in patients with acquired immunodeficiency syndrome. Ann Intern Med 104:511-514, 1986

58. Witt DJ, Craven DE, McCabe WR: Bacterial infections in adult patients with the acquired immune deficiency syndrome (AIDS) and AIDS-related complex. Am J Med 82:900-906, 1987

59. Yamaguchi E, Chaisson RE: Gram-negative bacteremias (GNB) in HIV-infected patients. Sixth International Conference on AIDS. (Abstract No. Th.B.539.) San Francisco, June 20-24, 1990

60. Yamaguchi E, Charache P, Chaisson RE: Increasing incidence of pneumococcal infections (PI) associated with HIV infection in an inner-city hospital, 1985-1989 (abstract). 1990 World Conference on Lung Health, May 20-24, Boston, Massachusetts. Am Rev Resp Dis 141:A619, 1990

23

MANAGEMENT OF HERPES VIRUS INFECTIONS (CMV, HSV, VZV)

W. LAWRENCE DREW, MD, PhD
WILLIAM BUHLES, PhD
KIM S. ERLICH, MD

CYTOMEGALOVIRUS

Infection with cytomegalovirus (CMV) is extremely common in patients with AIDS and can result in several clinical illnesses, including chorioretinitis, pneumonia, esophagitis, colitis, encephalitis, adrenalitis, and hepatitis.[2] Autopsy and clinical studies indicate that 90% of AIDS patients develop active CMV infection during their illness. Up to 40% of these individuals may experience life- or sight-threatening disease caused by this virus. Retinitis occurs in up to 25% of AIDS patients, whereas gastrointestinal disease and pneumonia occur in 5% to 10% and 5%, respectively. Not all patients with blood, urine, or tissue cultures positive for CMV have clinical illness related to the infection, and diagnosis of disease caused by CMV should be made by tissue biopsy with histologic evidence of virus-mediated damage. Detection of CMV antigen or nucleic acid in tissue is an alternative method for establishing that CMV is actually causing tissue infection. If viral culture is positive for CMV and no other pathogen is identified in tissue, the virus may be the cause of the clinical illness, and a therapeutic trial may be warranted. This section reviews these clinical syndromes and their treatment with ganciclovir (DHPG) or foscarnet.

Chorioretinitis

Ocular disease caused by CMV occurs only in patients with severe immunodeficiency and is especially common in patients with AIDS. Clinical evidence of CMV retinitis occurs in approximately 25% of AIDS patients, and autopsy series have revealed that CMV retinitis is present in up to 30% of patients. Retinitis is occasionally the presenting manifestation of AIDS, but it more commonly presents

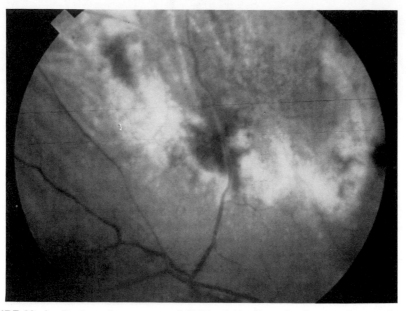

FIGURE 23–1. Funduscopic appearance of CMV retinitis, illustrating "cottage cheese and catsup" appearance resulting from perivascular exudates and hemorrhages. (Courtesy Dr. L. Schwartz, San Francisco.)

months to years after the diagnosis of AIDS has been established. Retinitis usually begins unilaterally, but progression to bilateral involvement is common because of the associated viremia. Systemic CMV infection also is frequently present, and other viscera may be simultaneously diseased. Decreased visual acuity, the presence of "floaters," or unilateral visual field loss is often the presenting complaint. Ophthalmologic examination typically reveals large creamy to yellowish-white granular areas with perivascular exudates and hemorrhages (referred to as a "cottage cheese and catsup" appearance) (Figure 23–1). These abnormalities may be found initially at the periphery of the fundus, but if left untreated, the lesions often progress to involve the macula and the optic disc. Histologic examination reveals coagulation necrosis and microvascular abnormalities.[1,64]

Differentiating suspected CMV retinitis lesions from "cotton wool spots" is essential. Cotton wool spots appear as small, fluffy, white lesions with indistinct margins and are not associated with exudates or hemorrhages.[1,64] They are common in AIDS patients, are usually asymptomatic, and probably result from microvascular lesions secondary to HIV infection. These lesions do not progress and often undergo spontaneous regression. Toxoplasmosis is the second most common opportunistic infection of the eye but is characterized by little if any hemorrhage. It is associated with cerebral toxoplasmosis in the majority of patients. Syphilis, herpes simplex, varicella-zoster virus (VZV), and tuberculosis are other infections with ocular findings.

Virtually all patients with CMV retinitis have CD4 lymphocyte counts <50 per mm^3, but it is not clear whether routine screening of patients should be performed when cell counts decline to this level. It is very important to inquire about visual

Table 23–1. Comparison of Course of CMV Disease in Ganciclovir-Treated versus Untreated Control Patients with AIDS

CMV SITE	NO. PATIENTS IMPROVED OR STABILIZED/TOTAL	
	GANCICLOVIR TREATED (%)	UNTREATED CONTROLS (%)
Retina	208/254 (82)	2/61 (3)
Gastrointestinal tract or colon	33/39 (85)	NA
Lung	18/23 (78)	1/7 (14)

NA, not available.

Table 23–2. Clinical Relapse of CMV Retinitis in Patients with AIDS

	MAINTENANCE GANCICLOVIR		
	NONE	LOW DOSE*	HIGH DOSE*
Number of patients	41	10	70
Mean cumulative induction dose (mg/kg)	162	155	167
Percent relapse free on day 120	14	0	58
Median days to relapse†	37	31	145

*Low dose, 10-20 mg/kg/wk; high dose, 25-35 mg/kg/wk.
†Kaplan-Meier estimate.

abnormalities and to examine the fundus carefully with pupillary dilatation and indirect ophthalmoscopy when there are complaints. Patients with suspected or confirmed CMV chorioretinitis should be considered for treatment with 9-(1,3,-dihydroxy-2-propoxymethyl) guanine (DHPG, ganciclovir) or foscarnet. These agents are effective in the treatment of CMV chorioretinitis, although lesions usually recur once therapy is discontinued.[3,29]

Initial "induction" treatment for CMV retinitis consists of 5 mg/kg twice daily for 14 days. The optimum dosage for maintenance therapy is approximately one half the induction dose (i.e., 5 mg/kg/day 7 days per week or 6 mg/kg/day for 5 days per week). Initial response (improvement or stabilization in vision or opthalmoscopic appearance) occurs in approximately 80% of treated patients. By comparison, the disease is relentlessly progressive in 90% of patients if left untreated (Table 23–1). Visual-field defects present at the onset of therapy do not reverse, but a decrease in visual acuity caused by edema of the macula may improve with treatment. Maintenance therapy throughout the life of the patient appears critical because the virus is only suppressed by ganciclovir and is not eliminated. Table 23–2 compares patients with CMV retinitis who received no maintenance therapy with those who received either low- or high-dose maintenance therapy. The data suggest that 25 to 35 mg/kg/week maintenance therapy is required for sustained remission. Toxicity, however, especially neutropenia, limits the dose and duration of maintenance therapy. Even with continued maintenance therapy, progression of CMV retinitis eventually occurs. This may result from viral resistance to the drug or from the patient's continued deterioration with progression of HIV infection. Retinal detachment may occur in later stages as the necrotic retina scars and thins.

Intravitreal injection has been used in certain special situations such as in patients in whom neutropenia limited the systemic use of the drug and in one series[7] appeared effective and relatively safe. Controlled, comparative studies are underway to determine efficacy and safety.

Central Nervous System Infection

Subacute encephalitis caused by CMV probably occurs in AIDS patients. Isolation and identification of CMV in brain tissue or cerebrospinal fluid has been reported[17,18,33] (see Chapter 13). CMV encephalitis in AIDS patients appears comparable to "subacute" encephalitis from other pathogens. Personality changes, difficulty concentrating, headaches, and somnolence are frequently present. The diagnosis can be confirmed only by brain biopsy, with evidence of periventricle necrosis, giant cells, intranuclear and intracytoplasmic inclusions, and isolation or other identification of the virus, for example, by antigen or nucleic acid.[33]

CMV may also cause myelitis or polyradiculopathy, which presents as a spinal cord syndrome with lower extremity weakness, spasticity, areflexia, and hypoesthesia. The cerebrospinal abnormalities are very unusual for a viral infection, namely, polymorphonuclear pleocytosis and a moderately low glucose concentration.[42] Administration of ganciclovir should be considered in AIDS patients with CMV encephalitis or polyradiculopathy, but no data on its efficacy are available.

Gastrointestinal Infection

Colitis

CMV colitis occurs in at least 5% to 10% of AIDS patients (see Chapter 12). Diarrhea, weight loss, anorexia, and fever are frequently present. The differential diagnosis includes infection caused by other gastrointestinal pathogens, including *Cryptosporidium, Giardia, Entamoeba, Mycobacterium, Shigella, Campylobacter,* and *Strongyloides stercoralis,* and involvement by lymphoma or Kaposi's sarcoma. Sigmoidoscopy reveals diffuse submucosal hemorrhages and diffuse mucosal ulcerations, although a grossly normal-appearing mucosa may be encountered in up to 10% of those with histologic evidence of CMV colitis (Figure 23–2). Biopsy reveals vasculitis, neutrophilic infiltration, CMV inclusions, and nonspecific inflammation.

Esophagitis

Clinically evident esophagitis in AIDS patients most commonly is due to either *Candida albicans* or herpes simplex virus (HSV), but CMV may also cause esophagitis (see Chapter 12). Patients with CMV esophagitis are apt to have pain on swallowing.

Treatment.   Patients with esophagitis or enterocolitis who do not have other pathogens detected by endoscopy, histology, or culture and who have CMV detected

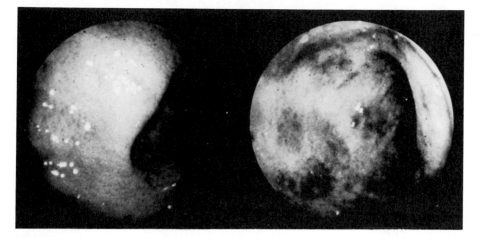

FIGURE 23–2. Sigmoidoscopic appearance of CMV colitis (two views), demonstrating diffuse submucosal hemorrhages and mucosal ulcerations. (Courtesy Dr. D. Dieterich, New York.)

by these methods may benefit from treatment with ganciclovir. The dosage for treating CMV colitis or esophagitis is usually 5 mg/kg twice daily for 14 to 21 days (depending on clinical response). It is uncertain whether maintenance therapy is necessary, although relapse or recurrences do occur.

The efficacy of ganciclovir treatment in patients with enterocolitis is not clear-cut. When compared to the effect with a placebo, a significant antiviral effect was observed, but a clinical benefit was less apparent. Diarrhea and abdominal discomfort were not relieved, but overall patients seemed to improve with this specific therapy. Also, none of the ganciclovir-treated patients developed CMV retinitis as did patients receiving placebo.[16] The response of CMV enterocolitis to foscarnet has not been systematically studied.

Pneumonia

Isolation of CMV from pulmonary secretions or lung tissue in AIDS patients with pneumonia who undergo bronchoscopy is common, but a true pathogenic role of the virus in the disease process is usually not apparent. Many patients with pulmonary disease and CMV isolation from the lung have concomitant infection with other pathogens, especially *Pneumocystis carinii*. Many of the patients respond to therapy directed at *P. carinii* pneumonia alone, raising the question of whether CMV is a true pulmonary pathogen. Patients with positive CMV cultures from lung tissue and no other pathogens identified on diagnostic bronchoscopy may have invasive CMV pneumonia. The diagnosis of CMV pneumonia is enhanced by a combination of factors, including positive CMV culture from lung tissue or pulmonary secretions, the presence of pathognomonic cells with intranuclear inclusion bodies, CMV antigen or nucleic acid in tissue, and the absence of other pathogenic organisms.

When CMV causes pulmonary disease in AIDS patients, the syndrome is that of an interstitial pneumonia. Patients often complain of gradually worsening shortness of breath, dyspnea on exertion, and a dry, nonproductive cough. The heart and respiratory rates are elevated, and auscultation of the lungs often reveals minimal findings with no evidence of consolidation. Chest radiograph shows diffuse interstitial infiltrates similar to those in patients with *P. carinii* pneumonia. Hypoxemia is invariably present.

Therapy with ganciclovir should be considered when a patient has documented CMV pulmonary infection as the only pathogen identified and a progressive deteriorating clinical course.[56] The treatment dosage is 5 mg/kg twice daily, although higher dosage may be necessary to produce a clinical response. Evidence suggests that the combination of ganciclovir with high-dose intravenous immunoglobulin is more efficacious than ganciclovir alone in treating CMV pneumonia in bone marrow transplant recipients.[23,49] No data support using this combination in AIDS patients, however.

Ganciclovir

Structure and Mechanism of Action

Ganciclovir (DHPG, Cytovene) is a nucleoside analog that differs from acyclovir (Zovirax) by a single carboxyl side chain. This structural change confers on the drug approximately 50 times more activity than acyclovir against CMV. Acyclovir has low activity against CMV since it is not well phosphorylated in CMV-infected cells. This is due to the absence of the gene for thymidine kinase (TK) in CMV. Ganciclovir, however, is active against CMV because it does not require TK for phosphorylation. Instead a viral-encoded phosphorylating enzyme apparently is present in CMV-infected cells. It is capable of phosphorylating ganciclovir and converting it to the monophosphate; then cellular enzymes convert it to the active compound, ganciclovir triphosphate. Ganciclovir triphosphate acts to inhibit the viral DNA polymerase.

Pharmacology and Dosage

Intravenous ganciclovir is the only form currently available for clinical use. Individual vials contain 500 mg per vial and contain 50 mg/ml when reconstituted in 10 ml sterile water. When administered by intravenous infusion over 1 hour in

Table 23–3. Dosage Adjustment for Ganciclovir Induction Treatment* in Patients with Impaired Renal Function

LEVEL OF RENAL FUNCTION	CREATININE CLEARANCE (ml/1.73 m²/min)	GANCICLOVIR DOSAGE (mg/kg)
Normal	>80	5.0 b.i.d.
Mild impairment	50-79	2.5 b.i.d.
Moderate impairment	25-49	2.5 once daily
Severe impairment	<25	1.25 once daily

*For maintenance therapy these recommendations should be halved.

the usual dosage of 5 mg/kg, peak blood levels are approximately 6 to 15 mg/ml, and the serum half-life is 2.9 hours. The drug is given two to three times daily during initial induction, whereas maintenance therapy consists of 5 to 6 mg/kg once daily or five to seven times per week. Since the drug undergoes renal excretion, the dosage must be reduced with impaired renal function. A formula for dose reduction is presented in Table 23–3. For maintenance therapy, these recommendations should be halved (see Chapter 9).

Clinical Use

Administration of ganciclovir is indicated for the treatment of acute CMV infection, but other herpes viruses (specifically, HSV-1, HSV-2, and VZV) are also susceptible to the drug in vitro. Since AIDS patients with severe CMV infection frequently have illnesses caused by other herpes viruses, a "bonus" of ganciclovir therapy may be an associated improvement of HSV and VZV infections. Ganciclovir is probably also active against Epstein-Barr virus, but this is not certain. Some investigators have reported that adenoviruses are also susceptible to ganciclovir.

Virologic Response to Ganciclovir

The results of CMV cultures of blood and urine in patients treated with ganciclovir are shown in Figure 23–3. Most of these patients had CMV retinitis, although AIDS patients with CMV infections of other organ systems are included. Of these patients, 87% had a complete virologic response (conversions of culture from positive to negative or a more than 100-fold reduction in CMV titer) in urine, and 83% had a complete response in blood culture. The median time until response was 8 days for both blood and urine cultures.

Resistance

Erice et al.[26] have reported about three Minnesota patients whose clinical course suggested the emergence of resistance and whose CMV isolates exhibited increases in the concentration of ganciclovir required to inhibit the virus in tissue culture by 90% (ID_{90}) over baseline determinations. We recently have documented that after 3 months of continuous ganciclovir therapy, approximately 10% of patients are excreting resistant strains of CMV (arbitrarily defined as strains that are only inhibited by four times or more the median concentration of ganciclovir required to inhibit a group of pretherapy isolates).[22] These strains remain sensitive to foscarnet, which may be used as alternate therapy.[37]

Toxicity

Toxicity frequently limits therapy with ganciclovir. The following primary organs are adversely affected.

Hematopoiesis. Neutropenia, defined as an absolute neutrophil count of

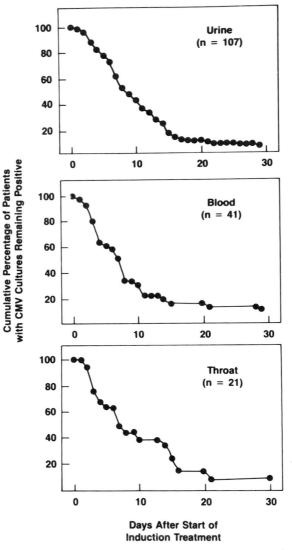

FIGURE 23–3. Time course of conversion of cytomegalovirus (CMV) cultures of specimens of urine, blood, or throat washings from the positive (before treatment) to negative (after treatment with ganciclovir). Cultures from individual patients were performed at various times after start of treatment. Numbers in parentheses are the number of patients in whom the particular body fluid or site was sequentially cultured. (From Buhles WC Jr, Mastre BJ, Tinker AJ, Strand V, Koretz SH, and the Syntex Collaborative Ganciclover Treatment Study Group: Ganciclovir treatment of life- or sight-threatening cytomegalovirus infection: Experience in 314 immunocompromised patients. Rev Infect Dis 10[suppl 3]:S495-S504, 1988.)

Table 23–4.   Comparison of Neutropenia and Thrombocytopenia in Patients with AIDS versus Those with Other Causes of Immunodeficiency

HEMATOLOGIC PARAMETER	UNDERLYING AIDS (%)	OTHER IMMUNODEFICIENCY (%)*
Nadir of absolute neutrophil count (ANC)†		
<500	16.2	13.3
<500 to <1000	24.3	10.7
≥1000	59.5	76.0
Nadir of platelet count		
<20,000	5.3	29.0
20,000 to <50,000	8.7	17.4
≥50,000	86.0	53.6

*Percentage of patients in each category. N = 462 patients on whom adequate hematologic data was available for neutropenia; N = 470 with thrombocytopenia.
†Counts are number of cells per microliter.

$<1000/mm^3$, occurs in nearly 40% of ganciclovir recipients (Table 23–4). Sixteen percent of patients receiving the drug develop neutrophil counts of $<500/mm^3$. Neutropenia usually occurs early (i.e., in the period of induction or during early maintenance treatment) but may occur later in therapy as well. The leukopenia is usually reversible, but at least five patients are known to have had irreversible suppression. Many AIDS patients have low white blood counts before beginning therapy, so the contribution of ganciclovir to leukopenia may not be entirely clear. Nonetheless, the dosage should be reduced when absolute neutrophil counts fall below $1000/mm^3$ or discontinued when severe leukopenia occurs (absolute neutrophil counts $<500/mm^3$). The drug may be resumed when neutrophil counts have risen to safe levels, preferably $>1000/mm^3$. It is not clear that neutropenia is dose related because many patients on high-dose maintenance therapy do not develop this adverse reaction. Nonetheless, reduction of dosage may bring about reversal of neutropenia. Discontinuation of therapy is necessary in patients whose neutrophils do not increase during dosage reduction. Thrombocytopenia (platelet count $<20,000/mm^3$) occurs in 9% of patients receiving the drug and is less likely to be seen in non-AIDS patients than AIDS patients (5% versus 29%).

Other Organ Systems.   Adverse effects on the central nervous system (CNS) occur in 17% of AIDS patients. Confusion is the most common symptom, occurring in 3% of patients, and 2% of patients experience convulsions, dizziness, headaches, or abnormal thinking. Overall, 15% of patients have gastrointestinal disturbances. Nausea is the most frequent complaint (5%), followed by vomiting (4%), abnormal liver function tests (3%), and diarrhea (2%).

Ganciclovir Plus Zidovudine (AZT).   Recent studies indicate that the combination of zidovudine and ganciclovir is more toxic than either agent alone even when zidovudine is given at a dose of 500 mg per day. It is now generally recommended that the two drugs not be given concurrently, although the use of granulocyte colony stimulating factor (G-CSF) may counter the neutropenia caused by these drugs. Newer antiretroviral agents with less hematologic toxicity such as dideoxyinosine (ddI) or dideoxycytidine (ddC) are now, or soon will be, available and, if tolerated, provide another means of maintaining antiretroviral activity while ganciclovir is being taken.

Gonadal Toxicity.   In preclinical animal studies it was determined ganciclovir is a potent inhibitor of spermatogenesis. Sperm counts in humans before and during ganciclovir therapy, however, have been performed too infrequently to provide meaningful information on spermatogenesis. Follicle-stimulating hormone (FSH) and luteinizing hormone (LH) have been measured in ganciclovir-treated patients, with increases occurring in approximately 30% of patients. This data may suggest end-organ toxicity. Unfortunately, control patients not receiving ganciclovir must also be studied to interpret these results accurately. Nonetheless, patients wishing to reproduce should use ganciclovir only for the strongest indications.

Premature Termination of Treatment.   Approximately one third of patients must discontinue or interrupt ganciclovir treatment. The most common cause of early interruption of therapy is neutropenia (65% of discontinuations). Adverse CNS reactions (11%) and thrombocytopenia (8%) account for most of the remaining interruptions.

Foscarnet

Foscarnet, also known as phosphonoformate, phosphonoformic acid, or PFA, is a pyrophosphate that inhibits the DNA polymerase of CMV. Specifically, the drug blocks the pyrophosphate-binding site of the viral DNA polymerase, preventing cleavage of pyrophosphate from deoxyadenosine triphosphate.[9] This action is relatively selective in that CMV DNA polymerase is inhibited at concentrations <1% of that required to inhibit cellular DNA polymerase. Unlike nucleosides such as acyclovir and ganciclovir, foscarnet does not require phosphorylation intracellularly to be an active inhibitor of viral DNA polymerases. This biochemical fact becomes especially important in regard to viral resistance since the principal mode of viral resistance to nucleoside analogs is a mutation that eliminates phosphorylation of the drug in virus-infected cells.

Pharmacology

The recommended initial therapy with foscarnet, 60 mg/kg administered intravenously every 8 hours, yields peak serum concentrations of 500 μm/L and trough concentrations of 40 μm/L (see Chapter 9). The intracellular concentration and half-life of antivirals are more important than serum levels, but the intracellular concentrations and half-life of foscarnet are unknown, although they probably exceed those of serum.

Cerebrospinal fluid (CSF) concentrations of foscarnet are approximately 40% of serum levels. Excretion is entirely renal without an hepatic component. Oral bioavailability is estimated at 12% to 22%, but it is poorly tolerated.

Adverse effects include renal impairment, anemia, hypocalcemia (especially ionized calcium), and hypophosphatemia. It is important to measure renal function frequently and adjust dosage accordingly to minimize toxicity.

Palestine et al.[47] recently reported a randomized control trial of foscarnet in the treatment of CMV retinitis in AIDS patients. Patients were assigned randomly to receive either no therapy or immediate treatment with intravenous foscarnet. The justification for the design was that the lesions were peripheral and not threatening visual acuity. The mean time to progression of retinitis was 3 weeks in the control group versus 13 weeks in the treatment group, thereby proving that foscarnet is effective therapy. Also, an excellent antiviral effect was achieved in the treatment group (i.e., 9 of 13 of the treated group had positive blood cultures for CMV at entry and all nine had cleared their blood by the end of the 3-week induction period). Adverse effects were seizures, hypomagnesemia, hypocalcemia, and elevated serum creatinine levels. In January 1992 a study comparing foscarnet with ganciclovir in the treatment of sight-threatening CMV retinitis was reported.[35] The two drugs were equivalently effective in treating retinitis; the mean time to progression of retinitis was approximately 56 days in both groups. The notable difference in the study was that patients treated with foscarnet had a 4-month longer survival time than those receiving ganciclovir. The explanation for the difference in survival time is not clear and does not seem entirely attributable to differences in the ability to take concurrent antiretroviral medications. However, this analysis was based on tabulating whether a patient had ever received any antiretroviral therapy (e.g., zidovudine, ddC, or ddI) and did not assess the quantitative ability of patients to take these medications. Presumably it was more difficult to continue a patient on concurrent zidovudine therapy while taking ganciclovir because of additive myelosuppression. Thus whether the survival benefit of foscarnet was due to these other medications or was an inherent effect of foscarnet therapy itself remains unclear. Now that cytokines (e.g., granulocyte macrophage colony stimulating factor [GM-CSF] and G-CSF) and ddI are available, it should be possible for patients to continue receiving antiretroviral medications while taking ganciclovir.

HERPES SIMPLEX VIRUS

Herpes simplex viruses types 1 and 2 (HSV-1, HSV-2) cause disease in both normal and immunocompromised hosts and are responsible for substantial morbidity in patients with AIDS. Many adult patients with AIDS have been prevously infected with HSV and are not susceptible to primary HSV infection. Primary HSV infection results in viral latency in nerve root ganglia that correspond to the site of initial infection. Latent HSV often reactivates in the immunosuppressed population and can cause severe recurrent HSV disease, with extensive tissue destruction and prolonged viral shedding in patients with AIDS. The prevalence of HSV infection in homosexual AIDS patients exceeds that of the general population and likely reflects the common risk factor for transmission of both HSV and HIV (sexual contact). Serologic studies have revealed that more than 95% of homosexual men with AIDS have been previously infected with HSV, allowing for viral reactivation and clinical illness later in life.[45,51] AIDS subgroups other than homosexual men such as hemophiliacs and transfusion recipients would be expected to have lower rates of previous HSV infection.

Clinical Presentation

Because most HIV-infected patients have been infected with HSV before the development of AIDS, recurrent HSV is much more common than primary HSV infection. HSV infection in AIDS patients is often atypical compared to infection in the normal host. The severity of the illness depends on several factors, including the site of initial infection, the degree of immunosuppression, and whether the episode represents initial-primary infection (no previous exposure to either HSV type), initial-nonprimary infection (previous exposure to the heterologous HSV type), or recurrent infection.

Large ulcerative lesions, without visceral or cutaneous dissemination, are frequent in HIV-infected patients and may result in a diagnosis of AIDS. In an individual with no other cause of underlying immunodeficiency or who has laboratory evidence of HIV infection, ulcerative HSV infection present for longer than 1 month is diagnostic of AIDS.[50]

Orolabial Infection

Orolabial HSV infection in adults with AIDS is usually due to recurrent disease. Primary orolabial HSV infection is more likely to occur in children with AIDS, however, because HIV infection in these patients may precede initial exposure to HSV.

The incubation period of primary HSV infection ranges between 2 and 12 days. In the normal host primary orolabial infection may be asymptomatic or result in a gingivostomatitis.[15,43,61] Immunocompromised patients apparently are at greater risk than normal hosts to develop a severe clinical illness during primary HSV-1 infection, with a painful vesicular eruption occurring along the lip, tongue, pharynx, or buccal mucosa. The vesicles rapidly coalesce and rupture to form large ulcers covered by a whitish yellow necrotic film.[61,63] Fever, pharyngitis, and cervical lymphadenopathy are frequently present in adults, whereas infants may display poor feeding and persistent drooling. Orolabial recurrences (fever blisters) in AIDS patients may increase in frequency and severity as immunosuppression increases. Alternatively, some AIDS patients will have only infrequent, mild, self-limiting recurrences throughout their disease.[2,48] Prodromal symptoms, consisting of tingling or numbness at the site of the impending recurrence, may be present from 12 to 24 hours before the onset of an actual HSV recurrence.

In the normal host orolabial herpes lesions usually heal in 7 to 10 days. By comparison, AIDS patients often have a prolonged illness with markedly delayed lesion healing. If left untreated, chronic ulcerative lesions with persistent viral shedding may occur for several weeks.[63]

Genital Infection

After a 2- to 12-day incubation period, local symptoms develop in the majority of individuals with primary genital herpes.[12] Small papules appear initially and rapidly evolve into fluid-filled vesicles, which are usually painful and tender to palpation. The vesicles ulcerate rapidly and, in the normal host, heal in 3 to 4 weeks by crusting and by reepithelialization. Tender inguinal adenopathy is common, and dysuria may be present even if the urethra is not infected. Systemic symptoms such as fever, headache, myalgias, malaise, and meningismus are also common during primary infection.[10,13]

In the normal host recurrent genital herpes is less severe than primary infection. Compared with primary infection, recurrent herpes typically results in fewer external lesions, a shorter duration of illness, and the absence of systemic symptoms.[12,13] In AIDS patients, however, the severity and duration of recurrent genital herpes may be more severe than that seen in normal hosts. Prolonged new lesion formation, with continued tissue destruction, persistent virus shedding, and severe local pain, is common. As with orolabial herpes, the frequency and severity of genital recurrences may increase with increasing immunosuppression, with symptoms lasting for several weeks.[2,70]

Asymptomatic genital shedding of HSV has been documented on 1% of the days on which cultures were obtained in nonimmunocompromised patients.[64] HIV-infected patients who are also infected with HSV would be expected to shed HSV at similar or even higher rates. All HSV-infected individuals (whether HIV infected or not) should be counseled about the possibility of asymptomatic HSV shedding and the possible risk of transmission of virus despite the absence of symptoms or visible lesions.

Anorectal Infection

Chronic perianal herpes was among the first reported oportunistic infections associated with AIDS. HSV is the most frequent cause of nongonococcal proctitis in sexually active homosexual men.[32,59] HSV proctitis usually results from primary HSV-2 infection but may also occur as a result of HSV-1 infection or recurrent disease caused by either viral type. Severe anorectal pain, perianal ulcerations, constipation, tenesmus, and neurologic symptoms in the distribution of the sacral plexus (sacral radiculopathy, impotence, and neurogenic bladder) are common findings of HSV proctitis and help differentiate it from proctitis resulting from other causes[32] (Figure 23–4). Anorectal or sigmoidoscopic examination in patients with HSV proctitis typically reveals a friable mucosa, diffuse ulcerations, and occasional intact vesicular or pustular lesions.[32]

Recurrent perianal lesions caused by HSV in the absence of true proctitis is also a common finding in patients with AIDS. Local pain, tenderness, itching, and pain on defecation are prominent symptoms of these lesions. Shallow ulcers in the perianal region are often visible on external examination, and ulcerative lesions frequently coalesce and extend along the gluteal crease to involve the area overlying the sacrum. These lesions are often atypical in appearance and may be confused with pressure decubiti (Color Plate II F). To prevent misdiagnosis, all perianal ulcerations and anal fissures should be cultured for HSV.

Esophagitis

Symptoms of HSV esophagitis typically include retrosternal pain and odynophagia (see Chapter 12). Dysphagia may be of acute onset or chronic and may be

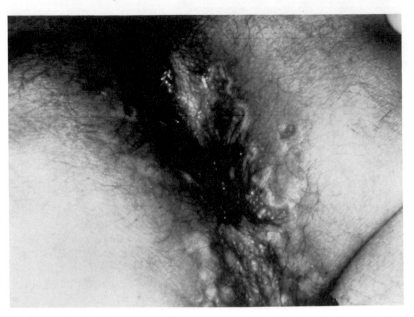

FIGURE 23–4.   Perianal ulcerations typical of herpes simplex. (Courtesy Dr. K. Erlich, Daly City, California.)

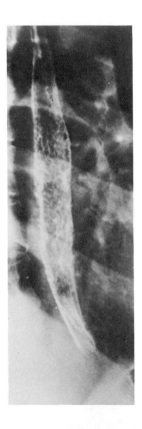

FIGURE 23–5.   Barium esophagram revealing a "cobblestone" appearance of the esophageal mucosa. These findings are typical in both HSV esophagitis and *Candida* esophagitis. (From Farthing CF, Brown SE, Staughton RCD: A Colour Atlas of AIDS and HIV Disease Slide Set, ed 2. London, 1989, Mosby–Year Book/Wolfe.)

severe enough to interfere with eating. Herpetic lesions in the oropharynx may not be present, and the clinical picture is often confused with *Candida* esophagitis. Radiographic contrast studies typically reveal a "cobblestone" appearance of the esophageal mucosa, although this finding is also present with *Candida* esophagitis (Figure 23–5). Definitive diagnosis of HSV esophagitis should be made by direct endoscopic visualizaton of the esophageal mucosa with positive viral culture and histopathologic evidence of invasive viral infection.

Encephalitis

HSV encephalitis occurs infrequently and is the most life-threatening complication of HSV infection in AIDS (see Chapter 13). Both HSV-1 and HSV-2 have been identified in brain tissue of AIDS patients, and simultaneous brain infection with HSV and CMV have been reported.[17,19] In adults with AIDS HSV encephalitis usually occurs as a complication of primary or reactivated orolabial HSV infection. In neonates the disease may occur as a result of primary HSV infection at the time of birth.[15]

The presentation of HSV encephalitis in adults with AIDS is often highly atypical. A subacute illness with subtle neurologic abnormalities is common in AIDS patients with HSV encephalitis, suggesting that host immune responses contribute to the clinical manifestations of the disease.[17,19] Headache, meningismus, and personality changes may develop gradually as the illness progresses. Alternatively, however, some AIDS patients develop acute HSV encephalitis. Abrupt onset of fever, headache, nausea, lethargy, and confusion may occur with temporal lobe abnormalities, cranial nerve defects, and focal seizures. Grand mal seizures, obtundation, coma, and death may eventually ensue.

The clinical diagnosis of HSV encephalitis may be extremely difficult because other CNS infections (including HIV encephalopathy, *Cryptococcus neoformans,* and *Toxoplasma gondii*) may present in an identical fashion. CSF usually reveals nonspecific findings, with elevated protein and a lymphocytic pleocytosis. Viral CSF cultures are usually negative.[44] Measurement of HSV antibody production in CSF has been evaluated as a means of diagnosis of HSV encephalitis but may have some limitations in patients with AIDS.[38] Computed tomography scan, radionuclide brain scan, or electroencephalography may reveal nonspecific abnormalities and are often helpful in identifying abnormal areas for brain biopsy. Diagnosis often requires brain biopsy and the recovery of virus or demonstration of viral antigens from tissue specimens.[44] The histopathologic abnormalities typically observed in normal hosts (hemorrhagic cortical necrosis and lymphocytic infiltration) may be absent in AIDS patients.[17,19] When diagnostic brain biopsy is contraindicated or refused, a trial of empiric antiviral chemotherapy may be warranted.

Acyclovir-Resistant HSV Infection

Since the initial description of acyclovir-resistant HSV infection in patients with AIDS, numerous additional reports have appeared in the literature.[25,27,28,41,54] The incidence of acyclovir-resistant HSV infections in immunocompromised hosts has been estimated as 4% to 5%,[25] but the exact incidence of this problem in the AIDS

Table 23–5. Dosage Adjustment of Intravenous Acyclovir in Patients with Renal Dysfunction

CREATININE CLEARANCE (ml/min/1.73 m²)	PERCENT OF STANDARD DOSE*	DOSING INTERVAL (hr)
>50	100	8
25-50	100	12
10-25	100	24
0-10	50	24

*Usually 5 mg/kg; 10 mg/kg is used for HSV central nervous system infections and in some instances for varicella-zoster virus infection.

population has not been determined. Most acyclovir-resistant HSV strains isolated from patients with AIDS have been deficient in the enzyme thymidine kinase. These mutated strains do not phosphorylate acyclovir to the active antiviral compound and are resistant to standard dosages of acyclovir. Although these thymidine kinase–deficient strains have not been isolated from nonimmunocompromised hosts and have reduced virulence in animal models, they remain capable of causing severe clinical illness in patients with AIDS.[28] Most reports of acyclovir-resistant HSV have cited localized chronic mucocutaneous infection, but cases of disseminated mucocutaneous disease,[41] meningoencephalitis,[31] and esophagitis[25] caused by these strains have been described.

Treatment

Acyclovir

The prompt administration of antiviral chemotherapy to AIDS patients with acute HSV infection reduces morbidity and the risk of serious complications. Acyclovir, the antiviral agent of choice for most HSV infections in AIDS patients, can be administered orally,[21,58,62,66] intravenously,[4,57,60,67] or topically.[14,70] The optimum route of administration, dosage, and duration of acyclovir therapy often depends on the site and severity of the acute HSV infection.

Acyclovir has a high therapeutic ratio as it undergoes selective phosphorylation by viral-induced thymidine kinase in HSV-infected cells. Acyclovir triphosphate acts by selective inhibition of viral DNA polymerase and early termination of DNA-chain synthesis. The drug has slightly higher activity against HSV-1 than HSV-2. Acyclovir distributes into all tissues, including the brain and CSF, and is cleared by renal mechanisms. The serum half-life in patients with normal renal function is 2 to 3 hours, and the intravenous dose should be reduced in patients with impaired renal function[40] (Table 23–5).

Foscarnet

Phosphonoformic acid (PFA, foscarnet, Foscavir), a pyrophosphate, has been approved by the Food and Drug Administration (FDA) as a treatment for CMV disease but also has activity against HSV infection. Unlike acyclovir, foscarnet does not require viral enzyme–mediated phosphorylation for activity; hence it remains an effective antiviral agent for treatment of acyclovir-resistant, thymidine kinase–deficient strains of HSV.[27] A recent study concluded that foscarnet is superior to vidarabine in the treatment of acyclovir-resistant HSV infections in AIDS.[54]

Management of HSV Infection (Table 23–6)

Most AIDS patients with primary or recurrent mucocutaneous HSV infections are not ill enough to require hospitalization and are suitable for outpatient treatment. The usual dose of acyclovir for outpatient therapy is 200 mg five times daily. Therapy can be started while awaiting results of viral culture (if the clinical suspicion is high) or when the diagnosis has been confirmed by the appropriate laboratory techniques.[58] Oral acyclovir should be continued until all external lesions are crusted.

Intravenous acyclovir should be reserved for patients with severe or extensive mucocutaneous HSV infection and for patients with viral dissemination, visceral organ infection (e.g., brain, esophagus, eye), or neurologic complications (atonic bladder, transverse myelitis). Treatment with intravenous acyclovir may also be indicated for AIDS patients who require specific antiviral chemotherapy but are unable to tolerate or absorb oral acyclovir because of nausea, dysphagia, or protracted diarrhea. The dose of intravenous acyclovir for patients with mucocutaneous HSV infection and normal renal function is 15 mg/kg/day in three divided doses.[67] Patients with life-threatening HSV infection (encephalitis, neonatal infection, disseminated infection) or visceral organ involvement (esophagitis, proctitis) should probably receive a higher dose—usually 30 mg/kg/day in three divided doses.[60,69] Treatment should last for a minimum of 10 days, but longer therapy in AIDS patients may be necessary. As noted above, the intravenous dose should be adjusted in patients with impaired renal function (Table 23–5). If prolonged therapy is required, oral acyclovir can be substituted for intravenous therapy when the patient is ready for hospital discharge.

Topical acyclovir is less effective than either oral or intravenous therapy, although comparative trials have not been performed. Although topical acyclovir decreases the duration of viral shedding in compromised hosts with mucocutaneous HSV infection, it does not reduce new lesion formation or the risk of dissemination.[14,70]

Table 23–6.   Management of HSV Infections in AIDS

CLINICAL PRESENTATION	TREATMENT
Mucocutaneous infection, mild	Acyclovir, 200 mg P.O. five times daily
Mucocutaneous infection, severe	Acyclovir, 15 mg/kg/day IV
Visceral organ infection	Acyclovir, 30 mg/kg/day IV
Recurrent mucocutaneous infection	Acyclovir, 200-400 mg t.i.d. or q.i.d.
Severe infection caused by acyclovir-resistant HSV	Foscarnet, 40 mg/kg IV t.i.d. (not FDA approved)
	Continuous infusion acyclovir, 1.5-2 mg/kg/hr (not FDA approved)

Modified from Drew WL: The medical management of AIDS. Infect Dis Clin North Am 2:505, 1988.

There is no apparent added benefit to the combination of topical acyclovir with either oral or intravenous acyclovir.[39] Topical acyclovir has little, if any, usefulness in the clinical setting.

Treatment with acyclovir should be continued until all mucocutaneous lesions have crusted or reepithelialized. Lesions may heal slowly in AIDS patients even with optimum antiviral chemotherapy. If lesion healing does not occur while the patient is receiving acyclovir, repeat viral cultures should be obtained, high-dose intravenous therapy (30 mg/kg/day) should be given, and acyclovir-resistant HSV infection should be ruled out. Antiviral susceptibility testing should be performed to determine whether acyclovir-resistant HSV infection is present.

Suppressive Acyclovir Therapy For HSV Infection

Many AIDS patients suffer from frequently recurring HSV infection or develop new HSV recurrences shortly after antiviral chemotherapy is discontinued. These patients can often be managed with suppressive acyclovir therapy.[21,62,66] AIDS patients requiring suppressive therapy should be treated initially with oral acyclovir, 200 mg q.i.d. or 400 mg b.i.d. Increase of daily dosage up to 400 mg q.i.d. may be necessary to control recurrences, but gastrointestinal intolerance to the drug may limit the amount that can be taken. "Breakthrough recurrences" that develop while the patient is receiving suppressive acyclovir therapy may be controlled by increasing the daily suppressive dose. Breakthrough recurrences may or may not represent the emergence of acyclovir-resistent strains.[46] Patients who demonstrate a good response to suppressive oral acyclovir at high doses may attempt a reduction in the daily suppressive dose. Although suppressive acyclovir therapy is approved for no longer than 12 months, patients have been maintained on daily acyclovir for up to 72 months with no evidence of adverse reactions or cumulative toxicity. Individuals maintained on long-term suppressive therapy should be cautioned, however, that recurrences likely will develop after discontinuation of therapy and that the first recurrence may be more severe than those previously experienced.[21,62,66] Many AIDS patients receiving acyclovir may also be taking zidovudine (AZT). There is no conclusive evidence that the combination of zidovudine and acyclovir results in synergistic activity against HIV. This combination may, however, be more myelosuppressive than treatment with zidovudine alone.

Management of Acyclovir-Resistant HSV Infection

With the increased incidence of acyclovir-resistant HSV infections observed in patients with AIDS, several studies have examined the utility of alternate antiviral agents and treatment regimens. Standard doses of intravenous or oral acyclovir have no clinical benefit if the HSV isolate is resistant to acyclovir ($ID_{50} > 3.0$ μg/ml) in vitro. Most acyclovir-resistant strains isolated from patients with AIDS have been thymidine kinase deficient and have remained susceptible in vitro to vidarabine, which is phosphorylated without thymidine kinase, and foscarnet, which does not require phosphorylation for activity. Initial uncontrolled reports suggested that foscarnet might have clinical use for acyclovir-resistant HSV.[27] A recent comparative trial confirmed that foscarnet is superior to vidarabine in the treatment of this disease and is much less toxic.[54] The dosage of foscarnet used for the treatment of acyclovir-resistant HSV infections in AIDS patients is 40 mg/kg every 8 hours (with reduction in dose for renal dysfunction), but the drug has not yet been approved by the FDA for this purpose.

Continuous infusion acyclovir therapy was effective in two patients with severe acyclovir-resistant HSV infection. Acyclovir was administered at a dosage of 1.5 to 2.0 mg/kg/hour for 6 weeks, and complete resolution of acyclovir-resistant HSV proctitis was observed.[24]

As with many opportunistic infections in AIDS patients, there is a high incidence of recurrent HSV disease after successful treatment for acyclovir-resistant HSV. Some (but not all) relapses in this setting have been due to acyclovir-resistant strains, suggesting that these mutant viruses may be capable of causing latency in the immunocompromised host. Chronic prophylaxis with daily acyclovir, 200 to 400 mg P.O. t.i.d., or foscarnet, 40 mg/kg/day intravenously, should be considered in patients who are treated successfully for acyclovir-resistant HSV.

VARICELLA ZOSTER VIRUS

Primary varicella zoster virus (VZV) infection is usually a childhood illness, with attack rates exceeding 90% in susceptible household contacts.[68] Most adults with AIDS have been previously infected with VZV and (as with HSV) are not susceptible to primary infection[51] (see Chapter 10).

AIDS patients develop recurrent VZV infection (zoster) more frequently than age-matched immunocompetent hosts. A retrospective review of 300 AIDS patients with Kaposi's sarcoma revealed that 8% of patients had at least one prior attack of zoster, an incidence seven times greater than expected by the age of the study group. Zoster also occurs with a higher-than-expected frequency in HIV-infected individuals who appear otherwise healthy. Additionally, some HIV-infected patients develop more than one episode of zoster in a relatively short period of time, an uncommon occurrence in competent hosts.[16,20,30,55,65]

Primary Infection—Varicella

Varicella in immunocompetent children is usually a benign illness. Adults, however, are more likely to develop complications during primary VZV infection; viral dissemination to visceral organs occurs in up to one third of immunocompetent adults with primary infection.[68] Although most adults with AIDS have been previously infected with VZV and are not susceptible to primary infection,[51] for those who are, a protracted and potentially life-threatening illness could follow.

Recurrent Infection—Zoster

Unlike primary VZV infection, recurrent VZV infection (zoster) is common in patients with AIDS. The illness usually begins with radicular pain and is followed by localized or segmented erythematous rash covering one to three dermatomes. Maculopapules develop in the dermatomal area, and the patient experiences increasing pain. The maculopapules progress to fluid-filled vesicles, and contiguous vesicles may become confluent with true bullae formation. In many HIV-infected patients the lesions remain confined in a dermatomal distribution and heal by crusting and reepithelialization.[10,11,30,55,65] Occasionally, however, widespread cutaneous or visceral dissemination may occur.[52] Extensive cutaneous dissemination may appear identical to primary varicella. Visceral dissemination to lung, liver, or the CNS may produce a life-threatening illness.

Reactivated infection involving the ophthalmic division of the trigeminal nerve often results in infection of the cornea (zoster ophthalmicus). The presence of vesicles on the tip of the nose is often associated with involvement of the eye. Although healing without sequelae may occur, untreated patients often develop anterior uveitis, corneal scarring, and permanent visual loss.[10,55]

Complications

Complications of VZV infection are common in immunocompromised patients and may cause prolonged morbidity and death.[20] Dissemination of virus to the lung, liver, and CNS has been associated with a mortality rate of 6% to 17%.

Varicella pneumonia may occur during primary VZV infection or during reactivated infection with visceral dissemination in immunocompromised patients. Symptoms are variable; many patients develop only mild respiratory symptoms, whereas others suffer from severe hypoxemia and succumb to respiratory failure. Radiographic abnormalities are usually out of proportion to the clinical findings, with diffuse nodular densities on chest radiograph and occasional pleural effusions.

Encephalitis is a rare complication of VZV infection in AIDS patients but may occur in association with visceral dissemination (see Chapter 13). The illness begins 3 to 8 days after the onset of varicella or 1 to 2 weeks after the development of zoster, but occasionally AIDS patients have developed progressive neurologic disease caused by VZV up to 3 months after the onset of localized zoster.[52] Headache, vomiting, lethargy, and cerebellar findings (ataxia, tremors, dizziness) are prominent findings. Diagnosis based on clinical criteria alone can be difficult, for other CNS infections can present in a similar fashion.

Management of VZV Infection (Table 23–7)

Oral acyclovir in the dosage used to treat herpes simplex infection (200 mg five times daily) does not result in serum drug levels adequate to inhibit VZV in tissue culture.[40] Higher doses of oral acyclovir (800 mg five times daily) have been approved by the FDA for the treatment of VZV infections.[34] This dose produces serum drug levels that inhibit the growth of VZV in vitro. Although somewhat effective clinically in the treatment of VZV infections, this higher-dose regimen may be poorly tolerated in some AIDS patients because of gastrointestinal side effects.

Management of primary or recurrent VZV infection in AIDS patients may require hospitalization and intravenous acyclovir therapy. Many AIDS patients with localized zoster will not be ill enough to require hospitalization, and the decision whether

Table 23–7.   Management of VZV Infections in AIDS

CLINICAL PRESENTATION	TREATMENT
Primary infection (varicella)	Acyclovir, 30 mg/kg/day IV, or acyclovir, 600-800 mg P.O. five times daily
Recurrent infection (localized zoster)	Acyclovir, 30 mg/kg/day IV, or acyclovir, 600-800 mg P.O. five times daily
Recurrent infection disseminated	Acyclovir, 30 mg/kg/day IV
Severe infection caused by acyclovir-resistant VZV	Foscarnet, 40 mg/kg t.i.d. IV (not FDA approved)

Modified from Drew WL: The medical management of AIDS. Infect Dis Clin North Am 2:507, 1988.

to hospitalize an individual patient must be based on several factors, including the severity of the infection, the immune status of the host, and whether visceral or cutaneous dissemination has occurred.

Immunocompromised hosts with primary or recurrent VZV infection treated with intravenous acyclovir have a reduction in the duration of viral shedding, new lesion formation, incidence of dissemination, and mortality rate.[4,57] All AIDS patients with disseminated VZV infection, either cutaneous or visceral, should be hospitalized and treated initially with intravenous acyclovir, 30 mg/kg/day in three divided doses (with dosage adjustments for renal dysfunction; see Table 23–4). Treatment should be continued for at least 7 days or until all external lesions are crusted. Oral acyclovir (800 mg five times daily) may be used for treatment of localized zoster in AIDS patients who do not require hospitalization and may prevent visceral or cutaneous dissemination.

Although some studies have suggested that the use of corticosteroids reduces the incidence of postherpetic neuralgia, other studies have failed to demonstrate a beneficial effect. Corticosteroids should be used cautiously in AIDS patients with zoster since the potential immunosuppressive effect of these drugs may outweigh any possible benefits.

Treatment of Acyclovir-Resistant VZV Infection

Acyclovir-resistant VZV has been identified in patients with AIDS. All strains have been isolated from patients previously treated with acyclovir for recurrent VZV or HSV infection.[36] These strains are sensitive to vidarabine and foscarnet in vitro. Foscarnet is clinically useful in this setting[53] but remains investigational.

SUMMARY

Herpes viruses (HSV, CMV, VZV) are common in AIDS patients and often exist in a chronic or progressive form. Clinically evident CMV retinitis occurs in approximately 10% of AIDS patients and can be effectively treated with the nucleoside analog ganciclovir (DHPG). Perianal ulcers, proctitis, and other clinical syndromes caused by HSV can be effectively treated with acyclovir, which administered daily can prevent HSV recurrence. Herpes zoster in a young adult may be the first indication of immune deficiency resulting from HIV. Since VZV is less susceptible to acyclovir than HSV is, intravenous acyclovir or high-dose oral therapy is required to achieve inhibitory blood levels.

REFERENCES

1. Akula SK, Mansell PWA, Ruiz R: Complications of the acquired immunodeficiency syndrome. Ann Intern Med 104:726-727, 1986
2. Armstrong D, Gold JWM, Dryjanski J, et al: Treatment of infections in patients with the acquired immunodeficiency syndrome. Ann Intern Med 103:738-743, 1985
3. Back MC, Bagwell SP, Knapp NP, et al. 9-(1,3-dihydroxy-2-propoxymethyl)guanine for cytomegalovirus infections in patients with the acquired immunodeficiency syndrome. Ann Intern Med 103:381-382, 1985
4. Balfour HH, Bean B, Laskin OL, et al: Acyclovir halts progression of herpes zoster in immunocompromised patients. N Engl J Med 308:1448-1453, 1983
5. Brock BV, Selke S, Benedetti J, et al: Frequency of asymptomatic shedding of herpes simplex virus in women with genital herpes. JAMA 263:418-420, 1990
6. Buhles WC Jr, Mastre BJ, Tinker AJ, et al: Ganciclovir treatment of life- or sight-threatening cytomegalovirus infection: Experience in 314 immunocompromised patients. Rev Infect Dis 10(suppl 3):S495-S504, 1988
7. Cantrill HL, Henry K, Melroe H, et al: Treatment of cytomegalovirus retinitis with intravitreal ganciclovir. Long term results. Ophthalmology 96:367-374, 1989
8. Chatis PA, Miller CH, Schrager LE, Crumpacker CS: Successful treatment with foscarnet of an acyclovir-resistant mucocutaneous infection with herpes simplex virus in a patient with acquired immunodeficiency syndrome. N Engl J Med 320:297-300, 1989
9. Chrisp, Clissold SP: Foscarnet: A review of its antiviral activity, pharmacokinetic properties and therapeutic use in immunocompromised patients with cytomegalovirus retinitis. Drugs 41:104-109, 1991
10. Cole EL, Meisler DM, Calabrese LH, et al: Herpes zoster ophthalmicus and acquired immune deficiency syndrome. Arch Ophthalmol 102:1027-1029, 1984
11. Cone LA, Schiffman HA: Herpes zoster and the acquired immunodeficiency syndrome (letter). Ann Intern Med 100:462, 1984
12. Corey L, Adams HG, Brown ZA, et al: Genital herpes simplex virus infections: Clinical manifestations, course, and complications. Ann Intern Med 98:958-972, 1983
13. Corey L, Homes KK: Genital herpes simplex virus infections: Current concepts in diagnosis, therapy, and prevention. Ann Intern Med 98:973-983, 1983
14. Corey L, Nahmias AJ, Guinan ME, et al: A trial of topical acyclovir in genital herpes simplex virus infections. N Engl J Med 306:1313-1319, 1982
15. Corey L, Spear PG: Infections with herpes simplex viruses (parts 1 and 2). N Engl J Med 314:686-691, 749-757, 1986
16. Dieterich DT, Rahmin M: Cytomegalovirus colitis in AIDS: Presentation in 44 patients and a review of the literature. J Acquir Immune Defic Syndr 4(suppl 1):S29-S35, 1991
17. Dix RD, Bredesen DE, Davis RL, Mills J: Herpesvirus neurological diseases associated with AIDS: Recovery of viruses from central nervous sytem (CNS) tissues, peripheral nerve, and cerebrospinal fluid (CSF) (Abstract 43). International Conference on AIDS, Atlanta, 1985
18. Dix RD, Bredesen DE, Erlich KS, et al: Recovery of herpes-viruses from cerebrospinal fluid of immunodeficient homosexual men. Ann Neurol 18:611-614, 1985
19. Dix RD, Waitzman DM, Follansbee S, et al: Herpes simplex virus type 2 encephalitis in two homosexual men with persistent adenopathy. Ann Neurol 17:203-206, 1985
20. Dolin R, Reichman RC, Mazur MH, et al: Herpes zoster and varicella infections in immunosuppressed patients. Ann Intern Med 89:375-388, 1978
21. Douglas JM, Critchlow C, Benedetti J, et al: Double blind study of oral acyclovir for suppression of recurrences of genital herpes simplex virus infection. N Engl J Med 310:1551-1556, 1984
22. Drew WL, Miner RC, Busch DF, et al: Prevalence of resistance in patients receiving ganciclovir for serious cytomegalovirus infection. J Infect Dis 163:716-719, 1991

23. Emanuel D, Cunningham I, Jules-Elysee K, et al: Cytomegalovirus pneumonia after bone-marrow transplantation successfully treated with the combination of ganciclovir and high-dose intravenous immune globulin. Ann Intern Med 109:777-782, 1988

24. Engel JP, Englund JA, Fletcher CV, Hill EL: Treatment of resistant herpes simplex virus with continuous-infusion acyclovir. JAMA 263:1662-1664, 1990

25. Englund JA, Zimmerman ME, Swierkosz EM, et al: Herpes simplex virus resistant to acyclovir: A study in a tertiary care center. Ann Intern Med 112:416-422, 1990

26. Erice A, Chou S, Biron K, et al: Ganciclovir (GCV) resistant strains of cytomegalovirus (CMV) in GCV-treated patients with AIDS. Fourth International Conference on AIDS. (Abstract 7190.) Stockholm, 1988

27. Erlich KS, Jacobson MA, Koehler JE, et al: Foscarnet therapy for severe acyclovir-resistant herpes simplex virus type-2 infections in patients with the acquired immunodeficiency syndrome (AIDS): An uncontrolled trial. Ann Intern Med 110:710-713, 1989

28. Erlich KS, Mills J, Chatis P, et al: Acyclovir-resistant herpes simplex virus infections in patients with the acquired immunodeficiency syndrome. N Engl J Med 320:293-296, 1989

29. Felsenstein D, D'Amico DJ, Hirsch MS, et al: Treatment of cytomegalovirus retinitis with 9-[2-hydroxy-l-(hydroxy-methyl) ethoxymethyl] guanine. Ann Intern Med 103:377-380, 1985

30. Friedman-Kien AE, Lafleur FL, Gendler E, et al: Herpes zoster: A possible early clinical sign for development of acquired immunodeficiency syndrome in high-risk individuals. J Am Acad Dermatol 14:1023-1028, 1986

31. Gateley A, Gander RM, Johnson PC, et al: Herpes simplex type 2 meningoencephalitis resistant to acyclovir in a patient with AIDS. J Infect Dis 161:711-715, 1990

32. Goodell SE, Quinn TC, Mkrtichian F, et al: Herpes simplex proctitis in homosexual men: Clinical, sigmoidoscopic, and histopathologic features. N Engl J Med 308:868-871, 1983

33. Hawley DA, Schaefer JF, Schulz DM, Muller J: Cytomegalovirus encephalitis in acquired immunodeficiency syndrome. Am J Clin Pathol 80:874-877,1983

34. Huff JC, Bean B, Balfour HH, et al: Therapy of herpes zoster with oral acyclovir. Am J Med 85(suppl 2A):84-89, 1988

35. Jobs D, and the Studies of Ocular Complications of AIDS Research Group, in collaboration with the AIDS Clinical Trial Group: Mortality in patients with the acquired immunodeficiency syndrome treated with either foscarnet or ganciclovir for cytomegalovirus retinitis. N Engl J Med 326:213-220, 1992

36. Jacobson MA, Berger TG, Fikrig S, et al: Acyclovir (ACV)-resistant varicella zoster virus (VZV) infection following chronic oral ACV therapy in patients with AIDS. Ann Intern Med 112:187-191, 1990

37. Jacobson MA, Drew WL, Feinberg J, et al: Foscarnet therapy for ganciclovir-resistant cytomegalovirus retinitis in patients with AIDS. J Infect Dis 163:1348-1351, 1991

38. Kahlon J, Chatterjee S, Lakeman FD, et al: Detection of antibodies to herpes simplex virus in the cerebrospinal fluid of patients with herpes simplex encephalitis. J Infect Dis 155:38-44, 1987

39. Kinghorn GR, Abeywickreme I, Jeavons M, et al: Efficacy of combined treatment with oral and topical acyclovir in first episode genital herpes. Genitourin Med 62:186-188, 1986

40. Laskin O: Acyclovir: Pharmacology and clinical experience. Arch Intern Med 144:1241-1246, 1984

41. Marks GL, Nolan PE, Erlich KS, Ellis MN: Mucocutaneous dissemination of acyclovir-resistant herpes simplex virus in a patient with AIDS. Rev Infect Dis 11:474-476, 1989

42. Miller RG, Storey JR, Greco CM: Ganciclovir in the treatment of progressive AIDS-related polyradiculopathy. Neurology 40:569-574, 1990

43. Nahmias AJ, Josey WE: Herpex simplex viruses 1 and 2. In Evans A (ed): Viral Infections of Humans: Epidemiology and Control, ed 2. New York, Plenum Press, 1982

44. Nahmias AJ, Whitley RD, Visintine AN, et al: Herpes simplex virus type 2 encephalitis: Laboratory evaluations and their diagnostic significance. J Infect Dis 146:829-836, 1982

45. Nerurkar L, Goedert J, Wallen W, et al: Study of antiviral antibodies in sera of homosexual men. Fed Proc 42:6109, 1983

46. Nusinoff-Lehrman S, Douglas JM, Corey L, et al: Recurrent genital herpes and suppressive oral acyclovir therapy: Relation between clinical outcome and in-vitro sensitivity. Ann Intern Med 104:786-790, 1986

47. Palestine AG, Polis MA, De Smet MD, et al: A randomized, controlled trial of foscarnet in the treatment of cytomegalovirus retinitis in patients with AIDS. Ann Intern Med 115:665-673, 1991

48. Quinnan GV, Masur H, Rook AH, et al: Herpes simplex infections in the acquired immune deficiency syndrome. JAMA 252:72-77, 1984

49. Reed EC, Bowden RA, Dandliker PS, et al: Treatment of cytomegalovirus pneumonia with ganciclovir and intravenous cytomegalovirus immunoglobulin in patients with bone marrow transplants. Ann Intern Med 109:783-788, 1988

50. Revision of the CDC Surveillance Case Definition for Acquired Immunodeficiency Syndrome. MMWR 36(suppl):1S-15S, 1987

51. Rogers MF, Morens DM, Stewart JA, et al: National case control study of Kaposi's sarcoma and *Pneumocystis carinii* pneumonia in homosexual men: Part 2, Laboratory results. Ann Intern Med 99:151-158, 1983

52. Ryder JW, Croen K, Kleinschmidt-DeMasters BK, et al: Progressive encephalitis three months after resolution of cutaneous zoster in a patient with AIDS. Ann Neurol 19:182-188, 1986

53. Safrin S, Berger TG, Gilson I, et al: Foscarnet therapy in five patients with AIDS and acyclovir-resistant varicella-zoster virus infection. Ann Intern Med 115:19-21, 1991

54. Safrin S, Crumpacker C, Chatis P, et al: A controlled trial comparing foscarnet with vidarabine for acyclovir-resistant mucocutaneous herpes simplex in the acquired immunodeficiency syndrome. N Engl J Med 325:551-555, 1991

55. Sandor E, Croxson TS, Millman A, et al: Herpes zoster ophthalmicus in patients at risk for AIDS. N Engl J Med 310:1118-1119, 1984

56. Shepp DH, Dandliker PS, de Miranda P, et al: Activity of 9-[2-hydroxy-1-(hydroxy-methyl) ethoxymethyl] guanine in the treatment of cytomegalovirus pneumonia. Ann Intern Med 103:368-373, 1985

57. Shepp DH, Dandliker PS, Meyers JD: Treatment of varicella zoster virus infection in severely immunocompromised patients. N Engl J Med 314:208-212, 1986

58. Shepp DH, Newton BA, Dandliker PS, et al: Oral acyclovir therapy for mucocutaneous herpes simplex virus infections in immunocompromised marrow transplant recipients. Ann Intern Med 102:783-785, 1985

59. Siegel FP, Lopez C, Hammer BS, et al: Severe acquired immunodeficiency in male homosexuals, manifested by chronic perianal ulcerative herpes simplex lesions. N Engl J Med 305:1439-1444, 1981

60. Skoldenberg B, Alestig K, Burman L, et al: Acyclovir versus vidarabine in herpes simplex encephalitis. Lancet 2:707-711, 1984

61. Spruance SI, Overall JC, Kern ER, et al: The natural history of recurrent herpes simplex labialis: Implications for antiviral therapy. N Engl J Med 297:68-75, 1977

62. Straus SE, Seidlin M, Takiff H, et al: Oral acyclovir to suppress recurring herpes simplex virus infections in immunodeficient patients. Ann Intern Med 100:522-524, 1984

63. Straus SE, Smith HA, Brickman C, et al: Acyclovir for chronic mucocutaneous herpes simplex virus infection in immunosuppressed patients. Ann Intern Med 96:270-277, 1982

64. Teich S, Orellana J: Retinal lesions in cytomegalovirus infection. Ann Intern Med 104:132, 1986

65. Verroust F, Lemay D, Laurian Y: High frequency of herpes zoster in young hemophiliacs (letter): N Engl J Med 316:166-167, 1987

66. Wade JC, Newton B, Flournoy N, et al: Oral acyclovir for prevention of herpes simplex virus reactivation after marrow transplantation. Ann Intern Med 100:823-828, 1984

67. Wade JC, Newton B, McLaren C, et al: Intravenous acyclovir to treat mucocutaneous herpes simplex virus infection after marrow transplantation. Ann Intern Med 96:265-269, 1982

68. Weller TH: Varicella and herpes zoster: Changing concepts of the natural history, control, and importance of a not-so-benign virus (parts 1 and 2). N Engl J Med 309:1362-1368, 1434-1440, 1983

69. Whitley RJ, Alford CA, Hirsch MS, et al: Vidarabine versus acyclovir therapy in herpes simplex encephalitis. N Engl J Med 314:144-149, 1986

70. Whitley RJ, Levin M, Barton N, et al: Infections caused by herpes simplex virus in the immunocompromised host: Natural history and topical acyclovir therapy. J Infect Dis 150:323-329, 1984

71. Whitley RJ, Soong SJ, Dolin R, et al: Adenine arabinoside therapy of biopsy proved herpes simplex encephalitis: National Institute of Allergy and Infectious Diseases collaborative antiviral study. N Engl J Med 297:289-294, 1977

24

MANAGEMENT OF SYPHILIS IN HIV-INFECTED PERSONS

GAIL BOLAN, MD

The management of syphilis in persons with coexisting HIV infection is an increasingly complex problem. Epidemiologic studies have demonstrated that a history of sexually transmitted diseases (STDs), including syphilis, is associated with an increased risk for HIV infection and AIDS and that STDs causing genital ulceration may be cofactors for acquiring HIV infection.[9,18,30] More recently isolated case reports have suggested that coexistent HIV infection may alter the natural history of syphilis and/or the dosage or duration of treatment required to cure syphilis.[3,31] Also, reports of false-negative serologic test results for syphilis in HIV-infected persons raise questions about the sensitivity of serologic diagnostic tests in such patients.[19,26,60] Questions about the efficacy of therapy for neurosyphilis and the significance of cerebrospinal fluid (CSF) abnormalities in patients with early syphilis may assume greater importance in the presence of HIV infection.[27,28,36,41-43]

Because data from prospective, controlled studies are not yet available to answer many of these questions, definitive recommendations for managing HIV-infected patients with syphilis are currently limited. Management options are presented here for clinicians to consider until more definitive recommendations can be made. Options to consider in treating HIV-infected patients include the following: (1) evaluating CSF for evidence of neurosyphilis earlier in the course of infection; (2) treating patients with penicillin regimens of longer duration, higher dose, and better CSF penetration; (3) obtaining biopsy specimens from suspicious lesions and using special stains for spirochetes in patients wtih serologic test results negative for syphilis; and (4) testing syphilitic patients for antibodies to HIV and testing HIV-infected patients for syphilis.

Our studies on the clinical management and therapy of syphilis in HIV-infected patients are supported by Public Health Service Grant No. H25/CCH 904371-02.

EPIDEMIOLOGY

Epidemiologic studies demonstrate that a history of an STD, including syphilis, is associated with an increased risk for HIV infection and AIDS among both homosexuals[9,30] and heterosexuals,[48] presumably because sexual behaviors that increase the risk for acquiring other STDs also increase the risk for acquiring HIV (see Chapter 1). Furthermore, STDs that cause genital ulcerations have been implicated as cofactors for acquiring HIV infection.[2] Therefore increases in the incidence of early syphilis in any population may presage future HIV-related disease.

Since 1982 the significant decreases seen in syphilis morbidity in the United States have occurred primarily among homosexual and bisexual men.[49] In areas reporting high rates of syphilis infection, the percentage of early syphilis cases occurring among homosexual and bisexual men decreased from 50% to 70% in the late 1970s to 5% to 15% in 1990.[49] These data presumably reflect changes in sexual practices that reduce the risk of HIV infection among homosexual and bisexual men. They suggest that education efforts encouraging safer-sex practices have been effective among homosexual men. However, safer-sex practices such as oral sex without ejaculation may reduce the risk of HIV infection but may not reduce the risk of syphilis unless a condom is used. In addition, because many patients with syphilis are not routinely tested for neurosyphilis or HIV infection and because these conditions (if diagnosed) are not reportable in many areas, the incidence of syphilis—especially neurosyphilis—in HIV-infected patients is unknown. Also, it is not known whether patients with HIV infection are at higher risk for syphilis than persons without HIV infection.

PATHOGENESIS

It is plausible that impairment of both cell-mediated and humoral immunity by HIV[4] could limit the host's defenses against *Treponema pallidum*, thereby altering the clinical manifestations and/or natural course of syphilis infection. Host immunity, especially cell-mediated immunity, plays an important role in protecting the host against syphilis.[45] In animal models selective impairment of cell-mediated immunity alters the host response to syphilis infection. Incubation time is shorter, lesions are more numerous and widespread, and healing time is slower.[44] Furthermore, HIV-induced meningeal inflammation may facilitate penetration of spirochetes into the central nervous sytem (CNS) and thus contribute to the development of symptomatic neurosyphilis.

CLINICAL MANIFESTATIONS AND COURSE

Recent case reports have suggested that the clinical manifestations of syphilis may be unusual and the course more rapid in patients with HIV infection.[31,43] These anecdotal reports have led to the hypothesis that in patients co-infected with HIV and *T. pallidum*, symptomatic neurosyphilis may be more likely to develop, the latency period before development of meningovascular syphilis may be shorter, and the efficacy of standard therapy for early syphilis may be reduced.

Neurosyphilis

Several cases of neurosyphilis have been reported in patients with HIV infection[31,32] (see Chapter 13). One patient presented with a diffuse maculopapular rash, hepatomegaly, and a unilateral facial palsy. Laboratory data were remarkable for transient elevation of serum transaminases, a rapid plasma reagin (RPR) titer of 1:512, and a positive fluorescent treponemal antibody-absorbed (FTA-abs) test result. CSF examination revealed mononuclear pleocytosis (66 cells/mm³), an elevated protein level (182 mg/dl), and a CSF-Venereal Disease Research Laboratory (VDRL) titer of 1:4. This case is consistent with secondary syphilis accompanied by acute syphilitic meningitis and cranial nerve involvement.

Another patient presented with a pure motor hemiplegia that appeared after a 2-month prodrome of fatigue, malaise, and headache. No previous history of syphilis or chancre was reported. Laboratory data were remarkable for transient elevation of serum transaminases, an RPR titer of 1:256, and a positive FTA-abs test result. CSF examination revealed lymphocytic pleocytosis (234 cells/mm³), an elevated protein level (94 mg/dl), hypoglycorrhachia (glucose, 33 mg/dl), and a CSF-VDRL titer of 1:1. This case is consistent with meningovascular syphilis. A third patient presented with posterior uveitis, neurosensory hearing loss, and meningovascular syphilis (pure motor hemiparesis) 4 months after the diagnosis of primary syphilis.

These case reports of neurosyphilis in HIV-infected persons are similar to cases reported before the AIDS epidemic.[39,53] Neurosyphilis may occur at any stage of syphilis. The clinical spectrum and time between primary infection and neurologic symptoms is well described.[53] Approximately 35% of persons with secondary syphilis have asymptomatic CNS involvement, with an abnormal cell count, protein level, glucose level, and/or reactive CSF-VDRL found on CSF examination. Acute syphilitic meningitis usually occurs within the first 2 years of infection; 10% of cases are diagnosed at the time of the secondary rash. Patients present with headache, meningeal irritation, and cranial nerve abnormalities. Typically, cranial nerves at the base of the brain (especially II, VII, and VIII) are involved. Meningovascular syphilis can occur a few months to 10 years after the primary infection (average, 7 years).

Unlike the sudden onset of thrombotic or embolic stroke syndromes, meningovascular syphilis is associated with prodromal symptoms for weeks to months before focal defects of a vascular syndrome are identified. Prodromal symptoms include headache, vertigo, insomnia, and psychiatric abnormalities such as personality changes. The focal defects initially are intermittent or progress slowly over a few days. In contrast, general paresis and tabes dorsalis are the parenchymatous forms of neurosyphilis that occur, in general, 10 to 30 years later. General paresis causes symptoms similar to those of any dementia, and syndromes similar to many psychiatric illness have also been described. Tabes dorsalis is associated with a triad of symptoms—lightning pains, dysuria, and ataxis—and a triad of signs—Argyll Robertson pupils, areflexia, and loss of proprioceptive sense.

The majority of symptomatic neurosyphilis cases reported among HIV-infected persons has presented with the early forms of neurosyphilis, namely acute syphilitic meningitis and meningovascular neurosyphilis. Tabes dorsalis was reported in one HIV-infected man who had been treated for primary syphilis 7 years earlier.[7] In addition, cases of syphilitic meningomyelitis with spastic paraparesis[57] and syphilitic polyradiculopathy with progressive leg pain and weakness[34] have been published.

Although it is clear that the neurosyphilis cases involving persons with concurrent HIV infection published to date do not represent unusual clinical manifestations, it is unknown if neurologic complications occur more frequently and earlier in HIV-infected patients. Until better data from controlled studies are available, the significance of these anecdotal case reports is difficult to determine, but the importance of a careful neurologic evaluation in any patient with syphilis is obvious. Of note, Lukehart et al.[36] found viable *T. pallidum* in the CSF of 12 of 40 patients with primary or secondary syphilis and no neurologic symptoms. In this study isolation of *T. pallidum* was associated with two or more abnormal CSF findings, including pleocytosis, elevated protein concentration, or a reactive CSF-VDRL test, but was not associated with coexisting HIV infection. These data suggest that asymptomatic CNS involvement at the time of early syphilis infection is common, but not more common in HIV-infected individuals.

Ocular and Otologic Syphilis

A number of case reports of ocular and otologic manifestations of syphilis in HIV-infected persons have been published recently.[2,17,35,38,55,59] The most common ocular findings in patients with concurrent HIV infection are uveitis, chorioretinitis, and retrobulbar neuritis. Retinitis or neuroretinitis, papillitis, vitreitis, and optic perineuritis have also been described. The most common presenting symptoms are decreased vision and/or eye pain. In addition to the abnormalities of the optic cranial nerve and the ocular motor nerves III and VI that can occur with acute syphilitic meningitis, these other ocular manifestations of syphilis have commonly been associated with the secondary stage of infection and CNS involvement. One case report of a gumma of the optic nerve has been published.[54]

Otologic syphilis is one of the few forms of sensorineural hearing loss that can be reversed if diagnosed and treated appropriately. Although the incidence of otologic symptoms in patients with HIV infection apparently is low, five cases of otosyphilis in persons with coexisting HIV infection have been reported by Smith and Canalis.[55] Otologic findings in these patients included progressive hearing loss, tinnitus, imbalance, and/or a sensation of ear fullness. Three patients had been treated for primary syphilis 2 to 5 years before the onset of symptoms. Only one patient with acute syphilis meningitis had evidence of CNS involvement coincidence with the diagnosis of otosyphilis.

These clinical manifestations of ocular and otologic syphilis among persons with concurrent HIV infection have also been described among persons without HIV infection. However, as is the case for neurologic complications, it is unknown if ocular and otologic findings occur more frequently in HIV-infected persons. Performing careful ophthalmologic and otologic examinations of symptomatic HIV-infected persons is essential.

Mucocutaneous Syphilis

Most HIV-infected patients with *T. pallidum* present with typical dermatologic clinical features of primary and secondary disease such as chancres and diffuse maculopapular rashes.[27] However, atypical chancres seen as fissures or abrasions have occurred in two patients in our clinic. Gummatous penile ulcerations have also been reported.[24,33] Case reports of unusual rashes include papular or nodular eruptions,[8,19] nodular or ulcerative lesions with necrotic centers (i.e., lues maligna),[19,52,61] and keratoderma.[46] These skin lesions have been characterized as more aggressive forms of secondary syphilis in HIV-infected persons, yet the same dermatologic presentations have been described in non–HIV-infected persons. Gummatous syphilis, a tertiary form of syphilis, has also been described in persons with HIV infection.[10] The frequency of these uncommon cutaneous findings cannot be determined by these case reports, and additional studies are needed to define the clinical spectrum of syphilis in both HIV-infected and non–HIV-infected populations.

DIAGNOSIS

Diagnosing syphilis may be more complicated in HIV-infected patients because of false-negative serologic test results and atypical clinical presentations in the presence of HIV infection. The diagnosis should be based on a number of factors, including the patient's history, the clinical findings, direct examination of lesion material for spirochetes, and the results of serologic tests for syphilis. The importance of a careful clinical examination of HIV-infected patients with syphilis cannot be overstated. CNS disease may occur during any stage of syphilis. Clinical evidence of neurologic involvement warrants examination of the CSF.

Dark-field examination or direct fluorescent antibody (DFA) staining of exudate from lesions suspected of being primary syphilis should always be done if feasible because in patients with suspicious lesions but negative serologies, a positive dark-field examination of DFA stain is diagnostic. Dark-field examination or DFA staining of selected secondary lesions should be used in establishing the diagnosis of secondary syphilis. It is important to confirm by DFA that the treponema seen in dark-field-positive oral lesions are *T. pallidum* since nonpathogenic spirochetes are found in the mouth.

Serologic tests for syphilis remain the cornerstone of diagnosing untreated syphilis infection—even in HIV-infected patients. Serum samples should be obtained from any patient in whom the diagnosis of syphilis is suspected. All patients with known HIV infection should also be screened for possible untreated syphilis infection. Nontreponemal antibody test results should be reported quantitatively and titered to a final end point.

A negative RPR or VDRL test result may not rule out syphilis in patients with HIV infection. Although the sensitivity of these serologic tests in diagnosing secondary syphilis is generally high, recent case reports of seronegative secondary syphilis in patients with HIV infection suggest that some patients fail to develop a normal antibody response to *T. pallidum*.[19,26,60] Even though these patients eventually seroconverted before treatment, more data are needed on the serologic response to *T. pallidum* in HIV-infected patients.

When clinical syndromes compatible with primary or secondary syphilis occur and when dark-field examinations and serologic test results are negative, the "prozone phenomenon" (i.e., falsely reading a nontreponemal serologic test as negative because the specimen was not tested after sufficient dilution so that the high concentration of antigen did not allow detectable antigen-antibody complex formation) should be ruled out. A biopsy should be performed on suspicious lesions, and such biopsy specimens should be evaluated for spirochetes, using special stains or isolation techniques or both. A silver stain such as the Steiner stain[58] has been used successfully. Specific DFA stains for *T. pallidum* can also be used. Because *T. pallidum* cannot be grown on artificial media, inoculation of laboratory animals (usually rabbit testicles) is the only method currently available to isolate the organism. This method is available only in a few research laboratories.

Clinicians should consult with infectious disease specialists or pathologists about special tests available in their areas. If spirochetes are not demonstrated on biopsy material or if special techniques are not available to identify spirochetes but clinical suspicion of syphilis remains high, clinicians may wish to treat HIV-infected patients presumptively for early syphilis. Such patients should be followed closely with serial serologic testing at 1 month, 2 months, 3 months, and 6 months to detect any delayed antibody response.

The specificity of the nontreponemal serologic tests for syphilis can be compromised in HIV-infected persons.[12] The nontreponemal tests detect antibodies directed against a cardiolipin-lecithin antigen. In patients with immunoglobulin abnormalities the RPR or VDRL test result may be false positive. Many persons with HIV infection have both anticardiolipin-lecithin antibodies and polyclonal gammopathy. Thus a positive RPR or VDRL test result may not represent active syphilis infection. However, it is best to assume reactive nontreponemal tests indicate active disease unless a serofast state has been well documented because reinfection is difficult to rule out and reactivation or relapse of a previously treated infection is also possible in a person with HIV infection.

Treponemal tests in HIV-infected patients previously treated for syphilis may not remain reactive after treatment. Haas et al.[21] demonstrated that seroreversion rates of treponemal tests were significantly associated with falling T-cell counts.[21] Rates of seroreversion were 7% for patients with asymptomatic HIV infection and 38% for patients with AIDS. More recently, Romanowski et al.[50] reported that seroreversion of treponemal tests also occurs in non–HIV-infected persons treated early in the course of their syphilis infection. In this study 13% of microhemagglutination-*Treponema pallidum* (MHA-TP) test results and 25% of FTA-abs test results were negative at 36 months following therapy for primary syphilis. Seroreversion was not found in patients treated for secondary or early latent syphilis. With progression of HIV disease, antitreponemal antibody reactivity may be lost in patients previously treated for syphilis; however, no data about the serologic response of treponemal tests in HIV-infected persons with active syphilis infection exist. Until additional data are available, the sensitivity of treponemal tests in HIV-infected individuals should be considered high in patients with syphilis infection of greater than 6 months. If asymptomatic patients have a positive nontreponemal test and a negative confirmatory treponemal test result, it is unlikely they have active syphilis.

Diagnosis of Neurosyphilis

The diagnosis of neurosyphilis is based on the CSF findings of cells, elevated protein concentration, and a positive CSF-VDRL test result. Even if the CSF-VDRL test result is negative, the finding of increased CSF leukocytes ($>5/mm^3$) and protein (>0.4 mg/ml) requires consideration of a diagnosis of neurosyphilis.[15] If the CSF-VDRL test result is negative, the diagnosis of neurosyphilis is complicated by the lack of another reliable diagnostic test and the difficulty of distinguishing between neurologic disease caused by *T. pallidum* and that caused by HIV or other CNS pathogens found in patients with AIDS.

The majority of symptomatic neurosyphilis cases among persons with coexisting HIV infection have a positive CSF-VDRL test result.[37] However, recent case reports of symptomatic neurosyphilis in HIV-infected patients whose initial CSF-VDRL test results were negative suggest that cases of neurosyphilis will go untreated if the CSF-VDRL is the only finding used to guide therapeutic decisions.[15] In these patients the CSF-VDRL test result became positive after penicillin therapy. These reports underscore the need for clinical judgment in establishing the diagnosis of active neurosyphilis in HIV-infected individuals. Better diagnostic tests for neurosyphilis are needed. Measurement of immunoglobulins or treponemal antigens and isolation of treponemes have been suggested, but they have not yet been adequately studied.[22] Detection of treponemal DNA using the polyermase chain reaction test is under development, and it may be a potentially useful test for diagnosing neurosyphilis.[6,23]

Indications for CSF Examination

It is currently unclear when to examine the CSF in patients with syphilis and concurrent HIV infection.[27,36,42,47,56] Examination of CSF for evidence of neurosyphilis should be performed in all HIV-infected patients (or patients at risk for HIV infection) who have any unexplained behavioral abnormalities, psychologic dysfunction, or ocular, auditory, or other neurologic symptoms or signs—especially those consistent with neurosyphilis. The CSF of HIV-infected patients also should be examined for evidence of neurosyphilis if they fail treatment for early syphilis (i.e., if the titer does not decrease appropriately—fourfold [two dilutions] decrease by 3 months and seronegative by 1 year for primary syphilis or fourfold by 6 months and seronegative by 2 years for secondary syphilis), if a fourfold or greater increase occurs, or if they are diagnosed with syphilis of greater than 1 year's duration.

Because of recent case reports of neurosyphilis or isolation of *T. pallidum* from the CSF of HIV-infected patients who had completed standard therapy for early syphilis, some experts believe that routine CSF examination in HIV-infected patients with syphilis of less than 1 year's duration is indicated and that therapy for neurosyphilis (see below) should be offered to those patients with a positive CSF-VDRL test result or with an abnormal cell count and protein concentration.[36,62,63] Other clinicians believe that all HIV-infected patients should be treated empirically with neurosyphilis regimens, even if the CSF examination is entirely normal. Many experts, however, believe that these isolated case reports do not yet justify the need for routine CSF examinations in patients with early syphilis and that additional studies are needed to determine the significance of these reports. The Centers for Disease Control (CDC) currently does not recommend routine CSF examination in patients with early syphilis.[56] Until data are available to address the need for evaluating the CSF in patients with early syphilis, the patients should be informed about the current dilemma, and their available treatment options should be discussed with them.

Indications for Screening for HIV Infection

Many of the diagnostic options discussed previously (e.g., lumbar punctures in patients with early syphilis) and the therapeutic options discussed below are recommended only for patients with coexisting HIV infection. Therefore it is important to know the HIV-antibody status of patients with syphilis when choosing diagnostic and therapeutic options. All patients with syphilis should be tested for HIV antibodies and counseled. If HIV antibody testing is not possible, the clinician should manage the patient, keeping in mind that HIV co-infection may be present.

TREATMENT FAILURES

Neurosyphilis

Several cases of neurologic relapse after benzathine penicillin G therapy for early syphilis have been reported in patients with HIV infection.[3,31,34,62] One patient was seen initially with eye pain, double vision, dizziness, and headache; 2 weeks later he was found in a stuporous state with hemiparesis, homonymous hemianopsia, and expressive aphasia. CSF evaluation revealed mononuclear pleocytosis (32 cells/mm^3), elevated protein level (92 mg/dl), and a CSF-VDRL titer of 1:4. This presentation is consistent with meningovascular syphilis. The patient had been treated for secondary syphilis 5 months before this neurologic event, and his serum VDRL titer had decreased from 1:256 to 1:16. Although a serum VDRL titer around the time of the stroke was 1:256, careful contact tracing and close follow-up after the initial treatment suggested that reinfection did not occur. Asymptomatic neurosyphilis (serum RPR titer of 1:8, normal CSF indices, and CSF-VDRL titer of 1:4) was also diagnosed in a patient with AIDS who was hospitalized for *Pneumocystis carinii* pneumonia. This patient had been treated for secondary syphilis 5 years before admission.

Neurologic relapse following penicillin therapy is not unique to HIV-infected patients[1,11,53] but is uncommon in non–HIV-infected patients. Additional studies are needed to determine the response of HIV-infected patients to currently recommended therapy.

Persistence of Treponemes

Lukehart et al.[36] found viable treponemes in the CSF of two of three HIV-infected patients with secondary syphilis 3 to 6 months after treatment with a single dose of 2.4 million units of benzathine penicillin G. In these two patients no signs or symptoms of neurologic relapse were reported, CSF-VDRL titers seroreverted, and the CSF white blood cell (WBC) count decreased, and in one patient the serum VDRL titer decreased. In another HIV-infected patient with early syphilis who was treated with a single dose of benzathine penicillin G, serum and CSF-VDRL titers were unchanged, but no treponemes were isolated 8 months after therapy. This patient also had no signs or symptoms of neurologic relapse. Long-term studies on larger numbers of patients are needed to determine whether persistence of treponemes is common and reflects inadequate therapy or whether the usual course after therapy is eventually to clear the CSF of organisms, albeit slowly.

Other Treatment Failure Issues

Clinicians have also reported slow resolution of skin lesions in patients with HIV infection after penicillin therapy, although the time period from treatment to resolution of the signs and symptoms of primary or secondary syphilis have never been well defined, even in patients without HIV infection. In addition, relapse of mucocutaneous signs and symptoms of secondary syphilis was documented in an AIDS patient treated for infectious syphilis 3 years earlier in our clinic. It is plausible that, in addition to neurologic relapse, other signs and symptoms of syphilis recur in HIV-infected individuals after treatment. Furthermore, the question of treatment failure has been raised about HIV-infected patients whose nontreponemal serologic titers fail to decrease following therapy for early syphilis.[12] As discussed previously, a positive RPR or VDRL test result may not represent active syphilis infection but rather a high serofast state. Additional studies are needed to determine the clinical and serologic response to currently recommended therapy among HIV-infected patients. Of note, treatment failures following erythromycin therapy have been reported in patients with concurrent HIV infection,[13] and failures with cephalosporins have also been observed.[42]

TREATMENT

The recent isolated case reports discussed previously have raised questions about the efficacy of current treatment recommendations for syphilis in the HIV-infected patient. Until further studies determine the optimum therapeutic regimen for early syphilis and neurosyphilis in HIV-infected patients and the significance of abnormal CSF findings in early syphilis, treatment in such patients will remain controversial.[16,27,36,42,47,56,65] The CDC currently recommends that penicillin regimens be used whenever possible for all stages of syphilis in HIV-infected patients (Table 24–1). Doxycycline should be avoided, erythromycin is not recommended, and no data about the efficacy of cephalosporins in treating syphilis in patients with HIV have been published. No proven alternative therapies to penicillin are available for treating patients with neurosyphilis, congenital syphilis, or syphilis in pregnancy. Therefore confirmation of penicillin allergy and desensitization is recommended for these patients. The following treatment recommendations are based on available data and the consensus recommendations published by the CDC.[56,65]

Treatment of Nonneurologic Syphilis of Less Than One Year's Duration

A careful clinical examination to rule out clinical evidence of neurologic involvement (e.g., optic and auditory symptoms and cranial nerve palsies) must be done before treatment of HIV-infected patients with syphilis of less than 1 year's duration.

Table 24–1.   Treatment of Syphilis in HIV-Infected Patients

Syphilis of Less Than 1 Year's Duration*
TREATMENT RECOMMENDED
Benzathine penicillin G, 2.4 million units intramuscularly (IM)
Unstudied Treatment Considerations
Benzathine penicillin G, 4.8 million units IM (administered as two doses of 2.4 million units IM
   weekly for 2 successive weeks)
Doxycycline, 100 mg P.O. twice a day for 14 days
Regimens for neurosyphilis as outlined below
Syphilis of Greater Than 1 Year's Duration†
TREATMENT RECOMMENDED
Benzathine penicillin G, 7.2 million units IM (administered as three doses of 2.4 million units IM
   weekly for 3 successive weeks)
Unstudied Treatment Considerations
Regimens for neurosyphilis as outlined below *plus*
Benzathine penicillin G, 7.2 million units IM (administered as three doses of 2.4 million units IM
   weekly for 3 successive weeks)
Neurosyphilis
TREATMENT RECOMMENDED
Aqueous crystalline penicillin G, 12 to 24 million units intravenously (IV) per day for 10 to 14 days
   (administered as 2 to 4 million units every 4 hours each day)
   or
Aqueous procaine penicillin G, 2.4 million units IM daily for 10 days, plus probenecid, 500 mg P.O.
   four times a day for 10 days
   plus
Benzathine penicillin G, 7.2 million units IM (administered as three doses of 2.4 million units IM
   weekly for 3 successive weeks)

---

*Incubating, primary, secondary, and early latent syphilis without clinical evidence of neurosyphilis.
†Late latent syphilis or syphilis of undetermined age but without clinical evidence of neurosyphilis.

For HIV-infected patients with incubating, primary, secondary, or latent syphilis of less than 1 year's duration and no clinical evidence of neurologic involvement, the same treatment regimen as for patients without HIV infection is recommended: 2.4 million units of benzathine penicillin G administered intramuscularly (IM) at a single session. In penicillin-sensitive patients allergy should be confirmed. If compliance and close follow-up are assured, use of doxycycline (100 mg orally two times a day for 2 weeks) may be considered if the patient refuses hospitalization. However, no data are available on the efficacy of tetracyclines in treating syphilis in HIV-infected patients, and if compliance and close follow-up cannot be assured in patients taking tetracyclines, desensitization to penicillin and management in consultation with an infectious disease expert are recommended.

Treatment of Nonneurologic Syphilis of More Than One Year's Duration

A careful clinical examination and CSF examination should precede and guide treatment of HIV-infected patients with syphilis of greater than 1 year's duration or of indeterminate duration. If CSF examination is not possible, patients should be treated for presumed neurosyphilis. If the CSF examination yields no evidence of neurosyphilis, administration of 7.2 million units of benzathine penicillin G total (administered as three doses of 2.4 million units by IM injection weekly for 3 successive weeks) is recommended. In penicillin-sensitive patients allergy should be confirmed, after which desensitization to penicillin and management in consultation with an infectious disease expert is recommended. Doxycycline is not recommended.

All patients should be warned about the possibility of a Jarisch-Herxheimer reaction before any treatment is given. In addition, HIV-infected patients should be informed that currently recommended regimens may be less effective for them than for patients without HIV infection and that close follow-up care is essential.

Treatment of Neurosyphilis

For HIV-infected patients with any type of symptomatic neurosyphilis (including ocular or otologic syphilis), aqueous crystalline penicillin G is the treatment of choice (12 to 24 million units intravenously [IV] per day [i.e., 2 to 4 million units every 4 hours for 10 to 14 days]). Penicillin-sensitive patients should be desensitized to penicillin.

If hospitalization is impossible, administration of aqueous procaine penicillin G is another option (2.4 million units IM daily plus probenecid 500 mg by mouth four times daily for 10 days). However, these injections are painful, and patient compliance may be difficult to assure. Many experts also recommend the addition of benzathine penicillin G (2.4 million units IM weekly for 3 successive weeks) after completion of aqueous crystalline or aqueous procaine penicillin G therapy.

Treatment Alternatives

Other outpatient regimens have been used in the treatment of neurosyphilis patients with normal immune function. These regimens include amoxicillin (2 g with probenecid, 500 mg, by mouth three times daily for 14 days),[14,25,40] although the minimum inhibitory concentrations (MICs) of the drug for *T. pallidum* are 10 to 20 times higher than that of penicillin, doxycycline (200 mg by mouth twice a day for 21 days),[64] and ceftriaxone (1 g IM daily for 14 days); however, tetracyclines and cephalosporins are less active than penicillin for syphilis therapy.[29] The efficacy of these regimens for treating syphilis in HIV-infected patients is unknown. For HIV-infected patients with symptomatic neurosyphilis or asymptomatic neurosyphilis and syphilis of greater than 1 year's duration, aqueous penicillin therapy is the treatment of choice.

Because of concerns about neurologic relapse and persistence of treponemes in the CSF in HIV-infected patients treated with benzathine penicillin G for early syphilis, some experts believe that until better data are available, HIV-infected patients with syphilis of less than 1 year's duration and abnormal CSF (i.e., with asymptomatic neurosyphilis) should be offered treatment regimens of longer duration, higher dosage, and better CSF penetration (e.g., the antibiotic regimens for neurosyphilis outlined previously).[36] Other experts emphasize that HIV-infected patients treated for syphilis who fail to respond (as defined below) to standard benzathine penicillin G therapy should also be offered antibiotic regimens of higher dose, longer duration, and better CSF penetration. Some clinicians believe that all HIV-infected patients with syphilis should be treated with penicillin regimens effective for neurosyphilis, an approach considered by others as of unproven benefit, impractical, and costly.[27] Still other experts suggest that HIV-infected patients with syphilis of less than 1 year's duration should receive a longer course of benzathine penicillin G therapy such as 2.4 million units IM weekly for 2 or 3 weeks.[16,42] Others have considered adding oral amoxicillin to the benzathine penicillin G regimen to supplement levels of penicillin in the blood.[63] The justification for using any of these alternative regimens is only theoretic. No studies comparing the efficacy of 2.4 million units of benzathine penicillin G with other treatment options for the treatment of syphilis in HIV-infected patients have been completed. Eradication of *T. pallidum* from patients with HIV infection may be impossible, and such patients may require chronic penicillin therapy to control their infection.

FOLLOW-UP

Until the efficacy of treatment regimens is better defined, the importance of closely following HIV-infected patients with syphilis cannot be overstated. All patients should be watched carefully for persistent or recurrent symptoms and for any signs of neurologic involvement.

Patients treated for syphilis of less than 1 year's duration should be examined and retested with a quantitative nontreponemal test at 1 to 2 weeks and at 1, 2, 3, 6, 9, and 12 months after treatment. The reasons for the follow-up intervals include verifying that the level of the nontreponemal test result peaks and then falls; documenting a Jarisch-Herxheimer reaction; monitoring resolution, persistence, or recurrence of clinical signs and symptoms and development of any new signs or symptoms, especially those involving the CNS; and assuring compliance with treatment, effective partner notification, and safer-sex practices. More frequent follow-up care may be necessary to characterize the peak level of the nontreponemal test titer in some cases. Patients should be followed longer if any questions about the adequacy of their clinical or serologic response exist. Patients must be followed using the same nontreponemal test because titers from the VDRL and RPR tests are not interchangeable. In the absence of HIV infection and no previous history of *T. pallidum* infection, treatment usually produces seronegativity within 1 year in patients with primary syphilis and within 2 years in patients with secondary syphilis. The serologic response in HIV-infected patients and patients with a history of syphilis infection is unknown.

Determining what constitutes a therapeutic cure of syphilis in patients with coexisting HIV infection is problematic because no simple test is available. Moreover, symptoms and signs of early syphilis may resolve even without treatment. Criteria defining treatment failure are currently based on curves of serologic response to treatment established in patients with normal immune function.[5,20,51] Treatment failure criteria include the following findings: (1) persistence or recurrence of signs or symptoms of syphilis; (2) a sustained, fourfold (two dilutions) increase in the titer of nontreponemal tests of greater than 2 weeks duration; or (3) failure of the initially high nontreponemal test titer in patients with early syphilis to decrease fourfold (two dilutions) by 3 months for primary syphilis and by 6 months for secondary syphilis. Until additional data on the serologic response in HIV-infected patients are available, the above criteria should also be used for determining treatment failures in HIV-infected patients.

For patients with neurosyphilis, repeat serologic testing as described previously and CSF examination at 6-month intervals are recommended until the findings have stabilized.[56] Abnormal CSF WBC counts and protein levels should decrease by 6 months if no coexisting CNS infections are present, but CSF-VDRL tests may not return to nonreactivity. If the CSF WBC count is not normal by 2 years, retreatment using an antibiotic regimen for neurosyphilis is recommended.

For HIV-infected patients treated for early syphilis whose serologic titers have not changed 1 year after therapy, a CSF examination is indicated. If there is no evidence of neurosyphilis, many clinicians are retreating the patient with 7.2 million units of benzathine penicillin G IM (i.e., 2.4 million units IM weekly for 3 weeks) and following the patient with repeat serologic testing every 6 months. Unless the patient has recurrent or new clinical signs or symptoms or a sustained fourfold increase in the serologic titer, no further therapy is offered. Other clinicians are not retreating such patients but simply are following them for evidence of relapse.

SEXUAL CONTACTS

An effort must be made to identify and treat any possible contacts of patients with early syphilis. In patients with primary syphilis all contacts for 3 months before the appearance of the chancre should be evaluated clinically and serologically. In patients with secondary syphilis and no history of a chancre contacts for the prior 6 months should be evaluated clinically and serologically. In patients with early latent syphilis and no history of symptoms or signs suggestive of primary or secondary syphilis, contacts for the prior 12 months should be evaluated clinically and serologically. Efforts should be made to establish a diagnosis of syphilis by history, clinical findings, and serologic testing before treating such contacts. However, persons exposed to a patient with early syphilis within the previous 3 months may be infected and seronegative and therefore should be treated presumptively for early syphilis, even without an established diagnosis.

Follow-up serologic tests should also be done at 1 week and 3 months to establish the diagnosis of syphilis in these contacts if they are HIV infected or at risk of HIV infection. All cases of infectious syphilis (primary, secondary, and early latent) must be reported to the local health department. In addition, some state and local health departments (e.g., in San Francisco) require that health care providers notify the Director of STD Control about HIV-infected patients who have (1) neurosyphilis confirmed by CSF examination (i.e., positive CSF-VDRL) or histopathology (DFA or special stains of biopsy material); (2) negative serologic test results for syphilis (nontreponemal [VDRL, RPR] or treponemal [FTA-abs, MHA-TP] tests) during secondary syphilis diagnosed by dark-field microscopy or histopathology of lesion material; or (3) failed treatment for syphilis as defined previously.

EDUCATION

All patients with syphilis and their contacts must be given education and counseling to reduce their risk of future STDs. Safer-sex messages should discuss reducing the numbers of sexual partners, knowing the health status of partners (if possible), avoiding unsafe sexual practices, and using condoms.

REFERENCES

1. Bayne LL, Schmidley JW, Goodin DS: Acute syphilitic meningitis: Its occurrence after clinical and serologic cure of secondary syphilis with penicillin G. Arch Neurol 43:137-138, 1986
2. Becerra LI, Ksiazek SM, Savino PJ, et al: Syphilitic uveitis in human immunodeficiency virus infected and noninfected patients. Ophthalmology 96:1727-1730, 1989
3. Berry CD, Hooton TM, Collier AC, Lukehart SA: Neurologic relapse after benzathine penicillin therapy for secondary syphilis in a patient with HIV infection. N Engl J Med 316:1587-1589, 1987
4. Bowen DL, Lane HC, Fauci AS: Immunopathogenesis of the acquired immunodeficiency syndrome. Ann Intern Med 103:704-709, 1985
5. Brown ST, Zaidi A, Larsen SA, Reynolds GH: Serologic response to syphilis treatment: A new analysis of old data. JAMA 253:1296-1299, 1985
6. Burstain JM, Frimprel E, Lukehart SA, et al: Sensitive detection of *Treponema pallidum* by using the polymerase chain reaction. J Clin Microbiol 29:62-69, 1991
7. Calderon W, Danville H, Nigro M, et al: Concomitant syphilitic and HIV infection: A case report. ACTA Neurol 45:132-137, 1990
8. Cusini M, Zerboni R, Muratori S, et al: Atypical early syphilis in a HIV-infected homosexual male. Dermatologica 177:300-304, 1988
9. Darrow WW, Echenberg DF, Jaffe HW, et al: Risk factors for human immunodeficiency virus (HIV) infections in homosexual men. Am J Public Health 77:479-483, 1987
10. Dawson S, Evans BA, Lawrence AG: Benign tertiary syphilis and HIV infection. AIDS 2:315-316, 1988
11. DiNubile MJ, Copare FJ, Gekowski KM: Neurosyphilis developing during treatment of secondary syphilis with benzathine penicillin in a patient without serologic evidence of human immunodeficiency virus infection. Am J Med 88:5-45N–5-48N, 1990
12. Drabick JJ, Tramont EC: Utility of the VDRL test in HIV-seropositive patients. N Engl J Med 322:271, 1990
13. Duncan WC: Failure of erythromycin to cure secondary syphilis in a patient infected with the human immunodeficiency virus. Arch Dermatol 125:82-84, 1989
14. Faber WR, Bos JD, Reitra PJ, et al: Treponemicidal levels of amoxicillin in cerebrospinal fluid after oral administration. Sex Transm Dis 10:148-150, 1983
15. Feraru ER, Aronow HA, Lipton RB: Neurosyphilis in AIDS patients: Initial CSF VDRL may be negative. Neurology 40:541-543, 1990
16. Fiumara N: Human immunodeficiency virus infection and syphilis. J Am Acad Dermatol 21:141-142, 1989
17. Gass JD, Braunstein RA, Chenoweth RG: Acute syphilitic posterior placoid chorioretinitis. Ophthalmology 97:1288-1297, 1990
18. Greenblatt RM, Lukehart SA, Plummer FA, et al: Genital ulceration as a risk factor for human immunodeficiency virus infection. AIDS 2:47-50, 1988
19. Gregory N, Sanchez M, Buchness MR: The spectrum of syphilis in patients with human immunodeficiency virus infection. J Am Acad Dermatol 22:1061-1067, 1990
20. Guinan ME: Treatment of primary and secondary syphilis: Defining failure at three- and six-month follow-up. JAMA 257:359-360, 1987
21. Haas JS, Bolan G, Larsen SA, et al: Sensitivity of treponemal tests for detecting prior treated syphilis during human immunodeficiency virus infection. J Infect Dis 162:862-866, 1990
22. Hart G: Syphilis tests in diagnostic and therapeutic decision making. Ann Intern Med 104:368-376, 1986
23. Hay PE, Clark JR, Taylor-Robinson D, Goldmeier D: Detection of treponemal DNA in the CSF of patients with syphilis and HIV infection using the polymerase chart reaction. Genitourin Med 66:428-432, 1990
24. Hay PE, Tam FWK, Kitchen VS, et al: Gummatous lesions in men infected with human immunodeficiency virus and syphilis. Genitourin Med 66:374-379, 1990
25. Hay PE, Taylor-Robinson D, Waldron S, Goldmeier D: Amoxicillin, syphilis, and HIV infection. Lancet 335:474-475, 1990
26. Hicks CB, Benson PM, Lupton GP, Tramont EC: Seronegative secondary syphilis in a patient infected with the human immunodeficiency virus (HIV) with Kaposi's sarcoma: A diagnostic dilemma. Ann Intern Med 107:492-495, 1987

27. Hook EW III: Syphilis and HIV infection. J Infect Dis 160:530-534, 1989
28. Hook EW III: Treatment of syphilis: Current recommendations, alternatives and continuing problems. Rev Infect Dis 11:S1511-S1517, 1989
29. Hook EW III, Baker-Zander SA, Moskovitz BL, et al: Ceftriaxone therapy for asymptomatic neurosyphilis. Case report and Western blot analysis of serum and cerebrospinal fluid IgG response to therapy. Sex Transm Dis (suppl 3):185S-188S, 1986
30. Jaffe HW, Choi K, Thomas PA, et al: National case-control study of Kaposi's sarcoma and *Pneumocystis carinii* pneumonia in homosexual men. Part 1. Epidemiologic results. Ann Intern Med 99:145-151, 1983
31. Johns DR, Tierney M, Felsenstein D: Alteration in the natural history of neurosyphilis by concurrent infection with the human immunodeficiency virus. N Engl J Med 316:1569-1572, 1987
32. Katz DA, Berger JR: Neurosyphilis in acquired immunodeficiency syndrome. Arch Neurol 46:895-898, 1989
33. Kitchen VS, Cook T, Doble A, Harris JR: Gummatous penile ulceration and generalized lymphadenopathy in homosexual man: case report. Genitourin Med 64:276-279, 1988
34. Lanska MJ, Lanska DJ, Schmidley JW: Syphilitic polyradiculopathy in a HIV-positive man. Neurology 38:1297-1301, 1988
35. Levy JH, Liss RA, Maguire AM: Neurosyphilis and ocular syphilis in patients with concurrent human immunodeficiency virus infection. Retina 9:175-180, 1989
36. Lukehart SA, Hook EW III, Baker-Zander SA, et al: Invasion of the central nervous system by *Treponema pallidum:* Implications for diagnosis and treatment. Ann Intern Med 109:855-862, 1988
37. Matlow AG, Rachlis AR: Syphilis serology in human immunodeficiency virus-infected patients with symptomatic neurosyphilis: Case report and review. Rev Infect Dis 12:703-707, 1990
38. McLeish WM, Pulido JS, Holland S, et al: The ocular manifestations of syphilis in the human immunodeficiency virus type-1 infected host. Ophthalmology 97:196-203, 1990
39. Merritt HH, Adams RD, Soloman HC: Neurosyphilis. New York, Oxford University Press, 1946
40. Morrison RE, Harrison SM, Tramont EC: Oral amoxicillin: An alternative treatment for neurosyphilis. Genitourin Med 61:359-362, 1985
41. Musher DM: How much penicillin cures early syphilis? Ann Intern Med 109:849-851, 1988
42. Musher DM: Syphilis, neurosyphilis, penicillin, and AIDS. J Infect Dis 163:1201-1206, 1991
43. Musher DM, Hamill RJ, Baughn RE: Effect of human immunodeficiency virus (HIV) infection on the course of syphilis and on the response to treatment. Ann Intern Med 113:872-881, 1990
44. Pacha N, Metzger M, Smogor W, et al: Effects of immunosuppressive agents on the course of experimental syphilis in rabbits. Arch Immunol Ther 27:45-51, 1979
45. Pavia CS, Folds JD, Baseman JB: Cell-mediated immunity during syphilis: A review. Br J Venereal Dis 54:144-150, 1978
46. Radolph JD, Kaplan RP: Unusual manifestations of secondary syphilis and abnormal humoral immune response to *Treponema pallidum* antigens in a homosexual man with asymptomatic human immunodeficiency virus infection. J Am Acad Dermatol 18:423-428, 1988
47. Recommendations for diagnosing and treating syphilis in HIV-infected patients. MMWR 37:600-602, 607-608, 1988
48. Risk factors for AIDS among Haitians in the United States. Evidence of heterosexual transmission. The Collaborative Study Group of AIDS in Haitian-Americans. JAMA 257:635-639, 1987
49. Rolfs RT, Nakashima AK: Epidemiology of primary and secondary syphilis in the United States: 1981-1989. JAMA 264:1432-1437, 1990
50. Romanowski B, Sutherland R, Fick GH, et al: Serologic response to treatment of infection syphilis. Ann Intern Med 144:1005-1009, 1991
51. Schroeter AL, Lucas JB, Price EV, Falcone VH: Treatment for early syphilis and reactivity of serologic tests. JAMA 221:471-476, 1972
52. Shulkin D, Tripoli L, Abell E: Lues maligna in a patient with human immunodeficiency virus infection. Am J Med 85:425-527, 1988
53. Simon RP: Neurosyphilis. Arch Neurol 42:606-613, 1985
54. Smith JL, Byrne SF, Cambron GR: Syphiloma/gumma of the optic nerve and human immunodeficiency virus seropositivity. J Clin Neuro Ophthalmol 10:175-184, 1990
55. Smith ME, Canalis RF: Otologic manifestations of AIDS: The otosyphilis connection. Laryngoscope 99:365-372, 1989
56. 1989 STD treatment guidelines. MMWR 38(suppl 8):5S-15S, 1989
57. Strom T, Schneck SA: Syphilis meningomyelitis. Neurology 41:325-326, 1991

58. Swisher BL: Modified Steiner procedure for microwave staining of spirochetes and non-filamentous bacteria. J Histotechnol 10:241-243, 1987
59. Tamesis RR, Foster CS: Ocular syphilis. Ophthalmology 97:1281-1287, 1990
60. Tikjob G, Russel M, Petersen CS, et al: Seronegative secondary syphilis in a patient with AIDS: Identification of *Treponema pallidum* in biopsy specimen. J Am Acad Dermatol 24:506-508, 1991
61. Tosca A, Starropoulos PG, Hatziolore E, et al: Malignant syphilis in HIV-infected patients. Int J Dermatol 29:575-578, 1990
62. Tramont EC: Persistence of *Treponema pallidum* following penicillin G therapy: Report of 2 cases. JAMA 236:2206-2207, 1976
63. Tramont EC: Syphilis in the AIDS era. N Engl J Med 316:1600-1601, 1987
64. Yim CW, Flynn NM, Fitzgerald FT: Penetration of oral doxycycline into the cerebrospinal fluid of patients with latent or neurosyphilis. Antimicrob Agents Chemother 28:347-348, 1985
65. Zenker PN, Rolfs RT: Treatment of syphilis, 1989. Rev Infect Dis 12:S590-S609, 1990

25

MALIGNANCIES ASSOCIATED WITH AIDS

LAWRENCE D. KAPLAN, MD
DONALD W. NORTHFELT, MD

Malignancies as a complication of immunodeficiency have been well described in the literature, being recognized long before the advent of the HIV epidemic.[29,50,54] The incidence of both Kaposi's sarcoma and non-Hodgkin's lymphoma are markedly increased in immunosuppressed allograft recipients. It is therefore not surprising that patients with HIV infection, who also have profound defects in cell-mediated immunity, also develop these two malignancies. The marked rise in the incidence of both Kaposi's sarcoma and B-cell lymphoma in populations at risk for HIV infection in the years since 1982 strongly suggests a causal relationship between immunodeficiency and the development of these malignancies.[48] As a result of this relationship, these neoplasms are included in the AIDS case definition established by the Centers for Disease Control (CDC).[9] Thus these neoplasms are referred to as "AIDS-defining" malignancies. They are listed in Table 25–1 with a variety of other malignancies that have been reported in HIV-infected individuals but for which no clear causal relationship has been established. In the case of cervical and anal carcinomas and interepithelial neoplasias, accumulating evidence suggests a relationship between immune function and the risk of invasive disease.[8,81]

Regardless of the causal relationship between various malignancies and the underlying immunodeficiency state, reports in the literature suggest that the natural history of cancer may be altered in the setting of HIV infection.[25,106,127] Patients tend to present with more advanced disease that is more rapidly progressive and responds less well to therapy than in the non–HIV-infected population.

Management of the HIV-infected patient with a malignancy imposes obstacles rarely encountered in the non–HIV-infected population. Poor bone marrow reserve and the risk of intercurrent opportunistic infections, problems frequently observed in this patient population, can compromise the delivery of adequate dose intensity. In addition, administration of chemotherapy may lead to further immunosuppression, resulting in a greater likelihood of opportunistic infection. Finally, toxicity responses to chemotherapeutic agents, antibiotics, and radiotherapy are excessive and often severe, further impairing the physician's ability to administer adequate therapy.

Table 25–1.   Malignancies in HIV Infection

AIDS DEFINING MALIGNANCIES	NON-AIDS DEFINING MALIGNANCIES	REFERENCE
Kaposi's sarcoma	Hodgkin's disease	55, 58, 115
B-cell lymphoma	Squamous carcinoma	15, 25, 42, 81, 127
	Head and neck	
	Anus	
	Cervix	
	Melanoma	126
	Plasmacytoma	127
	Adenocarcinoma colon	7
	Small cell lung carcinoma	42, 127
	Germ cell (testicular) tumor	125
	Basal cell tumor	51

This chapter focuses on the two AIDS-defining malignancies, Kaposi's sarcoma and non-Hodgkin's lymphoma, from primarily a clinical perspective. The natural history of these malignancies is presented along with various therapeutic options. Discussions of Hodgkin's lymphoma and cervical and anal interepithelial neoplasia have also been included.

KAPOSI'S SARCOMA

Kaposi's sarcoma (KS), once a rarely reported malignancy, is the most common neoplasm affecting HIV-infected individuals. It is seen primarily in homosexual men and has only rarely been reported in intravenous (IV) drug users or other risk groups.[87,113] The proportion of AIDS patients with KS as the initial AIDS diagnosis has changed since the first cases were reported in 1981.[16] In New York City KS was the initial AIDS diagnosis in 50% of non–IV-drug-using homosexual men diagnosed between 1981 and 1983. Between 1984 and 1987, however, this proportion had fallen to 30%. Similar trends have been reported from San Francisco.[112]

The pathogenesis of KS in HIV-infected patients remains uncertain. The decline in the incidence of KS in the homosexual male population during a period of time when sexual practices were changing and the nearly exclusive confinement of this neoplasm to the homosexual male population support the concept of another sexually transmitted agent's being involved in the pathogenesis of KS.[19] Other laboratory studies have implicated a variety of endothelial growth factors, including basic fibroblast growth factor, interleukin-1 (IL-1), tumor necrosis factor, and lymphotoxin in the etiology of KS.[20,91,114] The role of interleukin 6 (IL-6) has received particular attention. It recently has been demonstrated that HIV-associated KS tissue produces large amounts of immunoreactive IL-6 and that HIV-associated KS-derived cell lines produce and respond to IL-6 in an autocrine growth loop.[84] It has also been observed that male mice transgenic for the HIV-*tat* gene develop KS-like tumors.[129] Additional laboratory studies have demonstrated that the proliferation of KS spindle cells in vitro observed in response to HIV-*tat* is accompanied by an increase in IL-6 production by these same cells.[109] What the precise roles of these various factors may be in the pathogenesis and growth of KS in the clinical setting is currently the subject of investigation. A better understanding of the pathogenesis of this disease may have significant implications for future therapeutic strategies.

Clinical Presentation and Diagnosis

Unlike the more indolent, endemic form of KS, KS in the HIV-infected individual usually is an aggressive and unpredictable disease.[87,113] The skin is most commonly the first site of presentation. Palpable, firm, cutaneous nodules ranging from 0.5 to 2 cm in diameter are frequently observed. However, in early stages smaller, nonpalpable lesions may be seen. Some early lesions can appear like small ecchymoses. In more advanced disease cutaneous lesions can become confluent and form large tumor masses involving extensive cutaneous surfaces. In light-skinned individuals the lesions are typically violaceous in appearance (Color Plate I G), whereas in dark-skinned individuals, the lesions acquire a more hyperpigmented appearance, appearing brown or even black. Rather than being limited to a single cutaneous site as in endemic KS, KS in an individual with HIV infection can involve any cutaneous surface. Involvement of the head and neck is frequent, and the appearance of oral KS lesions is often the first sign of disease (Color Plate I H).

The natural history of KS associated with HIV infection more closely resembles that observed in immunosuppressed allograft recipients. The disease tends to progress with time and is associated with the appearance of larger and more numerous cutaneous lesions. However, the course of the disease is unpredictable. A patient may have relatively few lesions that remain stable over time. New cutaneous lesions may not appear for many months but may be followed by a sudden and rapid increase in disease activity. Visceral involvement with KS is extremely common and can involve almost any visceral site. Careful endoscopic examination will reveal gastrointestinal (GI) sites of disease in most patients.

Although KS is usually not a direct cause of death in HIV-infected patients, the morbidity associated with more advanced disease can be significant. Bulky cutaneous lesions may become painful and if large cutaneous surfaces are involved, can restrict movement. Lymphatic obstruction is common and can result in severe edema, most commonly involving the extremities (Color Plate I E) or the face. Visceral spread of KS is rarely symptomatic, particularly when it involves the GI tract. However, rare cases of obstruction, perforation, or GI bleeding have been reported.[27] In contrast, pulmonary KS may result in cough, bronchospasm, and dyspnea, and death caused by respiratory failure is not uncommon.[60,95] Finally, the social problems associated with this disfiguring neoplasm in the setting of an already socially stigmatizing disease cannot be overemphasized.

Careful examination of the skin and oral cavity at each clinic visit is the key to early diagnosis. Once lesions are identified, histologic confirmation should be obtained. This is particularly important because other cutaneous diseases, some of which can mimic KS, are common in the HIV-infected patient (see Chapter 10). For cutaneous lesions, a small punch biopsy specimen is generally obtained. Conventional biopsy techniques can be used at other sites. In patients with suspected pulmonary KS violaceous endobronchial lesions are typically observed on bronchoscopic examination. Unfortunately, attempts at endobronchial biopsy are frequently unsuccessful because of the submucosal nature of the lesions. However, bronchoscopic visualization of typical lesions is generally accepted for the purpose of diagnosis of pulmonary disease in patients who have known KS at other sites.[60]

Although historically the most common cause of death in individuals with HIV and KS is opportunistic infection, there is evidence that as survival is prolonged in individuals with HIV infection as a result of improvements in medical care, pulmonary involvement with KS is becoming an increasingly common cause of death.

Staging

Currently used staging systems are based primarily on tumor bulk. A modification of this staging system to include the presence or absence of constitutional symptoms is shown in Table 25–2. Unfortunately, these systems have not proved useful because a majority of patients fall into the most advanced stages. In addition, tumor bulk may not be the most important predictor of survival in this group of patients.

Analysis of data from 190 individuals with HIV-associated KS at UCLA Medical Center demonstrated the most important predictor of survival is the absolute CD4 + lymphocyte count[124] (Figure 25–1). Only 30% of patients with fewer than 100 CD4 lymphocytes survived for 1 year. Other features associated with a negative impact on survival in various studies have included prior history of opportunistic infection,[86] bulky tumor,[86,90] the presence of constitutional symptoms,[86,90] and initial presentation

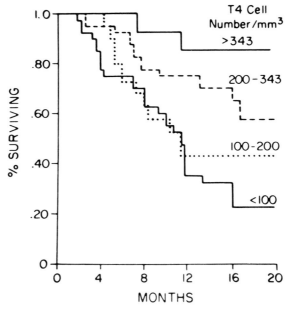

FIGURE 25–1. Relationship of various levels of T4 (CD4) cell numbers to survival in AIDS–Kaposi's sarcoma patients (Kaplan-Meier graph). (From Taylor J, et al.: Prognostically significant classification of immune changes in AIDS with Kaposi's sarcoma. Blood 67:666–671, 1986.)

Table 25–2.   Staging of Kaposi's Sarcoma

STAGE	CHARACTERISTICS
I	Limited cutaneous lesions (<10 or in one anatomic area)
II	Disseminated cutaneous lesions (>10 or in more than one anatomic area)
III	Visceral lesions only (gastrointestinal, lymph node)
IV	Cutaneous and visceral lesions
Subtypes	
A	No systemic signs or symptoms
B	Fevers >37.8° C unrelated to identifiable infection for >2 wk or weight loss >10% of body weight

From Mitsuyasu RT, Groopman JE: Biology and therapy of Kaposi's sarcoma. Semin Oncol 11:53-59, 1984.

Table 25–3.   Proposed Staging Classification for Kaposi's Sarcoma

GOOD RISK (0) ALL OF THE FOLLOWING	POOR RISK (1) ANY OF THE FOLLOWING
Tumor (T)	
Confined to skin and/or lymph nodes and/or minimum oral disease*	Tumor-associated edema or ulceration
	Extensive oral Kaposi's sarcoma (KS) lesions
	Gastrointestinal KS lesions
	KS lesions in other non-nodal viscera
Immune System (I)	
CD4 cells ≥200/μL	CD4 cells <200/μL
Systemic Illness (S)	
No history of OI or thrush	History of OI and/or thrush
No "B" symptoms†	B symptoms present
Karnofsky performance status ≥70	Karnofsky performance status <70
	Other HIV-related illness (e.g., neurologic disease, lymphoma)

Modified from Krown SE, Metroka C, Wernz J: Kaposi's sarcoma in the acquired immune deficiency syndrome: A proposal for uniform evaluation, response, and staging criteria. J Clin Oncol 7:9, 1201-1207, 1989.
*Minimum oral disease in non-nodular KS confined to the palate.
†"B" symptoms are unexplained fever, night sweats, >10% involuntary weight loss, or diarrhea persisting more than 2 wk.

that involves a mucosal surface or cutaneous site other than the lower extremities or the lymph nodes.[90]

Based on these known predictors of survival in patients with AIDS-associated KS, the Oncology Subcommittee of the National Institute of Health (NIH)-sponsored AIDS Clinical Trials Group (ACTG) has proposed a new staging classification, illustrated in Table 25–3. This system takes into account tumor bulk, immune function, and the presence of other systemic illness, including history of opportunistic infection by the presence of constitutional symptoms. It requires validation in future prospective clinical trials.

Treatment

Since most patients do not die as a direct result of KS, it would seem unlikely that therapy directed toward this neoplasm would have a significant impact on survival. Although the data are retrospective, a review of 194 cases of KS by Volberding, Kusick, and Feigal[131] suggests that this is, in fact, the case. There was no significant difference in median survival time between the group of patients treated with chemotherapy (or alpha interferon) and those who received no treatment.

Some patients with KS do require treatment. Subgroups of patients must be defined in terms of whom treatment will benefit most. The primary goals of therapy for patients with KS are palliation of symptoms and cosmesis. Achievement of good cosmetic results may not only improve appearance but significantly improve the patient's overall outlook.

Palliative therapy may be indicated in the following situations:

1. Painful or uncomfortable intraoral or pharyngeal lesions can interfere with eating or swallowing. Bulky KS can even result in airway compromise.

2. Lymphedema is a common complication of advanced KS. Because of its propensity for infiltrating lymphatics, obstruction and edema formation can occur relatively early. The face and the lower extremities are the sites most commonly affected. Lower-extremity edema can form as a result of bulky lymphadenopathy in the femoral, inguinal, or iliac regions; in the setting of confluent bulky cutaneous lesions; or even in the absence of bulky visible KS.

3. Painful or bulky lesions can occur at any site. Lesions involving the plantar surfaces of the feet may be particularly uncomfortable during ambulation.

4. Pulmonary KS is frequently symptomatic and can result in a variety of respiratory symptoms, which are becoming a more frequent complication of KS as patients survive for longer periods of time with the disease. Disease progression can be rapid, resulting in severe respiratory compromise and death.[35,60]

Another indication for therapy is rapidly progressive disease. Although it is impossible to prove benefit in the absence of a randomized trial, it is likely that without treatment, such patients will rapidly develop either symptomatic disease requiring palliative therapy or cosmetically problematic disease.

Treatment options include a variety of local and systemic therapies (Table 25–4). Systemic chemotherapy can result in subjective toxicities, myelosuppression, and immunosuppression, leaving the patient more susceptible to a variety of opportunistic infections. Thus the use of systemic chemotherapy should be approached cautiously. Local forms of therapy should be selected whenever possible.

**Table 25–4. Therapeutic Options for
Kaposi's Sarcoma**

Local Therapy	Systemic Therapy
Radiation	Chemotherapy
Cryotherapy	Interferon-α
Intralesional chemotherapy	
Laser surgery	

Local Therapy

Radiotherapy. Radiotherapy has been the most frequently used local therapeutic modality. A single dose of 800 cGy or the equivalent fractionated dose can be highly effective in achieving local palliation.[11,52]

Radiotherapy is not appropriate for the patient with widespread symptomatic disease but is best suited for the patient with a single or a few locally symptomatic areas. It is highly effective in relieving facial edema and can be applied to a field encompassing the whole face. It has also been frequently used, although less effectively, in the treatment of lower-extremity edema.[52] In addition, larger facial lesions, painful lesions, or other unsightly cutaneous lesions can be treated with radiotherapy. Intraoral and pharyngeal lesions are frequently treated with radiotherapy. However, a high frequency of severe mucositis occurrence has been observed in these patients.[52] As a result, laser surgery has been used more recently for treatment of some intraoral lesions at our institution.

Intralesional Chemotherapy. Small cutaneous lesions can be treated with intralesional chemotherapy for cosmetic purposes.[94] This is generally accomplished by intralesional injection of 0.01 mg of vinblastine in 0.1 ml sterile water using a tuberculin syringe. Repeated treatments may be necessary. A hyperpigmented area frequently remains after treatment.

Cryotherapy. Cryotherapy using liquid nitrogen has been successfully used for the treatment of isolated small KS lesions.[123] This treatment modality is particularly useful for the treatment of cosmetically unsightly lesions on the face.

Systemic Therapy

For the patient with more rapidly progressive disease or with advanced, widespread symptomatic disease, systemic therapy may be most appropriate. Several antineoplastic agents used alone or in combination are active against KS (Table 25–5).

Vincristine[85] and Vinblastine.[130] Vincristine and vinblastine have been used commonly for systemic therapy in patients with HIV-associated KS because each is subjectively well tolerated and the incidence of serious toxicity is low. However, when administered on a weekly basis, vinblastine can cause significant myelosuppression, necessitating dose reduction, and vincristine can cause significant peripheral neuropathy. The cumulative toxicities of each of these drugs can be reduced by administering each drug on an alternate-week basis.[57]

Etoposide (VP16). Etoposide is also an active agent in treating KS.[74] The frequent occurrence of alopecia in patients treated with etoposide makes it a poor choice for patients being treated primarily for cosmetic purposes. However, the more recent availability of an oral formulation of etoposide makes this an attractive agent for systemic therapy in other situations. When administered orally, etoposide is 50% bioavailable; therefore an appropriate oral dose is generally twice the standard IV dose. The use of daily administration of low-dose oral etoposide is currently under study.

Doxorubicin (Adriamycin). Doxorubicin may be the most active single agent against HIV-associated KS[36] and may be useful in the management of patients with more advanced disease or in those in whom prior therapy has failed to produce a

Table 25–5.   Chemotherapy in AIDS—Kaposi's Sarcoma

AGENTS	DOSE	REPORTED RESPONSE (%)	REFERENCE
Vincristine	2 mg/wk	20-59	85
Vinblastine	0.05-0.1 mg/kg/wk	25-30	130
Etoposide	150 mg/m² IV q.d. for 3 days every 3-4 wk or 50 mg P.O. q.d.	75	74
Doxorubicin (Adriamycin)	20 mg/m² every other week	53	36
Bleomycin	10-15 U/m² every 2 wk		
Combination Chemotherapy			
Vincristine *plus*	2 mg		
Vinblastine	0.1 mg/kg (alternate weeks)	45	57
Vincristine *plus*	2 mg		
Bleomycin	10 mg/m² (every 14 days)	100*	35
Doxorubicin *plus*	10-20 mg/m²		
Bleomycin *plus*	10 mg/m²		
Vincristine	2 mg (every 14 days)	87	36

*Results reported only for patients with pulmonary KS, N = 3.

response. A randomized trial has suggested that the combination regimen of doxorubicin, bleomycin, and vincristine (ABV) is more efficacious against KS than doxorubicin used as a single agent.[36] This regimen has been used successfully in patients with widespread, advanced KS, including those with peripheral edema and pulmonary involvement.[35] It is not unusual to see rapid improvement in peripheral edema or in respiratory symptoms after administration of this combination. The major short-term toxicity associated with doxorubicin is myelosuppression, which may require periodic dose reductions or the use of a myeloid growth factor.

The combination of vincristine and bleomycin has significant antitumor activity and may be especially useful for those patients with granulocytopenia, who are likely to be intolerant of more myelosuppressive regimens.[35,38,85]

The recent availability of the myeloid growth factors granulocyte colony-stimulating factors (G-CSF) and granulocyte-macrophage colony-stimulating factors (GM-CSF) may make administration of myelosuppressive chemotherapy easier in some individuals with KS. In patients who are severely symptomatic, particularly from pulmonary KS, with respiratory symptoms for which doxorubicin is believed strongly indicated but for whom a severely compromised hematologic reserve is a problem may be administered the three-drug (doxorubicin, bleomycin, vincristine) regimen, with growth factor support beginning on the day after chemotherapy administration.

Recently the use of liposome-encapsulated daunorubicin has been reported as showing promising results in a small pilot study.[117] Several ongoing trials currently are studying the use of liposome-encapsulated preparations of both daunorubicin and doxorubicin.

Interferon.   Alpha interferon is an attractive agent for use in the treatment of AIDS-associated KS because it possesses both antiproliferative[69] and apparent anti-HIV activity.[67,73] Alpha interferon used as a single agent in the treatment of HIV-associated KS has significant antitumor activity as demonstrated in a large number of clinical trials.[18,41,69,107,110,132,133] The importance of dose intensity in the administration of alphainterferon is demonstrated in Table 25–6. These data, compiled from several institutions,[41,110,107,133] demonstrate that high doses (>20 million units/ m²) of alpha interferon are more effective in inducing antitumor responses than are lower doses. Several studies have demonstrated that patients with better immune function (higher CD4 cell counts), without a prior history of opportunistic infection and without "B" symptoms, are more likely to respond to alpha interferon than those whose cellular immune function is more compromised and who have had a prior opportunistic infection and are symptomatic.[69,128]

Despite the frequency of objective responses and reports of long disease-free remissions, the use of alpha interferon in high doses as a single agent has been limited by its toxicity. With chronic administration, many patients experience a "flulike" syndrome, with low-grade fever, anorexia, malaise, myalgias, and weight loss. Although many patients develop tachyphylaxis to these symptoms during the first several weeks of treatment, these symptoms may persist and become sufficiently disabling to warrant either dosage reduction or discontinuation of the agent.

Most patients who go on to have significant antitumor response usually show evidence of tumor regression after 4 to 8 weeks of high-dose treatment. Often 6 or more months of therapy are required to achieve maximum tumor regression. Since tumor recurrence is usual after discontinuation of treatment, it is suggested that alpha interferon therapy be maintained for as long as the antitumor response persists.

Interferon-α and Zidovudine Combinations

The use of combinations of interferon-α and zidovudine has been investigated in several phase 1 trials, and continuing investigation in large clinical trials is currently underway. From the standpoint of antiretroviral therapy the combination of alpha interferon with zidovudine is an attractive one, for each of these agents

Table 25–6.   Interferon-α in AIDS-Related Kaposi's Sarcoma: Efficacy of Low-Dose Versus High-Dose Therapy

RESPONSE	LOW-DOSE <20 MILLION U/m²	HIGH-DOSE ≥20 MILLION U/m²
	N = 65	N = 105
Complete	1 (2%)	18 (17%)
Partial	3 (5%)	27 (26%)
Minor or stable	13 (20%)	17 (16%)
Progression	48 (74%)	43 (41%)

Data compiled from published studies at San Francisco General Hospital, the University of California at Los Angeles, Memorial Sloan-Kettering Cancer Center, the M.D. Anderson Hospital and Tumor Institute, and the National Cancer Institute. See text for references.

**Table 25–7.   Trials of Interferon-α with Zidovudine
for Kaposi's Sarcoma**

ALPHA INTERFERON	ALPHA INTERFERON DOSES OR RANGE	ZIDOVUDINE DOSES (mg q4h)	COMPLETE OR PARTIAL RESPONSE TOTAL (%)	REFERENCE
α-2A or α-nl	4, 5, 9, 18 million	100 or 200	17/37 (46)	70
α-2 or α-nl	9, 18, 27 million	100 or 200	20/43 (47)	23
α-nl	<5->25	50, 100, or 250	11/26 (42)	66
TOTAL			48/108 (45)	

appears to inhibit HIV-1 replication at a different stage of the viral life-cycle, and the combination has shown synergistic in vitro inhibition of HIV-1 replication.[49] Although zidovudine has failed to show any significant antitumor activity in patients with KS when used as a single agent,[72] the use of this agent is associated with improvement in immune function, a factor clearly associated with responsiveness of KS to interferon-α. Furthermore, the use of interferon-α is not associated with the decline in immune function normally associated with the use of standard cytotoxic chemotherapeutic agents.

The results of three clinical trials investigating the use of combination interferon-α with zidovudine are shown in Table 25–7. It appears that daily 600-mg doses of zidovudine can be safely combined with interferon-α doses of 4 to 18 million units daily. The most common dose-limiting toxicity has been neutropenia. Response rates of over 40% have been observed in all these trials and apparently are better at all levels of immune function when the results of treatment with these two agents are compared with historical data for the use of single-agent interferon-α. These response rates are particularly striking in view of the fact that interferon-α doses used in these trials were significantly lower than those known to have single-agent antitumor activity. The ability to use these lower doses of interferon-α may significantly reduce the incidence of subjective toxicities that frequently are dose limiting in patients treated with high-dose single-agent interferon-α.

Antiretroviral Agents

Zidovudine (ZDV) and Didanosine (Dideoxyinosine, ddI).   Zidovudine and didanosine are the only currently available antiviral agents with proven benefit in patients with HIV infection. Because of the possible occurrence of granulocytopenia in patients treated with zidovudine, the concurrent administration of potentially myelosuppressive chemotherapeutic agents is not recommended at this time. Although ddI is nonmyelosuppressive, there may be an increased risk of peripheral neuropathy when it is combined with vincristine; thus this combination should also be used with caution. However, because of demonstrated efficacy in a variety of stages of HIV infection, zidovudine or didanosine may benefit patients with limited and relatively stable KS who are not candidates for systemic therapy. Zidovudine may be safely administered along with radiotherapy or nonmyelosup-

Table 25–8. Kaposi's Sarcoma: Recommendations for Treatment

Minimal disease	
Stable or slowly progressive	1. Observation only
	2. Investigational agents
	3. Zidovudine with or without alpha interferon
Rapidly progressive	1. Vincristine and vinblastine
	2. Alpha interferon with or without zidovudine
Widespread symptomatic	1. Doxorubicin (Adriamycin)
	2. Adriamycin, bleomycin, vincristine (ABV)
Locally symptomatic	1. Radiotherapy
	2. Laser (oral lesions)
Local cosmesis	1. Intralesional chemotherapy
	2. Radiotherapy
	3. Cryotherapy
Cytopenic patients	1. Vincristine and/or
	2. Bleomycin

presive chemotherapeutic agents such as vincristine, provided that frequent hematologic evaluation is performed.

Therapeutic Recommendations

Table 25–8 summarizes the recommendations for treatment of patients with AIDS-associated KS. Patients with minimal disease (<25 cutaneous lesions), unless cosmetically unsightly or in pain, are generally not candidates for KS-directed therapy. They may benefit from zidovudine, ddI, or other antiretroviral therapy or from participation in clinical trials of investigational agents. Systemic therapy is recommended for patients with asymptomatic but rapidly progressive disease or for patients with widespread symptomatic disease.

The doxorubicin-containing regimens generally should be reserved for patients with more advanced disease or patients with previously unsuccessful therapy. Vincristine with or without bleomycin may benefit those patients with cytopenias. Alternatively, myeloid growth factors may be used to reduce myelotoxicity. Localized therapy, generally radiation, can palliate locally symptomatic disease. Local cosmetic problems can be treated successfully with radiotherapy, intralesional chemotherapy, or cryotherapy. Alpha interferon as a single agent is best reserved for those individuals with CD4 lymphocyte counts >200/mm^3, but for most patients the high doses required will prove too toxic. The use of low doses of alpha interferon with zidovudine may make this a much more tolerable treatment approach to the patient with systemic KS.

NON-HODGKIN'S LYMPHOMA

The non-Hodgkin's lymphomas (NHLs) are a heterogenous group of malignancies. Their biologic behavior ranges from indolent, requiring no therapy, to aggressive malignancies with few long-term survivors. Approximately 70% of NHL originate in B cells, and another 20% derive from T cells.

In the most commonly used classification system for the NHLs,[93] these malignancies are divided into three major categories: low grade, intermediate grade, and high grade, according to pathologic characteristics of involved lymph nodes and morphologic criteria of the lymphoma cells.

The first cases of NHL in homosexual men were reported in 1982,[135] and increasing numbers of cases have been reported since that time. The finding of an intermediate or high-grade B-cell NHL in an HIV-infected individual constitutes an AIDS diagnosis as defined by the CDC.[9] Advanced extranodal disease is commonly found at presentation, and median survival times have been short.

Epidemiology

The incidence of NHL has increased markedly in individuals with impaired cell-mediated immunity.[29,54] The best described of these groups is immunosuppressed allograft recipients, a group in which the incidence of NHL is 30 to 50 times that of the general population.[54,99,100] Similarly, Harnly et al.[48] have demonstrated a statistically significant increase in the incidence of NHL among never-married men ages 25 to 44 years in San Francisco between the years 1980 to 1985. The increase in census tracks with a high incidence of AIDS was greater than the increase in other San Francisco census tracts. In 1985 the incidence of NHL was five times greater than the rate in 1980. However, increases in incidence rates were not observed for other malignancies. Similar trends have been observed for New York City.[68]

Despite suggestions that the incidence of NHL in HIV-infected individuals receiving long-term antiretroviral therapy may be as high as 46% at 36 months, in a small group of patients with HIV disease data as yet do not indicate a rise in incidence out of proportion to the rising incidence of new AIDS diagnoses.[104] There are indications, however, that as treatment for the underlying HIV disease becomes more successful and as patients survive for longer periods of time in the absence of opportunistic infections, more cases of lymphoma will appear in this patient population. It has been estimated that by 1992 HIV-associated NHL will account for 8% to 27% of all NHL diagnosed in the U.S.[30] A recent large prospective observational study indicates an incidence of approximately 1.6% per year that is constant over time in a population with advanced HIV infection treated with zidovudine.[89] Undoubtedly, the most reliable information about the incidence of NHL in the setting of HIV infection comes from a Danish study in which all cases of HIV-associated NHL in the country, including both primary and secondary diagnoses, were reported to a central registry.[44] These data indicate a total of 27 cases of NHL diagnosed in 356 cases of AIDS (8%) through December of 1988.

Pathogenesis

The etiology of NHL in patients with HIV infection is not known. In immunosuppressed allograft recipients molecular data have implicated Epstein-Barr virus (EBV) as a potential causative agent in the development of NHL. Several studies have documented the presence of EBV-DNA sequences in the vast majority of B-cell lymphomas from transplant recipients.[46,99,118] The majority of lymphomas described in this population has been classified as immunoblastic lymphomas. However, in this patient population aggressive lymphoproliferative processes have also been described that apparently are polyclonal by both immunologic and morphologic criteria.[28,46,47] In some of these cases a typical monoclonal lymphoma has subsequently developed.[45]

Although the finding of chromosome t (8;14) translocations, like those seen with Burkitt's lymphoma, and the finding of EBV nuclear antigen in some tumors[4,10,40,102] suggested that EBV might also be implicated in the etiology of HIV-associated lymphomas, more recent observations indicate that EBV-DNA sequences are present in a minority of patients with HIV-associated lymphoma.[59,82,119,122] However, there is also information suggesting that EBV-DNA sequences may be present in a majority of primary central nervous system (CNS) lymphomas in patients with HIV infection.[80,82] In addition, evaluation of immunoglobulin gene rearrangements using Southern blot hybridization techniques demonstrates that, although many of the B-cell tumors observed in this patient population have clonal immunoglobulin gene rearrangements, clonal rearrangements are not observed in other lymphomas.[82,119] These tumors may represent "polyclonal" processes not unlike those observed in allograft recipients.[47] This heterogeneity of molecular characteristics, including the clonality and the presence or absence of EBV, suggests that lymphomagenesis may occur through several different mechanisms. Although EBV may be involved in the pathogenesis of some HIV-associated lymphomas, other viruses, spontaneous genetic changes, cytokines, or even the underlying immune disregulation itself may give rise to NHL.

Clinical Characteristics

Like the molecular features of the lymphomas themselves, the individuals presenting with HIV-associated NHL are also a heterogeneous group. Individuals with HIV-associated NHL are not all severely immunocompromised. Patients seen at San Francisco General Hospital with peripheral (as opposed to primary CNS) NHL have exhibited a wide-range of CD4 lymphocyte counts, with a mean value of $200/mm^3$ (N = 95). Over one third of these individuals had CD4 lymphocyte counts $>200/mm^3$. NHL was the initial AIDS-defining diagnosis in 70%. Patients with primary CNS lymphoma represent a very different patient population. These individuals are almost universally severely immunocompromised with CD4 lymphomcyte counts $<50/mm^3$.[77]

The vast majority of the NHLs observed in patients with HIV infection are classified as B-cell malignancies.[76,134] A small number of NHLs of other histologic and immunologic subtypes have been observed, including T-cell lymphoma[59,92,105] and others of uncertain lineage.[65] Of 327 cases reported in the literature from five centers, 73% of the lymphomas were classified as high grade, 24% as intermediate grade, and 3% as low grade.[3,34,59,64,79,134] Most B-cell lymphomas in these individuals are classified as diffuse large-cell tumors of either intermediate-grade type or the high-grade immunoblastic type (Color Plate II *G*). In addition, approximately one third of patients present with tumors of the high-grade, small, noncleaved cell variety (Color Plate II *H*).

Widespread disease involving extranodal sites is the hallmark of AIDS-associated lymphoma at the time of diagnosis. Ziegler et al.[134] reported that 95% of patients had evidence of extranodal disease; 42% of patients had CNS disease; and 33% had bone marrow involvement. In a series of 89 patients diagnosed at New York University, 87% had extranodal disease at presentation.[64] The most common sites of disease included the GI tract, CNS, bone marrow, and liver. At San Francisco General Hospital two thirds of the patients had stage IV disease, and 31% had extranodal disease alone, with no identifiable site of nodal disease.

As observed in other immunosuppressed patients with NHL, unusual extralymphatic presentations are common. Sites of disease have included the rectum,[6] heart and pericardium,[1,43] and common bile ducts.[56] GI involvement has been reported in up to 27% of individuals with lymphoma,[27] and virtually any site in the GI tract or hepatobiliary tree can be involved. In the San Francisco General Hospital series other unusual sites of disease included subcutaneous and soft tissue, epidural space, appendix, gingiva, parotid gland, and paranasal sinus.[59]

NHL confined to the CNS frequently has been reported in association with HIV infection.[2,24,37,121] The most common presenting symptoms have been confusion, lethargy, and memory loss. Other symptoms have included hemiparesis, aphasia, seizures, cranial nerve palsies, and headache. Single or multiple discreet lesions are the most common findings on computed tomographic (CT) or magnetic resonance imaging (MRI) scans of the brain. The lesions are frequently hypodense and contrast enhancing. Both clinical presentation and CT or MRI scan findings are frequently indistinguishable from those associated with toxoplasmosis.

Given the similarity in clinical presentation and radiographic findings to other CNS disorders, the diagnosis of primary CNS lymphoma can be difficult to make. Patients presenting with neurologic symptoms should be evaluated promptly with CT or MRI scans of the brain. Lumbar puncture should be performed if not contraindicated by the CT findings. A serum specimen from patients with focal lesions should be sent for cryptococcal antigen and toxoplasma titers. Since toxoplasmosis is rare in individuals with negative toxoplasma serologies,[39] brain biopsy should be performed in a timely fashion in this group of patients. Individuals with focal intracerebral lesions and positive serologic studies for toxoplasma are typically started on antitoxoplasma therapy and observed closely for signs of improvement or deterioration.

Treatment and Prognosis

The use of multiagent chemotherapeutic regimens for the treatment of intermediate and high-grade NHL in the non-HIV-infected individual has resulted in a dramatic improvement in prognosis for this group.[17] A complete response rate as high as 86% and long-term survival rates as high as 65% have been reported in patients treated for aggressive, large cell lymphomas.[12]

In HIV-infected individuals, however, the use of similar chemotherapeutic regimens has not resulted in as favorable an outcome (Table 25–9). Complete response rates are lower than the corresponding rates in the non–HIV-infected population, and these responses are usually of short duration. In a retrospective review by Ziegler et al.[134] of patients treated at multiple institutions, 53% of 66 patients who could be evaluated achieved complete response to combination chemotherapy; however, 54% of the complete responders subsequently relapsed. In a series of patients

Table 25–9. Response to Chemotherapy and Survival Times in HIV-Associated Non-Hodgkin's Lymphoma

INSTITUTION	NO.	TREATMENT REGIMEN	COMPLETE RESPONSE (%)	MEDIAN SURVIVAL TIME (MO)	REFERENCE
USC	22	m-BACOD and others	45	NA	34
NYU	83	Various	33	5.0	64
UCSF	65	Various	54	5.5	59
MSKCC	30	Various	56	6.0	79
Pacific Medical Center	31	CHOP and MACOP-B	39	7.0	3
MultiCenter	66	Various	53	NA	134
ACTG	36	m-BACOD	42	NA	78
Italian Cooperative Group	72	Various	35	4.0	55

NA, not applicable; USC, University of California; NYU, New York University; UCSF, University of California, San Francisco; MSKCC, Memorial Sloan-Kettering Cancer Institute; ACTG, AIDS Clinical Trial Group, National Institutes of Health; Multicenter: UCSF, USC, NY Hospital/Cornell, University of Texas/M.D. Anderson, NYU/Kaplan Cancer Center, and MSKCC; m-BACOD, methotrexate, bleomycin, doxorubicin, cyclophosphamide, vincristine, and dexamethasone; CHOP, cyclophosphamide, doxorubicin, vincristine, and prednisone; MACOP-B, methotrexate, doxorubicin, cyclophosphamide, vincristine, prednisone, and bleomycin.

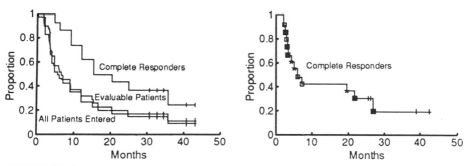

FIGURE 25–2. *Left,* Overall survival in patients with AIDS-related lymphoma. Tick marks indicate patients who are alive at the given time interval. *Right,* Event-free survival in 16 complete responders. Tick marks indicate patients who are still alive in continuous complete remission; dark boxes, development of intercurrent HIV-related illness; open boxes, development of relapse of lymphoma; asterisks, death from unknown cause. Event-free survival is taken from the time of achievement of complete remission to the time of relapse, HIV-related illness, or death. (From Levine AM, Wernz JC, Kaplan L, et al: Low-dose chemotherapy with central nervous system prophylaxis and zidovudine maintenance in AIDS-related lymphoma. JAMA 266:84–88, 1991. Copyright 1991 American Medical Association.)

from San Francisco General Hospital 54% of 59 patients who could be evaluated and who were treated with a variety of combinations of chemotherapeutic regimens had complete responses.[59] Twenty-three percent of these complete responders subsequently relapsed (Figure 25–2).

Morphologic subtype appeared to predict response to chemotherapy in one series of patients reported from New York University.[64] The best complete response rate was reported for those patients classified as having a large, noncleaved cell lymphoma (52%), whereas those having a small, noncleaved cell and immunoblastic lymphoma had response rates of 26% and 21%, respectively. One group has reported a 64% complete response rate in a series of 11 patients treated with the methotrexate, doxorubicin, cyclophosphamide, vincristine, prednisone, bleomycin (MACOP-B) regimen.[3] However, it cannot be determined from this small number of patients whether this represents significant improvement in the complete response rate over that observed in other series of patients.

Survival times from a number of large series of patients reported in the literature are shown in Table 25–9. Median survival times in these groups range from 4 to 7 months. In the series of 23 patients who received chemotherapy at the Pacific Medical Center, the median survival time was 20 months in those patients achieving complete response to therapy.[3]

Although overall survival times in patients with AIDS-associated NHL are disappointing, subgroups of patients can be identified in which the therapeutic outcome is significantly better than for other groups of patients. Morphologic subtypes predictive of response to therapy in patients treated at New York University were also predictive of survival in this same series.[64] Patients with intermediate-grade, large-cell lymphoma had the longest median survival time (7.5 months); those with small, noncleaved cell lymphoma had a median survival time of 5.5 months; and those with immunoblastic lymphoma had a median survival time of only 2 months.

In the San Francisco General Hospital series median survival time for all patients receiving chemotherapy (N = 65) was only 5.5 months. However, life-table analysis for subgroups within this population illustrates the importance of prognostic features (Table 25–10). Those features identified as being predictive of significantly improved survival time included an absolute CD4 + lymphocyte count >100 cells/mm^3, absence of a prior AIDS diagnosis, Karnofsky performance score ≥70%, and the absence of an extranodal site of disease.

Evaluation of newly diagnosed patients for these prognostic features may help determine how to approach therapy in the individual with this disease. The patient without a prior AIDS diagnosis whose immune function is relatively good is a much better candidate for therapy than is a patient whose diagnosis of lymphoma comes after a history of multiple opportunistic infections. Since many patients will fall between these extremes, these prognostic characteristics can only serve as rough guidelines in determining which patients to treat.

Table 25–10. Predictors of Survival in Chemotherapy-Treated HIV-Associated Non-Hodgkin's Lymphoma (n = 65)

CHARACTERISTICS	MEDIAN SURVIVAL TIME	p VALUE
CD4 count		.01
<100/mm^3	4.1	
>100/mm^3	24	
Prior AIDS		.0001
Yes	2.2	
No	8.3	
Karnofsky performance scale		.03
<70%	3.8	
≥70%	6.8	
Extranodal disease		.01
Yes	4.2	
No	12.2	

What the most appropriate therapeutic regimen will be for a given patient also must be individualized, for there is no known "best" regimen. Poor bone marrow reserve and the occurrence of opportunistic infections often result in dose reductions and delays in therapy. In addition, the risk of further immunosuppression when treating HIV-infected patients with aggressive combination chemotherapy must be considered.

Contrary to the belief that more intensive chemotherapy is associated with improved clinical outcome in non–HIV-associated lymphoma, retrospective data from two centers have suggested that in HIV-infected individuals with NHL, survival may be improved in those treated with less aggressive regimens. Survival data from the San Francisco General Hospital cohort of chemotherapy-treated patients with NHL revealed that patients receiving chemotherapy regimens containing ≥ 1 g/m^2 of cyclophosphamide had a median survival time of only 4.6 months compared to those treated with regimens containing <1 g/m^2 of cyclophosphamide who had a median survival time of 12.2 months ($p = .02$).[59] Similarly, in a study of nine patients treated with a novel, more aggressive, chemotherapeutic regimen consisting of high-dose cytosine arabinoside, L-asparaginase, vincristine, prednisone, cyclo-phosphamide (high dose), methotrexate and leucovorin, only three patients achieved complete remission.[34] This intensive regimen was associated with a high risk of mortality caused by opportunistic infection.

Two different approaches to therapy have been studied and recently reported. In the first of these clinical trials patients were treated with a modification of the standard methotrexate, bleomycin, doxorubicin, cyclophosphamide, vincristine, and dexamethasone (m-BACOD) regimen. Instead of administering cyclophospha-mide at 600 mg/m^2 and doxorubicin at 45 mg/m^2, these two agents were admin-istered at 300 mg/m^2 and 25 mg/m^2, respectively. All patients received CNS prophylaxis and zidovudine maintenance after the completion of chemotherapy. Complete remission was observed in 16 of 35 individuals (46%), and the median survival time for the 35 patients who could be evaluated was 6.5 months. These results are not significantly different from those previously reported using a variety of more standard chemotherapeutic regimens; however, these results were achieved at the expense of significantly less hematologic toxicity, with only 10% of che-motherapeutic cycles complicated by an absolute neutrophil count of <500/mm^3. Fifteen cycles (12%) were delayed because of neutropenia. The survival curves shown in Figure 25–2 demonstrate that durable, complete remissions were achieved in some individuals, with a median survival time of 15 months in the 16 complete responders.

In a second approach to therapy more standard doses of cyclophosphamide, doxorubicin, vincristine and prednisone (CHOP) chemotherapy were used in a trial in which patients receiving chemotherapy were randomized either to receive con-current therapy with GM-CSF or no further adjunctive treatment.[61] Table 25–11 demonstrates that individuals receiving GM-CSF had significantly higher mean nadir of absolute neutrophil counts than did those in the control group and those receiving GM-CSF had a significantly shorter duration of life-threatening neutropenia com-pared with those in the control group. As a result, those patients who received GM-CSF spent a mean time of 5.9 days in the hospital for febrile neutropenic episodes through the course of their treatment compared with a mean of 18.6 days in the control group. This small clinical trial was not designed to evaluate response or survival, but it clearly demonstrated that one of the most significant morbidities

Table 25-11. Hematologic Variables in Patients Receiving rGM-CSF vs Control

	TREATMENT GROUP				
	CONTROL (n = 10)		rGM-CSF (n = 11)		
	NO.	(RANGE)	NO.	(RANGE)	p*
Total number of chemotherapy cycles	42		41		
Nadir of absolute neutrophil count (ANC), mean (range)	0.360	(0-1.90)	0.886	(0-4.70)	.009
Days ANC <0.5 × 10^9/L, mean (range)	5.0	(0-26)	1.3	(0-12)	.02
Nadir platelet count,‡ mean (range)	129	(16-302)	106	(13-210)	.1
Peak eosinophil count,‡ mean (range)	0.105	(0-0.60)	1.37	(0-5.70)	.001

From Kaplan LD, Kahn JO, Crowe S, et al: Clinical and virologic effects of recombinant human granulocyte-macrophage colony-stimulating factor in patients receiving chemotherapy for human immunodeficiency virus-associated non-Hodgkin's lymphoma: Results of a randomized trial. J Clin Oncol 9:929-940, 1991.
*Control versus delayed rGM-CSF.
†Control versus early rGM-CSF.
‡Expressed as cells × 10^9/L.

associated with chemotherapy in this patient population can be reduced with the adjunctive use of a myeloid growth factor.

These two different approaches to therapy—low dose versus standard dose—are currently being compared directly in an ongoing randomized trial through the ACTG program. It is hoped that clinical trials like this one will determine which treatment approach is optimal in terms of both reduced toxicity and prolonged survival. It is clear, however, that these more standard approaches probably will not have a major impact on survival. In the presence of the underlying immunodeficiency state, more novel approaches using nonmyelosuppressive and nonimmunosuppressive treatment modalities, either alone or as an adjunct to cytotoxic therapy, are needed. Clinical trials are being initiated that use monoclonal immunotoxins directed toward cell-surface determinants that are unique to HIV-associated NHLs. It is hoped that as we continue to learn more about the biology of the HIV-associated lymphomas, we can develop more rational and effective treatment modalities that take advantage of the unique molecular characteristics of these tumors.

Treatment of Primary Central Nervous System Lymphoma

Primary CNS lymphoma has been particularly difficult to treat. Many cases have been diagnosed at autopsy,[134] and those presenting antemortem often have had advanced immunodeficiency and have suffered multiple previous bouts of opportunistic infections.[2]

In the largest published series of treated patients reported in the literature Baumgartner et al.[2] observed that 76% of 29 patients treated with 4000 cGy of whole brain radiotherapy showed evidence of significant clinical improvement, and 69% demonstrated complete or partial radiographic response. Similar results have been reported in smaller series from other institutions. In a series reported by Formenti et al.[24] complete responses to cranial irradiation occurred in six of the 10 patients. Despite this good response rate, survival times remain short, with median survival time for treated patients reported as between 2 and 5 months.[2,24] In patients with CNS lymphoma opportunistic infection has been the most common cause of death.[2,24] In Formenti's series[24] 50% of the patients died of opportunistic infection, and only two died of recurrent lymphoma. In Baumgartner's series[2] of those patients undergoing postmortem examination, the only patient who died as a result of uncontrolled lymphoma developed a site of disease outside of the radiation portal in the cervical spinal cord.

Since most CNS lymphoma patients have severe immunodeficiency, they are highly susceptible to a variety of opportunistic infections, especially *Pneumocystis carinii* pneumonia. At the present time, there is little justification for more aggressive approaches for treating CNS lymphoma since so few patients actually die of recurrent lymphoma. It is not known, however, whether the adjunctive use of both antiretroviral and antibiotic prophylaxis against opportunistic infection will affect survival rates by reducing the frequency of this common cause of death.

Treatment Recommendations

In selecting therapy for patients with HIV-associated NHL, emphasis should be placed on individualized therapy. Although standard-dose chemotherapy may be appropriate for the patient with good immune function and without a prior opportunistic infection, a lower-dose treatment regimen might be selected for the patient with more severe immunologic compromise, marginal performance score, and a history of opportunistic infection. For some patients who are severely ill, a decision may be made to withhold therapy altogether. These decisions must take into account not only the patient's history and present condition, but also the patient's own desires for a given therapeutic approach. Regardless of the chemotherapeutic approach used, it is strongly recommended that all patients treated with chemotherapy receive adjunctive antibiotic prophylaxis against *P. carinii* pneumonia. Clinical trials investigating the use of less immunosuppressive treatment approaches are currently in progress.

HODGKIN'S DISEASE

As discussed previously, Hodgkin's disease is not an AIDS-defining illness. The precise relationship of this malignancy to the underlying immunodeficiency state is unclear. Hodgkin's disease has rarely been reported in patients with primary immunodeficiency disorders[29] and has not been reported in immunosuppressed transplant recipients.[54] The observation that the frequency of Hodgkin's disease in the single male population aged 20 to 49 years in San Francisco has not increased in the years since 1979 when HIV seroprevalence markedly increased[58,68] argues against a direct causal relationship between HIV-related immunodeficiency and the occurrence of Hodgkin's disease in this population. This is in striking contrast to the earlier sharp rise in the frequency of NHL observed in the same population during the same time period.[48,68]

Clinical observations suggest that Hodgkin's disease in a patient with HIV infection has a different natural history and therapeutic outcome when compared to cases of Hodgkin's disease in the general population. The clinical features and therapeutic outcome in 14 homosexual men with Hodgkin's disease diagnosed at San Francisco General Hospital have been compared with those in a group of 35 single men 20 to 49 years of age diagnosed with Hodgkin's disease between the years 1973 to 1979.[58] Mixed cellularity was the most common histologic pattern among the 14 risk-group patients, whereas nodular sclerosis was significantly more common in the control population. All but one of the risk-group patients presented with advanced (stage III or IV) disease. Bone marrow and liver were the most common sites of extranodal disease.

The outcome of therapy in these patients has been disappointing. Of 12 patients treated at San Francisco General Hospital who could be evaluated, seven were complete responders to either nitrogen mustard, vincristine, procarbazine, and prednisone (MOPP) or MOPP with doxorubicin (Adriamycin), bleomycin, vinblastine, and decarbizine (MOPP-ABVD).[58] Six of these seven complete responders subsequently relapsed. Eight patients (62%) developed *P. carinii* pneumonia during treatment. None of these patients are currently living. One half of the patients died with advanced Hodgkin's disease, and the remaining patients died as a result of opportunistic infections. Median survival time was less than 1 year in this population, compared with 12 years in the control population. There were no differences in either response or survival time between those patients treated with MOPP alone and those treated with MOPP-ABVD.

The mean dose intensity of chemotherapy delivered to our patients was only 41% of the planned therapeutic dose. This was a result of the need for frequent dose reductions and delays in chemotherapy because of poor bone marrow reserve and intercurrent opportunistic infections. The very low-dose intensity of chemotherapy may account for the high relapse rate observed in complete responders.

The Italian cooperative group for AIDS-related tumors more recently reported on 35 cases of Hodgkin's disease occurring in HIV-infected individuals.[55] Eighty-nine percent of these patients were IV drug abusers, 3% were homosexual males, and 9% were IV drug–using homosexual males. Fifty-three percent of the patients presented with mixed-cellularity histologic type, 31% with nodular sclerosis, and 16% with lymphocyte depletion. Seventy-eight percent of patients presented with either stage III or IV disease. Seventeen patients were treated with either MOPP, ABVD, ABV, or MOPP alternating with ABVD. Only eight patients (30%) achieved complete remission. Of 13 patients who died, 7 (54%) died of opportunistic infections, 3 died of progression of Hodgkin's disease, and 2 died of disseminated intravascular coagulation. In one patient the cause of death could not be determined. The median survival time of these patients with Hodgkin's disease was 15 months.

Any illness can be complicated by coexisting HIV infection without a cause-and-effect relationship. Although frequency data from San Francisco do not support the development of Hodgkin's disease as a direct result of HIV infection, those Hodgkin's disease patients who are HIV seropositive are more likely to present with advanced stage and poor prognosis histologic pattern. They are more likely to have a poor therapeutic outcome and to develop AIDS-associated opportunistic infection during therapy. These observations suggest that HIV serologic testing can provide important prognostic information in selected patients with Hodgkin's disease.

As is the case for NHLs in HIV-seropositive patients, experience thus far does not suggest that survival with Hodgkin's disease will be improved with more aggressive chemotherapeutic regimens. Poor bone marrow reserve and the occurrence of opportunistic infections have made it difficult to administer full doses of standard Hodgkin's disease chemotherapy to these patients. Preliminary results of a clinical trial using a relatively nonmyelosuppressive combination chemotherapeutic regimen for patients with Hodgkin's disease in patients with HIV infection were recently reported and were encouraging.[62] This treatment regimen used a combination of bleomycin, vincristine, streptozocin, and etoposide. Of the first five patients treated with this regimen, four of five had complete responses to chemotherapy alone, and a fifth had a complete response following completion of both chemotherapy and radiotherapy. Myelosuppression was not observed, and all patients remain alive and well. Future therapeutic approaches will focus on the use of more standard chemotherapeutic regimens with hematopoietic growth factors. Since a significant proportion of these patients will die as a result of opportunistic infection, prophylaxis against *P. carinii* pneumonia is strongly encouraged during chemotherapy.

HUMAN PAPILLOMAVIRUS INFECTION AND ANOGENITAL NEOPLASIA

Recently published reports suggest that HIV-induced immunodeficiency may also promote the development of neoplasia in the cervical and anal mucosa. Cervical and anal cancers probably will become increasingly common manifestations of HIV disease as patients with profound immunodeficiency who would have succumbed to opportunistic infections earlier in the epidemic survive for extended periods of time because they receive more effective antiretroviral, prophylactic, and antimicrobial therapies. The resulting state of prolonged, severe immunodeficiency provides the necessary milieu for the emergence of diseases that develop after longer latency such as anogenital carcinomas.

HPV Infection, Immunosuppression, and Anogenital Neoplasia

Anogenital neoplasia has a recognized association with chronic immunodeficiency. Studies of cohorts of immunosuppressed organ transplant recipients, for example, have demonstrated a 100-fold increase in incidence of vulvar and anal carcinomas and a fourteenfold increase in the incidence of cervical carcinoma as compared with controls.[98,101]

Considerable evidence links the development of anogenital carcinoma to human papillomavirus (HPV) infection. The so-called "oncogenic" HPV genotypes (HPV-16, HPV-18, and HPV-31) have been detected in 80% to 90% of cervical intraepithelial neoplasia (CIN) grade 3 lesions and invasive cervical cancers.[103] HPV infection has been presumed to play a similar causative role in the development of anal carcinoma as suggested by the presence of HPV DNA and mRNA in tumor tissues from that site.[33] The high incidence of anogenital cancer in immunosuppressed transplant recipients is probably a consequence of the high prevalence of detectable anogenital HPV infection in that population. The prevalence of HPV infection is five to 17 times greater in immunosuppressed transplant recipients than in the general population.[120]

HIV Infection and Cervical Neoplasia

Over the past 5 years, a number of anecdotal reports have appeared about the possible connection between HIV-induced immunodeficiency and cervical neoplasia (see Chapter 28). In one study cytologic preparations of cervicovaginal smears from 35 HIV-infected women and 23 uninfected women were examined by one cytologist who was blinded to the individuals' HIV status.[116] Thirty-one percent of HIV-infected women had cytologic squamous atypia, compared to 4% of HIV-seronegative women ($p = .019$). Twenty-six percent of HIV-infected women had cytologic or histopathologic findings suggestive of genital HPV infection, compared to 4% of HIV-seronegative women ($p = .072$).

Feingold et al.[21] extended these observations by obtaining molecular evidence of HPV infection in the cervicovaginal epithelium of women with HIV infection using Southern blot hybridization. Forty-nine percent of the HIV-infected women studied had HPV infection, compared with 25% of a group of non-HIV-infected women with similar sociodemographic and behavioral characteristics ($p < .05$). Forty percent of the HIV-infected women had squamous intraepithelial lesions on cervical cytology, compared with 9% of the non-infected women ($p < .01$). Women with concurrent HIV and HPV infection were 42 times more likely to have a cytologic abnormality than were women without evidence of either virus. In addition, 50% of women with symptomatic HIV infection (AIDS, persistent generalized lymphadenopathy, oral candidiasis) had a cytologic abnormality, whereas only 23% with asymptomatic HIV infection were cytologically abnormal. These data suggest that more prolonged and/or severe immunosuppression may allow progression of HPV-mediated cytologic abnormalities.

An important report by Maiman et al.[81] described a cohort of HIV-infected women in New York with invasive and preinvasive cervical neoplasia. In comparison to a group of non–HIV-infected women from the same institution, cervical neoplasia in HIV-infected women was more advanced at presentation, was more likely to recur, was associated more commonly with perianal involvement, and was associated more often with cytologic or histologic evidence of HPV infection (97% versus 56%, $p < .01$). The authors concluded that HPV-related neoplasia is having a significant impact in HIV-infected women whom they serve.

Despite the apparent high prevalence of cervical neoplasia in HIV-infected women, only a few cases of invasive cervical cancer have been reported.[81,88,108] However, experience with immunosuppressed transplant recipients suggests that a prolonged period of immunosuppression (mean, 88 months) may be necessary to permit development of anogenital cancer.[98] Most patients with HIV infection die of opportunistic infections much earlier in the course of symptomatic HIV disease and therefore may not survive long enough to develop cervical cancer. Improvements in survival times are being achieved currently through the use of effective antiretroviral, prophylactic, and antimicrobial therapies.[31,75] These successes may permit the emergence of cervical carcinoma among HIV-infected women with a high prevalence of cervical neoplasia.

HIV Infection and Anal Neoplasia

The relationship of HIV infection, HPV infection, and anal neoplasia has also been described. Although an association of anal neoplasia and HPV infection in homosexual men has been recognized for some time,[14,53] it is now apparent that HIV-infected, immunosuppressed men are particularly at risk for the development of HPV-related anal neoplasia.

Several early investigations provided preliminary evidence of the relationship of HIV infection, HPV infection, and anal neoplasia. Two small studies demonstrated HPV in neoplastic anal lesions of homosexual men by histopathologic and/or immunohistochemical techniques.[13,32] One individual in each study had a diagnosis of AIDS at the time that anal neoplasia was found. Frazer et al.[26] examined a larger cohort of homosexual men, using anorectal cytologic smears, HIV antibody testing, and T-lymphocyte phenotyping. They found that HIV seropositivity, lower CD4 + T-lymphocyte counts, and lower CD4 + :CD8 + ratios were significantly associated with more pronounced cytologic atypia.

More recently Palefsky et al.[97] assessed the prevalence of anal HPV infection and precancerous abnormalities of the anal epithelium in 97 severely immunodeficient, HIV-infected homosexual men. Thirty-nine percent of the men had abnormal anal cytology, and 54% had HPV DNA in their anal cytologic specimens. Abnormalities on anal cytologic smear were significantly associated with the presence of HPV DNA (risk ratio, 4.6), and median CD4 + T-lymphocyte counts of men with abnormal cytologic findings were significantly lower than those of men with normal findings ($p = .05$).

Another cohort of 105 homosexual men, including men with and without HIV infection, took part in a similar study conducted by Caussy et al.[8] HPV DNA was found in anal cytologic specimens from 53% of HIV-infected men, compared to 29% of non–HIV-infected men ($p = .012$). Anal neoplasia was also present more frequently in HIV-infected men (24% versus 7%; $p = .03$). Multivariate logistic regression analysis of data from the HIV-infected men showed low CD4 + T-lymphocyte count was an independent risk factor for detection of HPV DNA ($p = .04$). Similar findings have been reported from a study of 120 Danish homosexual men[83] and from a study of 101 homosexual men attending a sexually transmitted diseases clinic in Seattle.[63]

Clinical Implications of HIV-Related Anogenital Neoplasia

The studies cited previously demonstrate that anogenital HPV infection and neoplasia are common in persons with HIV infection. Information on the natural history of these conditions is limited, but it should be presumed that these lesions are precancerous and likely to evolve into invasive cancer over time. Early detection of preinvasive or minimally invasive cancers of the anogenital region can provide the opportunity to cure these diseases, as has been demonstrated by the successful use of Papanicolaou (Pap) smears in screening programs in the general population. It therefore seems reasonable that some patients with HIV infection, particularly those with relatively better prognosis (higher CD4 + T-lymphocyte count, no prior

Table 25–12. Proposed Guidelines for Management of HIV-Associated Anogenital Neoplasia

Screening for Cervical Neoplasia
All HIV-infected women
Annual Papanicolaou (Pap) smear of cervix
Consider baseline colposcopy
HIV-infected women at high risk for HPV infection*
Pap smear every 6 months
Careful inspection of vulvar, vaginal, and anal epithelium
Treatment for Cervical Neoplasia
Refer to a gynecologist for standard treatment
Screening for Anal Neoplasia
HIV-infected men with history of anal intercourse
Anal Pap smear†
Anoscopy on a routine basis
Biopsy of any abnormality identified on anoscopy
Frequent anoscopic follow-up if abnormalities were identified previously
Treatment for Anal Neoplasia
Anal intraepithelial neoplasia
Electrocautery or cryotherapy
Invasive Cancer
Surgical excision and/or radiotherapy

*Those with a history of multiple sexual partners or sexual partners with HIV infection.
† Studies evaluating the use of anal Pap smears currently are underway.

opportunistic infections or malignancies) would benefit from early detection and treatment of anogenital neoplasia. Dr. Joel Palefsky of the University of California, San Francisco,[96] has proposed guidelines (Table 25–12) for management of cervical and anal neoplasia in HIV-infected persons.

A study is currently underway in which a large population of HIV-infected men will be examined with anal Pap smears and biopsies to validate the use of the Pap smear as a screening tool in this setting (J. Palefsky, personal communication). Recommendations about the widespread use of the anal Pap smear for population screening must await the results of this or similar studies.

Cervical cancer and anal cancer are likely to become more common problems in patients with HIV-induced immunodeficiency as the epidemic progresses. Observations about the development of malignancies in other states of immunosuppression suggest that these cancers will become more frequent as therapeutic interventions prolong survival. Strategies for prevention, detection, and treatment of HIV-associated anogenital malignancies will be needed.

SUMMARY

Patients with HIV infection, like immunosuppressed transplant recipients, are at high risk for the development of both Kaposi's sarcoma (KS) and B-cell non-

Hodgkin's lymphoma. Although other malignancies may occur in the HIV-infected patient, epidemiologic evidence does not suggest a causal relationship between the underlying immunodeficiency state and the subsequent development of malignancy. Whether causally related or not, however, any malignancy occurring in a patient with HIV infection is likely to have a more aggressive course and to be associated with short survival time.

KS is the most common malignancy seen in HIV-infected patients. The etiology of KS is uncertain, as are the reasons for its nearly exclusive confinement to the homosexual male population with HIV infection. Prognosis is related to the extent of the disease, immune function, and the presence of systemic and local symptoms. A variety of local and systemic therapeutic modalities are available, including radiotherapy, cryotherapy, chemotherapy, and interferon-α. Which treatment approach is most appropriate for an individual depends on the extent of disease, the presence of local symptoms, including pain or edema, or the presence of cosmetically unsightly disease. Early studies suggest that the concurrent use of interferon-α and zidovudine may make the use of lower doses of interferon-α possible. The concurrent use of zidovudine with other chemotherapeutic regimens currently is being explored.

Patients with B-cell lymphoma tend to present with advanced extranodal disease, and primary lymphoma of the CNS frequently has been reported as well. Not unlike B-cell lymphoma seen in allograft recipients, lymphoma in the presence of HIV infection appears to arise out of background of polyclonal B-cell activation. Although a viral cause has been suspected, the cause of lymphoma in these patients remains unknown. Response to therapy in these patients has been disappointing. Response rates to chemotherapy have been lower than those observed in other lymphoma patients, and treatment has been complicated by lack of adequate bone marrow reserve and by occurrence of frequent opportunistic infections. Although overall survival times have been short, factors predictive of improved survival time include better immune function, absence of a prior AIDS diagnosis, good performance score, and absence of an extranodal site of disease. Experience suggests that in some patients more aggressive chemotherapy may be associated with shortened survival time. Recent clinical trials have demonstrated that either the use of reduced dosage chemotherapeutic regimens or the use of myeloid growth factors can reduce the morbidity associated with chemotherapy for this disease. Determining which of these treatment approaches will be of the greatest benefit with respect to response and survival time must await the results of ongoing clinical trials.

Cervical and anal neoplasia related to HPV infection can also occur as a consequence of HIV-induced immunodeficiency. Longstanding, profound immunodeficiency increases the risk of developing HPV-related anogenital neoplasia, as has been described in transplant recipients requiring prolonged immunosuppression. As the survival time of patients with HIV infection is extended through the use of more effective antiretroviral, prophylactic, and antimicrobial therapies, the resulting state of profound, prolonged immunodeficiency will provide the necessary milieu for the emergence of anogenital neoplasia.

Treatment of the patient with an HIV-associated malignancy imposes obstacles and challenges that are unique in medicine. For this reason it is especially important that treatment be individualized carefully, with the patient playing an important role in determining which therapeutic alternative is most appropriate.

REFERENCES

1. Balasubramanyam A, Waxman M, Kazal HL, Lee MH: Malignant lymphoma of the heart in acquired immunodeficiency syndrome. Chest 90:243-246, 1986
2. Baumgartner J, Rachlin J, Beckstead J, et al: Primary central nervous system lymphomas: Natural history and response to radiation therapy in 55 patients with acquired immunodeficiency syndrome. J Neurosurg 73:206-211, 1990
3. Bermudez M, Grant K, Rodvien R, Mendes F: Non-Hodgkin's lymphoma in a population with or at risk for acquired immunodeficiency syndrome: Indications for intensive chemotherapy. Am J Med 86:71-76, 1989
4. Bernheim A, Berger R: Cytogenetic studies of Burkitt lymphoma-leukemia in patients with acquired immunodeficiency syndrome. Cancer Genet Cytogenet 32:67-74, 1988
5. Brooks JJ: Kaposi's sarcoma: A reversible hyperplasia. Lancet 2:1309-1311, 1986
6. Burkes RL, Meyer PR, Gill PS, et al: Rectal lymphoma in homosexual men. Arch Intern Med 146:913-915, 1986
7. Cappell MS, Yao F, Cho KC: Colonic adenocarcinoma associated with the acquired immunodeficiency syndrome. Cancer 62:616-619, 1988
8. Caussy D, Goedert JJ, Palefsky J, et al: Interaction of human immunodeficiency and papilloma viruses: Association with anal intraepithelial abnormality in homosexual men. Int J Cancer 46:214-219, 1990
9. Centers for Disease Control: Revision of the case definition of acquired immunodeficiency syndrome for national reporting—United States. MMWR 4:373-374, 1985
10. Chaganti R, Jhanwar S, Koziner B, et al: Specific translocations characterize Burkitt's-like lymphoma of homosexual men with the acquired immunodeficiency syndrome. Blood 61:1269-1272, 1983
11. Chak LY, Gill PS, Levine AM, et al: Radiation therapy for AIDS-related Kaposi's sarcoma. J Clin Oncol 6:863-867, 1988
12. Connors JM, Klimo P: MACOP-B chemotherapy for malignant lymphomas and related conditions: 1987 Update and additional observations. Semin Hematol 25(suppl 2):41-46, 1988
13. Croxson T, Chabon AB, Rorat E, Barash IM: Intraepithelial carcinoma of the anus in homosexual men. Dis Colon Rectum 27:325-330, 1984
14. Daling JR, Weiss NS, Hislop TG, et al: Sexual practices, sexually transmitted diseases, and the incidence of anal cancer. N Engl J Med 317:973-977, 1987
15. Daling JR, Weiss NS, Klopfenstein LL, et al: Correlates of homosexual behavior and the incidence of anal cancer. JAMA 247:1988-1990, 1982
16. Des Jarlais DC, Stoneburner R, Thomas P: Declines in proportion of Kaposi's sarcoma among cases of AIDS in multiple risk groups in New York City. Lancet 2:1024-1025, 1987
17. DeVita VT, Hubbard SM, Young RC, Longo DL: The role of chemotherapy in diffuse aggressive lymphomas. Semin Hematol 25(suppl 2):2-10, 1988
18. deWit R, Schatenkerk JKME, Boucher CAB, et al: Clinical and virological effects of high-dose recombinant interferon-α in disseminated AIDS-related Kaposi's sarcoma. Lancet 2:1214-1217, 1988
19. Drew WL, Mills J, Hauer LB, et al: Declining prevalence of Kaposi's sarcoma in homosexual AIDS patients paralleled by fall in cytomegalovirus transmission. Lancet 1:66, 1988
20. Ensoli B, Nakamura S, Salahuddin SZ, et al: AIDS-Kaposi's sarcoma-derived cells express cytokines with autocrine and paracrine growth factors. Science 243:223-226, 1989
21. Feingold AR, Vermund SH, Burk RD, et al: Cervical cytologic abnormalities and papillomavirus in women infected with human immunodeficiency virus. J Acquir Immune Defic Syndr 3:896-903, 1990
22. Fischl MA, Richman DD, Greico MH, et al: The efficacy of azidothymidine (AZT) in the treatment of patients with AIDS and AIDS-related complex. A double-blind, placebo-controlled trial. N Engl J Med 317:185-191, 1987
23. Fischl MA, Uttamchandani R, Resnick L, et al: A phase I study of recombinant human interferon alfa-2 or human lymphoblastoid interferon alfa-n1 and concomitant zidovudine in patients with AIDS-related Kaposi's sarcoma. J Acquir Immune Defic Syndr 4:4-10, 1991
24. Formenti SC, Gill PS, Rarick M, et al: Primary central nervous system lymphoma in AIDS: Results of radiation therapy. Cancer 63:1101-1107, 1989
25. Frager DH, Wolf EL, Competiello LS, et al: Squamous cell carcinoma of the esophagus in patients with acquired immunodeficiency syndrome. Gastrointest Radiol 13:358-360, 1988

26. Frazer IH, Crapper RM, Medley G, et al: Association between anorectal dysplasia, human papillomavirus, and human immunodeficiency virus infection in homosexual men. Lancet 2:657-660, 1986

27. Friedman SL: Gastrointestinal and hepatobiliary neoplasms in AIDS. Gastroenterol Clin North Am 17:465-486, 1988

28. Frizzera G, Hanto DW, Gajl Peczalkska K, et al: Polymorphic diffuse B-cell hyperplasias and lymphomas in renal transplant recipients. Cancer Res 41:4262-4279, 1981

29. Frizzera G, Rosai J, Dehner LP, et al: Lymphoreticular disorders in primary immunodeficiencies: New findings based on an up-to-date histologic classification of 35 cases. Cancer 46(4):692-699, 1980

30. Gail MH, Pluda JM, Rabkin CS, et al: Projections of the incidence of non-Hodgkin's lymphoma related to acquired immunodeficiency syndrome. J Natl Cancer Inst 83:695-701, 1991

31. Gail MH, Rosenberg PS, Goedert JJ: Therapy may explain recent deficits in AIDS incidence. J Acquir Immune Defic Syndr 3:296-306, 1990

32. Gal AA, Meyer PR, Taylor CR: Papillomavirus antigens in anorectal condyloma and carcinoma in homosexual men. JAMA 257:337-340, 1987

33. Gal AA, Saul SH, Stoler MH: In situ hybridization analysis of human papillomavirus in anal squamous cell carcinoma. Mod Pathol 2:439-443, 1989

34. Gill P, Levine A, Krailo M, et al: AIDS-related malignant lymphoma: Results of prospective treatment trials. J Clin Oncol 5:1322-1328, 1987

35. Gill PS, Akil B, Colletti P, et al: Pulmonary Kaposi's sarcoma: Clinical findings and results of therapy. Am J Med 87:57-61, 1989

36. Gill PS, Krailo M, Slater L, et al: Randomized trial of ABV (adriamycin, bleomycin and vinblastine) vs A (adriamycin) in advanced Kaposi's sarcoma (KS) (abstract). Am Soc Clin Oncol, New Orleans, 1988, p 11

37. Gill PS, Levine A, Meyer P, et al: Primary central nervous system lymphoma in homosexual men. Am J Med 78:742-748, 1985

38. Glaspy J, Miles S, McCarthy S: Treatment of advanced stage Kaposi's sarcoma with vincristine and bleomycin (abstract). Am Soc Clin Oncol, Los Angeles, 1986, p 10

39. Grant I, Gold J, Armstrong D: Risk of CNS toxoplasmosis in patients with acquired immune deficiency syndrome. Proceedings Interscience Conference on Antimicrobial Agents and Chemotherapy. (Abstract 441.) New Orleans, 1986

40. Groopman J, Sullivan J, Mulder C, et al: Pathogenesis of B-cell lymphoma in a patient with AIDS. Blood 67:612-615, 1986

41. Groopman JE, Gottlieb MS, Goodman J, et al: Recombinant alpha-2 interferon therapy for Kaposi's sarcoma associated with the acquired immunodeficiency syndrome. Ann Intern Med 100:671-676, 1984

42. Groopman JE, Mayer K, Zipoli T, et al: Unusual neoplasms associated with HTLV-III infection. Proc Am Soc Clin Oncol 5:14, 1986

43. Guarner J, Brynes RK, Chan WC, et al: Primary non-Hodgkin's lymphoma of the heart in two patients with the acquired immunodeficiency syndrome. Arch Pathol Lab Med 111:254-256, 1987

44. Hamilton-Dutoit SF, Pallesen G, Franzman MB, et al: AIDS-related lymphoma. Histopathology, immunophenotype and association with Epstein-Barr virus as demonstrated by in situ nucleic acid hybridization. Am J Pathol 138:149-163, 1991

45. Hanto DW, Frizzera G, Gajl-Peczalkska K, et al: Epstein-Barr virus induced B-cell lymphoma after renal transplantation. N Engl J Med 306:913-918, 1982

46. Hanto DW, Frizzera G, Purtilo, et al: Clinical spectrum of lymphoproliferative disorders in renal transplant recipients and evidence for the role of Epstein-Barr virus. Cancer Res 41:4253-4261, 1981

47. Hanto DW, Gajl-Peczalkska KJ, Frizzera G, et al: Epstein-Barr virus induced polyclonal and monoclonal B-cell lymphoproliferative disease occurring after renal transplantation. Ann Surg 198:356-369, 1983

48. Harnly ME, Swan SH, Holly EA, et al: Temporal trends in the incidence of non-Hodgkin's lymphoma and selected malignancies in a population with a high incidence of acquired immunodeficiency syndrome (AIDS). Am J Epidemiol 128:261-267, 1988

49. Hartshorn KL, Vogt MW, Chou TC, et al: Synergistic inhibition of human immunodeficiency virus *in vitro* by azidothymidine and recombinant interferon alpha-A. Antimicrobial Agents Chemother 31:168-172, 1987

50. Harwood AR, Osoba D, Hofstader SL, et al: Kaposi's sarcoma in recipients of renal transplants. Am J Med 67:759-765, 1979

51. Heyer DM, Desmond S, Volberding P, Kahn J: Changing prevalence of malignancies in men at San Francisco General Hospital during the HIV epidemic (Abstract WBO 19). Proc V Int Conf AIDS 5:206, 1989

52. Hill DR: The role of radiotherapy for epidemic Kaposi's sarcoma. Semin Oncol 14(suppl 3):1207, 1987

53. Holly EA, Whittemore AS, Aston DA, et al: Anal cancer incidence: Genital warts, anal fissure or fistula, hemorrhoids, and smoking. J Natl Cancer Inst 81:1726-1731, 1989

54. Hoover R, Fraumeni JF: Risk of cancer in renal transplant recipients. Lancet 2:55-57, 1973

55. Italian Cooperative Group for AIDS-related Tumors: Malignant lymphomas in patients with or at risk for AIDS in Italy: Reports. J Natl Cancer Inst 80:855-860, 1988

56. Kaplan L, Kahn J, Jacobson M, et al: Primary bile duct lymphoma in the acquired immunodeficiency syndrome (AIDS). Ann Intern Med 110:162, 1989

57. Kaplan LD, Abrams D, Volberding P: Treatment of Kaposi's sarcoma in acquired immunodeficiency syndrome with an alternating vincristine-vinblastine regimen. Cancer Treat Rep 70:1121-1122, 1986

58. Kaplan LD, Abrams DA, Volberding PA: Clinical course and epidemiology of Hodgkin's disease in homosexual men in San Francisco (abstract). International Conference on AIDS, Washington, DC, June 1-5, 1987

59. Kaplan LD, Abrams DI, Feigal E, et al: AIDS-associated non-Hodgkin's lymphoma in San Francisco. JAMA 261:719-724, 1989

60. Kaplan LD, Hopewell PC, Jaffe H, et al: Kaposi's sarcoma involving the lung in patients with the acquired immunodeficiency syndrome. J Acquir Immune Defic Syndr 1:23-30, 1988

61. Kaplan LD, Kahn JO, Crowe S, et al: Clinical and virologic effects of recombinant human granulocyte-macrophage colony-stimulating factor in patients receiving chemotherapy for human immunodeficiency virus-associated non-Hodgkin's lymphoma: Results of a randomized trial. J Clin Oncol 9:929-940, 1991

62. Kaplan L, Kahn D, Northfelt D, et al: Novel combination chemotherapy for Hodgkin's disease (HD) in HIV-infected individuals. Paper presented at American Society of Clinical Oncology Annual Meeting, 1991, p 33

63. Kiviat N, Rompalo A, Bowden R, et al: Anal human papillomavirus infection among human immunodeficiency virus-seropositive and -seronegative men. J Infect Dis 162:358-361, 1990

64. Knowles DM, Chamulak G, Subar M, et al: Lymphoid neoplasia associated with the acquired immunodeficiency syndrome (AIDS). Ann Intern Med 108:744-753, 1988

65. Knowles DM, Inghirami G, Ubraico A, Dalla-Favera R: Molecular genetic analysis of three AIDS-associated neoplasms of uncertain lineage demonstrates their B-cell derivation and the possible pathogenic role of Epstein-Barr virus. Blood 73:792-799, 1989

66. Kovacs JA, Deyton L, Davey R, et al: Combined zidovudine and interferon-α therapy in patients with Kaposi's sarcoma and the acquired immunodeficiency syndrome (AIDS). Ann Intern Med 111:280-286, 1989

67. Kovacs JA, Lance HC, Masur H, et al: A phase III, placebo-controlled trial of recombinant alpha interferon in asymptomatic individuals seropositive for the acquired immunodeficiency syndrome. Clin Res 35:479A, 1987

68. Kristal AR, Nasca PC, Burnett WS, Mikl J: Changes in the epidemiology of non-Hodgkin's lymphoma associated with epidemic human immunodeficiency virus (HIV) infection. Am J Epidemiol 128:711-718, 1988

69. Krown SE: The role of interferon in the therapy of epidemic Kaposi's sarcoma. Semin Oncol 14(suppl 3):27-33, 1987

70. Krown SE, Gold JWM, Niedzwiecki D, et al: Interferon-α with zidovudine: Safety, tolerance, and clinical and virologic effects in patients with Kaposi sarcoma associated with the acquired immunodeficiency syndrome (AIDS). Ann Intern Med 112:812-821, 1990

71. Krown SE, Metroka C, Wernz JC: Kaposi's sarcoma in the acquired immunodeficiency syndrome: A proposal for uniform evaluation, and staging criteria. J Clin Oncol 7:1201-1207, 1989

72. Lane HC, Falloon J, Walker RE, et al: Zidovudine in patients with human immunodeficiency virus (HIV) infection and Kaposi's sarcoma. Ann Intern Med 111:41-50, 1989

73. Lane HC, Feinberg J, Davery V, et al: Anti-retroviral effects of interferon-alpha in AIDS-associated Kaposi's sarcoma. Lancet 2:1218-1222, 1988

74. Laubenstein LJ, Krigel RL, Odajnyk CM, et al: Treatment of epidemic Kaposi's sarcoma with etoposide or a combination of doxorubicin, bleomycin and vinblastine. J Clin Oncol 2:1115-1120, 1984
75. Lemp GF, Payne SF, Neal D, et al: Survival trends for patients with AIDS. JAMA 263:402-406, 1990
76. Levine A, Meyer P, Begandy M, et al: Development of B-cell lymphoma in homosexual men. Ann Intern Med 100:7-13, 1984
77. Levine AM, Sullivan-Halley J, Pike MC, et al: AIDS-related lymphoma: Prognostic factors predictive of survival. Cancer (in press)
78. Levine AM, Wernz JC, Kaplan L, et al: Low-dose chemotherapy with central nervous system prophylaxis and zidovudine maintenance in AIDS-related lymphoma. JAMA 266:84-88, 1991
79. Lowenthal D, Straus D, Campbell S, et al: AIDS-related lymphoid neoplasia. The Memorial Hospital Experience. Cancer 61:2325-2337, 1988
80. MacMahon EME, Glass JD, Hayward SD, et al: Epstein-Barr virus in AIDS-related primary central nervous system lymphoma. Lancet 338:969-973, 1991
81. Maiman M, Fruchter RG, Serur E, et al: Human immunodeficiency virus infection and cervical neoplasia. Gynecol Oncol 38:377-382, 1990
82. Meeker TC, Shiramizu B, Kaplan L, et al: Evidence for molecular subtypes of HIV-associated lymphoma: Division into peripheral monoclonal, polyclonal and central nervous system lymphoma. AIDS 5:669-674, 1991
83. Melbye M, Palefsky J, Gonzales J, et al: Immune status as a determinant of human papillomavirus detection and its association with anal epithelial abnormalities. Int J Cancer 46:203-206, 1990
84. Miles SA, Rezai AR, Logan D, et al: AIDS Kaposi's sarcoma-derived cells produce and respond to interleukin 6. Sixth International Conference on AIDS. (S.A.66.) San Francisco, 1990, p 113
85. Mintzer DM, Real FX, Jovino L, Krown SE: Treatment of Kaposi's sarcoma and thrombocytopenia with vincristine in patients with the acquired immunodeficiency syndrome. Ann Intern Med 102:200-202, 1985
86. Mitsuyasu R, Taylor J, Glaspy J, et al: Heterogeneity of epidemic Kaposi's sarcoma. Implications for therapy. Cancer 57:1657-1661, 1986
87. Mitsuyasu RT, Groopman JE: Biology and therapy of Kaposi's sarcoma. Semin Oncol 11:53-59, 1984
88. Monfardini S, Vaccher E, Pizzocaro G, et al: Unusual malignant tumors in 49 patients with HIV infection. AIDS 3:449-452, 1989
89. Moore RD, Kessler H, Richman DD, et al: Non-Hodgkin's lymphoma in patients with advanced HIV infection treated with zidovudine. JAMA 265:2208-2211, 1991
90. Myskowski PL, Niedzweicki D, Shurgot BA, et al: AIDS-associated Kaposi's sarcoma: Variable associated with increased survival. J Am Acad Dermatol 18:1299-1306, 1988
91. Nakamura S, Salahuddin SZ, Biberfeld P, et al: Kaposi's sarcoma cells: Long-term culture with growth factor from retrovirus-infected CD4 + T cells. Science 42:426-430, 1988
92. Nasr S, Brynes R, Garrison C, Chan W: Peripheral T-cell lymphoma in a patient with acquired immunodeficiency syndrome. Cancer 61:947-951, 1988
93. National Cancer Institute: NCI-sponsored study of classifications of non-Hodgkin's lymphoma. Summary and description of a working formulation for clinical usage. The Non-Hodgkin's Lymphoma Pathologic Classification Project. Cancer 49:2112-2135, 1982
94. Newman SB: Treatment of epidemic Kaposi's sarcoma (KS) with intralesional vinblastine injection (IL-VLB) (abstract). American Society of Clinical Oncology, New Orleans, 1988, p 5
95. Ognibene FP, Steis RG, Macher AM, et al: Kaposi's sarcoma causing pulmonary infiltrates and respiratory failure in acquired immunodeficiency syndrome. Ann Intern Med 102:471-475, 1985
96. Palefsky J: Human papillomavirus infection among HIV-infected individuals. Hematol Oncol Clin North Am 5:357-370, 1991
97. Palefsky JM, Gonzales J, Greenblatt RM, et al: Anal intraepithelial neoplasia and anal papillomavirus infection among homosexual males with group IV HIV disease. JAMA 263:2911-2916, 1990
98. Penn I: Cancers of the anogenital region in renal transplant recipients: Analysis of 65 cases. Cancer 58:611-616, 1986
99. Penn I: Lymphomas complicating organ transplantation. Transplant Proc 15(suppl 1):2790-2797, 1983

100. Penn I: The incidence of malignancies in transplant recipients. Transplant Proc pp 323-326, 1975
101. Penn I: Tumors of the immunocompromised patient. Ann Rev Med 39:63-73, 1988
102. Petersen JM, Tubbs RR, Savage RA, et al: Small non-cleaved B-cell Burkitt-like lymphoma with chromosome t(8;14) translocation and Epstein-Barr virus nuclear-associated antigen in a homosexual man with acquired immune deficiency syndrome. Am J Med 78:141-148, 1985
103. Pfister H: Relationship of papillomaviruses to anogenital cancer. Obstet Gynecol Clin North Am 14:349-361, 1987
104. Pluda JM, Yarchoan R, Jaffe ES, et al: Development of non-Hodgkin's lymphoma in a cohort of patients with severe human immunodeficiency virus (HIV) infection on long-term antiretroviral therapy. Ann Intern Med 113:276-282, 1990
105. Presant CA, Gala K, Wiseman C, et al: Human immunodeficiency virus-associated T-cell lymphoblastic lymphoma in AIDS. Cancer 60:1459-1461, 1987
106. Ravalli S, Chabon AB, Khan AA: Gastrointestinal neoplasia in young HIV-positive patients. Am J Clin Pathol 91:458-461, 1989
107. Real FX, Oettgen HF, Krown SE: Kaposi's sarcoma and the acquired immunodeficiency syndrome: Treatment with high and low doses of leukocyte A interferon. J Clin Oncol 4:544-551, 1986
108. Rellihan MA, Dooley DP, Burke TW, et al: Rapidly progressing cervical cancer in a patient with human immunodeficiency virus infection. Gynecol Oncol 36:435-438, 1990
109. Rezai A, Martinez-Maza O, Gaynor R, et al: HIV-Tat increases production by and proliferation of AIDS-KS derived cells. Annual meeting of American Society of Clinical Oncology, 1991, p 33
110. Rios A, Mansell PWA, Newell GR, et al: Treatment of acquired immunodeficiency syndrome-related Kaposi's sarcoma with lymphoblastoid interferon. J Clin Oncol 3:506-512, 1985
111. Rogo KO, Kavoo-Linge: Human immunodeficiency virus seroprevalence among cervical cancer patients. Gynecol Oncol 37:87-92, 1990
112. Rutherford GW, Schwarcz SK, Lemp GF, et al: The epidemiology of AIDS-related Kaposi's sarcoma in San Francisco. J Infect Dis 159:569-572, 1989
113. Safai B: Pathophysiology and epidemiology of epidemic Kaposi's sarcoma. Semin Oncol 2(suppl 3):7-12, 1987
114. Salahuddin SZ, Nakamura S, Biberfeld P, et al: Angiogenic properties of Kaposi's sarcoma-derived cells after long-term culture *in vitro*. Science 242:430-433, 1988
115. Schoeppel SL, Hoppe RT, Dorfman RF, et al: Hodgkin's disease in homosexual men with generalized lymphadenopathy. Ann Intern Med 102:68-70, 1985
116. Schrager LK, Friedland GH, Maude D, et al: Cervical and vaginal squamous abnormalities in women infected with human immunodeficiency virus. J Acquir Immune Defic Syndr 2:570-575, 1989
117. Sharma D, Muggia F, Lucci L, et al: Liposomal daunorubicin (VS103): Tolerance and clinical effects in AIDS-related Kaposi's sarcoma (KS) during a phase I study. American Society of Clinical Oncology, 1990, p 4
118. Shearer WT, Ritz J, Finego MJ, et al: Epstein-Barr virus-associated B-cell proliferations of diverse clonal origins after bone marrow transplantation in a 12-year-old patient with severe combined immunodeficiency. N Engl J Med 312:1151-1159, 1985
119. Shiramizu B, Herndier B, Meeker T, et al: Molecular and immunophenotypic characterization of AIDS-associated EBV-negative polyclonal lymphoma. J Clin Oncol (in press)
120. Sillman FH, Sedlis A: Anogenital papillomavirus infection and neoplasia in immunodeficient women. Obstet Gynecol Clin North Am 14:537-558, 1987
121. So YT, Beckstead J, Davis R: Primary central nervous system lymphoma in acquired immunodeficiency syndrome: A clinical and pathological study. Ann Neurol 20:566-572, 1986
122. Subar M, Neri A, Inghirami G, et al: Frequent c-*myc* oncogene activation and infrequent presence of Epstein-Barr virus genome in AIDS-associated lymphoma. Blood 72:667-671, 1988
123. Tappero JW, Berger TG, Kaplan LD, et al: Cryotherapy for cutaneous Kaposi's sarcoma (KS) associated with acquired immune deficiency syndrome (AIDS): A phase II trial. J AIDS 4:839-846, 1991
124. Taylor J, Afrasiabi R, Fahey JL, et al: Prognostically significant classification of immune changes in AIDS with Kaposi's sarcoma. Blood 67:666-671, 1986
125. Tessler AN, Catanese A: AIDS and germ cell tumors of testis. Urology 30:203-204, 1987
126. Tindal B, Finlayson R, Mutimer K, et al: Malignant melanoma associated with human immunodeficiency virus infection in three homosexual men. J Am Acad Dermatol 20:587-591, 1989

127. Tirelli V, Vaccher E, Sinicco A, et al: Forty-nine unusual HIV-related malignant tumors (Abstract WCP 50). Proc V Int Conf AIDS 5:600, 1989
128. Vadhan-Raj S, Wong G, Gnecco C, et al: Immunological variables as predictors of prognosis in patients with Kaposi's sarcoma and the acquired immunodeficiency syndrome. Cancer 46:417-425, 1986
129. Vogel J, Hinrichs SH, Reynolds RK, et al: The HIV *tat* gene induces dermal lesions resembling Kaposi's sarcoma in transgenic mice. Nature 335:606-611, 1988
130. Volberding PA, Abrams DA, Conant M, et al: Vinblastine therapy for Kaposi's sarcoma in the acquired immunodeficiency syndrome. Ann Intern Med 103:335-338, 1985
131. Volberding PA, Kusick P, Feigal D: Effects of chemotherapy for HIV associated Kaposi's sarcoma on longterm survival (abstract). Proc ASCO 8:12, 1989
132. Volberding PA, Mitsuyasu R: Recombinant interferon alpha in the treatment of acquired immune deficiency syndrome-related Kaposi's sarcoma. Semin Oncol 2(suppl 5):2-6, 1985
133. Volberding PA, Mitsuyasu RT, Golando JP, et al: Treatment of Kaposi's sarcoma with interferon interferon alfa-2b (Intron A). Cancer 59:620-625, 1987
134. Ziegler J, Beckstead J, Volberding P, et al: Non-Hodgkin's lymphoma in 90 homosexual men. Relation to generalized lymphadenopathy and the acquired immunodeficiency syndrome. N Engl J Med 311:565-570, 1984
135. Ziegler JL, Drew WL, Miner RC, et al: Outbreak of Burkitt's-like lymphoma in homosexual men. Lancet 2:631-633, 1982

IV

SPECIAL ASPECTS OF AIDS

26

THE CHEST FILM IN AIDS

PHILIP C. GOODMAN, MD

The variety of opportunistic infections and neoplasms reported in patients with AIDS has changed little since the initial descriptions of this disease in the summer of 1981.[8,9] The chest radiographic features of these entities may overlap, discouraging some from using the chest film as means of distinguishing between diseases. Nevertheless, some differences in appearance have proved fairly constant and, if recognized, permit an ordering of diagnoses into a most probable sequence. This chapter reviews the chest film abnormalities observed with the more usual opportunistic infections and neoplasms seen in patients with AIDS. Less commentary is given to the infrequently observed diseases associated with the syndrome.

OPPORTUNISTIC INFECTIONS

Pneumocystis carinii Pneumonia

Pneumocystis carinii pneumonia (PCP) is the most common opportunistic infection seen in patients with AIDS.[44] Chest film abnormalities are frequently present, yet in approximately 5% to 10% of cases, the chest radiograph is normal.[26] The diagnosis in this setting is suggested by clinical and laboratory findings such as shortness of breath, lowered Po_2, decreased diffusing capacity, and occasionally an abnormal gallium lung scan. The diagnosis is confirmed by observing *P. carinii* in induced sputum, bronchoalveolar lavage, or lung biopsy samples (see Chapter 17).

In the great majority of patients with PCP, chest films are abnormal and reveal diffuse bilateral and usually fairly symmetric, fine reticular heterogeneous opacities[15,22,28] (Figure 26–1). Variations in this pattern occur frequently and include unilateral or focal lung opacities of the same quality or rarely focal alveolar consolidation[24] (Figure 26–2). Occasionally the interstitial pattern is medium to coarse, and on rare occasions a miliary pattern is observed (Figure 26–3). Focal nodules with or without cavitation have also been attributed to *P. carinii* infection[2] (Figure 26–4). The cavity walls are generally thicker than those observed with pneumatoceles.[35] The outer margins may be irregular or smooth. Cavitary nodules of PCP are usually solitary and fairly pathognomonic. Occasionally cavitary nodules of *Cryptococcus* infection have a similar appearance.

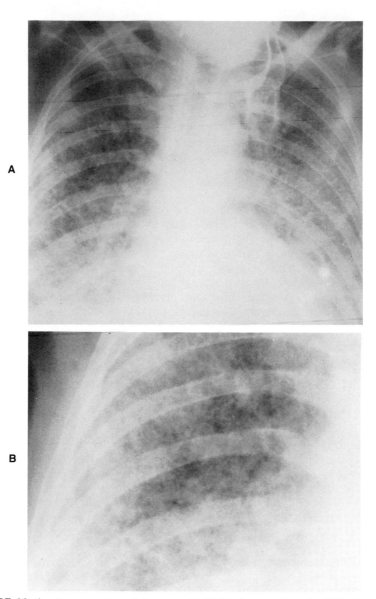

FIGURE 26–1.   *Pneumocystis carinii* pneumonia (PCP). **A,** Anteroposterior (AP) chest film demonstrates moderate to severe bilateral reticular heterogeneous densities. **B,** Close-up of the right midlung demonstrates the fine nature of the reticular density seen in PCP. In the peripheral areas of the lung, coalescence of these densities has produced a more homogeneous consolidation as seen in severe episodes of infection.

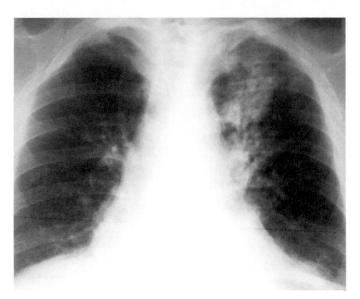

FIGURE 26–2. *Pneumocystis carinii* pneumonia (PCP). Posteroanterior (PA) chest film demonstrates a focal area of fairly homogeneous consolidation in the left upper lobe. Air bronchograms are seen in this region of alveolar density.

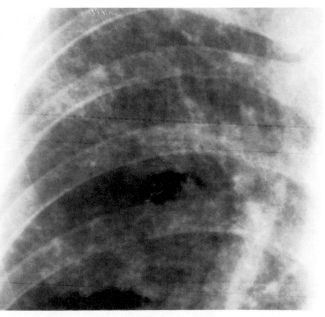

FIGURE 26–3. *Pneumocystis carinii* pneumonia (PCP). Close-up of a PA chest film demonstrates a fine to medium nodular or miliary pattern in the right upper and middle lobes.

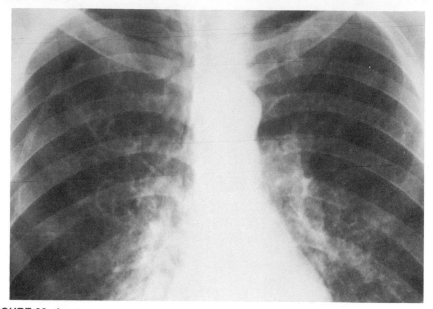

FIGURE 26–4. *Pneumocystis carinii* pneumonia (PCP). PA chest film demonstrates a solitary thick-walled cavity in the right upper lobe. PCP may appear in this fashion secondary to ischemic necrosis of affected lung.

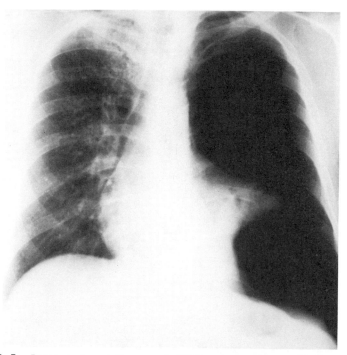

FIGURE 26–5. *Pneumocystis carinii* pneumonia (PCP) and pneumothorax. PA chest film demonstrates large, left-sided tension pneumothorax. The right lung and in particular the right upper lobe demonstrates a medium reticulonodular pattern.

With appropriate therapy, improvement in the radiographic findings is expected within 7 to 10 days. Without therapy, rapid progression to a worsened, diffuse heterogeneous, and in later stages severe bilateral homogeneous consolidation may occur. Therapy with intravenous trimethoprim-sulfamethoxazole may lead to worsening of the chest film abnormalities within 4 days of the institution of treatment. This most likely is caused by pulmonary edema due to the large amount of fluid required for intravenous therapy with this antibiotic and does not necessarily indicate worsening of pneumonia.[64] If warranted, diuretic therapy will often result in rapid improvement in the patient's radiographic and clinical state. Eventually complete resolution of radiographic abnormalities is expected, although in some instances residual interstitial densities are observed.[52] Recently adjunctive therapy with corticosteroids has been recommended for patients with moderate to severe PCP.[4] Rapid improvement may be observed in the chest film following this regimen.[29,53]

A few interesting complications of PCP have been recognized with some frequency in the last 4 to 5 years. Spontaneous pneumothorax has been observed in many patients with PCP (Figure 26–5). The size of pneumothorax has varied from

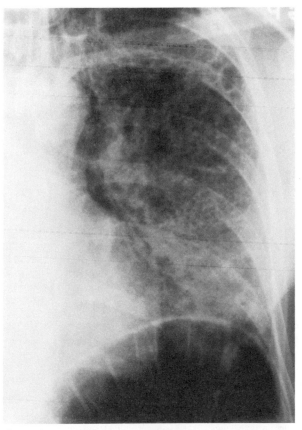

FIGURE 26–6. *Pneumocystis carinii* pneumonia (PCP) and pneumatoceles. Close-up of a PA chest film demonstrates heterogeneous medium interstitial densities in the left lung. In the periphery of the left upper lobe, small thin-walled, air-filled structures representing pneumatoceles are demonstrated. These usually resolve in 3 to 6 months but occasionally lead to pneumothorax.

small to extremely large, and it may require tube thoracostomy. Although somewhat controversial, the timing of the pneumothoraces is probably not related to treatment but apparently is due to infection with *P. carinii* itself.[55,62] In some instances pneumatoceles precede the appearance of pneumothorax (Figure 26–6). In one series 10% of patients with PCP had pneumatoceles.[54] These thin-walled air-containing structures are solitary or multiple and may increase or decrease in size rapidly (Figure 26–7). Resolution is generally seen in 3 to 6 months. In rare instances air-fluid levels have been noted within the pneumatoceles. These abnormalities have not been observed in AIDS patients with infections other than PCP. The mechanism for pneumatocele formation in this setting is unclear, and, although it may be due to a check valve mechanism, there is little pathologic proof this occurs in these patients.[49] Others suggest that necrosis in subpleural locations of the lung may result in pneumatoceles and subsequent pneumothorax.[17] Premature formation of bullae as seen by computed tomography (CT) has been described in patients with AIDS.[37]

The distribution of PCP can be altered by prophylactic therapy with inhaled pentamidine. In a number of patients who have undergone this therapeutic regimen, new cases of PCP are preferentially located in the upper lobes[5,38,57] (Figure 26–8). The reason for this probably is poor coverage of the upper lobes by pentamidine taken in aerosolized form. These unprotected areas are thus more likely to harbor *P. carinii* and to be selectively involved in pneumonia. With this therapy other unusual features, including pneumothorax and pleural fluid, have also been reported.[16]

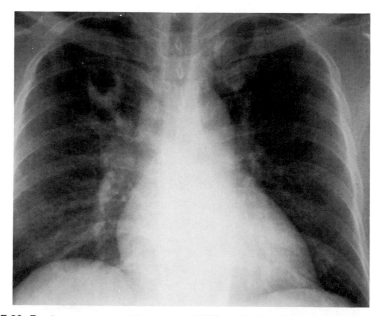

FIGURE 26–7. *Pneumocystis carinii* pneumonia (PCP). A PA chest film demonstrates multiple thin-walled pneumatoceles in both lungs. These will generally resolve over months. A pneumothorax is noted in the right hemithorax.

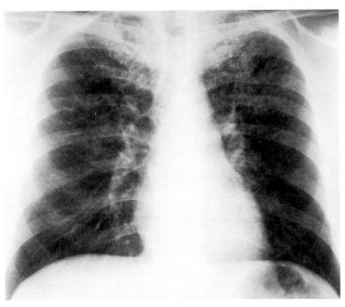

FIGURE 26–8. *Pneumocystis carinii* pneumonia (PCP). PA chest film demonstrates predominantly upper lobe medium reticular densities. This distribution of PCP may be the result of prior prophylactic aerosolized pentamidine therapy and mimics the distribution of reactivation tuberculosis.

Mycobacterial Infections

Various mycobacterial species have been responsible for pulmonary infections in patients with AIDS.[7,28,33] Clearly the majority of infections have been caused by *Mycobacterium tuberculosis* and *M. avium* complex (MAC) (see Chapter 18). The radiographic appearance of tuberculosis in this setting depends on the stage of HIV infection.[32,50] Early in the course of infection tuberculosis appears as it does in otherwise non-immune-suppressed individuals; that is, patients with reactivation tuberculosis, considered the most common pathogenesis of tuberculosis in these patients, will present with heterogeneous nodular and cavitary infiltrates in the superior segments of the lower lobes and apical and posterior segments of the upper lobes (Figure 26–9). These radiographic findings are not seen later in HIV infection, when diffuse and somewhat coarse interstitial densities are observed with or without the presence of hilar or mediastinal adenopathy[25] (Figure 26–10). Adenopathy itself may occur with different frequency within different AIDS risk groups. Thus lymphadenopathy was found in a higher percentage (approximately 80%) of intravenous drug abusers or Haitian patients with HIV infection and tuberculosis than in HIV-infected homosexual males with tuberculosis (approximately 20%).[10,59,61] The overall incidence of tuberculosis in AIDS patients has been reported as high as 24%.[48] Conversely, nearly 30% of adult non-Asian patients with tuberculosis had HIV infection.[6] Late in the course of HIV infection, tuberculosis has only rarely if ever resulted in cavitation.[15] Pleural fluid is seen with varying incidence (9% to 22%).[25]

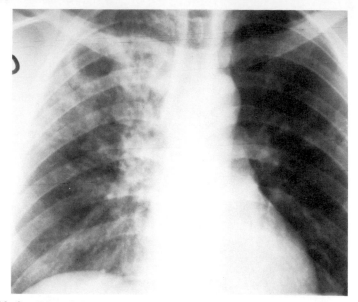

FIGURE 26–9. Tuberculosis. PA chest film demonstrates heterogeneous medium to coarse reticular densities in the right upper lobe. A large cavity is seen in this area. Minimal left upper lobe heterogeneous changes are seen. This pattern is typical of reactivation tuberculosis seen in the early stages of HIV infection.

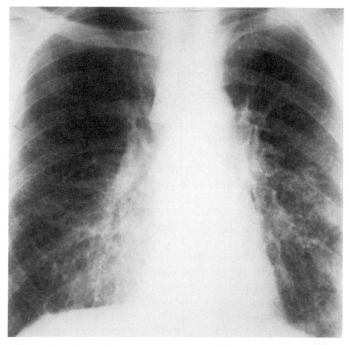

FIGURE 26–10. Tuberculosis. PA chest film demonstrates right paratracheal adenopathy and a diffuse fine to medium reticulonodular infiltrate. This is the pattern seen in patients with late-stage HIV infection and tuberculosis. Since adenopathy is not associated with PCP, it should not be considered a likely cause of disease in this patient.

The presence of adenopathy, pleural fluid, or a coarse bilateral heterogeneous infiltrate is much more typical of tuberculosis than of PCP.

Antituberculosis therapy should result in chest film improvement, paralleling a clinical response by the patient.[58] Within weeks, the radiographic abnormalities seen with this infection should begin to resolve. Worsening of a chest film while a patient is receiving appropriate medication should prompt a workup for an alternate infection.

Typically MAC is seen in lymph nodes, liver, bone marrow, blood, and urine of patients with AIDS. Involvement of pulmonary parenchyma results in diffuse, heterogeneous interstitial patterns with or without lymphadenopathy.[24] No definite features distinguishing between this species or other species of mycobacterial infection and tuberculosis have been observed on chest films. Recently a comparison of chest films in AIDS patients with tuberculosis or MAC disease revealed that with the latter infection, approximately 50% had interstitial disease, 11% had adenopathy, and none had pleural fluid.[43]

Fungi

A variety of fungal infections have been observed in patients with AIDS. In regions endemic for *Histoplasma capsulatum* and *Coccidioides immitis*, these organisms have been responsible for a number of opportunistic pneumonias in HIV-infected individuals[1,3,39,59,65] (see Chapter 20). The radiographic appearance of these pneumonias is similar. Commonly, a diffuse, bilateral, poorly defined, small nodular infiltrate is noted (Figure 26–11). Lymphadenopathy is reported with variable incidence with both of these fungal infections. Other manifestations, including

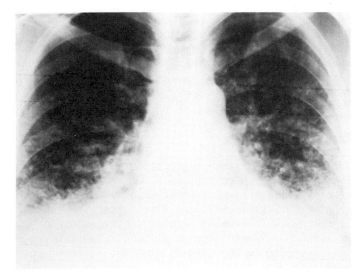

FIGURE 26–11. Histoplasmosis. Diffuse, bilateral, fairly coarse nodular densities are seen in both lungs. This pattern is commonly reported in patients with disseminated histoplasmosis and coccidioidomycosis. Adenopathy is also associated with these diseases in patients with AIDS.

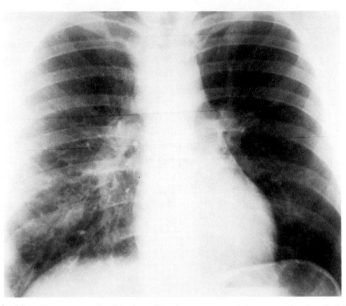

FIGURE 26–12. Cryptococcosis. PA chest film demonstrates right paratracheal and right hilar adenopathy. Occasionally parenchymal lung nodules and reticular interstitial densities are also seen in patients with intrathoracic cryptococcosis.

cavitation, alveolar consolidation, and pleural fluid, have been reported but are less frequently observed.[19,40]

Cryptococcal infections of AIDS patients generally affect the central nervous system, but some cases of cryptococcal pneumonia have been reported (see Chapter 19). The radiographic appearance is variable and includes single or multiple well-defined nodules with or without cavitation, diffuse reticular interstitial infiltrates, pleural fluid, and hilar or mediastinal adenopathy[11,12,61] (Figure 26–12). A miliary pattern may also be seen with this and other fungal infections[42] (see Chapter 19).

Cytomegalovirus

Cytomegalovirus (CMV) pneumonia was reported as one of the initial opportunistic infections seen in patients with AIDS. However, our experience suggests that this organism, although frequently observed in patients with AIDS, may not be responsible for pathologic lung changes. Consequently, our policy is to put less emphasis on this diagnosis compared with the other opportunistic infections. In those patients reported to have CMV pneumonia, a diffuse, fine to medium reticular interstitial pattern appears on chest films.[60] However, ascertaining that the radiographic abnormalities have been caused by this organism is difficult since other opportunistic agents frequently coexist. CMV as the sole pathogen responsible for pneumonia is extremely rare[41,63] (see Chapter 23).

PYOGENIC INFECTION

Pneumonias caused by pyogenic organisms such as *Streptococcus pneumoniae* and *Haemophilus influenzae* have been reported with increasing frequency in patients with AIDS[18,46,51] (see Chapter 22). It has been well established that both T-cell and B-cell immune function is compromised in these patients, thus accounting for the increased frequency of pyogenic infections. The radiographic features are similar to those seen in non-immune-suppressed individuals.[66] Air-space consolidation resulting in homogeneous density in a segment or lobe of lung is frequently observed (Figure 26–13). Parapneumonic effusions are also seen. Generally patients with pyogenic pneumonia do not have concomitant infection with opportunistic organisms such as *P. carinii*. Response to appropriate antibiotics is similar to that of non-immune-suppressed hosts so that radiographic improvement is seen within 1 to 2 weeks. It is important to consider bacterial pneumonias in differential diagnosis lists because they may significantly affect patient morbidity and mortality.[46]

Bronchitis caused by pyogenic organisms has also been seen with moderate frequency in patients with AIDS. Radiographically it is manifested by peribronchial thickening and "tram tracking" (Figure 26–14). The latter finding is caused by bronchial mucosal edema and peribronchial inflammation and is seen as thin, parallel, linear densities following the expected course of bronchi. This is not a feature of the pneumonia caused by *P. carinii*.

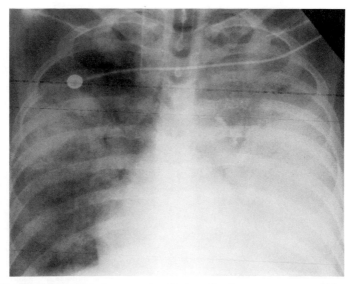

FIGURE 26–13.   Pneumococcal pneumonia. AP chest film demonstrates a severe bilateral air-space consolidation, worse on the left than on the right. The findings are typical of severe pyogenic pneumonia.

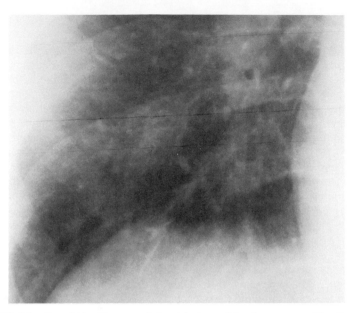

FIGURE 26–14.   Bronchitis. Close-up of the right lower lobe demonstrates thin, linear densities paralleling the course of segmental bronchi. This finding is called "tram tracking" and has been seen in AIDS patients with clinical bronchitis.

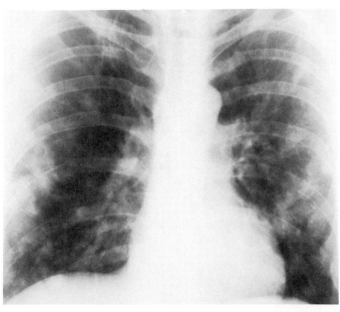

FIGURE 26–15.   Kaposi's sarcoma (KS). Scattered, poorly defined nodules are seen in both lungs. This is a classic presentation of pulmonary KS. Other manifestations include pleural fluid and coarse linear interstitial densities.

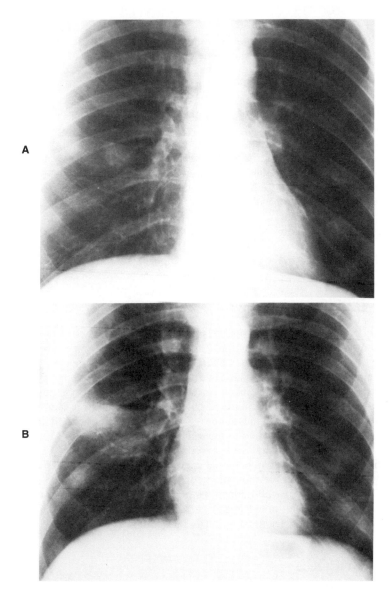

FIGURE 26–16. Kaposi's sarcoma (KS). **A,** PA chest film demonstrates two poorly defined nodules in the right middle lobe and one poorly defined nodule in the left retrocardiac area. These findings are typical of KS. **B,** The same patient 2 weeks later. At this time more homogeneous consolidation is seen in the lower lobe and right middle lobe. This type of rapid change is most likely due to hemorrhage in the sites of pulmonary KS.

NEOPLASMS

Kaposi's Sarcoma

The radiographic features of Kaposi's sarcoma are somewhat distinctive.[14,21,26,34,56] Pulmonary parenchymal involvement is manifested by coarse, poorly defined nodular densities scattered throughout the lungs (Figure 26–15) (see Chapter 25). Concomitant coarse, linear densities usually distributed in a perihilar location are also frequent. Pleural fluid is reported in 35% to 50% of patients with Kaposi's sarcoma and is probably the result of pleural metastases. Kaposi's nodules generally increase slowly in size over several months. Rapid change in size of a suspected Kaposi's sarcoma pulmonary nodule with progression to lung consolidation should suggest the possibility of hemorrhage in the region of these highly vascular lesions (Figure 26–16). Hilar and mediastinal adenopathy may be observed but is uncommon (approximately 8%).[45] CT findings in patients with Kaposi's sarcoma reflect what is seen on chest films, with poorly marginated nodular and coarse perihilar densities being most common.[45]

In patients with a history of intravenous drug abuse, differentiating Kaposi's sarcoma nodules from septic emboli may be impossible. However, within a few days, septic emboli tend to cavitate, whereas Kaposi's sarcoma nodules will not.

Non-Hodgkin's Lymphoma

General differences in the lymphomas seen in patients with AIDS as compared to those seen in the general population include a greater stage of involvement at the time of initial discovery, greater aggressiveness of the neoplasm, an almost exclusive tendency for the lymphomas to be non-Hodgkin's variety, and a decreased frequency of intrathoracic involvement[31] (see Chapter 25). An early study of AIDS patients with non-Hodgkin's lymphoma revealed that only 10% of patients had chest manifestations.[67] The radiographic features of non-Hodgkin's lymphoma in this setting include unilateral and bilateral pleural effusions in nearly half the patients. Hilar or mediastinal adenopathy is observed on nearly one fourth of chest films (Figure 26–17). Pulmonary parenchymal involvement is manifested by reticulonodular interstitial infiltrates or alveolar consolidation in nearly one quarter of patients. The appearance of well-defined parenchymal nodules remarkable for their rapidity of growth has been noted in rare instances (Figure 26–18). Cavitation of these nodules may occur after therapy but is rare.[31]

MISCELLANEOUS

Lymphocytic Interstitial Pneumonitis

Lymphocytic interstitial pneumonitis (LIP) is a disease of unknown etiology that is characterized by an accumulation of lymphocytes and plasma cells in the pulmonary interstitial space (see Chapter 27). Although even distribution is usually demonstrated, focal collections of lymphocytes may be observed.[13,23] This entity is recognized as an index diagnosis for AIDS in the pediatric patient. Chest films

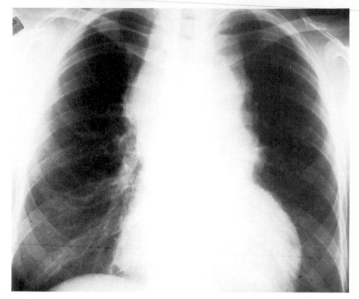

FIGURE 26–17. Non-Hodgkin's lymphoma. PA chest film demonstrates severe mediastinal adenopathy. Intrathoracic involvement in AIDS patients with non-Hodgkin's lymphoma has been observed approximately 10 percent of the time. Adenopathy, pleural fluid, and nodular parenchymal disease have been noted.

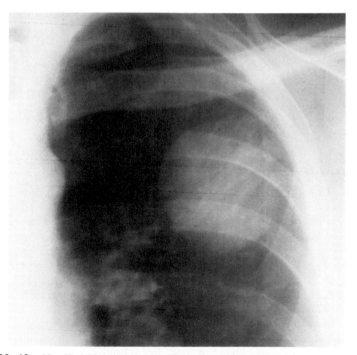

FIGURE 26–18. Non-Hodgkin's lymphoma. This large, well-defined nodule appeared over a period of 6 weeks. A needle biopsy was unrevealing, but an open lung procedure demonstrated a large non-Hodgkin's lymphoma lesion.

447

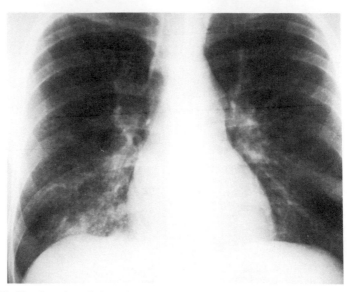

FIGURE 26–19. Lymphocytic interstitial pneumonia (LIP). PA chest film demonstrates bibasilar fine to medium reticular interstitial densities indistinguishable from PCP. An open lung biopsy revealed LIP.

of these individuals are indistinguishable from those seen in patients with PCP. They typically demonstrate diffuse or focal, fine to medium reticular interstitial infiltrates[47] (Figure 26–19). Some reports indicate a tendency toward small nodular densities that correlate well with pathologic findings.[20] The chest radiographs remain stable initially but worsen over weeks to months. Lymphadenopathy may be seen in the late stages of disease.[30] Open lung biopsy is required for definitive diagnosis. Steroid therapy may result in rapid radiographic improvement.

SUMMARY

The task of interpreting chest radiographs in patients with AIDS will be made easier, it is hoped, by applying the information contained in this chapter. Although the various infections and neoplasms seen with this syndrome occasionally have similar appearances on chest films, some patterns should allow construction of a limited differential diagnosis list. Indeed, some findings are nearly specific for certain processes. For example, in this setting pneumatocele formation is seen exclusively in those with PCP. The finding of poorly defined nodular densities with associated pleural effusions is almost pathognomonic for Kaposi's sarcoma. On the other hand, some radiographic findings should dissuade one from considering certain diagnoses. For example, pleural fluid and lymphadenopathy are rarely if ever encountered in patients with PCP alone; thus other entities such as non-Hodgkin's lymphoma, tuberculosis, or fungal infection should be considered. With experience, a more confident interpretation of the chest film will lead to better patient management.

REFERENCES

1. Abrams DI, Robia M, Blumenfeld W, et al: Disseminated coccidioidomycosis in AIDS. N Engl J Med 310:986, 1984
2. Barrio JL, Suarez M, Rodriguez JL, et al: *Pneumocystis carinii* pneumonia presenting as cavitating and non-cavitating solitary pulmonary nodules in patients with the acquired immunodeficiency syndrome. Am Rev Respir Dis 134:1094, 1986
3. Bonner JR, Alexander WJ, Dismukes WE, et al: Disseminated histoplasmosis in patients with the acquired immune deficiency syndrome. Arch Intern Med 144:2178, 1984
4. Bozzette SA, Satler FR, Chiu J, et al: A controlled trial of early adjunctive treatment with corticosteroids for *Pneumocystis carinii* pneumonia in the acquired immunodeficiency syndrome. N Engl J Med 323:1451, 1990
5. Case Records of the Massachusetts General Hospital Case 9-1989. N Engl J Med 320:582, 1989
6. Centers for Disease Control: Advisory Committee for Elimination of Tuberculosis. Tuberculosis and human immunodeficiency virus infection. MMWR 38:236, 1989
7. Centers for Disease Control: Diagnosis and management of mycobacterial infection and disease in persons with human immunodeficiency virus infection. Ann Intern Med 106:254, 1987
8. Center for Disease Control: Kaposi's sarcoma and *Pneumocystis* pneumonia among homosexual men: New York City and California. MMWR 30:305, 1981
9. Centers for Disease Control: *Pneumocystis* pneumonia—Los Angeles. MMWR 30:250, 1981
10. Chaisson RE, Schecter GF, Theuer CP, et al: Tuberculosis in patients with the acquired immunodeficiency syndrome: Clinical features, response to therapy, and survival. Ann Rev Respir Dis 136:570, 1987
11. Chechani V, Camholz SL: Pulmonary manifestations of disseminated cryptococcosis in patients with AIDS. Chest 98:1060, 1990
12. Clark RA, Greer DL, Valaines GT, et al: *Cryptococcus neoformans* pulmonary infection in human immunodeficiency virus-1–infected patients. J Acquir Immune Defic Syndr 3:480, 1990
13. Conces DJ, Tarver RD: Noninfectious and non-malignant pulmonary disease in AIDS. J Thorac Imaging 6:53, 1991
14. Davis SD, Henschke CI, Chamides BK, et al: Intrathoracic Kaposi sarcoma in AIDS patients: Radiographic-pathologic correlation. Radiology 163:495, 1987
15. DeLorenzo IJ, Huang CT, Maguire GP, et al: Roentgenographic patterns of *Pneumocystis carinii* pneumonia in 104 patients with AIDS. Chest 91:323, 1987
16. Edelstein H, McCabe RE: Atypical presentations of *Pneumocystis carinii* pneumonia in patients receiving inhaled pentamidine prophylaxis. Chest 98:1366, 1990
17. Feuerstein IM, Archer A, Pluda JM, et al: Thin-walled cavities, cysts and pneumothoraces in *Pneumocystis carinii* pneumonia: Further observations with histopathologic correlation. Radiology 174:697, 1990
18. Fimberkoff MS, El Sadr W, Schiffman G, et al: *Streptococcus pneumoniae* infections and bacteremia in patients with acquired immune deficiency syndrome with report of a pneumococcal vaccine failure. Am Rev Respir Dis 130:1174, 1984
19. Garay SM, Belenko M, Fazzini E, et al: Pulmonary manifestations of Kaposl's sarcoma. Chest 91:39, 1987
20. Goldman HS, Ziprowski MN, Charytan M, et al: Lymphocytic interstitial pneumonitis in children with AIDS: A perfect radiographic-pathologic correlation (abstract). AJR 145:868, 1985.
21. Goodman PC: Kaposi's sarcoma. J Thorac Imaging 6:43, 1991
22. Goodman PC. *Pneumocystis carinii* pneumonia. J Thorac Imaging 6:16, 1991
23. Goodman PC: Pulmonary disease in children with AIDS. J Thorac Imaging 6:60, 1991
24. Goodman PC: Pulmonary manifestations of AIDS. Curr Probl Diagn Radiol 17:81, 1988
25. Goodman PC: Pulmonary tuberculosis in patients with the acquired immunodeficiency syndrome. J Thorac Imaging 5:38-45, 1990
26. Goodman PC, Broaddus VC, Hopewell PC: Chest radiographic patterns in the acquired immunodeficiency syndrome. Am Rev Respir Dis 129:26, 1984
27. Goodman PC, Daley C, Minagi H: Spontaneous pneumothorax in AIDS patients with *Pneumocystis carinii* pneumonia. AJR 147:29, 1986
28. Goodman PC, Gamsu G: Radiographic findings in the acquired immunodeficiency syndrome. Postgrad Radiol 7:3, 1987
29. Groskin SA, Stadnick ME, DuPont PG: *Pneumocystis carinii* pneumonia: Effect of corticosteroid treatment on radiographic appearance in a patient with AIDS. Radiology 180:423, 1991

30. Haney PJ, Yale-Loehr AJ, Nussbaum AR, et al: Imaging of infants and children with AIDS. AJR 152:1033, 1989
31. Haskal ZJ, Lindan C, Goodman PC: Lymphoma in the immunocompromised patient. Radiol Clin North Am 28:885, 1990
32. Hopewell PC: Tuberculosis and human immunodeficiency virus infection. Semin Respir Infect 4:111, 1989
33. Hopewell PC, Luce JM: Pulmonary manifestations of the acquired immunodeficiency syndrome. Clin Immunol Allergy 6:489, 1986
34. Kaplan L, Hopewell PC, Jaffe H, et al: Kaposi's sarcoma involving the lung in patients with the acquired immunodeficiency syndrome. J AIDS 1:23, 1988
35. Klein JS, Warnock M, Webb WR, et al: Cavitating and noncavitating granulomas in AIDS patients with *Pneumocystis* pneumonitis. AJR 152:753, 1989
36. Kovacs A, Forthal DN, Kovacs JA, et al: Disseminated coccidioidomycosis in a patient with acquired immune deficiency syndrome. West J Med 140:447, 1984
37. Kuhlman JE, Knowles MC, Fishman EK, et al: Premature bullous pulmonary damage in AIDS: CT diagnosis. Radiology 173:23, 1989
38. Lowery S, Fallat R, Feigal DW, et al: Changing patterns of *Pneumocystis carinii* pneumonia on pentamidine aerosol prophylaxis. Abstracts from Fourth International Conference on AIDS 1:419, 1988
39. Mandell W, Goldberg DM, Neu HC: Histoplasmosis in patients with the acquired immune deficiency syndrome. Am J Med 81:974, 1986
40. Marshall BC, Cox JK Jr, Carroll KC, et al: Case report: Histoplasmosis as a cause of pleural effusion in the acquired immunodeficiency syndrome. Am J Med Sci 300:98, 1990
41. Miles PR, Baughman RP, Linnemann CC Jr: Cytomegalovirus in the bronchoalveolar lavage fluid of patients with AIDS. Chest 97:1072, 1990
42. Miller WT Jr, Edelman JM, Miller WT: Cryptococcal pulmonary infection in patients with AIDS: Radiographic appearances. Radiology 175:725, 1990
43. Modelevsky T, Sattler FR, Barnes PF: Mycobacterial disease in patients with human immunodeficiency virus infection. Arch Intern Med 149:2201, 1989
44. Murray JF, Garay SM, Hopewell PC, et al: Pulmonary complications of the acquired immunodeficiency syndrome: An update. Am Rev Respir Dis 135:504, 1987
45. Naidich DP, Tarras M, Garay SM, et al: Kaposi's sarcoma: CT radiographic correlation. Chest 96:723, 1989
46. Nichols L, Balogh K, Silverman M: Bacterial infections in the acquired immunodeficiency syndrome. Am J Clin Pathol 92:787, 1989
47. Oldham SAA, Castillo M, Jacobson FL, et al: HIV-associated lymphocytic interstitial pneumonia: Radiologic manifestations and pathologic correlation. Radiology 170:83, 1989
48. Page JW, Liautaud B, Thomas F, et al: Characteristics of the acquired immunodeficiency syndrome (AIDS) in Haiti. N Engl J Med 309:945, 1983
49. Panicek DM: Cystic pulmonary lesions in patients with AIDS. Radiology 173:12, 1989
50. Pitchenik AE, Burr J, Suarez M, et al: Human T-cell lymphotropic virus-III (HTLV-III) seropositivity and related disease among 71 consecutive patients in whom tuberculosis was diagnosed. Am Rev Respir Dis 135:875, 1987
51. Polsky B, Gold JWN, Whimbey E, et al: Bacterial pneumonia in patients with the acquired immunodeficiency syndrome. Ann Intern Med 104:38, 1986
52. Ramaswany G, Jagadha V, Tchnentkoff V: Diffuse alveolar damage and interstitial fibrosis in acquired immunodeficiency syndrome. Patients without concurrent pulmonary infection. Arch Pathol Lab Med 109:408, 1985
53. Rankin JA, Pella JA: Radiographic resolution of *Pneumocystis carinii* pneumonia in response to corticosteroid therapy. Am Rev Respir Dis 136:182, 1987
54. Sandhu JS, Goodman PC: Pulmonary cysts associated with *Pneumocystis carinii* pneumonia in patients with AIDS. Radiology 173:33, 1989
55. Scannell KA: Pneumothoraces and *Pneumocystis carinii* pneumonia in two AIDS patients receiving aerosolized pentamidine. Chest 97:479, 1990
56. Sivit CJ, Schwartz AM, Rockoff SD: Kaposi's sarcoma of the lung in AIDS. Radiologic pathologic analysis. AJR 148:25, 1987
57. Small P, Goodman PC, Montgomery AB: Case 9-1989: AIDS and a cavitary pulmonary lesion (letter). N Engl J Med 321:395, 1989

58. Small P, Hopewell PC, Schecter GF, et al: Chest radiographs in HIV-infected patients with pulmonary tuberculosis: Initial abnormalities and evolution with therapy. (In preparation.)
59. Stansell JD: Fungal disease in HIV-infected persons: Cryptococcosis, histoplasmosis, and coccidioidomycosis. J Thorac Imaging 6:28, 1991
60. Stover DE, White DA, Romano PA, et al: Spectrum of pulmonary diseases associated with the acquired immune deficiency syndrome. Am J Med 78:429, 1985
61. Suster B, Akerman M, Orenstein M, et al: Pulmonary manifestations of AIDS: Review of 106 episodes. Radiology 161:87, 1986
62. Toronto aerosolized pentamidine study group: Aerosolized pentamidine and spontaneous pneumothorax in AIDS patients. Chest 97:510, 1990
63. Wallace JM, Hannah J: Cytomegalovirus pneumonitis in patients with AIDS. Chest 92:198, 1987
64. Wharton J, Coleman DL, Wofsy CB, et al: Trimethoprim-sulfamethoxazole or pentamidine for *Pneumocystis carinii* pneumonia in the acquired immunodeficiency syndrome. Ann Intern Med 105:37, 1986
65. Wheat IJ, Slama TG, Zeckel ML: Histoplasmosis in the acquired immune deficiency syndrome. Am J Med 78:203, 1985
66. White S, Tsou E, Waldhorn R, et al: Life threatening bacterial pneumonia in male homosexuals with laboratory features of the acquired immunodeficiency syndrome. Chest 87:486, 1985
67. Zieler JL, Beckstead JA, Volberding PA, et al: Non-Hodgkin's lymphoma in 90 homosexual men. N Engl J Med 311:565, 1984

27

PEDIATRIC AIDS

MOSES GROSSMAN, MD

EPIDEMIOLOGY

AIDS in children presents many special problems for the infected child, for his or her family, for the physicians involved with the child's care, and for society.

The number of infected children appears small when compared with the epidemic affecting adults in the United States (see Chapter 1). As of July 1, 1991, approximately 3000 cases of AIDS had been reported in children under the age of 13, representing approximately 2% of all reported cases. The disease has almost certainly been under reported for a variety of reasons,[15] but even at this level of reporting, it is already the most common cause of childhood immunodeficiency and one of the 10 leading causes of death in children. Some 75% to 80% of HIV infections are acquired perinatally; the percentage will increase in the future because blood and blood products have been screened since 1985 and that route of acquiring the infection will dwindle to a trickle over the next few years.

The important issue epidemiologically concerns the number of HIV-infected children (as opposed to children with AIDS) and the number and prevalence of HIV-infected childbearing women. The cord blood studies being conducted by the Centers for Disease Control (CDC) and others show widely ranging rates in different geographic areas, from a low of 0.03% positive antibodies in cord blood (reflecting maternal infection) to a high of 8%.[14,18] The majority of births in infected women is in the racial minority groups (48% in blacks and 22% in Hispanics), and they occur predominantly in innercity areas associated with poverty and drug abuse.[28] As the number of affected children increases, more and more physicians will find themselves confronted with HIV-infected children as patients. Thus all physicians treating children must be acquainted with the approach to diagnosis and the principles of management of this infection.

PERINATAL HIV INFECTION: APPROACH AND DIAGNOSIS

The key to prevention of HIV infection and AIDS in children is the prevention of infection in childbearing women. Thus a vigorous and continued educational effort is needed among that population group. Minority women residing in inner urban areas and drug users in particular are at the highest risk of infection. Programs that will reach these women effectively need the highest priority. Women at risk must be taught how to protect themselves against infection and must be encouraged to have their own HIV-antibody status tested before considering a pregnancy.

It is currently customary to recommend testing the HIV-antibody status only in pregnant women who find themselves in one of the high-risk categories.[40] This testing should be done as early as is feasible so that the expectant mother who is HIV-antibody positive can be counseled and an informed decision made about continuing or interrupting the pregnancy. There is a serious debate at the present time about whether HIV-antibody testing should be restricted to women in the so-called "high-risk categories" or whether all pregnant women should be offered the HIV-antibody test routinely.[4] Experience with hepatitis B during the perinatal period has shown that 40% of women who are surface antigen positive and thus capable of transmitting infection to their infants are missed when testing is restricted to high-risk categories.[35] As a result, the current CDC recommendation is that **all** pregnant women be tested for hepatitis B surface antigen. Although the epidemiology of HIV infection is similar to that of hepatitis B, it is not identical; the prevalence of HIV infection is less than that of hepatitis B at the present time, but certain similarities can be drawn between the two.

Another argument for routine testing of all pregnant women is that such a policy would diminish the stigma of performing the test (suggesting that the patient is at increased risk of HIV infection and possibly jeopardizing health or life insurance). The most important argument in favor of routine testing of all pregnant women is the evolving standard for management of babies born to HIV-positive mothers. *Pneumocystis carinii* pneumonia (PCP) prophylaxis must be started very early (sometimes at 1 month of age),[9] and protocols are being studied for initiation of antiviral therapy both during pregnancy and at birth.[36] The other side of the argument is that routine testing and particularly proper counseling of all pregnant women will increase the cost of pregnancy, a cost that may not yet be justified by the current national prevalence, certainly not in all areas of the United States. I believe that, at the very least, the issue of HIV infection should be brought to the attention of all pregnant women. One large health maintenance group (Kaiser-Permanente, Northern California) already has a policy in place requiring all pregnant women to view a very well-done videotape on the subject of HIV infection at the first prenatal visit.

Strictly routine testing is precluded by ethical considerations and statutory laws in some states (e.g., California). Nevertheless, I advocate the routine offering of the HIV-antibody test to all pregnant women.

A serious unresolved problem is when during pregnancy the vertical transmission to the fetus actually occurs. HIV infection of the fetus can occur as early as the twentieth week of gestation.[15] What proportion of infection occurs across the placenta as opposed to intrapartum is not known. In addition, infection can be transmitted through breast milk.[27] In fact, an uninfected mother can herself be infected by feeding an infected infant.[44] Thus breast-feeding by known infected HIV mothers is not recommended.

The current reported rates of maternal-fetal transmission average 25% to 30% in the United States, with a low rate of 12.9% reported by the European Collaborative Study Group and 45% reported from Nairobi, Kenya.[14,41] At the present time it is not clear which infants get infected, why some get infected but others do not, and when during pregnancy and/or delivery the infection occurs. Infection can occur very early in pregnancy, but which percentage occurs at that stage is not clear. Some suggest that timing of maternal HIV infection in relation to pregnancy, the presence of maternal antibodies (e.g., to the V3 loop of HIV gp120), and the maternal plasma viral load may be important determinants of whether infection will occur.[31]

The delivery of an HIV-positive mother must be approached with full attention to body substance precautions, as should every delivery. Once the infant has had his or her first bath and maternal blood and secretions are washed off, caring for the infant does not require any precautions except when handling blood.

At the time of birth it is impossible to tell clinically which infant will be infected. At the same time some medical and societal considerations require that the HIV status of the infant be determined as rapidly as possible.

Serologic diagnosis, which is the mainstay of diagnosis in adults, is fraught with problems in infants[15] (see Chapter 3). Initially all infants will reflect the presence of maternal IgG and will be antibody positive whether they are infected or not. The majority of infants will begin to synthesize their own IgG and will remain antibody positive after the maternal IgG dissipates (around 1 year of age). However, a small percentage of infected infants are unable to synthesize IgG by the age of 1 year, and these infants will become HIV-antibody negative.[16,43] Infected babies do not uniformly synthesize anti-HIV IgM; thus this test, which is useful in many vertically transmitted perinatal infections, is not reliable and not usable in detecting HIV infection.[38] In infected infants p24 antigen is not uniformly present. Thus a positive p24 test is meaningful; a negative test does not rule out infection. Culture for the presence of HIV virus is the "gold standard" at the present time but is not generally available to the practicing physician.

Culturing the virus takes a long time. Additionally, only approximately 50% of infants who will be infected are culture positive in the first 2 months of life.

Polymerase chain reaction (PCR), a method that amplifies the small amount of viral DNA that may be present, is a very promising new methodology for the early diagnosis of the infected newborn.[38,39] This test is more widely available than culture and probably has similar sensitivity and specificity. However, it must be performed meticulously because a minute amount of contamination with maternal DNA will get amplified and produce a positive test.

Another recent suggestion is the determination of anti-HIV IgA antibody in the newborn infant.[23] This antibody is not transmitted across the placenta. Thus finding anti-HIV IgA in the infant means that the infant is infected. However, like the other tests, this one may not be positive in the first few months of life.

Another technique in development for early infant diagnosis is an in vitro antibody production assay.[1] This assay detects the presence of antibody-producing B lymphocytes. Several methods have been described, but none of them is ready for clinical use.

In summary, using current methodology, there is every likelihood of identifying an HIV-infected infant by 6 months of age, but it is still very difficult to do so in the first 1 to 2 months of life—a time when important management decisions must be made.

Most of the available diagnostic tests are summarized in Table 27–1.

Negative serology in the presence of a **totally healthy** infant by 18 months of age can be taken as firm evidence of lack of HIV infection.

Table 27–1. Diagnostic Tests Available for Determining Infant Infection

HIV viral culture	Gold standard; specific; not 100% sensitive, particularly in very young infants
Anti-HIV IgG (ELISA, Western blot, or immunoassay)	Positive result indicates *maternal* antibody in first 9 mo of life
Anti-HIV IgM	Specific; only 65% sensitive
p24 Antigen	Specific; only 65% sensitive
Polymerase chain reaction (PCR)	Very sensitive, promising test; may rival HIV culture; requires meticulous performance; not very sensitive in first 2 mo of life
Anti-HIV IgA	Specific, but not very sensitive in first few months of life
In vitro antibody production	Experimental; detects presence of antibody-producing B cells in infant

ELISA, enzyme-linked immunosorbent assay.

CLINICAL SYNDROME

HIV-infected infants are typically asymptomatic at birth. Although the onset of symptoms is variable in the United States, the average age of onset of severe immunodeficiency ranges from 5 to 10 months, with 50% to 90% of infants becoming ill by their first birthday; few vertically infected infants remain asymptomatic beyond the third year of life.[6,20]

The principal signs and symptoms of pediatric HIV infection are listed in Table 27–2. Many of them are nonspecific. Lymphadenopathy, hepatosplenomegaly, and failure to thrive are the most frequent, although nonspecific, presenting manifestations of HIV infection. Repeated common infections in young infants (e.g., invasive *Haemophilus influenzae* infections) should arouse suspicion about underlying HIV infection. Thrush and candidal dermatitis are common in HIV-infected children, but they occur in many normal children also. Failure to thrive is another very common manifestation of HIV infection.

In a child whose background puts him or her at risk for AIDS (e.g., baby of an intravenous drug user), these nonspecific signs and symptoms should lead to early suspicion of HIV disease and to laboratory investigation.

Some manifestations are very suggestive of HIV infections. Foremost among them is lymphocytic interstitial pneumonia (LIP), which occurs in 35% to 40% of

Table 27–2. Principal Signs and Symptoms of Pediatric Aids

Failure to thrive	Neurologic involvement
Diarrhea	Developmental delay
Frequent otitis media	Loss of attained milestones
Frequent other common pediatric infections	Dementia
Invasive or disseminated infections	Encephalopathy
Thrush	Acquired or congenital microcephaly
Opportunistic infections	Lymphadenopathy
Lymphocytic interstitial pneumonia	Hepatosplenomegaly
Skin diseases (*Candida* and seborrhea)	Cardiomyopathy
Parotid swellings	Chronic eczematoid rash

Table 27–3.   CDC Classification for HIV-Infected Children

P-0	Indeterminate infection in perinatally exposed children younger than 15 months
P-1	Asymptomatic infection
P-2	Symptomatic infection (causes other than HIV excluded)
	A Nonspecific findings
	B Progressive neurologic disease
	C Lymphocytic interstitial pneumonia (LIP)
	D Secondary infectious diseases

Abbreviated from Centers for Disease Control: MMWR 36:225-236, 1987.

children with AIDS. Children develop nodular peribronchial lymphoid infiltrates, often with hilar adenopathy. The definitive diagnosis of LIP is histologic; experienced radiologists can make an accurate radiologic diagnosis of the condition, but in diagnosing LIP it is important to **exclude** other forms of lung pathology (see Chapter 26). LIP causes ventilatory compromise, and clubbing may occur.

Salivary gland enlargement (particularly of the parotid glands) is a unique manifestation in childhood. All body organs are subject to pathology secondary to HIV infection that may become clinically manifest; cardiomyopathy, hepatitis, pancreatitis, thrombocytopenia, and hemolytic anemia have all been described.

Neurologic disease, namely encephalopathy, is a common and devastating clinical finding in most HIV-infected children[5,7] (see Chapter 13). Classically it causes developmental delay and the loss of developmental milestones that already have been acquired. Progression may be slow, rapid, or intermittent. Acquired microcephaly is common. Computed tomographic (CT) scans and magnetic resonance imaging (MRI) show brain atrophy, ventricular enlargement, attenuation of white matter, and calcification of basal ganglia.

Many other neurologic manifestations have been described. The neurologic manifestations are compounded and confounded by frequent maternal substance abuse, prematurity, and a difficult social setting.

Opportunistic infections occur in children as they do in adults. *Pneumocystis* pneumonia is the most common of them, occurring in approximately 50% of children with AIDS. Most other opportunistic infections have been described in children, notably *Mycobacterium avium-intracellulare* infections and candidal infections.[15]

Children with vertically transmitted HIV infection have a very poor prognosis. The median survival time after the diagnosis of AIDS is made using CDC criteria is 9 months.[36] Children diagnosed in the first year of life have an even shorter survival time.

The CDC defines AIDS in the pediatric population, a definition with which physicians seeing children should be familiar,[37] and it has a classification system for HIV-infected children, briefly summarized in Table 27–3.[10]

LABORATORY FEATURES

The diagnosis of AIDS can be made clinically, but it depends heavily on laboratory confirmation. The diagnosis of HIV infection is based on laboratory findings. The principal laboratory findings are listed in Table 27–4. HIV-infected children have early and major B-cell involvement; this often manifests as polyclonal hypergam-

Table 27–4.   Principal Laboratory Findings in Pediatric HIV Infection

Presence of anti-HIV antibody (confirmed by Western blot or radioimmunoassay)
Isolation of HIV virus
Polymerase chain reaction
Polyclonal hypergammaglobulinemia
Reduced CD4 count and CD4:CD8 ratio
Loss of cell-mediated immunity (anergy)
Poor antibody response to antigen challenge
Positive cerebrospinal fluid findings (pleocytosis, elevated protein level)
Anti-HIV IgA
Thrombocytopenia
Leukopenia
Positive Coombs' test for anemia

maglobulinemia and poor antibody response to specific antigens.[15] T-cell involvement is a cardinal feature of this infection, and the best means of following the progress of the disease is to measure CD4 counts (CD4 counts are normally higher in infants; they are also less predictive of illness than they are in adults). Many other measures of immune function and organ system function are also abnormal.

ADOLESCENT HIV INFECTIONS

Adolescents (ages 13 to 18 years) present special problems and special concerns within the pediatric HIV spectrum of disease.[17] The number of actual reported cases of AIDS in this group is small (approximately 1% of all reported cases). However, several recent seroprevalence studies have revealed seroprevalence rates in urban areas of up to 4.7%.[12]

The probability is high that young adults presenting with clinical AIDS in their early twenties acquired the infection as teens. There is currently a surge in the incidence of other sexually transmitted diseases among teens, and that may be an ominous sign for HIV infections as well. It is urgent and imperative that all teenagers be exposed to intensive culturally and age-appropriate education about HIV infection and its prevention. Centers for counseling and testing adolescents must be organized; adult centers often lack the experience and orientation for counseling adolescents.

The legal and ethical issues concerning consent by teens need clarification. Adolescents may legally give consent in all issues involving sexually transmitted diseases. HIV is sexually transmitted, but consent in this case involves far weightier issues than consent for the treatment of gonorrhea. Can an adolescent refuse the physician permission to disclose his or her HIV infection to the parents? Is such a refusal legally binding? Can the adolescent consent to treatment with an experimental, highly toxic drug? These are the issues needing further clarification. Finally, most current HIV-treatment protocols are for individuals over the age of 18 or for young children. Adolescents have been excluded in part because there are not enough of them in any one location to make a valid series, in part because of the issues mentioned previously, and in part because of the resultant increased liability for these decisions. It is urgent that we address the adolescent issues in our country and in our communities.

MANAGEMENT

The principal management issues are listed in Table 27–5. Management must be interdisciplinary; these children have social and emotional problems of extraordinary complexity in addition to their medical problems. Many have parents who are dead, ill, or unable to function by virtue of disease or drug addiction. Many need foster care; thus they are involved with both the social service system and the juvenile justice system.[34]

Physicians cannot and should not try to manage these children without an appropriate team. Many of these children are poor, and access to care is a problem. The state of California has made an enlightened decision: medical care for all babies of HIV-positive mothers is paid for by entitlement through California Children Services. This ensures that financing and case management of the early and difficult period when it is not clear whether the infant is infected will be paid for, as will the care of the symptomatic child with AIDS. These children may receive their care from physicians around the state but **must** be seen in consultation in approved pediatric centers capable of dealing with this infection. This scheme also ensures that children will have access to treatment protocols as they develop.

HIV-infected children need diligent **primary care.** Minor symptoms can be signs of serious, even life-threatening infections. Febrile episodes must be taken seriously. Cough may be the first manifestation of serious pulmonary disease. Nutrition is important; every effort must be made to supply adequate calories and proteins.

Timely immunization is also important (Table 27–6). Current recommendations call for the use of the normal immunization schedule (DPT, MMR, HbCV) with the single exception that killed polio vaccine (Salk) is recommended instead of the live attenuated product (Sabin),[3,19] since the recipient and other family members might be immunocompromised by virtue of their HIV infections and thus susceptible to paralysis by the attenuated vaccine strain. For the same reason, the other children in the household should also not receive live attenuated polio vaccine. These children should receive conjugated *H. influenzae* vaccine. Immunizations with pneumococcal polysaccharide vaccine should also be considered; unfortunately, administering this vaccine is not possible before the age of 24 months at the present time. Finally, children over 6 months of age should be immunized with the appropriate influenza vaccine.

Children who are known or suspected of being HIV-infected must have a supportive and knowledgeable primary care physician in addition to close supervision at a recognized pediatric HIV center. Most such centers have a protocol detailing

Table 27–5.   Management of an HIV-Infected Child

Access to care
Continued health supervision
Vigorous therapy of common pediatric infections
Aggressive and early therapy of opportunistic infection
Immunization
Attention to caloric intake
Provision of an opportunity for social and emotional development
Prevention of *Pneumocystis carinii* infection (prophylactic therapy)
Prevention of common infections (intravenous immunoglobulin)
Antiretroviral therapy

Table 27–6. Recommendations for Routine Immunization of HIV-Infected Children

VACCINE	AGE
Diphtheria, tetanus, pertussis (DTP)	Routine schedule
Inactivated polio vaccine (IPV)	Routine schedule
Measles, mumps, rubella, live attenuated (MMR)	15 mo
Conjugated *Haemophilus influenzae* type b vaccine (HbCV)	2 mo
Pneumococcal polysaccharide vaccine	24 mo
Influenza vaccine	6 mo

Modified from American Academy of Pediatrics Report of Committee on Infectious Diseases.

the different physical and laboratory evaluations to perform at different ages. An example of such a protocol can be found in the guidelines of the New York Health Department.[25]

Management of Bacterial Infections

Unlike adults, HIV-infected children are subject to frequent and serious bacterial infections (encapsulated bacteria and *Salmonella* are particularly common), usually involving common microbial pathogens; these infections often occur before the first opportunistic infection and may be the early manifestation of clinical AIDS. Such bacterial infections must be treated promptly, preferably by using bactericidal antimicrobials and ensuring compliance with oral medications (see Chapter 22).

In an attempt to prevent such bacterial infections, a number of investigators and clinicians have administered monthly intravenous immunoglobulin. A recently published multicenter study[26] concluded that the use of 400 mg/kg of intravenous immunoglobulin on a monthly basis in symptomatic HIV-infected children significantly increased the time free from bacterial infections for those entering treatment with CD4+ lymphocyte counts $>0.2 \times 10^9/L$.

Management of Opportunistic Infections

The two principal opportunistic infections affecting children are *P. carinii* pneumonia and candidal infections; however, the entire spectrum of such infections affecting adults has been seen in children. The medications and approaches to therapy in children are similar to those used in adults.[15,35] The most common clinical problem is the presentation of a child with pulmonary infiltrates. This clinical situation presents the physician with a broad differential: *Pneumocystis* pneumonia, LIP, or bacterial or viral or mycobacterial infection. Radiologic appearance of the lungs is often helpful but not foolproof. Rapid clinical onset with cough and rapidly developing hypoxia suggest *Pneumocystis* pneumonia, and specific diagnosis and early therapy for this infection are urgent because of the rapid progression of the disease[11] (see Chapter 17). Bronchoscopy and bronchoalveolar lavage with examination of the stained specimens usually provide the best approach. Therapy includes the use of trimethoprim-sulfamethoxazole, 20 mg TMP and 100 mg SMX/kg/day,

**Table 27–7. Pediatric Guidelines for
P. carinii Pneumonia Prophylaxis**

All infected children with documented previous episode of PCP.
Seropositive infants (indeterminate infection) 1-12 mo of age with CD4 count <1500/mm^3
All infected children with the following:
  1-12 mo of age with CD4 count <1500/mm^3
  12-24 mo of age with CD4 count <750/mm^3
  24-72 mo of age with CD4 count <500/mm^3
  Over 6 years of age with CD4 count <200/mm^3

divided into four doses orally or intravenously, whichever is appropriate, for 14 to 21 days; or pentamidine isethionate, 4 mg base/kg/day intravenously for 14 days. Corticosteroids have been used with success as adjunctive therapy in HIV-infected adults with moderate to severe PCP. There is insufficient data to decide on the use of this therapy in younger children and infants. A recent survey of practitioners favored the use of methylprednisolone in a dose of 0.5 to 1 mg/kg given intravenously every 6 to 12 hours for 5 to 14 days in patients with severe disease.[21]

PCP prophylaxis is of particular concern in very young infants because PCP has been reported often in infants younger than 2 years with CD4 counts as high as 1500/mm^3.[22] It is often the first clinical presentation of HIV infection in infants. For these reasons recent CDC guidelines suggest a more aggressive approach for prophylaxis[9] (Table 27–7). In some instances this form of management will result in placement of a child on prophylaxis before the presence of HIV infection has been diagnosed with certainty. The standard drug is trimethoprim-sulfamethoxazole, 150 mg/m^2/day of trimethoprim and 750 mg/m^2 of sulfamethoxazole, given orally once or twice a day for 3 consecutive days of each week. Alternate prophylactic regimens include aerosolized or parenteral pentamidine or oral dapsone (see Chapter 17).

The use of antiviral, antifungal, and antimycobacterial agents is described elsewhere in this volume.

LIP need not be treated unless it interferes with ventilation and oxygenation. If it does, other causes of pulmonary pathology must be excluded first. The current approach to treating LIP is to use glucocorticoids[26]; unfortunately, there are no controlled treatment trials for guidance in determining optimum dosage or duration of therapy.

ANTIRETROVIRAL THERAPY

Zidovudine (AZT, azidothimidine, marketed as Retrovir) was released by the U.S. Food and Drug Administration for use in adult patients in 1987 and is in widespread use today (see Chapter 7). Experimental use of zidovudine in children has lagged far behind adult usage. In October 1989 zidovudine was approved for the treatment of children outside of research protocols. The preliminary results of several uncontrolled studies using oral doses of 180 mg/m^2 every 6 hours (roughly equivalent to 200 mg every 4 hours in adults) showed improvements in both virologic and immunologic parameters and in the clinical status of infected children.[24]

Pizzo et al.,[33] at the National Cancer Institute, performed a particularly interesting study. They treated a group of children with a constant intravenous infusion of zidovudine (0.9 to 1.4 mg/kg/hour). The analysis of the study showed that the patients had significant and occasionally sustained improvement in their encephalopathy. Many of these children also showed significant improvement in their intelligence quotient scores.

Current AIDS Clinical Trial Group (ACTG) protocols are designed to compare the efficacy and toxicity of oral zidovudine at 90 versus 180 mg/m² four times daily.[36] There are no controlled studies or firm recommendations about when to begin zidovudine therapy in infants and children. A recent poll indicated that many clinicians initiate zidovudine therapy in infants and children who have symptomatic HIV infection (class P-2) and in asymptomatic children whose CD4 count is less than 500/mm³. We strongly recommend that every physician encourage each patient to enroll in one of the many available ACTG protocols so that answers to some of the current issues can be forthcoming. A particularly interesting current protocol offers zidovudine (or placebo) to HIV-infected pregnant women to see if vertical transmission can be interrupted.[36] Information about available protocols and enrollment can be obtained by calling the AIDS Clinical Trial Information Service (1-800-TRIALS A) or by calling a regional pediatric ACTG (see reference 36 for a list of regional centers).

Zidovudine is available in a 10 mg/ml, raspberry flavored, well-tolerated syrup. It has significant hematologic toxicity, requiring periodic blood counts (every 2 weeks at first, then monthly). Dosage reduction may be necessary because of anemia or neutropenia. Whether the addition of erythropoietin or granulocyte colony-stimulating factor will ameliorate bone marrow toxicity has not yet been determined.

Both dideoxyinosine (ddI, didanosine, Videx) and dideoxycytidine (ddC, HIV-CID) have completed phase I and II testing in pediatric patients.[8,30,32] The former has been licensed for use in children. A recently completed study showed that ddI used in symptomatic children in the dose of 60 to 540 mg/m²/day orally given every 8 hours produced results similar to those with zidovudine. Ongoing randomized trials use dosages of 100 to 300 mg/m²/day divided into three doses. Videx is now available as chewable dispersible tablets or as a pediatric powder to make into oral solution. No neuropathy was observed in this study, but pancreatitis did occur when higher doses were used. Antacids are now used routinely with oral ddI.

DdI and ddc, alone or in combination with zidovudine, must be tested to establish optimum regimens for use in children.

SOCIAL-SOCIETAL ISSUES

The importance of general supportive care for the HIV-infected child has already been emphasized. Such support systems must be extended beyond strict health matters. Access to health care, both financially and geographically, has been discussed. Many infected children require foster care because of parental inability to provide the needed care. Arrangements for foster care normally are left to departments of social services. However, in the case of HIV-infected children real teamwork is needed between the health and social services components. Prospective foster parents must be recruited, supported with continued in-service training, provided access to a health professional, and given higher compensation and a smaller number of children for which to care than foster parents normally receive. Permission for testing and for experimental drug regimens must be obtained from Juvenile Courts.[40]

Many infected children would benefit from the stimulation they are likely to receive in a day care center. The concern about placing these children in day care is their over-exposure to many infections, both gastrointestinal and respiratory, that tend to spread when children in diapers are commingled.[2] There is no concern about spreading HIV infection since such horizontal spread by casual contact has not been demonstrated.[42] Thus the decision about day care should be made about each child individually, balancing the gain of stimulation against the risk of acquired nosocomial infection.

Early in the epidemic the CDC stated that children with AIDS would benefit by normal classroom schooling and that they did not pose a hazard to their classmates.[13] Although initially controversial, this position has been widely accepted. The reality is that few children with vertically transmitted infection will live long enough to go to school; those whose infection was transmitted through blood products encompass youngsters of all ages, but they will be an ever-diminishing number.

One very high-risk group for acquiring HIV infection consists of runaway adolescents who live on the street and often subsist by engaging in prostitution. This group of teens has very few support systems. They are usually school dropouts and have severed their family connections. We need to plan the care of this group of youngsters, some of whom inevitably will develop AIDS.

The key to preventing further spread of HIV transmission is education, and this education needs to begin during childhood. Age and culturally appropriate curricula have been designed and currently are in use in many communities. It is our obligation to see to it that the communities in which we live and practice incorporate the education of youth in their community AIDS planning.

REFERENCES

1. Amadori A et al: Diagnosis of human immunodeficiency virus infection in infants; In vitro production of virus specific antibody in lymphocytes. Pediatr Infect Dis J 9:26, 1990
2. American Academy of Pediatrics Committee on Infectious Disease: Health guidelines for the attendance in day care and foster care settings of children infected with human immunodeficiency virus. Pediatrics 79:466-471, 1987
3. American Academy of Pediatrics Report of Commitee on Infectious Disease 1991. Elk Grove Village, Ill.
4. Barbacci M, Quinn T, Kline R, et al: Failure of targeted screening to identify pregnant women. Johns Hopkins University. Fifth International Conference of AIDS. (Abstract MBP5.) Montreal, June 1989
5. Belman A, Diamond G, Dickson D, et al: Pediatric acquired immunodeficiency syndrome: Neurologic syndrome. Am J Dis Child 142:29-35, 1988
6. Blanche S, Ramzioux C, Muscato M-LG, et al: A prospective study of infants born to women seropositive for human immunodeficiency virus type 1. N Engl J Med 320:1643-1648, 1989
7. Brouwers P, Belman AL, Epstein LG: Central nervous system involvement. In Pizzo PA, Wilfert CM: Pediatric AIDS. Baltimore, Williams & Wilkins, 1991, pp 318-338
8. Butler KM, Husson RN, Balis FM, et al: Dideoxyinosine in children with symptomatic human immunodeficiency virus infection. N Engl J Med 324:137-144, 1991
9. Centers for Disease Control: Guidelines for prophylaxis against *Pneumocystis carinii* pneumonia for children infected with human immunodeficiency virus. JAMA 256:1637-1644, 1991

10. Classification system for human immunodeficiency virus (HIV) infection in children under 13 years of age. MMWR 36:225-236, 1987
11. Connor E, Bagarazzi M, McShery G, et al: Clinical and laboratory correlates of *Pneumocystis carinii* pneumonia in children infected with HIV. JAMA 365:13, 1693-1697, 1991
12. D'Angelo LJ, Getson PR, Luban NLC, Gayle MD: Human immunodeficiency virus in urban adolescents: Can we predict who is at risk. Pediatrics 88:982-986, 1991
13. Education and foster care of children infected with human T lymphotropic virus type III. MMWR 34:521, 1985
14. European Collaborative Study: Children born to women with HIV-1 infection: Natural history and risk of transmission. Lancet 337:8736, 254-260, 1991
15. Falloon J, Eddy T, Wiener L, Pizzo P: Human immunodeficiency virus infection in children. J Pediatr 114:1-30, 1989
16. Goetz DW, Hall SE, Harbinson RW, Reid MJ: Pediatric acquired immunodeficiency syndrome with negative human immunodeficiency virus antibody response by enzyme-linked immuno-sorbent assay and Western blot. Pediatrics 81:356-359, 1988
17. Hein K: Risky business: Adolescents and human immunodeficiency virus. Pediatrics 88:1052-1054, 1991
18. Hutto C, Parks WP, Lai S, Mastrucci MT, et al: A hospital-based prospective study of perinatal infection with human immunodeficiency virus type 1. J Pediatr 118:3, 347-353, 1991
19. Immunization of children infected with human immunodeficiency virus: Supplementary ACIP statement. MMWR 37:181-183, 1988
20. Johnson JP, Nair P, Hines SE, et al: Natural history and serologic diagnosis of infants born to HIV infected women. Am J Dis Child 143:1147-1153, 1989
21. Kline M, Shearer WT: A national survey on the care of infants and children with HIV infection. J Pediatr 118:817-821, 1991
22. Kovacs A, Frederic T, Church J, et al: CD4 T-lymphocyte counts and *Pneumocystis carinii* pneumonia in pediatric HIV infection. JAMA 265:13, 1698-1703, 1991
23. Martin NL, Levy JA, Legg H, et al: Detection of infection with human immunodeficiency virus (HIV) type 1 in infants by an anti-HIV immunoglobulin A assay using recombinant proteins. J Pediatr 118:3, 354-358, 1991
24. McKinney RE, Maha MA, Connor EM, et al: A multicenter trial of oral zidovudine in children with advanced immunodeficiency virus disease. N Engl J Med 324:15, 1018-1025, 1991
25. Mendez H: Ambulatory care of HIV seropositive infants and children. J Pediatr 119:514-517, 1991
26. National Institute of Child Health and Human Development Intravenous Immunoglobulin Study Group: Intravenous immunoglobulin for the preventing of bacterial infections in children with symptomatic human immunodeficiency virus infection. N Engl J Med 325:73-90, 1991
27. Oxtoby MJ: Human immunodeficiency virus and other viruses in human milk: Placing the issue in broader perspective. Pediatr Infect Dis J 7:825-835, 1988
28. Oxtoby MJ: Perinatally acquired human immunodeficiency virus infection. Pediatr Infect Dis J 9:609, 1990
29. Pizzo PA: Pediatric AIDS: Problems within problems. J Infect Dis 161:316-325, 1990
30. Pizzo PA: Treatment of HIV infected infants and young children with dideoxynucleosides. Am J Med 88:5B-165, 1990
31. Pizzo PA, Butler KM: In the vertical transmission of HIV, timing may be everything. N Engl J Med 325-329, 652-654, 1991
32. Pizzo P, Butler K, Balis F, et al: Dideoxycytidine alone and in an alternating schedule with zidovudine in children with symptomatic human immunodeficiency virus infection. J Pediatr 117:799-808, 1990
33. Pizzo PA, Eddy J, Fallon J, et al: Effect of continuous intravenous infusion of zidovudine (AZT) in children with symptomatic HIV infection. N Engl J Med 319:889-896, 1988
34. Pizzo PA, Wilfert CM: Treatment considerations for children with human immunodeficiency virus infection. Pediatr Infect Dis J 9:690, 1990
35. Prevention of perinatal transmission of hepatitis B virus: Prenatal screening of all pregnant women for hepatitis B surface antigen. MMWR 37:341-346, 1988
36. Prober CG, Gershon AA: Management of newborns and infants born to HIV seropositive mothers. Pediatr Infect Dis J 10:684-695, 1991
37. Revision of the CDC surveillance case definition for acquired immunodeficiency syndrome. MMWR 36:15-155, 1987

38. Rogers MF, Chin-Yih DV, Kilbourne B, Schochetman G: Advances and problems in the diagnosis of human immunodeficiency virus infection in children. Pediatr Infect Dis J 10:523-531, 1991

39. Rogers MF, Ou C-Y, Rayfield M, et al: Use of polymerase chain reaction for early detection of proviral sequences of HIV in infants born to seropositive mothers. N Engl J Med 320:1649-1654, 1989

40. Rutherford GW, Oliva GE, Grossman M, et al: Guidelines for the control of perinatally transmitted HIV infection and care of infected mothers, infants and children. West J Med 147:104, 1987

41. Ryder RW, Nsa W, Hassig SE: Perinatal transmission of the human immunodeficiency virus type I to infants of seropositive mothers in Zaire. N Engl J Med 320:1637-1642, 1989

42. Sande MA: Transmission of AIDS: The case against casual contagion. N Engl J Med 314:380-382, 1986

43. Senturia YD, Peckham CS, Ades AE: Seronegativity and paediatric AIDS. Lancet 1:1151-1152, 1987

44. Van de Perre P, Simonon A, Msellati P, et al: Postnatal transmission of human immunodeficiency virus type-1 from mother to infant. N Engl J Med 325:9, 593-598, 1991

28

THERAPEUTIC ISSUES IN WOMEN WITH HIV DISEASE

CONSTANCE B. WOFSY, MD

Women constitute the fastest growing population of persons with AIDS in the United States, with 11% of all reported cases of AIDS in adults occurring in women.[7] Overall, 50% of women have contracted AIDS from their own personal intravenous (IV) drug use, 18% from sex with an IV drug user, 11% from heterosexual transmission, and 10% from transfusion and other blood products, and 11% remain unidentified or not fully evaluated. Thus IV drug use directly or indirectly accounts for a minimum of 68% of HIV in women, with implications for intervention and drug treatment.[1,8] Currently in the United States there are approximately 18,000 women with AIDS and an estimated 140,000 who are HIV infected.[37] Of those with AIDS, 74% are black and Hispanic. The same population has a very high incidence of sexually transmitted diseases, including syphilis (especially congenital syphilis), and high rates of tuberculosis, which raises the specter of the multidrug-resistant tuberculosis now seen sporadically in metropolitan cities on the eastern seaboard of the United States and in the prison system of New York City.[9] AIDS is the fifth leading cause of death in women nationally and is the leading cause of death in women of child-bearing age in New York City.[12] Heterosexual transmission is the fastest growing risk group nationally, increasing from 3% of all AIDS cases among women in 1983 to 1984 to 16% in 1989 to 1990.[3] Reports suggest that within the heterosexual transmission group, up to 50% did not know that they had been exposed to HIV even when closely questioned.[7,27] HIV could be isolated from 30% of semen specimens from HIV-infected men with early disease, and zidovudine did not affect sperm morphology or seminal characteristics.[25] Transmission of HIV occurs increasingly in the general population of women and does not provide a point focus on which to target outreach and intervention measures such as those instituted for groups with specific behaviors in common such as IV drug use or homosexuality.

Among HIV discordant couples (those with only a single HIV-positive partner), heterosexual transmission is more efficient from male to female, and most infections have occurred by the vaginal route, although rectal sex is associated with increased risk.[39] The cumulative incidence of transmission between discordant couples sug-

Table 28–1.   Factors Associated with Heterosexual Transmission of HIV

FACTOR	MALE TO FEMALE	FEMALE TO MALE
Lack of condom	Yes	Yes
Anal intercourse	Yes	No
Sex during menses	No	Yes
Number of sexual contacts	Yes	Yes
Advanced disease state*	Yes	Yes
Zidovudine decreases risk	Possibly	Unknown
Genital sores, infections, or inflammation	Yes	Yes
Oral contraceptives†	Yes	Unknown
Intrauterine contraceptive device (IUD) use	Possibly	Unknown

Modified from Padian N: Epidemiology of AIDS and heterosexually transmitted HIV in women. AIDS File 5:1-2, 1991.
*As measured by CD4, p24 antigen, or AIDS diagnosis.
†Whether oral contraceptives are protective or increase the likelihood of transmission is controversial.

gests a 20% risk of transmission from male to female after unprotected sex over a sustained period in a fixed partnership; other studies suggest a range of 7% to 50%. Female-to-male transmission is less efficient; a recent study showed only one out of 72 male partners of HIV-infected females became infected.[40] Other studies have suggested a nearly equal efficiency of transmission between men and women. Factors associated with increased transmission include lack of condom use, anal intercourse, number of contacts, advanced disease state (measured by CD4 and p24 antigen or AIDS diagnosis), genital ulcerative disease and other sexually transmitted diseases, and intrauterine contraceptive device (IUD) use[21,38,41] (Table 28–1). A recent African study suggests cervical ectopy is associated with risk of acquisition; this is of particular note since this condition is seen with greatest frequency in the extremes of age, particularly adolescence.[33] The prevalence of HIV in adolescent 16- and 17-year-old women Job Corps applicants is 2.3 per 1000 compared to 1.5 per 1000 in males and among black and Hispanic students from large Northeast cities; seroprevalence reached 24.8 per 1000 by 21 years of age.[46] Sexually transmitted disease, HIV, and crack cocaine are indelibly associated.[19,34]

CLINICAL MANIFESTATIONS

Opportunistic Infections and HIV-Associated Infections

By the current Centers for Disease Control (CDC) definition of AIDS, *Pneumocystis* remains the leading AIDS-defining diagnosis in women.[37] Lack of access to care, minimal self-motivation, attention to the health care of the child in favor of committed self-care, and the large proportion of disenfranchised women all contribute to less early detection and intervention and probably a concomitant sustained high frequency of *Pneumocystis*. AIDS-defining diagnoses seen with particular frequency from data combined from a number of small cohorts are *Pneu-*

mocystis carinii pneumonia, esophageal Candida, disseminated Mycobacterium avium, and mucocutaneous herpes simplex virus. Women are not protected from any of the other AIDS-defining opportunistic infections. Bacterial infections, especially respiratory infections with encapsulated organisms such as Diplococcus pneumoniae and Haemophilus influenzae, occur more frequently in IV drug users than in homosexual men.[49]

In a cohort of 200 HIV-infected Rhode Island women followed at regular intervals, the initial clinical manifestation of HIV infection in 117 symptomatic women were Candida vaginitis (n = 43), lymphadenopathy (n = 17), bacterial pneumonia (n = 15), acute retroviral syndrome (n = 8), and constitutional symptoms such as unexplained weight loss of 10 pounds or more or diarrhea for 4 weeks or more (n = 8). The remainder had syndromes that would suggest to most clinicians a consideration of HIV infection (i.e., thrush, tuberculosis, hairy leukoplakia, herpes zoster, P. carinii pneumonia [PCP], AIDS encephalopathy, and cytomegalovirus [CMV] retinitis).[5] The more frequent nonspecific presentations of vaginitis pneumonia and constitutional symptoms of retroviral syndrome or AIDS-related complex (ARC) would not suggest to any other than the most alert clinician the possibility of HIV disease. In a review of AIDS in women reported to the CDC by December 1990, 73% of women with AIDS were residents of large metropolitan areas of over 1 million population, mostly on the Atlantic seaboard, suggesting a target for interventions; the other 26% were from smaller cities, making it harder to target a specific population.[16]

Factors that may influence the presentation or response to therapy include pharmacokinetics of drugs, due either to gender or interference with commonly associated drugs such as methadone or oral contraceptive pills, and possible differences in the immune system since autoimmune diseases are traditionally more frequent in women than in men. To date, gender-specific immunologic abnormalities have not been identified. Early symptoms of HIV in women, as in men, are extremely nonspecific, including night sweats, diarrhea, yeast infection, cough, and weight loss.[16] Since women frequently use emergency rooms, family planning clinics, sexually transmitted disease clinics, youth guidance centers, jail clinic facilities, and drug treatment units, these are the sites at which to target efforts at early diagnosis and use of early intervention with antiviral and prophylactic therapies.

Malignancies (see Chapter 25)

Kaposi's sarcoma, seen frequently in homosexual men, is found in less than 2% of HIV-infected women as an initial AIDS diagnosis and occurs infrequently in heterosexual men. There may be a sexually transmitted cofactor associated with angiogenesis,[2] and when Kaposi's sarcoma has been seen in women, it has been associated with sex with a bisexual man.[39] Non-Hodgkin's lymphoma, an AIDS-defining diagnosis, is too infrequently encountered in women to judge whether it is more or less frequent in HIV-infected women or men[20]; however, it does constitute an AIDS-defining diagnosis in either group. Growing evidence suggests increased occurrence and aggressiveness of cervical cancer. To date, increased frequency of breast cancer, lung cancer, or other malignancies is not seen as compared to occurrence in the general population.

Gynecologic Manifestations

Much attention has been given to three disorders that may be more frequent, more severe, and less responsive to therapy in HIV-infected women, particularly those with advanced immunosuppression, than in HIV-uninfected women.[11,17,28,29] They are human papilloma virus, vaginal warts, and associated cervical disorders such as CIN II and III, *Candida* vaginitis, and pelvic inflammatory disease.

Cervical Disorders

An increased frequency of abnormal Papanicolaou (PAP) smear results has been noted in women attending HIV, methadone maintenance, and cervical dysplasia clinics, but well-conducted prospective trials with appropriate controls have not been undertaken.[7,11,17] In one study 40% of 35 HIV-positive women had squamous intraepithelial lesions on cervical cytology compared with 9% of 32 HIV-negative women.[17] Of additional concern is the potential inadequacy of a PAP smear as routine screening measure in women with HIV. In a study of 32 HIV-infected women, 78% had a normal PAP smear result, with 3% having cytologic findings suggesting cervical intraepithelial neoplasia. However, colposcopy associated with biopsy disclosed that 41% had cervical abnormalities.[29] This discovery has profound implications since colposcopy is more time consuming and requires highly trained personnel because the interpretation of the associated staining of the cervix can be very subjective and is not subject to simple standardization. Cervical neoplasia is also more likely with an advanced stage of immunosuppression.[28,29] All women are advised to have a pelvic examination and PAP smear yearly, and the CDC has applied the same guidelines for HIV-infected women with normal cervical cytology. Because CIN is more frequent and more aggressive in women with severe immunosuppression, a PAP smear may be recommended every 6 months, particularly for women with more advanced immunodeficiency.[11,30] Although colposcopy would be the most sensitive and specific diagnostic tool, the general lack of availability and standardization suggests that assiduous attention to appropriate PAP smear tests and follow-up comprises the most relevant approach available at this time. The recognition of the enhanced sensitivity of colposcopy may make it more widely used in the future.

Vaginal Candida

Vaginal candidiasis is a frequent disorder in women and is especially prevalent in HIV-infected women,[5,23,42] and with the next CDC definition revision it is expected to become a designated HIV-associated symptomatic disorder.[10] Although there have been no prospective controlled trials, a study in a large cohort of HIV-infected women in Rhode Island showed that *Candida* vaginitis in HIV-infected women developed when only mild immunosuppression was present.[23] Women with HIV and vaginal *Candida* had a mean CD4 count of 506 in contrast to those with esophageal *Candida* from the same population in whom the mean CD4 count was 30. *Candida* vaginitis occurred in 44 of 200 prospectively followed, HIV-infected women and, in fact, was the most frequent symptomatic disorder that first heralded a change in health and early HIV disease in this population. Strikingly, in no instance did new, recurrent, or more refractory *Candida* prompt the initial examining physician to evaluate or offer HIV testing.[23]

Response of vaginal *Candida* to therapy using topical antifungals such as clotrimazole (Gyne-Lotrimin) is usually very good. Since this preparation is available over the counter, it is important to provide the information that new and unexpected or more frequent or more refractory *Candida* in the absence of antibiotics should prompt affected women and their clinicians to consider HIV testing. For more refractory cases the use of ketoconazole (400 mg/day for 14 days, followed by 5-day courses each month for 6 months, with monitoring of liver function tests) or for most refractory cases, fluconazole, can be extremely effective[30]; however, both are substantially more expensive than topical therapy and require a doctor's prescription. Physicians seeing women with recurrent or refractory vaginal candidiasis should offer HIV counseling and testing.

Genital Ulcerative Disease and Pelvic Inflammatory Disease

Severe ulcerative genital herpes was the AIDS-defining diagnosis in 18% of 44 women prospectively followed who developed AIDS.[5] Genital herpes simplex virus infections are very prevalent in the population at large and may be particularly refractory in HIV-infected men and women. Recommended treatment is an initial course of acyclovir of 200 mg 5 times per day for 10 days and with suppression a course of 400 mg b.i.d. for those who have more than six outbreaks a year. Infrequent acyclovir-resistant herpes has been reported in severely immunocompromised persons with severe genital ulcer disease.[28] Although these infections may respond to foscarnet, the therapy may be teratogenic and should be avoided in HIV-infected pregnant women.[43] Genital ulcerative disease is a well-described risk factor for transmission of HIV, particularly in studies in Africa where sexually transmitted diseases are more prevalent.[21] HIV is prevalent in women with pelvic inflammatory disease (PID), and there are inferences that PID is more prevalent and may be more severe with advanced HIV disease. There are no prospective studies, and treatment guidelines would not differ; however, close surveillance is necessary.[22,44]

Menstrual Disorders

Anecdotal reports suggest that menstrual disorders are seen with greater frequency in HIV-infected women. A New York study of IV drug-using women compared 39 HIV-positive women to 39 HIV-negative women and identified more menstrual abnormalities in the HIV-positive ones—41% versus 24% in the negative ones.[48] Amenorrhea and between-period bleeding were noted particularly; however, further documentation of the specific types of menstrual irregularity, the frequency, and the gynecologic hormone interaction is needed. These disorders are relevant not only for personal discomfort but also because they indicate unsuspected pregnancy masquerading as delayed periods or amenorrhea because of the teratogenicity of therapies of early intervention and treatment of opportunistic infections. Menstrual irregularities make prediction of time of fertility difficult for those wishing to conceive or avoid pregnancy and allow for the potential increased exposure to menstrual blood for a partner.

Progression of Disease

Studies of disease progression in women are limited and when available, are derived from three principle sources: large national data bases, which usually include the diagnosis of AIDS and the date of death with little additional interval information; small-to-moderate sized cohort studies of 50 to 200 women, often followed less than 3 years; and large cohort studies conducted in other regions (e.g., Africa) from which the inferences, because economic, sociologic, and medical and public health conditions there differ so much from those in the United States, may not be applicable to the United States or Western Europe. Reports from the CDC suggest that survival time of women and heterosexual men is similar. Studies of cohorts in other cities suggest shortened survival time for women. A recent study of survival time in San Francisco, California, suggests it is similar in men and women receiving HIV antiretroviral therapy, but in those not receiving antiretroviral therapy, men survived longer than women. In the Bronx, New York, impact of access to or adherence to follow-up care strongly influenced survival time, with it substantially shortened in women who had no prior care before a severe HIV-related infection.[1,4,5]

GUIDELINES FOR TREATMENT OF HIV AND ASSOCIATED ILLNESSES IN WOMEN

Guidelines established for now-licensed antiretroviral therapies, specifically zidovudine (AZT) and dideoxyinosine (ddI), and prophylaxis against PCP are derived from large national studies conducted on men and women. Although men predominate in these studies, the results of these studies led to licensure and now establish recommendations for persons of both genders. Data on two large national studies from the AIDS Clinical Trials Group (ACTG 016 and 019) comparing zidovudine versus placebo in mildly symptomatic HIV-infected patients and AIDS in ACTG 016 and asymptomatic HIV-infected persons in ACTG 019 have recently been analyzed and suggest no difference in benefit from zidovudine for women or for persons of color.[15,18,26,47]

In the absence of data to the contrary, women, like men, are advised to take zidovudine (500 to 600 mg/day) when CD4 counts fall below $500/mm^3$ and to start prophylaxis for PCP when CD4 count falls below $200/mm^3$, particularly in those women with ancillary symptoms such as fever, hairy leukoplakia, and thrush. Potential issues affecting treatment with antiretrovirals or PCP prophylaxis include the lower mean body weight in women, lower mean hemoglobin level, with the potentially complicating effect of zidovudine or dapsone in further inducing anemia, and absence of established controls for CD4 counts in men versus women. The more recently licensed antiretroviral, ddI, has been evaluated using even smaller numbers of patients (see Chapter 7). The most frequent toxicities of ddI or the not-yet-licensed ddC are rash, pancreatitis, peripheral neuropathy, and diarrhea. None of these toxicities has a predictable or obvious female-related toxicity.

Tuberculosis, bacterial endocarditis, and sepsis are seen more frequently in IV drug users. Treatment guidelines do not differ by gender, and the clinical presentation is not expected to have gender-related differences exclusive of infection of the reproductive organs. A drug-related interference in individuals taking both rifampin and methadone replacement is frequently encountered. Rifampin alters the metabolism of many drugs, including methadone, and can result in wide swings of dose requirement in someone who may previously have been on a well-established methadone program. The issue of treatment is doubly compounded by the high prevalence of infection and large numbers of uninsured persons receiving care at municipal hospitals in large metropolitan cities, with an increasingly reluctant and exhausted population of care providers. New York City has recently experienced a 28.2% decline in matches of U.S. graduating medical students and residency programs.[16,35]

Treatment of HIV Disease and Opportunistic Infections in Pregnancy

Early studies suggested an adverse effect of pregnancy on progression of HIV disease. More recently small studies reported in abstracts from cities in the United States and Europe suggest no difference in progression or immunologic state or clinical end points after 2 to 3 years; however, immunosuppressed pregnant women are at risk for serious infections, especially pneumonias, bacterial and *Pneumocystis*.[4,5,32] Women IV drug users at a methadone clinic had a mean of 2.5% live births, and 60% had had an abortion.[45] When pregnancy termination choices were examined in 28 HIV-infected pregnant women compared to 36 HIV-seronegative women, all of whom were in drug treatment, 50% and 44%, respectively, chose abortion, and their choice was dictated by previous experience with abortion, not by their HIV infection or other factors.[6]

Zidovudine

The package insert included with zidovudine places it in pregnancy category C, with the description "Animal studies demonstrate fetal risk but there are no human trials and neither human nor animal studies are available." The recommendation further states that "it is not known whether zidovudine can cause fetal harm when administered to a pregnant woman or can affect reproductive capacity. Zidovudine should be given to pregnant women only if clearly needed." To aid in evaluating the fetal risk from zidovudine, a registry of women who have by choice or inadvertently received zidovudine during pregnancy is kept by the drug manufacturers. To date, no specific adverse effect to mother or child[17] has been reported. Pharmacologic studies in humans do not suggest excessive accumulation of zidovudine in the placenta or fetal tissue and obstetric and gynecologic specialists in HIV now strongly recommend zidovudine therapy for women with fewer than 200 CD4 cells, and many recommend zidovudine for those with 200 to 500 CD4 cells, although there are regional differences of opinion in attempting to balance the issue of maternal benefit and potential fetal risk. When prescribed, doses are the same as for nongravid women.[30]

Prophylaxis for Pneumocystis carinii *Pneumonia*

No prophylactic therapies have been endorsed or approved by the Food and Drug Administration (FDA) for use in pregnancy. However, based on past therapies and the growing body of community practice dictated by necessity, trimethoprim (TMP)-sulfamethoxazole (SMX) has become the standard PCP prophylactic regimen used in pregnancy.[30,31] Although conventional dictum suggests that TMP-SMX therapy should be avoided in the third trimester of pregnancy because of kernicterus, cases of this complication have not been reported, and TMP-SMX can be used through delivery in those women who can tolerate it.[30,31] Dapsone has been used in pregnancy in women who have dermatitis herpetiformis and leprosy, conditions which necessitate daily and long-term therapy with dapsone, without major problems.[24] However, because of the risk of interference with dihydrofolate reductase, dapsone should be used with caution and necessitates obtaining a careful baseline glucose-6-phosphate dehydrogenase level. Aerosol pentamidine has the advantage of little systemic absorption, but evaluation of pulmonary distribution in women with a gravid uterus has not been undertaken. It is less effective than TMP-SMX in clinical trials, and aerosol pentamidine does not protect against extrapulmonary PCP.[36]

PCP may be particularly severe during pregnancy.[30,32] For treatment of active disease, TMP-SMX is the most attractive therapeutic option. IV pentamidine should be avoided, and dapsone should be held in reserve after careful risk to benefit assessment.

Treatment of other opportunistic infections in pregnancy may be particularly problematic.[13] Of 26 therapies for common opportunistic disorders or HIV disease that may occur during pregnancy, no drugs are classified as category A, in which controlled clinical trials in women have demonstrated no fetal risk. The clinician is left with a very difficult professional choice about treatment options, and common sense and inference from animal studies and use of the drug for treatment of other diseases must be incorporated in making such a decision. Data from animal studies may be useful in decision making but should be interpreted with care. Even if extensive anecdotal experience suggests that a drug is well tolerated in the pregnant woman, the decision to use the drug still must be considered on an individual basis. The patient should be informed in as simple terms as possible about the state of knowledge and the best situation tailored to the specific infection that can be made at that time. Table 28–2 indicates the FDA pregnancy category and some very general guidelines for therapy, mostly from anecdotal experience of use of these therapies in serious or life-threatening disease. Although published guidelines in this emerging field are sparse, several excellent reviews address this issue and provide counseling and testing indications for pregnant women.[4,30,50]

Clinical Research and Access to Care

Women currently comprise 11% to 12% of the total AIDS population. In 1990 a group of researchers from the ACTG of the National Institutes of Health noted that 6.7% of clinical trial subjects were women (at a time when women nationally comprised 9.8% of those with AIDS diagnoses).[14] Women most frequently were enrolled in studies of early stage disease in large antiviral trials, which suggests that these studies are more accessible and/or more acceptable to women who may

Table 28–2. Treatment Options During Pregnancy

DRUG	FDA PREGNANCY CATEGORY	USE IN SERIOUS DISEASE*
Acyclovir	C	Yes
Amikacin	D	Avoid in early pregnancy
Amphotericin B	B	Yes
Ciprofloxacin	C	Avoid
Clindamycin	N/A	Yes
Clofazimine	C	No experience
Clotrimazole oral troche	C	Yes
Clotrimazole vaginal suppository or cream	B	Yes
Dapsone	C	Yes
Dideoxycytidine (ddC)	N/A	No experience
Didanosine (ddI)	N/A	No experience
Ethambutol	N/A	Yes
Fluconazole	C	No experience
Ganciclovir	C	No experience
Isoniazid	N/A	Yes
Pentamidine IV	N/A	Avoid in preference to alternative
Pentamidine inhaled	C	Little systemic absorption; no experience
Primaquine	N/A	Avoid
Pyrazinamide (PZA)	N/A	Avoid
Pyrimethamine	C	Possibly
Rifampin	C	Yes
Sulfadiazine	N/A	Yes
Trimethoprim	C	Seldom indicated alone
Trimethoprim-sulfamethoxazole	C	Yes
Zidovudine (AZT)	C	Yes

From Coleman RL: Treatment during pregnancy. AIDS File, 5:6, 1991.
*For life-threatening condition or serious condition.
 Risk categories: N/A, classification not available; A, controlled studies in women demonstrate no risk; B, animal studies demonstrate no fetal risk, but there are no human trials, *or* animal studies demonstrate a risk not corroborated by human trials; C, animal studies demonstrate fetal risk but there are no human trials, *or* neither human nor animal studies are available; D, evidence exists for fetal risk in humans, but benefit may outweigh the risk; E, evidence exists for fetal risk in humans, but benefit is clearly outweighed by risk.

associate access to clinical trials with access to clinical care. Every effort should be undertaken to include substantial numbers of women in upcoming clinical trials and to establish guidelines for enrollment of pregnant women, standard enrollment guidelines, female-specific end points, and guidelines about dose, body weight, and laboratory measurements standardized for women.

REVISED CDC DEFINITION OF AIDS

The CDC has reevaluated the applicability of the original CDC definition of AIDS, which was revised in 1987. The key changes in the definition that are expected to become effective with the next CDC definition revision are that AIDS may be defined either by the existing surveillance definition, using designators of opportunistic infections, malignancies, and constitutional deterioration, or the newly incorporated definition of a CD4 count <200. In addition, there will be three clinical categories: (1) asymptomatic HIV with persistent generalized lymphadenopathy and acute HIV infection; (2) symptomatic conditions, which include several that are particularly prevalent in women, including bacterial endocarditis, meningitis, pneumonia, or sepsis, and constitutional symptoms such as fever >38.5° C or diarrhea lasting longer than 1 month; *Mycobacterium tuberculosis*—pulmonary; and several that relate to the female reproductive tract such as persistent candidiasis vulvovaginal, severe cervical dysplasia or carcinoma, and pelvic inflammatory disease; and (3) infections and malignancies in the 1987 surveillance definitions. Additionally, the issue of disability is expected to be disassociated from the specific CDC definition. Many believe that cervical carcinoma, more frequent and severe in HIV-infected women, should constitute an AIDS-defining diagnosis rather than a symptomatic, HIV-associated condition. It is estimated that its inclusion would increase the number of women meeting the new AIDS surveillance case definition by approximately 50% and that the focus on more nonspecific presentations might stimulate offering of HIV testing and would emphasize the importance of the gynecologic examination.[10]

SUMMARY

The increasing frequency of HIV in women emphasizes the more extensively reviewed issues of epidemiology, transmission, and perinatal infection and opens the next avenues of clinical management of HIV-infected pregnant and non-pregnant women—the pathogenesis, infections, and malignancies of the female reproductive tract, methods of enrolling women in epidemiologic and clinical trials to achieve statistically significant results in end point, mortality, and natural history, and the role of HIV as a sexually transmitted disease in the heterosexual population, particularly among women.

REFERENCES

1. Allen JR, Setlow VP: Heterosexual transmission of HIV—A view of the future (editorial). JAMA 266:1695-1696, 1991
2. Beral V, Peterman TA, Berkelman RL, Jaffe HW: Kaposi's sarcoma among persons with AIDS: A sexually transmitted infection? Lancet 335:123-128, 1990
3. Berkelman R, Fleming P, Chu S, et al: (Abstract W.C. 102.) Women and AIDS: The increasing role of heterosexual transmission in the United States. Seventh International Conference on AIDS. Florence, Italy, June 1991
4. Brettle RP, Leen CLS: The natural history of HIV and AIDS in women. AIDS 5:1283-1292, 1991
5. Carpenter CJ, Mayer KH, Stein MD, et al: Human immunodeficiency virus infection in North American women: Experience with 200 cases and a review of the literature. Medicine 70:307-325, 1991
6. Carter RJ, Schoenbaum EE, Robertson VJ, et al: Knowledge of HIV antibody status and decisions to continue or terminate pregnancy among intravenous drug users. JAMA 3367-3571, 1989
7. Centers for Disease Control: AIDS in women—United States. MMWR 47:845-846, 1990
8. Centers for Disease Control: HIV/AIDS survey. September 1991
9. Centers for Disease Control: Nosocomial transmission of multidrug-resistant tuberculosis among HIV-infected persons—Florida and New York, 1988-1991. MMWR 40:585-591, 1991

10. Centers for Disease Control: 1992 revised classification system for HIV infection and expanded AIDS surveillance case definition for adolescents and adults (draft).

11. Centers for Disease Control: Risk for cervical disease in HIV-infected women, New York City. MMWR 39:826-849, 1990

12. Chu SY, Buehler JW, Berkelman RL: Impact of the human immunodeficiency virus epidemic on mortality in women of reproductive age, United States. JAMA 264:225-229, 1990

13. Coleman R: Treatment during pregnancy. AIDS File 5:6, 1991

14. Cotton D, Feinberg J, Finkelstein D, ACTG SDAC: Participation of women in a multicenter HIV clinical trials program in the United States. (Tu.D. 114.) Seventh International Conference on AIDS. Florence, Italy, June 1991

15. Easterbrook PJ, Keruly JC, Creah-Kirk T, et al: Racial and ethnic differences in outcome in zidovudine-treated patients with advanced HIV disease. JAMA 266:2713-2718, 1991

16. Ellerbrock TV, Bush TJ, Chamberland ME, Oxtoby MJ: Epidemiology of women with AIDS in the United States, 1981 through 1990. JAMA 265:2971-2975, 1991

17. Feingold PR, Vermund SH, Burk RA, et al: Cervical cytologic abnormalities and papilloma virus in women infected with human immunodeficiency virus. J AIDS 3:896-903, 1990

18. Fishl MA, Richman DD, Grieco MH, et al: The efficacy of azidothymidine (AZT) in the treatment of patients with AIDS and AIDS-related complex: A double-blind, placebo-controlled trial. N Engl J Med 317:185-191, 1987

19. Fullilove RE, Fullilove MT, Bowser BP, Gross SA: Risk of sexually transmitted disease among black adolescent crack users in Oakland and San Francisco, Calif. JAMA 263:851-855, 1990

20. Gail MH, Pluda JM, Rabkin CS, et al: Projections of the incidence of non-Hodgkin's lymphoma related to acquired immunodeficiency syndrome. J Natl Cancer Inst 83:695-701, 1991

21. Greenblatt RM, Lukehart SA, Plummer FA, et al: Genital ulceration as a risk factor for human immunodeficiency virus infection. AIDS 2:47-50, 1988

22. Hoegsberg B, Abulafia O, Sedlis A, et al: Sexually transmitted disease and human immunodeficiency virus infection among women with pelvic inflammatory disease. Am J Obstet Gynecol 163:1135-1139, 1990

23. Imam W, Carpenter CJ, Mayer K, et al: Hierarchial pattern of mucosal *Candida* infections in HIV seropositive women. Am J Med 89:142-146, 1990

24. Jacobus Pharmaceutical: Dapsone USP. In Physicians' Desk Reference. Crandall, NJ, Medical Economics Co, 1991, p 1107

25. Krieger JN, Coombs RW, Collier AC, et al: Fertility parameters in men infected with human immunodeficiency virus. J Infect Dis 164:464-469, 1991

26. Lagakos S, Fischl MA, Stein DS, et al: Effects of zidovudine therapy in minority and other subpopulations with early HIV infection. JAMA 266:2709-2712, 1991

27. Landesman S, Minkoff H, Holman S, et al: Serosurvey of human immunodeficiency virus infection in parturients. JAMA 258:2701-2703, 1987

28. Maiman M, Fruchter RG, Segur E, et al: Human immunodeficiency virus and cervical neoplasia. Obstet Gynecol 38:377-382, 1991

29. Maiman M, Tarricons N, Viera J, Suarez J: Colposcopic evaluation of human immunodeficiency virus seropositive women. Obstet Gynecol 78:84-88, 1991

30. Minkoff HL, DeHovitz JA: Care of women infected with the human immunodeficiency virus. JAMA 266:2253-2258, 1991

31. Minkoff HL, Moreno J: Drug prophylaxis for human immunodeficiency virus infected pregnant women: Ethical considerations. Am J Obstet Gynecol 163:1111-1113, 1990

32. Minkoff HL, Willoughby A, Mendez H, et al: Serious infections during pregnancy among women with advanced immunodeficiency virus infection. Am J Obstet Gynecol 162:30-34, 1990

33. Moss GB, Clemetson D, D'Costa L, et al: Association of cervical ectopy with heterosexual transmission of human immunodeficiency virus: Results of a study of couples in Nairobi, Kenya. J Infect Dis 164:588-591, 1991

34. Nelson KE, Vlahov D, Cohn S, et al: Sexually transmitted diseases in a population of intravenous drug users: Association with seropositivity to the human immunodeficiency virus. J Infect Dis 164:157-163, 1991

35. Ness RB, Kelly JV, Killian CD: House staff recruitment to municipal and voluntary New York City residency programs during the AIDS epidemic. JAMA 266:2843-2846, 1991

36. NIAID/NIH: Important therapeutic information on prevention of recurrent *Pneumocystis carinii* pneumonia in persons with AIDS. Executive Summary, October 11, 1991

37. NIAID/NIH and NIH Centers for Disease Control: Clinical Courier 9(6), 1991

38. Padian NS: Epidemiology of AIDS and heterosexually transmitted HIV in women. AIDS File 5:1-2, 1991

39. Padian NS, Marquis L, Francis DP, et al: Male to female transmission of human immunodeficiency virus. JAMA 258:788-790, 1987

40. Padian NS, Shiboski SCn, Jewell NP: Female to male transmission of human immunodeficiency virus. JAMA 266:1664-1667, 1991

41. Plummer FA, Simones JN, Cameron DW, et al: Cofactors in male-female sexual transmission of human immunodeficiency virus type 1. J Infect Dis 163:233-239, 1991

42. Rhoads JL, Wright C, Redfield RR, Burke DS: Chronic vaginal candidiasis in women with human immunodeficiency virus infection. JAMA 257:3105-3107, 1987

43. Safrin S, Assaykeen T, Follansbee S, Mills J: Foscarnet therapy for acyclovir-resistant mucocutaneous herpes simplex virus infection in 26 AIDS patients: Preliminary data. J Infect Dis 161:1078-1084, 1990

44. Safrin S, Dattel BJ, Haver L, Sweet RL: Seroprevalence and epidemiologic correlates of infection in women with acute pelvic inflammatory disease. Obstet Gynecol 75:666-670, 1990

45. Schoenbaum, Hartel D, Selwyn PA, et al: Risk factors for human immunodeficiency virus infections in intravenous drug users. N Engl J Med 147:104-108, 1987

46. St. Louis ME, Conway GA, Hayman CR, et al: Human immunodeficiency virus infection disadvantaged adolescents—Findings from the US Job Corps. JAMA 266:2387-2391, 1991

47. Volberding PA, Lagakos SW, Koch MA, et al: Zidovudine in asymptomatic human immunodeficiency virus infections: A controlled trial in persons with fewer than 500 CD4-positive cells per cubic millimeter. N Engl J Med 322:941-949, 1990

48. Warne PA, Ehrhardt A, Schochter D, et al: Menstrual abnormalities in HIV + and HIV − women with a history of intravenous drug use. (M.C. 3113.) Seventh International Conference on AIDS. Florence, Italy, June 1991

49. Witt DJ, Craven DE, McCabe WR: Bacterial infections in adult patients with the acquired immunodeficiency syndrome (AIDS) and AIDS-related complex. Am J Med 82:900-906, 1987

50. Working Group on HIV Testing of Pregnant Women and Newborns: HIV infection, pregnant women, and newborns. JAMA 264:2416-2420, 1990

29

AIDS LITIGATION FOR THE PRIMARY CARE PHYSICIAN

JOHN McDOUGALL KERN, JD
BONNI BROWNLEE CROY, MPH

Since 1984 the number and variety of legal actions related to HIV disease have kept pace with the epidemic. Although transfusion-associated AIDS litigation and the new legal challenges surrounding the HIV-positive health care provider have claimed much of the attention of trial counsel and the media, descriptions of other lawsuits directed at physicians who care for patients with HIV may help others learn from their colleagues' experience.

In November 1986, for example, a young man was wheeled into the operating room for débridement of an earlier surgical wound that would not heal. After general anesthesia had been administered, the surgeon and anesthesiologist discussed whether the patient's wound-healing difficulty might be secondary to AIDS. During the operation the surgeon allegedly ordered, and the anesthesiologist allegedly drew, a blood sample.

The blood sample arrived in the hospital's histocompatibility laboratory with an order for HIV testing. The result was sent only to the surgeon and read, "HTLV-III antibody ELISA Positive. This test is not diagnostic of AIDS. False positives and false negatives may occur." The laboratory slip was placed in the patient's file in the surgeon's office, and although the surgeon notified the patient's internist of the result, the patient was never notified.

More than a year later, the patient applied for disability insurance and sent a signed consent to the surgeon's office, allowing disclosure of his medical records. The insurance carrier received the records and denied the patient's application based on the fact that—unknown to the patient—he was positive on a single HIV-antibody screening test, unconfirmed by Western blot.

The resulting class-action lawsuit named the surgeon, the anesthesiologist, and the hospital, alleged 11 different legal theories, and sought to review every HIV

This chapter does not present legal advice in regard to particular situations. For advice about specific circumstances, a lawyer should be consulted.

test ever performed at the hospital to determine if the hospital regularly engaged in the "deceptive" practice of testing without consent.

This is just one of the many types of lawsuits brought by patients with HIV disease against the professionals attempting to care for them. Suits now pending generally fall into six major categories: misdiagnosis; treatment; refusal to treat; consent; confidentiality and sexual partners; and fear of AIDS.

MISDIAGNOSIS

In a Massachusetts trial that resulted in a $750,000 jury verdict, a 28-year-old mother of two complained to her physician of skin lesions, respiratory difficulty, and enlarged lymph nodes. He diagnosed these symptoms as secondary to stress, cigarette smoking, and a lack of exercise. Two years later, she tested positive for antibody to HIV and began zidovudine (AZT) treatment. The jury's verdict implied that earlier diagnosis would have made a difference, not only in the length of her life, but in its quality. The verdict also revealed the jury's anger toward the physician.[1]

Another case presents the flip side of a failure to diagnose.* In 1984 a young man was diagnosed with AIDS based on biopsy-proven Kaposi's sarcoma. He resigned from his employment and notified family members that he was homosexual and had AIDS. He then took a trip around the world while he was still able to do so. On his return, he was informed that further pathologic evaluation had shown that the lesion was not Kaposi's sarcoma, and subsequent HIV-antibody testing was repeatedly negative.

In April 1991 a San Francisco jury awarded $228,000 to a man mistakenly diagnosed with AIDS-related complex (ARC) on the basis of laboratory tests belonging to another patient.[2] The plaintiff suffered the emotional distress of believing that he was HIV infected for 6 months until subsequent testing revealed the error. The testing laboratory, the hospital, and the doctor were held liable.

Another testing case involved a child who tested HIV-positive by enzyme-linked immunosorbent assay (ELISA), confirmed by immunofluorescent assay (IFA). The parents were fully informed of the prognosis of HIV disease and chose to enroll the child in an experimental protocol using a recombinant therapy. After more than a year of treatment, the child tested HIV negative. The lawsuit seeks recovery for the parents' emotional distress from the misdiagnosis and for injury to the child from the unnecessary treatment.

The lesson from all these cases is clear: physicians should never rely on laboratory results until blood samples repeatedly test positive by ELISA and are confirmed by Western blot. Although this is normal procedure in most testing laboratories today, the clinician needs to know the basis of the positive result. In addition, the testing data must be correlated with clinical history, risk factors, and physical condition since samples can be mislabeled or contaminated. Attempts to resolve a questionable result with a p24 antigen or polymerase chain reaction (PCR) test, which will identify the presence of the human immunodeficiency virus in proviral DNA, have caused further difficulty based on indeterminate results, particularly in children

---

*We do not refer by citation to actions that have not yet been filed or that are in litigation but have not received the attention of the public news media.

younger than 1 year of age. The best advice to the clinician is to **never** act on a single ELISA result and to consult a specialist in laboratory medicine to resolve conflicts.

TREATMENT

Regrettably, even AIDS researchers and clinicians who have prolonged and ameliorated the clinical course of AIDS patients have become targets in lawsuits. One case involves an AIDS patient afflicted with toxoplasmosis, a parasitic invasion of the muscles and the brain. Toxoplasmosis is treated by the synergistic effect of two drugs (pyrimethamine and sulfadiazine), and although clinical improvement is often noted, relapse and mortality statistics are high.

In this case the patient sought (but did not receive) $750,000 from his treating physician, the hospital, and pharmacy when he was given the wrong medication because of pharmacy error. The patient experienced unpleasant side effects and unilaterally discontinued all medications for toxoplasmosis. The plaintiff alleged that the incorrect medication caused depression and hallucinations, which forced him to stop all medications. There was no notation of his divulging this information to his physician. Depression is not uncommon in AIDS patients, and this patient had a past history of hallucinations secondary to alcoholism. Unfortunately, however, the patient went 2 months with no treatment for toxoplasmosis. He then saw another physician, who restored effective treatment the same day with a new prescription of the proper sulfa drug.

Treating AIDS patients has become one of the classic challenges of internal medicine because clinical management requires expertise in the many physiologic systems that can be secondarily involved through the effect of HIV infection. In addition, new pharmaceutical applications are evolving so rapidly that treatment innovations are published weekly. For all but the AIDS specialist at a research center, these circumstances require constant consultation to avoid a charge of failure to provide treatment consistent with the rapidly changing "standard of care." Since the number of patients with HIV disease continues to mount, physicians undertaking the care of AIDS patients in their private practices should develop a professional relationship with a specialist at an established HIV/AIDS treatment center.

REFUSAL TO TREAT

In one pending lawsuit an indigent man in need of hernia repair allegedly received surreptitious HIV testing along with his normal blood work. After a positive result, he was referred to a major AIDS treatment center for the hernia operation since it could not be accomplished in a "timely manner" at the referring hospital. The ruse resulted in a lawsuit against the hospital and surgeon after word of the patient's positive HIV status spread throughout the small town. The strength of this lawsuit is based on the disclosure of the patient's HIV status, but it also raises a "failure to treat" claim, which must be based on specific antidiscrimination laws.

Failure to treat patients in a federally funded institution has resulted in actions in federal court under the discrimination clause of Section 504 of the Vocational Rehabilitation Act of 1973.[3] The recent passage of the Americans with Disabilities Act will add protections.

In one action a residential treatment program excluded HIV-positive substance-abuse patients because of the likelihood of "unsupervised and uncontrollable sexual activity among participants."[4] The lawsuit caused modifications of admission policies; similar cases are pending.[5]

On November 1, 1990, the United States District Court for the District of Massachusetts ruled that a Rehabilitation Act lawsuit for refusal to treat may continue even after the patient's death.[6]

Although the American Medical Association has clearly taken the position that the physician has an ethical duty to treat AIDS patients,[7] individual physicians contend that they are not legally obligated to do so. Lawsuits against groups of physicians for refusing to treat patients with HIV disease continue on many legal grounds. In one pending case the plaintiff is suing under five separate code sections for failure to provide medical care.[8] These federal, state, and local laws specifically prohibit discrimination against persons with HIV disease.

The only practical legal advice to physicians wishing to isolate themselves from the HIV patient population is that refusing to treat puts them legally at risk. Therefore they should develop (and document the existence of) a referral system that ensures the patient receives prompt and appropriate medical care. Like a victim of "patient dumping" (who is refused medical care based on inability to pay), an AIDS patient with a treatable medical condition who continues to suffer because of a refusal to give care is an emotionally sympathetic plaintiff to a jury.

CONSENT, CONFIDENTIALITY, AND SEXUAL PARTNERS

Standing outside a patient's half-opened door, a physician turned to the patient's sexual partner and broke the news that the patient was HIV positive. After counseling the sexual partner about the consequences and urging testing, the physician entered the room to find the patient absent. Hours later the patient's body was found on an awning several stories below the open window of his room. The physician's major legal problem, in addition to the suicide, was the violation of the patient's confidentiality rights under a then-existing **criminal** statute.

Several state laws once required a written, specifically worded consent for HIV testing signed by the "subject of the blood test," and provided criminal penalties for disclosure of the result to any "third party" by the physician who ordered the test. Health care workers could not even be told whether they were treating an HIV-positive patient, and the patient's spouse or sexual partner could not be told of the test result, even in circumstances in which there was a continuing risk of exposure.

In 1989 new legislation passed in one jurisdiction avoided some of the hardships imposed by the original statutes but maintained the goal of confidentiality, without which, proponents argue, continued testing and research might not be possible.

In obtaining the patient's consent for HIV testing, the previous requirement of a specific, printed consent has been modified to require the same informed consent necessary for surgery.[9]

The test result may now be known not only by the physician ordering the test, but also by the other members of the health care team who provide treatment[10]; the

HIV-antibody test result may now be included in the patient's medical record[11] and need not hide between the lines of a progress note.

The major problem remains for the medical records department, which must eliminate references to HIV-antibody status before providing a copy of the chart to third parties such as health insurance carriers. Especially in large centers, a complex system must be developed to avoid inadvertent disclosures.

Physicians can now tell sexual partners that they are at risk without chancing a lawsuit. After attempting to obtain the patient's consent, the physician may notify the spouse or sexual partner of the patient, even if the patient refuses consent,[12] but the doctor does **not** incur liability for **not** doing so.[13] No physician has a duty to notify.[14]

Several states have passed laws requiring mandatory HIV testing of prisoners, prostitutes, and other "suspect" populations. The recent Centers for Disease Control (CDC) recommendations on HIV-positive health care providers has caused intense disagreement. As the policy and ethical debates continue, the United States military uses mandatory testing to ensure the health of its service personnel, whereas general public resistance has halted attempts to require HIV testing to obtain a marriage license or—in the most extreme suggestion to date—as a mandatory enclosure with every income tax return.

One case has suggested that, under some circumstances, there may be constitutional violations inherent in mandatory testing. The United States Court of Appeals for the Eighth Circuit found that mandatory testing of employees working with retarded children with aggressive or violent behavior (to protect the children) was a search and seizure, which must comply with the reasonableness standards of the Fourth Amendment. Although the State argued that the test was necessary, the Court barred the mandatory testing program, finding the risk of transmission "trivial."[15]

One California court considered the same issue after the passage of Proposition 96,[16] which allows testing of a criminal defendant at the request of the victim and the State.[17] An appellate court has now upheld this form of mandatory testing.[18]

FEAR OF AIDS

Anyone who received a blood transfusion before March 1985 or has a possible exposure in any setting has a "fear of AIDS." On February 17, 1989, a Los Angeles jury returned a verdict against the estate of Rock Hudson in the amount of $21,750,000 in the case of a man who has had several negative test results for the antibody to HIV but has a fear of AIDS based on 160 post-diagnosis sexual encounters with a now-deceased AIDS patient.[19] Judge Bruce Geernaert termed that concern, ". . . an ongoing fear of death which is very substantial whether measured in quantity or quality."

Although this case and its result are unusual in many respects, any medical negligence action in which the patient is exposed to blood or body fluids of a health care professional or another patient may now include an emotional distress cause of action based on a fear of AIDS theory.

Unlike "fear of cancer" cases, in which the genuineness of a claim of emotional distress must be based on showing an objective fact of exposure to a carcinogen, an actual physical injury, or precancerous condition,[20] the basis for an objective fear of AIDS is factually ascertainable by HIV testing. Although plaintiffs cannot be forced to submit to HIV testing in many states, allowing someone to sue for a fear of AIDS claim at trial when a simple blood test would determine whether there is any basis for that fear is clearly unreasonable. The issue has been litigated. A motion sought an order either compelling a child-plaintiff's consent to HIV testing or, in the alternative, precluding admission of fear of AIDS evidence at trial. When the child tested HIV negative by PCR, the $1.2 million demand evaporated.

Finally, fear of AIDS based on exposure to HIV-positive health care professionals, even without actual transmission of the virus, poses one of the major legal challenges of the epidemic. A single surgeon can generate cases by several thousand people, each claiming a fear of AIDS. Such cases do have limits, however.

One court decision recently held that a surgeon must inform a patient of the surgeon's positive HIV-antibody status before an operation as part of informed consent.[21] The same court upheld a medical center's right to require a special consent form advising patients of the surgeon's HIV-antibody status, based on a small risk of HIV transmission and a substantial risk that any patient would have a fear of AIDS if the information were divulged after surgery. The same judge ruled that the medical center had breached the surgeon's confidentiality when his HIV test result became widely known at the hospital, which ended his practice. In the end the medical center paid the surgeon for his lost earnings because of the breach of confidentiality. In a state that forbids disclosure of an HIV result, the compelled consent issue might have been resolved differently.

Although this ruling appears to have been based on the absolute certainty that the patient would have a fear of AIDS, even though the likelihood of transmission is remote, another court has dismissed similar lawsuits by patients based on fear of AIDS. In two cases Judge Joseph H.H. Kaplan dismissed lawsuits by surgical patients of Almaraz,[22] an otolaryngologist, who died of AIDS-related disease in November 1990. Both patients were HIV-antibody negative more than 6 months after potential exposure. The Court held that the patients could not recover for fear of AIDS that had not occurred.

CONCLUSION

The tragedy, social stigma, and fatal prognosis of AIDS have led to an epidemic of lawsuits by its victims, and the unfortunate targets of these actions are often the highly visible health care professionals. Cases continue to be pressed to trial. The results of these trials over the coming years will determine whether AIDS litigation is destined to be another footnote to the epidemic or a substantial new area of professional liability for all health care professionals.

REFERENCES

1. *Elizabeth Ramos v. Harvard Community Health Plan, Inc.*, MA Superior Court, Middlesex County, No. 86-4114
2. *Welenken v. SmithKline Bio-Science Laboratories, Ltd.*, San Francisco Sup. Ct. No. 881107
3. 29 U.S.C. § 794, Denial of equal health services based on handicap
4. *John Doe v. Centinela Hospital, et al*, U.S.D.C. (C.D. Cal.) No. 87-2514 PAR
5. *Jane Doe v. Lankenan Hospital, et al*, U.S.D.C. (E.D. Pa.) No. 88-8007
6. *Glanz v. Vernick*, No. 89-0748-MA
7. Council on Ethics and Judicial Affairs: Ethical issues involved in the growing AIDS crisis. JAMA 259:1360, 1988
8. *State of California v. Health America Corp.*, San Francisco Superior Court No. 899466. Violations were alleged of (1) Health and Safety Code Section 1386(b)(7); (2) 10 Calif. Code Reg. Section 1300.67.10; (3) Unruh Civil Rights Act, Civil Code Sections 51, *et seq.;* (4) San Francisco Police Code Section 3305; and (5) San Francisco Police Code Section 3805
9. Cal. H. & S. C. A. § 199.2(a)
10. Cal. H. & S. C. A. § 199.24(c)
11. Cal. H. & S. C. A. § 199.2(1)
12. Cal. H. & S. C. A. § 199.25(b)
13. *Tarasoff v. Regents*, 17 Cal.3d 425 (1976)
14. Cal. H. & S. C. A. § 199.25(c)
15. *Glover v. Eastern Nebraska Office of Retardation, et al*, No. 88-1678 (8th Cir. 1989)
16. Cal. H. & S. C. A. § 199.95-199.99
17. *Rice v. Municipal Court*, Santa Clara County No. 678770
18. *Johnson v. Municipal Court, City and County of San Francisco*, Cal. Ct. of App. 1st Dist. Div. 5, No. A045336, March 31, 1989. The case was remanded to the Superior Court to determine whether HIV can be transmitted by saliva and whether Ms. Johnson had blood in her saliva, which was transmitted to a deputy sheriff she allegedly bit. This statute, as well as laws allowing testing of prostitutes and allowing jail guards to know the HIV-antibody status of prisoners, has thus far been upheld.
19. *Marc Christian v. Wallace Sheft, Executor of the Estate of Rock Hudson*, L.A. Sup. No. 574153. On April 21, 1989, the Superior Court reduced the verdict to $5,500,000, and the case is now on appeal on the legal issues.
20. *Ferraro v. Galluchio*, 152 N.E.2d 149 (1958); *Lorenc v. Chemirad Corporation*, 179 A.2d 401 (1962); *Adams v. Johns-Manville Sales Corp.*, 783 F.2d 589 (5th Cir. 1986); *Arnett v. Dow Chemical Co.*, March 21, 1988 Order, San Francisco Master File No. 729586, Judicial Council Coordination Proceedings No. 954
21. *Behringer v. The Medical Center at Princeton*, NJ Sup. Ct. Law Div., Mercer County No. L88-2550 (April 25, 1991)
22. *Perry Rossi v. Rudolf Almaraz, MD, and Johns Hopkins Hospital*, Baltimore City Cir. Ct. No. 90344028; *Sonja Faya v. Rudolf Almaraz, M.D., and Johns Hopkins Hospital*, Baltimore City Cir. No. 90345011

30

SUPPORTING HEALTH CARE WORKERS IN TREATMENT OF HIV-INFECTED PATIENTS

MOLLY COOKE, MD

IMPACT OF AIDS ON HEALTH CARE WORKERS

The psychologic and emotional impact of caring for HIV-infected patients has been recognized, at least in areas in which HIV infection is prevalent, since the beginning of the epidemic. In 1981 in San Francisco and New York, doctors, nurses, laboratory technologists, and dietary workers discussed the new disease and speculated about its transmissibility. By 1982 health care workers in the cities associated with the outbreak were familiar with colleagues who refused to do autopsies, failed to admit ill patients to the hospital, and provided inadequate emergency room care. In San Francisco where both local television and newspapers gave prompt and thorough attention to the new disease, anxiety among health care workers waxed and waned in part as a function of the volume and nature of media coverage. The recognition in 1983 of AIDS cases associated with the therapeutic administration of blood products confirmed the suspicion that the disease was potentially transmissible by occupational exposures to body fluids. In addition, many physicians were confronted by the realization that treatments they had ordered with the intention of benefiting their patient had resulted in the acquisition of a lethal infection. By 1984 national media were covering AIDS; Perri Klass, then a medical student in Boston, described her response and that of her colleagues in an article in the *New York Times* with the headline, "The age-old fear of contagion arises when treating an AIDS patient."

Consternation about the risk associated with the treatment of HIV-infected patients increased in the summer of 1987 when the Centers for Disease Control (CDC) described three cases in which the virus apparently was transmitted to health care workers by skin and mucous membrane exposures. Several surgeons announced that they would not operate on HIV-infected patients, regardless of the consequences to the patient. The American Nursing Association, the American College of Physicians, and ultimately the American Medical Association all issued statements

Reprinted from Cooke M: Supporting Health Care Workers in Treatment of HIV-Infected Patients. Primary Care 19(1):245-256, 1992.

reminding their constituents of the obligation of health care professionals to care for the sick. Despite these exhortations, many health care workers, including a possibly disproportionate number of physicians, continue to resist the care of HIV-infected patients. An article in the *New York Times* in April 1990, "AIDS War Shunned by Many Doctors," began, "Nine years into the AIDS epidemic, most of the nation's physicians are still failing to take part in the fight to treat and control the deadly disease." The report in August 1990 of apparent transmission of HIV from an infected dentist to one or more of his patients has raised new issues for health care workers: the possibility of mandatory HIV screening and restriction of practice.

The HIV epidemic has raised a variety of issues that are stressful and some even threatening for health care workers. Themes include occupational risk, fear, anger, conflict among providers, concerns about professional competence, sexuality, stigma, reproductive rights, illegal drug use, grief, and burnout.[4] Despite 10 years' experience with the disease, these issues remain very challenging, even in hospitals and clinical programs that are considered models for AIDS care.[2] This chapter reviews the phenomenon of AIDS avoidance, the stresses experienced by health care workers committed to the care of HIV-infected individuals, and strategies for supporting health care providers of AIDS care.

AIDS AVOIDANCE

Prevalence of Reluctance to Treat

Anecdotal descriptions of health care workers who refuse to care for HIV-infected patients abound. Actual data on the extent of the problem are predictably much more difficult to obtain. To some extent the prevalence of AIDS avoidance depends on how the question is phrased. Many more health workers agree with the statement "I would like to have the option to decline to care for AIDS patients" than with the statement "I have on occasion refused to care for an AIDS patient." With that caveat, a variety of surveys suggests that 33% to 65% of physicians are reluctant to treat HIV-infected patients. The prevalence of reluctant providers among medical students has been estimated at 40%, among nurses, 50%, and among dentists, 75% before the report of apparent transmissions from a Florida dentist.[5,6,9,12,13,15,19]

There has been considerable speculation about the impact of the HIV epidemic on the availability of nurses and internists. Clearly, career decisions are complex, and there was evidence of declining popularity of internal medicine before the advent of the AIDS pandemic. However, information on the influence of AIDS on career decisions made by health care workers is available from several studies. In a study of internal medicine residents, 24% indicated that they had deliberately sought a low AIDS-prevalence residency, and a comparable percentage intentionally will seek a low AIDS-prevalence area for their post-training practice. Only 17% of the residents indicated a strong commitment to working with HIV-infected patients at the completion of training, and only 3% planned to seek a high AIDS-prevalence area for post-training practice. Overall, studies of internists in training suggest that 10% to 15% have a strong commitment to AIDS work, 25% are actively AIDS avoidant, and the remainder are making career decisions independent of the epidemic.

The prevalence of AIDS avoidance and the evidence that the HIV epidemic is affecting the career decisions of at least a proportion of students in the vital patient care fields of internal medicine, family practice, and nursing raise concerns about the availability of medical care to HIV-infected patients.[20] The problem is intensified by the spread of the epidemic into populations that already experience severe difficulty accessing medical care. The interaction of psychologic reluctance to treat HIV on the part of health professionals with the social and economic barriers to receiving medical care that underserved, inner-city populations face may result in de facto denial of care for many inner-city HIV patients. There is already evidence that the HIV epidemic is having an especially marked effect on the ability of publicly funded, municipal hospital residencies to attract trainees, compared to that of university training programs with a comparable AIDS volume.[3] It will be critical to understand both reluctance to treat and the stresses of AIDS work to motivate health care workers to care for the increasing numbers of people who have become and will become ill from HIV and to support those providers who undertake to care for people with AIDS.

Fear of Contagion and Occupational Risk

Occupational risk and fear of contagion have dominated the discussion of reluctance to treat AIDS.[8] Virtually all media coverage of health care workers declining to care for AIDS patients and much of the formal research on provider attitudes have assumed that people who are willing to treat AIDS patients are for some reason less concerned with the risk of occupational infection than "non-treaters." This hypothesis does not withstand careful examination, however. Very early in the epidemic, it was noted that women health care workers appeared less uneasy working with AIDS patients than their male colleagues, at least when homosexual intercourse was the predominant risk behavior. Much larger studies have continued to show a marked difference in AIDS avoidance between men and women. When injection drug use is the most common risk behavior, this difference in the attitudes of men and women health care workers is not seen. Even in the earliest days when very little was known about the infective agent and the level of occupational risk, there was no basis for believing men and women health care workers faced different probabilities of occupational infection. Therefore the differential suggests that factors other than simple differences in the estimations of occupational risk mediate reluctance to treat.[10,19]

Health care workers in high HIV-prevalence settings retain a healthy respect for and considerable apprehension about occupational transmission.[15] This concern is well placed; in a large study of internal medicine residents, 22% of the residents training in institutions in which AIDS is prevalent and the population is injection drug using have had needle sticks from HIV-positive patients, compared to 7% of residents training in AIDS-prevalent areas where the population is primarily homosexual and to 5% of residents training in "low-AIDS" institutions. On a scale measuring "fear of contagion," the residents at "high AIDS/drug-user prevalent" programs were the most fearful, yet they had the greatest commitment to working with HIV-infected people at the completion of training. In fact, it makes little sense to believe that health care providers who work in settings where HIV is prevalent and have the greatest chance of exposure to HIV-positive body fluids and ultimately of occupational seroconversion would not be fearful. Other factors must explain the variations in willingness to treat people with AIDS.

Factors Associated with AIDS Avoidance

A negative opinion of homosexuality and negative attitudes toward homosexuals are the most frequently identified characteristics of health care workers who are reluctant to treat HIV-infected patients.[5,7,13] Other factors that appear to influence the willingness of health care workers to treat people with AIDS include attitudes toward injection drug users, level of comfort with a terminal care or hospice mode of treatment, and the individual health care worker's sense of the duty of medical professionals.[14,19] In a study of medical residents these four factors accounted for more than 50% of the variance between residents with a strong intention to treat HIV-infected patients at the completion of training and those with little or no commitment to AIDS care. The decisions of practicing physicians about treating people with AIDS are presumably influenced by the same factors but are also subject to some practical considerations. In low AIDS-prevalence areas, concerns about professional competence and unwillingness to undertake medical care that is perceived as complex and demanding and for which the provider has had no formal training are frequently cited as rationales for referring HIV-infected patients. In high AIDS-prevalence areas practicing physicians have other concerns. In a 1987 survey of community physicians in Queens, New York, 35% were caring for people with HIV-spectrum disease. However, 32% of the respondents indicated that they would not accept new patients with HIV.[28] Again, fear of contagion did not distinguish practitioners providing care from those who did not. Rather, the belief that seeing HIV-infected patients is bad for one's practice (by making it difficult to hire office staff and increasing the risk of losing other patients) was significantly associated with non-treatment. It is likely that additional factors influence the willingness of other professionals and paraprofessionals in health care to work with an HIV-infected population, but groups other than physicians and nurses are essentially unstudied.

CONCERNS OF HEALTH CARE WORKERS PROVIDING AIDS CARE

Characteristics of Professionals Providing AIDS Care

HIV infection has become sufficiently dispersed in the population of the United States that a large number of health care workers have had at least some limited experience in the care of infected patients, and it is not possible to generalize about the characteristics of providers as a whole.[25] However, some observations about the health care workers with the highest degree of commitment to AIDS care can be made. Medical residents with a strong intention to work with HIV-infected patients at the completion of training are characterized by a relative absence of prejudicial attitudes about homosexuality and injection drug use, a strong sense of professional responsibility, and relative comfort with the hospice mode of some AIDS care, negotiating the ethical dilemmas raised by AIDS and meeting both psychosocial and technical medical needs. These attributes are also found in many practitioners in primary care fields; perhaps not surprisingly, residents in training programs specifically identified as "primary care" internal medicine residencies are much more likely to indicate a strong commitment to HIV care than residents in categorical internal medicine programs. Although AIDS care has been associated with a few "model" programs and often is delivered in academic settings in conjunction with clinical research, it increasingly is becoming a "primary care" disease, both because the numbers of infected individuals requires it and because primary care clinicians bring the appropriate skills and commitment.

Persistence of Concerns About Occupational Infection

As discussed previously, apprehension about occupational risk does not disappear among committed providers. Regarding health care workers who are providing care to HIV patients as fearless or unconcerned about occupational transmission does not do justice to the tension that these professionals feel between their commitment to helping their patients and the justifiable desire to preserve their own health and safety and that of their families. Despite the frequent comparisons of occupational risk associated with hepatitis B and that associated with HIV, health care workers tend to perceive them as qualitatively different because of the latter's uniformly high fatality rate. Practitioners in high prevalence areas alternate between finding reassurance in the published statistics on seroconversion rates after needle-stick injuries and finding the same statistics worrisome (see Chapter 4). Concern about occupational infection fluctuates; certain events—either in the practice setting or outside events reported in the media—can lead to reappearance of fear. The impact of the CDC's announcement of "splash seroconversions" in 1987 is an example; the unfolding story of Dr. Hacib Aoun's occupational infection and media coverage of litigation in New York relating to an occupational accident to a resident that resulted in her HIV seroconversion are others.

More recently the announcement of the apparent infection of five dental patients by an HIV-infected dentist has had a significant impact on the climate in which all health care workers care for their HIV-infected patients (see Chapter 1). The documentation of transmission from practitioner to patient, which is generally regarded as much more rare than transmission in the other direction, serves as a reminder of the real risks of caring for people who are HIV infected. Discussion of mandated HIV-antibody screening, proposals to fine or imprison HIV-infected health care workers who do not divulge their antibody status to patients, recommendations regarding restriction of practice of some or all health care workers who are found HIV infected, and most recently the promulgation of the CDC recommendations on management of infected health care workers have increased the anxiety of many medical professionals about occupational HIV infection and its consequences (see Chapter 4). Many physicians and nurses are frankly angry, believing that society is disregarding the considerable personal risk health care workers have faced over the past 10 years of HIV care. This type of collective increase in concern prompted by some event covered in the media is likely to become less common as time passes and medical workers and society accommodate to the pandemic but will not disappear entirely.

AIDS STRESS AND BURNOUT

Stressful situations are ones that an individual considers important or significant in which the challenges may exceed the individual's capabilities. Many stresses are associated with AIDS care in addition to the concern about occupational infection. Some are generic and associated with all kinds of medical work; others are particularly associated with caring for young patients with a lethal prognosis and still others related more specifically to the behaviors commonly associated with HIV transmission[22] (Table 30–1). Different occupations within the general field of health care are associated with markedly different levels and sources of stress. Appreciation of the specific stressors for health care workers in different occupations may permit the development of more focused and effective interventions for the various professionals providing AIDS care.

Individuals working with HIV-infected patients experience a number of stresses typical of virtually all health care work. A very rapid work pace and the sense of exponentially increasing patient volume are burdensome for all AIDS providers. In addition, physicians are frequently troubled by concerns about professional competence, the necessity to make important decisions with incomplete information, and an onerous sense of responsibility for patient outcomes.[11,18] Although nurses share the stress of responsibility for patient outcomes, their characteristic stressors are unmeetable patient needs, conflict with other staff, and a low level of control

Table 30–1. Stresses of AIDS Care

Generic Stressors in Health Care
Overwork
Low control over working conditions
Concerns about competence
Responsibility for patient well-being
Decision making under uncertainty
Staff conflict
Patient needs, especially unmeetable ones
Stressors Associated with Diseases with Poor Prognosis
Daily confrontation with death
Therapeutic impotence
Role confusion
"Grief overload"
Stressors Typical of AIDS
Fear of contagion/occupational risk
Reactions to stigmatized behaviors
Over-identification
Conflicts between family and homosexual support system
Youth of patients
Dementia and neurologic deterioration of patients
Destructiveness of disease-wasting syndrome and Kaposi's sarcoma

Modified from Pleck JH, O'Donnell L, et al: AIDS-phobia, contact with AIDS, and AIDS-related job stress in hospital workers. J Homosex 15:41, 1988.

over the work place. Because low level of control over the working environment is a major source of job stress, nurses characteristically report the most job stress among health care professionals. Other health care workers (e.g., pharmacists and respiratory therapists) may associate job stress with lack of recognition from physician and nursing colleagues and poor opportunities for professional advancement.[30] Recognition of the diverse sources of stress in the medical workplace can improve communication and working relations between medical professionals.

"Burnout" is a subjective response to chronic job stress. Although in a formal sense the syndrome may not be entirely distinguishable from depression, many health care workers in high-intensity AIDS care environments describe an emotional state experienced primarily as physical and emotional depletion rather than sadness.[1,26,27] The elements of burnout include loss of idealism, enthusiasm, and purpose; physical and emotional exhaustion; the development of negative attitudes toward work; and a loss of empathy for patients.[24] Health care workers who experience this depletion typically have poor relations with coworkers, are unable to deal with patients and their friends and family in a caring way, and ultimately leave the work setting that produced the burnout.[17]

Many AIDS organizations from clinical programs to community-based providers of various social supports are reporting increased personnel turnover, difficulty recruiting new staff, and burnout among remaining providers.[21] The origins of these phenomena are complex and include an AIDS-related reduction in the numbers of healthy homosexual men available to work as paid staff and volunteers, accumulated grief, and simple overwork. Whatever the cause, the toll burnout takes on providers who have to quit and the health care workers they leave behind and burnout's profoundly destructive effect on the workplace atmosphere militate for the development of innovative and effective programs for its prevention.

STRATEGIES FOR SUPPORTING HEALTH CARE WORKERS

Motivating Reluctant Providers

Most health care workers are neither intensely AIDS-avoidant nor profoundly committed to the care of HIV-infected patients. To prevent the entire burden of AIDS care from falling on a small number of deeply committed providers, additional health care workers must be encouraged to participate. In this regard the statements of professional organizations indicating an expectation that their constituents will provide care have been useful. The American Nurses' Association promulgated one of the earliest statements of this type; the American College of Physicians, the American Association of Medical Colleges, and the American Medical Association subsequently developed statements. At the local level, institutional policy and the consequences of avoiding AIDS care should be clearly stated to prospective and current staff. Rather than being perceived as authoritarian, this approach reduces divisive perceptions that some staff are receiving special privileges and promotes a communitarian sense of teamwork. For medical staffs, inclusion of a specific statement in hospital bylaws indicating that attending physicians are expected to care for all patients whose primary complaint falls within the physician's expertise, regardless of intercurrent medical problems, may be useful.

Table 30–2.   Managing the Stress of AIDS Care

Institutional Policies and Procedures
Continuing education addressing competency concerns and professional growth
Explicit procedures for occupational HIV exposures
Disability insurance and medical benefits
Work Environment
Secure financing and good job security
Democratic management style
Multidisciplinary patient care teams
Opportunities for flexible scheduling
Active approaches to conflict resolution
Individual Approaches and Strategies
Mixed HIV and non-HIV practice
Opportunities for professional growth
Reasonable expectations of self
Self-care, including exercise and time off

For the very apprehensive professional who is reluctant to care for HIV-infected patients, individual discussion and counseling may be useful. Counseling should explore the reasons for reluctance. To the extent that concern about occupational transmission underlies reluctance to provide care, staff who are exposed to blood and other potentially infective body fluids should be told that their concerns are valid. It is inappropriate (and ineffective) to dismiss concerns about occupational transmission of HIV. However, discussion should refocus the attention and concern of the apprehensive provider on careful infection control procedures rather than on avoidance of AIDS patients. All staff members deserve up-to-date and accurate information about workplace risks and ready access to the devices and supplies needed to practice safely (Table 30–2).

Retaining Committed Providers: Institutional Modifications and Interventions

An open, positive, and committed attitude toward AIDS care on the part of institutional leaders is an important first step in creating an organizational culture that is supportive of frontline AIDS providers. This attitude should be accompanied by an active and appropriate educational program so that health care workers can stay current with management and, when appropriate, research developments in this rapidly moving field. Anxiety about competency of care is demoralizing[9,29]; programs to maintain and increase competency can be an important source of enthusiasm for providers.

A significant source of concern for even the most committed AIDS providers has involved employment benefits, specifically medical and disability coverage in the event of occupational seroconversion. This is less of a problem for fully trained physicians, who typically carry adequate disability coverage and health insurance, than it is for medical students and non-physician health care workers. The Workers' Compensation system provides lifetime medical coverage for work-related injuries. Therefore institutions that facilitate reporting of needle sticks and completion of the "First Report of Injury" forms are assisting employees who may seroconvert get access to good medical coverage. Since staff members may acquire HIV infection through non-occupational transmission, it is important that employees know whether their employer will respond to claims of occupational injury with an investigation of life-style (see Chapter 4).

Health care institutions can also help frontline health care workers deal with the stresses of AIDS care through the provision of psychologic support and particular administrative structures and approaches.[1,27] Opportunities for professional development help staff members increase their sense of mastery and confidence; since the same situation may be perceived as either challenging or stressful, depending on the worker's preparation, institutional assistance may be extremely important. A democratic management style decreases stress attributable to perceived low level of control over the work environment. Staffing schedules that permit health care workers to vary the length and frequency of their shifts and to work with patients of different levels of acuity allow providers to rest and renew themselves. A multidisciplinary team structure decreases the sense of overwhelming responsibility for all their patients' needs with which committed providers may suffer. Sharing responsibility for patient care can promote a sense of connection between staff members, which is very rewarding in its own right. Finally, opportunities for staff to get together, on the employer's time, to share their thoughts and feelings and to discuss meaningful patient care experiences and strategies for renewal can be restorative and inspiring.

Individual Strategies and Approaches

Many personal approaches to the stresses of AIDS care have been advocated without a clear consensus on successful strategies. Self-awareness, including the ability to recognize the personal impact of AIDS care, and a commitment to self-care, the discipline of taking time away from patients to read, exercise, be with friends, or do whatever else a health care worker finds restorative, have been cited as attributes of successful or "hardy" clinicians.[16,23,27] Social support may be useful as well, provided the caregiver's supports endorse AIDS work. When a health care worker's personal supports have significant anxiety about occupational HIV transmission, discussion of AIDS care will increase the caregiver's stress. An individual's style of coping with stress likely is important. Work with coping styles in other contexts would suggest that avoidant and resigned emotional responses ("I'm not going to think about that," "AIDS care is tough for everyone") are much less successful over time than strategies that emphasize opportunities for growth ("What can I learn about my responses to difficult situations from this experience?").

SUMMARY _____

The care of HIV-infected patients is demanding, raising concerns among health care workers about safety, competence, and emotional endurance. Many health care workers are reluctant to undertake this challenging work. For many professions within health care (e.g., nursing), there is a clearly articulated responsibility to treat all ill individuals. However, there has been and still is less unanimity on this point among physicians. Clearly, a first issue is to continue the discussion of the nature of physicians' professional responsibility and to convey an understanding of the duties of physicians to medical students and to those considering careers as doctors. Meanwhile, efforts must continue to recruit individuals in all areas of health care to work with HIV-infected people. To some extent, this process will happen as a natural consequence of the evolution of the epidemic and its decreasing geographic and demographic restriction. However, "mainstreaming" AIDS care will also require continuing attention to important issues such as acquiring and maintaining the requisite professional competence in the management of HIV-related illnesses, ensuring the availability of support services required for the comprehensive care of HIV complications, and continuing education on and proactive monitoring of infection control practices. All of these activities assist in the creation of a positive environment for the care of AIDS patients. In addition, the emotional consequences of caring for HIV-infected people should be directly addressed, although there is less information on which strategies are useful. A supportive working environment, characterized by some meaningful element of control by all health care workers, not just the medical staff, nonauthoritarian management, explicit and responsive processes for approaching the inevitable ethical dilemmas that arise in the care of HIV-infected patients, and a recognition of both the emotional and psychologic aspects of medical care and the technical areas are the sine qua non. In such an environment health care providers will be able to develop and institute programs that address their particular needs. Strategies that have been helpful are diverse and include support groups, rotation of clinical assignments, part-time work, social activities away from the workplace, and collective spiritual activities.

REFERENCES

1. Bolle JL: Supporting the deliverers of care: Strategies to support nurses and prevent burnout. Nurs Clin North Am 23:843, 1988
2. Cooke M: Physician risk and responsibility in the HIV epidemic. West J Med 152: 57, 1990
3. Cooke M, Sande MA: Sounding board: The HIV epidemic and training in internal medicine—Challenges and recommendations. JAMA 260:519, 1988
4. Cotton DJ: The impact of AIDS on the medical care system. JAMA 260:519, 1988
5. Currey CH, Johnson M, Ogden B: Willingness of health-professions students to treat patients with AIDS. Acad Med 65:472, 1990
6. Feldmann TB, Bell RA, et al: Attitudes of medical school faculty and students toward acquired immunodeficiency syndrome. Acad Med 65:464, 1990
7. Ficarrotto TJ, Grade M, et al: Predictors of medical nursing students' levels of HIV-AIDS knowledge and their resistance to working with AIDS patients. Acad Med 65:470, 1990
8. Gerbert B, Maguire B, Badner V, et al: Why fear persists: Health care professionals and AIDS. JAMA 260:3481, 1988
9. Hayward RA, Shapiro MF: A national study of AIDS and residency training: Experiences, concerns, and consequences. Ann Intern Med 114:23, 1991
10. Herek GM: Heterosexuals' attitudes toward lesbians and gay men: Correlates and gender differences. J Sex Res 25:451, 1988
11. Horstman W, McKusick L: The impact of AIDS on the physician. In McKusick L (ed): What To Do About AIDS: Physicians and Mental Health Professionals Assess the Issues. Los Angeles: Los Angeles University Press, 1986, p 64
12. Imperato PJ, Feldman JG, et al: Medical students' attitudes towards caring for patients with AIDS in a high incidence area. NY State J Med 233, 1988
13. Kegeles SM, Coates TJ, et al: Perceptions of AIDS: The continuing saga of AIDS-related stigma. AIDS 3:S253, 1989

14. Kelley JA, St. Lawrence SJ, et al: Stigmatization of AIDS patients by physicians. Am J Public Health 77:798, 1987
15. Link RN, Feingold AR, et al: Concerns of medical and pediatric house officers about acquiring AIDS from their patients. Am J Public Health 78:455, 1988
16. Martin CA, Julian RA: Causes of stress and burnout in physicians caring for the chronically and terminally ill. Hospice 3:121, 1987
17. McCranie EW, Brandsma JM: Personality antecedents of burnout among middle-aged physicians. Behav Med 14:30, 1988
18. McKusick L, Horstman W, Abrams D, et al: The physiological impact of AIDS on primary care physicians. West J Med 144:751, 1986
19. Merrill JM, Laux L, Thornby JI: AIDS and students' attitudes. South Med J 82:426, 1989
20. Ness RN, Killian CD, et al: Likelihood of contact with AIDS patients as a factor in medical students' residency selections. Acad Med 64:588, 1989
21. Ouellette Kobasa SC: AIDS and volunteer associations: Perspectives on social and individual change. Milbank Q 68:281, 1990
22. Pleck JH, O'Donnell L, et al: AIDS-phobia, contact with AIDS, and AIDS-related job stress in hospital workers. J Homosex 15:41, 1988
23. Quill TE, Williamson PR: Healthy approaches to physician stress. Arch Intern Med 150: 1857, 1990
24. Ray EB, Nichols MR, Perritt LJ: A model of job stress and burnout. Hospice 3:3, 1987
25. Rizzo JA, Marder WD, Willke RJ: Physician contact with and attitudes toward HIV-seropositive patients. Med Care 28:251, 1990
26. Ross MW, Seeger V: Short communications determinants of reported burnout in health professionals associated with the care of patients with AIDS. AIDS 2:395, 1988
27. Scott CD, Jaffe DT: Managing occupational stress associated with HIV infection: Self-care and self-management skills. Occup Med State Art Rev 4:85, 1989
28. Somogyi A, Watson-Abady JA, Mandel FS: Attitudes toward the care of patients with acquired immunodeficiency syndrome. Arch Intern Med 150:50, 1990
29. Tesch BJ, Simpson DE, Kirby BD: Medical and nursing students; Attitudes about AIDS issues. Acad Med 65:467, 1990
30. Wolfgang AP: Job stress in the health professions: A study of physicians, nurses, and pharmacists. Behav Med 14:43, 1988

31

CLINICAL CARE OF PATIENTS WITH AIDS
Developing a System

PAUL A. VOLBERDING, MD

Physicians caring for patients with AIDS appreciate that the epidemic has thrust them into the middle of an intense public debate. Much more than just a medical problem, the AIDS epidemic poses important political and social dilemmas. For the medical profession and especially for the hospital involved in the care of patients with AIDS, the disease forces a reexamination of care structures and calls for new approaches to the many difficulties in the care of AIDS patients. These issues are especially germane given current widespread financial distress, with shifts of un-insured and underinsured patients to the public health sector. This is particularly true as the demographics of the HIV epidemic continue to shift to more disadvantaged populations.

In this chapter some implications of AIDS care are addressed by first considering briefly the experience at San Francisco General Hospital and by then attempting to make generalizations from this experience to providers and medical centers with a more limited involvement with this epidemic. Limitations in generalizing from the local situation are pointed out.

AIDS IMPACT AT SAN FRANCISCO GENERAL HOSPITAL

The history of AIDS at San Francisco General Hospital began with early and unrecognized cases of opportunistic infections in 1980 and early 1981. The first patient with Kaposi's sarcoma was admitted to the hospital in June 1981, and with the first report of epidemic Kaposi's sarcoma and *Pneumocystis carinii* pneumonia came the awareness that the hospital was already seeing patients with this new epidemic disease.

The clinical experience with AIDS patients at San Francisco General Hospital increased, and in early 1983 patient volume warranted establishment of an outpatient clinic dedicated to the care of these individuals. By the middle of 1983 the hospital averaged eight to 10 inpatients with AIDS. Because of this and problems in appropriately educating nursing, medical, and other staff in all areas of the hospital, San Francisco General Hospital established the world's first inpatient unit, which opened in June 1983.[13] An academic division of AIDS care and research was formed in the department of medicine in 1984 to help coordinate the growing volume of patients and clinical studies.

Demographic characteristics of AIDS patients at San Francisco General Hospital were an important factor in determining the overall structure and success of our program. In contrast to AIDS patients in many other parts of the country and in particular on the Eastern Seaboard, AIDS patients at San Francisco General Hospital were predominantly homosexuals rather than users of intravenous drugs and were usually not from racial or ethnic minority groups. As determined from San Francisco Department of Public Health reports of AIDS cases from July 1981 to November 1989, more than 90% of San Francisco AIDS patients were homosexual and 85% were white. Because San Francisco General Hospital is a public facility caring for the medically indigent and because of a continuing increase in HIV disease in this group, our hospital demographics are rapidly changing. Persons of color, the homeless, and injection drug users now represent a significant fraction of patients. Inpatients at San Francisco General Hospital in most cases have Centers for Disease Control (CDC)-defined AIDS, either known at the time of admission or established during their stay. Outpatients in the AIDS clinic also usually have CDC-defined AIDS, although approximately one third of the clinic census is composed of the initial group of patients with severe earlier disease stages. The relatively homogeneous background of patients and the visible nature of the homosexual community in San Francisco made it relatively easy for San Francisco General Hospital to work with community organizations representing the bulk of the AIDS patient burden. However, with this relative homogeneity changing, it has become more critical for us to find new ways to interact with other organizations.

The volume of AIDS care at San Francisco General Hospital has expanded continually with the epidemic. When the AIDS inpatient unit was formed in mid-1983, the average inpatient census was approximately eight patients and the outpatient unit was handling approximately 100 to 120 appointments per month. Currently the outpatient HIV clinic registers 2000 visits per month, the largest volume of any single outpatient clinic at the hospital. The inpatient AIDS census on some days is greater than 50 patients on a medical-surgical service of fewer than 200 beds.

BASIC COMPONENTS OF HIV DISEASE CARE

The structure of the care of patients with HIV disease at San Francisco General Hospital has already been mentioned. This structure can be seen as a triangle, the points of which are the dedicated outpatient clinic, the AIDS inpatient unit, and community-based organizations with hospital-focused services. For reasons detailed later in the chapter, the care of the AIDS patients at San Francisco General Hospital has involved many medical and surgical subspecialties and a wide array of psychosocial services.

Psychosocial services are provided by a variety of individuals and organizations. The AIDS Health Project provides professional counseling for patients with AIDS, and employees of this organization are included in the AIDS clinic at San Francisco

General Hospital. Finally, professional counseling and psychiatric care are provided in both inpatient and outpatient settings by full-time faculty and staff.

COMPLEXITIES OF AIDS CARE

A central challenge facing medical institutions in the care of patients with AIDS- and HIV-associated illnesses derives from the enormous medical complexity of these diseases. Manifestations of HIV infection can affect any organ system in the body, and the patients commonly have several critical illnesses at the same time. In treating these illnesses, physicians more frequently encounter the toxic effects of drugs than when the same drugs are used in the care of non-AIDS patients,[5,7,9] and the toxicity of one required drug may overlap with the toxicity of a second drug also required for the care of that patient. Some common HIV-associated illnesses such as cryptosporidiosis have no effective treatment, and many drugs required in the care of patients with HIV-associated illnesses are difficult to obtain or cumbersome to administer. This is especially obvious with drugs still considered experimental, which is true of more drugs used in the care of AIDS patients than in other complex diseases. This problem is well known to AIDS medical care providers. For example, until several years into the AIDS epidemic, pentamidine required individual applications for drug release on a compassionate basis from the CDC, and foscarnet, a drug now approved for the care of sight-threatening cyto-megalovirus (CMV) retinitis, had to be obtained on an individual, case by case, basis.[2]

In addition to being cumbersome, the use of experimental or nonapproved drugs in AIDS patients may pose administrative difficulties. Although these drugs can be obtained from the manufacturer, hospitals or practitioners must provide the clerical and administrative staff to maintain records of the drug use, and reimbursement for the drug's use or even for the hospital admission required for drug administration may be difficult or impossible to obtain. In our experience insurance sources, Medicaid in particular, often disallow the costs of entire hospital stays if any experimental agent is administered. Recent changes, both in place and proposed, are only now altering this situation. Various new mechanisms—the "treatment investigational new drug (IND) and parallel track"—have been established to broaden the distribution of new drugs for AIDS before the completion of formal clinical trials. Yet even here, the administrative requirements for drug prescription may be daunting.

A final complexity in the case of AIDS patients arises from the poor prognosis of the underlying disease. Patients with advanced HIV illnesses may express a desire for less intense care or less aggressive diagnostic procedures. Physicians may likewise elect to limit therapy because of an underlying poor prognosis. Although in many situations this is an appropriate response to severe underlying disease, this limitation in care frequently poses ethical dilemmas for AIDS care providers.

The medical complexities of the diseases caused by HIV infection are reflected in the administrative burden of coordinating the involvement of relevant health professionals. At San Francisco General Hospital, for example, AIDS clinical re-search is being conducted by at least seven divisions within the department of internal medicine (oncology, AIDS, infectious disease, gastroenterology, nephrol-ogy, endocrine, pulmonary) and by many other departments, including psychiatry, pediatrics, obstetrics and gynecology, epidemiology and international health, surgery, microbiology, and biochemistry. Although such involvement is understandable and encouraging from the perspective of our understanding this disease, it does require that hospitals and medical centers develop some means of coordinating care and clinical research.

It has seemed important to us at San Francisco General Hospital to deliver care to the fullest possible spectrum of HIV-exposure backgrounds and to patients with all stages of HIV disease. To these ends, novel changes are being initiated. For example, the AIDS clinic staff is providing care for HIV-infected clients in the methadone maintenance clinic. Also, because patients with early HIV disease (those still asymptomatic) are still employed, we are opening evening clinic hours. To address the growing needs of women and children, we are actively collaborating in the establishment of augmented services in the AIDS clinic and in separate dedicated facilities. In these and similar ways we seek to keep AIDS clinic providers most current in the aspects of the epidemic that are changing most rapidly.[3,10,14]

PSYCHOSOCIAL NEEDS IN AIDS

In addition to the medical and administrative complexities in AIDS care as discussed, patients have clear and often nearly overwhelming psychosocial needs. Patients with AIDS and HIV infection are commonly young and have limited experience in dealing with medical insurance policies. In fact, many HIV-infected persons, because of their recent entrance into the labor force, are employed by small companies with limited health care benefits or none at all. Thus financial assistance in the form of reviewing insurance status and processing applications for additional coverage are often paramount early in the patient's disease course. With advancing disease, issues of housing and personal assistance may become at least as large a source of concern to the patient as the medical problems. Patients with AIDS are often evicted from housing or forced by reasons of economy or convenience to change their residence during their illness. Patients with AIDS, facing the loss of intellectual capacity and mobility caused by HIV-associated illnesses, may require assistance in such activities as housecleaning and shopping to remain in a community-based environment.

COUNSELING SERVICES

Counseling is also important for patients with HIV infection.[1] Although such patients may require a variety of counseling services during the course of their illness, the most important points are services required at the time of diagnosis and those required as patients enter the terminal phase. Early in the disease course, nonprofessional counseling is often more effective and appropriate. In many cases this remains true as the disease accelerates, although more intensive and individualized approaches may also be required, as may prescription of psychotropic medications. For these reasons we have found it important to have a support staff that can assess the need for and provide aid ranging from the concrete to psychiatric and both nonprofessional and professional psychotherapeutic assistance.

STRESS IN AIDS CARE PROVIDERS

Health professionals who care for AIDS patients experience enormous personal stress. This stress arises from a number of sources, including the medical complexity of the disease, the stigma of AIDS, and AIDS risk behaviors. Other factors contributing to the stress are that AIDS patients are often disfigured by the disease, that they are young, and that death from AIDS often appears inevitable to both the patient and the physician. In many organizations those who provide AIDS care are relatively isolated from their colleagues and peers and receive little external recognition for their efforts.

Several approaches to reducing the stress in AIDS care providers can be considered. Organizations should consider providing staffing levels for AIDS care adequate to the acuity level as well as to the patient volume, although this is increasingly seen as an unaffordable "luxury," especially in financially pressed public institutions. Health professionals, including physicians, nurses, and others, may require more flexible schedules or a smaller proportion of time involved in the direct provision of AIDS care to reduce accumulated AIDS stress. In addition, physicians and other health professionals should be encouraged to discuss issues of grief and loss in a safe environment. At San Francisco General Hospital we have begun small meetings of AIDS clinic personnel in a group therapy format to approach some of these issues and have found the experience to be extremely rewarding.

Even after administrative and organizational attempts to reduce stress are made, stress should be expected to continue. Organizations should anticipate a higher-than-average staff turnover. This should, in general, not be considered to represent programmatic problems but rather to reflect unavoidable and chronic stress. In addition to the concerns of direct providers of AIDS care, questions can be anticipated from other hospital staff. Often this concern is stated in the general question, "Why are we getting involved in AIDS?" This issue, often an expression of fear, might be dealt with by an aggressive program of education. All staff members should be included in a regular program of education conducted on a repeating basis to reinforce the information and to update it as understanding of the HIV infection changes. Because much of the fear is of occupational transmission, surgeons and nurses—the professionals most likely to receive occupational injuries—should be invited to participate at all levels of the development of educational programs and infection control policies. Hospitals must develop a comprehensive and clearly stated set of policies regarding AIDS, which include infection control aspects, the ethical response and professional responsibility to care for AIDS patients, and guidelines for testing in the hospital setting. These guidelines developed in conjunction with input from surgery and nursing staff members should be widely communicated in writing to minimize the frequent misconception that fear of occupational infection with HIV has not been addressed at the administrative level. Certainly such policies should also delineate the problem of the HIV-infected health care worker (e.g., occupational restrictions, if any).

Fear from non-AIDS patients in the hospital must also be considered as they recognize that AIDS patients are in the hospital and may also be concerned that this will put them at risk for infection with HIV or associated infections.[4] The lack of risk to other patients must be stressed along with a clear statement that AIDS patients are in need of medical care and that policies ensuring the safety of other patients have been addressed and enforced. This education of non-AIDS patients should also stress the positive advantages of newer methods of infection control that help protect them from non-AIDS-related nosocomial infections at least as much as from HIV-associated problems (see Chapter 4).

STRATEGIES FOR ORGANIZING AIDS CARE

AIDS presents a unique set of problems that require a fresh look at the organization of medical services. Most AIDS patients require the services of many medical subspecialties, especially infectious disease, oncology, and pulmonary medicine, at some point in their disease course. If the case volume warrants doing so, a hospital may benefit from bringing these subspecialties together in a dedicated AIDS outpatient facility. If the volume or the medical structure does not permit this, another approach is to formalize a network of relevant disciplines to minimize miscommunication and duplication of clinic visits and laboratory testing.

Along with subspecialists, generalists in both internal medicine and family practice can be used effectively in the care of patients with AIDS. The medical problems of AIDS patients, although complex, are somewhat predictable. Between acute episodes, when subspecialists may be required, the bulk of AIDS care can, and perhaps should, be delivered by a physician with a more general orientation. To be most effective, generalists must be given additional training and clinical experience with AIDS and recognition of the importance of their role by the hospital center.

In public facilities such as San Francisco General Hospital the development of explicit guidelines for the primary care of HIV-infected patients in all associated clinics might also be considered. This, to us, will be increasingly necessary to distribute the large burden of the epidemic.

A system of AIDS care must also include social services, both counseling and financial assistance, for the reasons described. The precise nature of these services and background of the disciplines involved (clinical psychology, psychiatry, or social work) may vary considerably from hospital to hospital. These staff members, in addition to providing the aforementioned services, should be prepared to work with the physicians to minimize the problems of obtaining experimental drugs and reimbursement for their use.

A final important component for the organization of AIDS care concerns the many ethical dilemmas that can be anticipated. Issues of patients' competency to consent to medical care, given HIV dementia, and the extent to which care should be continued in the face of terminal disease make the establishment and active use of a medical ethics committee essential. This committee should be invited to participate actively in regular conferences regarding patient care and to assist in evaluation in specific cases. It should be urged to provide a practical response to ethical problems in the hope that the AIDS provider staff members will gradually become more skilled in addressing these often uncomfortable situations and preventing them from developing.

CONTROLLING THE COST OF AIDS CARE

AIDS patients require the complete set of services anticipated for any patient group with a difficult, progressive, and ultimately fatal disease. This includes treatment in a hospital's acute care unit and outpatient facilities, community-based services, and some acute and extended care. The cost of AIDS care has been estimated to be $50,000 to $150,000 from diagnosis to death.[6,11,12] Most estimates are still crude and may vary considerably among regions and patient groups. Our experience in San Francisco suggests that a well-conceived system of medical care for AIDS patients, with a focus as described on community-based services, can reduce these costs. At San Francisco General Hospital, we have, for example, found that our lifetime medical cost for AIDS patients is approximately $50,000.[11] We have achieved this cost by intentionally reducing the average length of stay for AIDS patients and by assembling community-based services that can deliver comprehensive yet cost-effective care, which, moreover, our patients prefer over hospitalization for acute care.

One way that AIDS costs have been unexpectedly reduced at San Francisco General Hospital concerns the use of intensive care facilities. Although we have never explicitly attempted to limit the use of intensive care for patients with AIDS, we have found that a more aggressive program of education about the outcome of ventilator support has caused fewer patients to request this form of treatment. A survey of our experience showed that only 10% to 15% of patients given ventilator support survived that hospitalization. When our patients were informed of this, the majority declined this intervention, and despite an increasing census in the hospital, we have seen a decrease in intensive care admissions.[15] The wisdom at this approach is underscored by reports that more selective initiation of ventilator support increases survival rates in intensive care units.[8]

Reducing the rate and duration of hospitalization is the principal means of controlling AIDS cost. To do this, we must closely examine outpatient services and facilities. Outpatient transfusions, antibiotics, and chemotherapeutic infusions are obvious ways to reduce hospitalizations; more aggressive outpatient management of *P. carinii* pneumonia, the most common opportunistic infection in AIDS, also is critical. Outpatient therapy and prophylaxis for *P. carinii* pneumonia have been more possible since the development of regimens of oral trimethoprim-sulfamethoxasole, of dapsone and trimethoprim, and of primaquine and clindamycin. Similar attempts in outpatient therapy for cryptococcal meningitis with amphotericin B or fluconazole, and for CMV-associated retinitis with ganciclovir and foscarnet are also worth considering. Yet these newer therapies are often extremely expensive, and more attention is required to monitor and control their overusage.

In summary, several steps can be used to control the cost of AIDS. Hospitals and medical centers can develop systems that concentrate service as the volume of AIDS patients allows and that focus on outpatient and community-based care. Hospitals should closely monitor the use of intensive care and educate patients and staff to reduce this expensive and frequently unneeded medical treatment. Hospitals can maximize their use of community-based care by explicitly inviting community organizations to participate in the establishment of AIDS care systems, in some cases as full-time staff members within the hospital. Finally, as the medical center is able to shift more care to the outpatient setting, it must seek reimbursement for these services, which may require staff members who are specifically devoted to this activity.

The impact of AIDS can be further limited by public and private hospitals' working together to ensure that the burden of AIDS care is well distributed rather than being unfairly concentrated at one or a small number of facilities. In all facilities criteria of effectiveness such as average length of stay and use of intensive care should be monitored and reported regularly to hospital administrators. Finally, the increased use of physician extenders such as nurse practitioners and physician's assistants may prove valuable in controlling the impact of AIDS on the physician and community.

THE POSITIVE SIDE OF AIDS CARE

AIDS patients are often young, well educated about their disease, and extremely compliant with their medical care. Furthermore, they are often extremely appreciative of expert care that is both comprehensive and socially sensitive. AIDS is at the cutting edge of many issues central to medicine and society, and working directly with AIDS patients allows the medical system to participate in a vital debate, which may well change the face of American medicine for decades to come. The final and most obvious reason for physicians and medical systems to become more involved in AIDS care is the clear need of all HIV-infected patients for expert, comprehensive, and efficient care. Given the long tradition of response to these issues in the setting of other diseases, a similar response from the medical system to this epidemic is expected.

REFERENCES

1. Abrams DI, Dilley WJ, Maxey LM, et al: Routine care and psychosocial support of the patient with acquired immunodeficiency syndrome. Med Clin North Am 70:707-720, 1986
2. Felsenstein D, D'Amico DJ, Hirsch MS, et al: Treatment of cytomegalovirus retinitis with 9-[2-hydroxy-1-(hydroxy-methyl) ethoxymethyl] guanine. Ann Intern Med 103:377-380, 1985
3. Francis DP, Anderson RE, Gorman ME, et al: Targeting AIDS prevention and treatment toward HIV-1-infected persons: The concept of early intervention (special communication). JAMA 262:2572-2576, 1989
4. Gerbert B, Maguire BT, Hulley SB, et al: Physicians and acquired immunodeficiency syndrome: What patients think about human immunodeficiency virus in medical practice. JAMA 262:1969-1972, 1989
5. Gordin FM, Simon GL, Wofsy CB, et al: Adverse reactions to trimethoprim-sulfamethoxazole in patients with the acquired immunodeficiency syndrome. Ann Intern Med 100:495-499, 1984
6. Hardy A, Rausch K, Echenberg DF, et al: The economic impact of the first 10,000 cases of AIDS in the United States. JAMA 225:209-211, 1986
7. Jaffe HS, Abrams DI, Ammann AJ, et al: Complications of co-trimoxazole in treatment of AIDS-associated *Pneumocystis carinii* pneumonia in homosexual men. Lancet 2:1109, 1983
8. Luce JM, Wachter RM: Intensive care for patients with the acquired immune deficiency syndrome. Intensive Care Med 15:481-482, 1989
9. Mitsuyasu R, Groopman J, Volberding P: Cutaneous reaction to trimethoprim-sulfamethoxazole in patients with AIDS and Kaposi's sarcoma (letter). N Engl J Med 308:1535-1536, 1983
10. Rhame F, Maki D: The case for wider use of testing for HIV infection. N Engl J Med 11:1248-1254, 1989
11. Scitovsky AA, Rice DP, Showstack J, et al: Estimating the direct and indirect economic costs of the acquired immunodeficiency syndrome 1985, 1986 and 1990. Task order 282-85-0061, No 2, 1986. Atlanta, Centers for Disease Control

12. Seidman RL, Williams SJ, Mortensen LM: Assessing the economic impact of AIDS in local communities: Current and projected costs for San Diego County. West J Med 151:467-471, 1989
13. Steinbrook R, Lo B, Tirpack J, et al: Ethical dilemmas in caring for patients with the acquired immunodeficiency syndrome. Ann Intern Med 103:787-790, 1985
14. Volberding PA: HIV infection as a disease: The medical indications for early diagnosis (editorial). J AIDS 2:421-425, 1989
15. Wachter RM, Luce J, Lo B, et al: Life-sustaining treatment for patients with AIDS. Chest 95:647-652, 1989

INDEX

Note: page numbers in *italics* indicate a figure; page numbers followed by the letter t indicate a table.